Motor Control

THEORY AND PRACTICAL APPLICATIONS

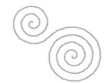

Motor Control

THEORY AND PRACTICAL APPLICATIONS

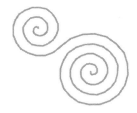

Anne Shumway-Cook, Ph.D.

Research Coordinator
Department of Physical Therapy
Northwest Hospital
Seattle, Washington

Marjorie H. Woollacott, Ph.D.

Professor
Department of Exercise and Movement Science
Institute of Neuroscience
University of Oregon
Eugene, Oregon

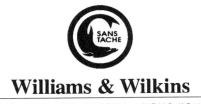

Williams & Wilkins

BALTIMORE • PHILADELPHIA • HONG KONG
LONDON • MUNICH • SYDNEY • TOKYO

A WAVERLY COMPANY

Editor: John P. Butler
Development Editor: Nancy H. Evans
Copy Editor: Judith F. Minkove
Designer: Wilma E. Rosenberger
Illustration Planner: Ray Lowman
Production Coordinator: Charles E. Zeller
Photographer: David Trees

Copyright © 1995
Williams & Wilkins
428 East Preston Street
Baltimore, Maryland 21202, USA

Printed in the United States of America

Library of Congress Cataloging in Publication Data

Shumway-Cook, Anne, 1947–
    Motor control : theory and practical applications / Anne Shumway-Cook, Marjorie H. Woollacott.—1st ed.
        p.   cm.
    Includes index.
    ISBN 0-683-07757-0
    1. Physical therapy. 2. Motor learning.   I. Woollacott, Marjorie H., 1946–   .   II. Title.
    RM701.S55   1995
    612.7—dc20   94-26889
                                                                         CIP

                                                                    97 98 99
                                                              3 4 5 6 7 8 9 10

It is with great love and gratitude that we dedicate this book to the many people, including professional colleagues, reviewers, and patients, who have contributed to the development of the ideas presented here. We gratefully acknowledge the divine source of our enthusiasm, wisdom, and joy. We dedicate this book, as we do all our actions, to the One who set it before us to do and provided us steadfast wisdom and support throughout its creation.

Photographs by David Trees, Education and Training Department, Northwest Hospital.

PREFACE

In recent years there has been a tremendous interest among clinicians regarding new theories of motor control and the role of these theories in guiding clinical practice. The explosion of new research in the field of neuroscience and motor control has widened the gap between research/theory and clinical practices related to helping patients regain motor control. This book is an attempt to bridge the gap between theory and practice. The book stresses the scientific and experimental basis of new motor control theories, and explains how principles from this science can be applied to clinical practice. While many theories of motor control are discussed, the major thrust of the book is to present a **systems theory** of motor control and a clinical approach to assessment and treatment of motor control problems based on a systems model. We refer to this clinical approach as a "task oriented approach." The book is divided into four sections. Section I, entitled "Theoretical Framework," reviews current theories of motor control, motor learning, and recovery of function following neurological insult. The clinical implications of various theories of motor control are discussed. In addition, this section reviews the physiological basis of motor control and motor learning. Finally, this section includes a chapter that presents a suggested conceptual framework for clinical practice.

This first section leads into the major thrust of the book which addresses motor control issues as they relate to the control of posture and balance (Section II), mobility (Section III), and upper extremity manipulatory functions (Section IV). The chapters included in each of these sections follow a standard format. The first chapter discusses issues related to normal control processes. The second (and in some cases third) chapter describes age-related issues. The third chapter presents research on abnormal function, while the final chapter discusses the applications of current research to the assessment and treatment of motor dyscontrol in each of the three functional areas.

We envision that this text will be of use in both undergraduate and graduate courses on normal motor control, motor development across the life span, and rehabilitation in the areas of physical and occupational therapy as well as kinesiology.

Motor Control: Theory and Practical Applications seeks to provide a framework that will enable the clinician to incorporate theory into practice. More importantly it is our hope that this book will serve as a springboard for developing new, more effective, approaches to assessing and treating patients with motor dyscontrol.

CONTENTS

Section I

THEORETICAL FRAMEWORK

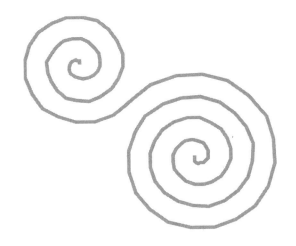

Chapter 1

THEORIES OF MOTOR CONTROL

INTRODUCTION

What Is Motor Control?

In this textbook we define motor control as the study of the nature and cause of movement. When we talk about motor control, we are actually talking about two issues. The first issue deals with stabilizing the body in space, that is, motor control as it applies to postural and balance control. The second issue deals with moving the body in space, that is, motor control as it applies to movement. Thus, the term motor control is defined broadly here to encompass the control of both movement and posture.

STUDY OF ACTION

Movement is often described within the context of accomplishing a particular action. As a result, motor control is usually studied in relation to specific actions or activities. For example, motor control physiologists might ask: how do people walk, run, talk, smile, reach, or stand still? Researchers often study movement control within the context of a specific activity, like walking, hoping that understanding control processes related to this activity will provide insight into principles for how all of movement is controlled. So the study of motor control includes the study of *action*.

STUDY OF PERCEPTION

Unfortunately, the term motor control in itself is somewhat misleading, since movement arises from the interaction of multiple processes, including perceptual, cognitive, and motor processes. Perception is essential to action, just as action is essential to perception. Actions are performed within the context of an environment. Sensory-perceptual systems provide information about the body and the environment, and are clearly integral to the ability to act effectively within an environment (1). Thus, understanding motor control requires the study of *perception*.

STUDY OF COGNITION

In addition, since movement is not usually performed in the absence of intent, cognitive processes are essential to motor control. In this book we define cognitive processes broadly to include attention, motivation, and emotional aspects of motor control that underlie the establishment of intent or goals. Motor control includes perceptual and action systems, which are organized to achieve specific goals or intents. Thus, the study of motor control must include the study of **cognitive processes** as they relate to the control of perception and action.

INTERACTION OF INDIVIDUAL, TASK, AND ENVIRONMENT

While each of these aspects of motor control—perception, action, and cognition—can be studied in isolation, we believe a true picture of the nature of motor control cannot be achieved without a synthesis of information from all three.

However, motor control research that focuses only on processes within individuals without taking into account the environments in which they move, or the tasks they are performing, will produce an incomplete picture. Accordingly, in this book our discussion of motor control will focus on the interaction of the individual, the task, and the environment. Figure 1.1 illustrates this concept that movement emerges from an interaction between these three factors.

Why Should Clinicians Study Motor Control?

Why should clinicians be concerned with the study of motor control? They spend a considerable amount of time retraining motor dyscontrol in patients who have functional limitations. Clinicians have been referred to as

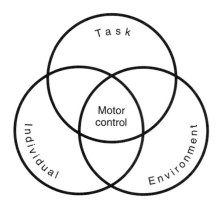

Figure 1.1. Motor control emerges from an interaction between the individual, the task, and the environment.

"applied motor control physiologists" (2). Their actions are based on the belief that movement control is important, even essential, to the achievement of functional competence. Since motor control is the study of the nature and cause of movement, understanding motor control is essential to clinical practice.

Understanding motor control is easier said than done. This is because there is not a universal agreement among scientists or clinicians about the nature and cause of movement. There is no single theory of motor control that everyone accepts. Among the many theories that will be discussed in this chapter, each has made specific contributions to the field of motor control and each has implications for the clinician retraining motor dyscontrol.

WHAT IS A THEORY OF MOTOR CONTROL?

A *theory* of motor control is a group of abstract ideas about the nature and cause of movement. Theories are often, but not always, based on models of brain function.

What is a *model*? A model is a representation of something, usually a simplified version of the real thing. The better the model, the better it will predict how the real thing will behave in a real situation. Why is a model of brain function needed? Because the brain is so complex, a model can represent and to some extent simplify complex concepts. A model of brain function, related to motor control, is a simplified representation of the structure and function of the brain as it relates to the coordination of movement. Theories of motor control and models of brain function then go hand in hand.

The idea that there may be more than one theory of motor control may be a new concept to many therapists. Different theories of motor control reflect philosophically different views about how the brain controls movement. These theories often reflect differences in opinion about the relative importance of various neural components of movement. For example, some theories stress peripheral influences, others may stress central influences, while still others may stress the role of information from the environment in controlling behavior. Thus, motor control theories are more than just an approach to explaining action. Often they stress different aspects of the organization of the underlying neurophysiology and neuroanatomy of that action. Some theories of motor control look at the brain as a black box and simply study the rules by which this black box interacts with changing environments.

What Is the Relationship Between Theory and Practice?

Do theories really influence what therapists do with their patients? YES! Rehabilitation practices reflect the theories, or basic ideas, we have about the cause and nature of function and dysfunction (3). In general, then, the actions of therapists are based on assumptions that are derived from theories. The specific practices used to assess and treat the patient with motor dyscontrol are determined by underlying assumptions about the nature and cause of movement. Thus, motor control theory is part of the *theoretical* basis for clinical practice.

What are the advantages and disadvantages of using theories in clinical practice? Theories provide:

- a framework for interpreting behavior;
- a guide for clinical action;

- new ideas; and
- working hypotheses for assessment and treatment.

FRAMEWORK FOR INTERPRETING BEHAVIOR

Theory can help therapists to interpret the behavior or actions of patients they treat. Theory allows the therapist to go beyond the behavior of one patient, and broaden the application to a much larger number of cases (3).

Theories can be more or less helpful depending on their ability to predict or explain the behavior of an individual patient. When a theory and its associated assumptions does not provide an accurate interpretation of a patient's behavior, it loses its usefulness to the therapist. Thus, theories can potentially limit a therapist's ability to observe and interpret movement problems in patients.

For example, look at the patient pictured in Figure 1.2. Mrs. Johnson is a 67-year-old woman referred for rehabilitation following a cerebral vascular accident, which has produced motor dyscontrol in her left side. The patient habitually sits with her left arm flexed and drawn close to her body. When asked to extend her left arm, she cannot actively extend at the elbow. If you try to extend her arm, there is resistance. In addition, when she walks, her knee is stiff and hyperextended, and she uses a toe-heel pattern.

Prior to deciding how to retrain arm function and gait, as her therapist, you must decide what the underlying problems are. What is preventing her from actively extending her arm? Why is she unable to walk with a heel-toe gait? You might assume the patient's inability to extend her arm is the result of spasticity in the elbow flexors. In addition, her inability to walk heel-toe is the result of spasticity in the gastrocnemius muscle. This assumption might be based on a theory of motor control that suggests that **reflexes** are an important part of movement control, and that abnormal reflexes are a major reason patients cannot move normally. Based on this theory, you might attribute the loss of arm

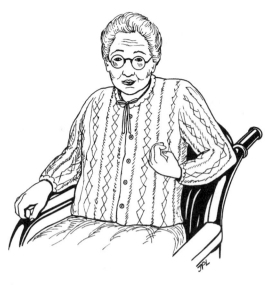

Figure 1.2. Mrs. Johnson is a 67-year-old woman referred for therapy because of a right cerebral vascular accident resulting in a left hemiparesis. Pictured is her habitual sitting posture.

function, specifically the inability to actively extend the elbow, to be primarily the result of **spasticity**, defined as *a release of the stretch reflex*, in the elbow flexors.

Has your theoretical framework helped you to correctly interpret this patient's behavior? Only if this patient's problems are in fact solely the result of spasticity. The theory has not helped you as a clinician if it has limited your ability to explore other possible explanations for your patient's behavior. What are some of the other factors that potentially impair arm function in your stroke patient? Later in this chapter we will discuss other theories of motor control that will provide alternative explanations for loss of function.

GUIDE FOR CLINICAL ACTION

Theories provide therapists with a possible guide for action. Clinical practices designed to treat the patient with motor dyscontrol are based on an understanding of the nature and cause of normal movement, as well as an understanding of the basis for abnormal movement. Therapeutic strategies aimed at retraining motor control reflect this basic understanding. In the above example, spasticity

is assumed to be a major determinant of abnormal function. As a result, numerous approaches have been developed to assess and treat spasticity in the course of retraining function. However, because there are many different theories about the nature and cause of movement, there are potentially many other therapeutic approaches for retraining motor dyscontrol.

NEW IDEAS: DYNAMIC AND EVOLVING

Theories are dynamic, and change to reflect greater knowledge relating to the theory. How does this affect clinical practices related to retraining motor dyscontrol? Changing and expanding theories of motor control need not be a source of frustration to clinicians. Expanding theories can broaden and enrich the possibilities for clinical practice. New ideas for the assessment and treatment of motor dyscontrol will evolve to reflect new ideas about the nature and cause of movement.

WORKING HYPOTHESES FOR ASSESSMENT AND TREATMENT

A theory is not directly testable, since it is abstract. Rather, theories generate hypotheses, which are testable. Information gained through hypothesis testing is used to validate or invalidate a theory. This same approach is useful in clinical practice. So-called *hypothesis-driven clinical practice* (4) transforms the therapist into an active problem solver. Using this approach to retrain motor dyscontrol calls for the therapist to generate multiple hypotheses (explanations) for why patients move (or don't move) in ways to achieve functional independence. During the course of therapy the therapist will test various hypotheses, discarding some, and generating new explanations that are more consistent with their results.

THEORIES OF MOTOR CONTROL

There is tremendous enthusiasm among therapists for critically examining the models upon which much of clinical practice is based. Therapists are recognizing the limitations of past theories and the expanding possibilities of new solutions based on new models of motor control and recovery of function.

In this section we will review theories of motor control and explore some of their limitations and possible clinical implications. It is important to understand that all models are unified by the desire to understand the nature and cause of movement. The difference is in the approach. It is not unlike the story of the five men trying to understand the nature and function of an elephant. One carefully and systematically studies the trunk, and learns everything there is to know about the nature and function of the trunk. Another studies the nature and function of the feet; another, the tail. Each in his own way has provided essential information about the elephant. However, a true understanding about the nature and function of an elephant is only possible by combining information from all sources. In this spirit, we approach the following section on theories of motor control, their limitations, and possible clinical applications.

Reflex Theory

Sir Charles Sherrington, a neurophysiologist in the late 1800s and early 1900s, wrote the book *The Integrative Action of the Nervous System* in 1906. His research formed the experimental foundation for a classic reflex theory of motor control. For Sherrington, reflexes were the building blocks of complex behavior. Reflexes worked together, or

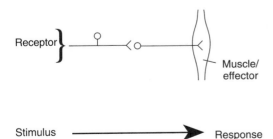

Figure 1.3. The basic structure of a reflex consists of a receptor, a conductor, and an effector.

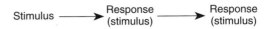

Figure 1.4. Reflex chaining as a basis for action. A stimulus leads to a response, which becomes the stimulus for the next response, which becomes the stimulus for the next response.

in sequence, to achieve a common purpose (5).

Sherrington performed elegant experiments with cats, dogs, and monkeys to show the existence of the reflex, and to carefully describe and define reflexes. The conception of a reflex requires three different structures, as shown in Figure 1.3: a receptor, a conducting nervous pathway, and an effector. The conductor consists of at least two nerve cells, one connected to the effector, the other connected to the receptor. The reflex arc then consists of the receptor, the conductor, and the effector (6).

Sherrington went on to describe complex behavior in terms of compound reflexes, and their *successive combination* or *chaining* together. Sherrington gave the following example of a frog capturing and eating a fly. Picture Mr. Toad sitting in the sun on his lily pad. Along comes the fly; seeing the fly (stimulus) results in the reflex activation of the tongue darting out to capture the fly (response). If he is successful, the contact of the fly on the tongue causes reflex closure of the mouth, and closure of the mouth results in reflex swallowing.

Sherrington concluded that with the whole nervous system intact, the reaction of the various parts of that system, the simple reflexes, are combined into greater actions, which constitute the behavior of the individual as a whole. Figure 1.4 represents this concept of reflex chaining. Sherrington's view of a reflexive basis for movement persisted unchallenged for 50 years, and continues to influence thinking about motor control today.

LIMITATIONS

Because Sherrington looked primarily at reflexes, and asked questions about the central nervous system (CNS) related to reflexes, he drew a picture of the CNS and motor control that was skewed towards reflex control. There are a number of limitations of a reflex theory of motor control (1).

The reflex cannot be considered the basic unit of behavior if both spontaneous and voluntary movements are recognized as acceptable classes of behavior, since the reflex must be activated by an outside agent.

Another limitation of the reflex theory of motor control is that it does not adequately explain and predict movement that occurs in the absence of a sensory stimulus. More recently, it has been shown that animals can move in a relatively coordinated fashion in the absence of sensory input (7).

Yer another limitation is that the theory does not explain fast movements, that is, sequences of movements that occur too rapidly to allow for sensory feedback from the preceding movement to trigger the next. For example, an experienced and proficient typist moves from one key to the next so rapidly that there isn't time for sensory information from one keystroke to activate the next.

An additional limitation is that the reflex chaining model fails to explain the fact that a single stimulus can result in varying responses depending on context and descending commands. For example, there are times when we need to override reflexes to achieve a goal. For example, normally touching something hot results in the reflexive withdrawal of the hand. However, if our child is in a fire, we may override the reflexive withdrawal to pull the child out.

Finally, reflex chaining does not explain the ability to produce novel movements. Novel movements put together unique combinations of stimuli and responses according to rules previously learned. A violinist, who has learned a piece on the violin, and also knows the technique of playing the cello, can play that piece perfectly on the cello without necessarily having practiced the piece on the cello. The violinist has learned the rules for playing the piece and has applied them to a novel or new situation.

CLINICAL IMPLICATIONS

How might a reflex theory of motor control be used to interpret a patient's behavior, and serve as a guide for the therapist's actions?

If chained or compounded reflexes are the basis for functional movement, clinical strategies designed to test reflexes should allow therapists to predict function. In addition, a patient's movement behaviors would be interpreted in terms of the presence or absence of controlling reflexes. Finally, retraining motor control for functional skills would focus on enhancing or reducing the effect of various reflexes during motor tasks. Applying a reflex theory to interpreting motor dyscontrol was shown in our previous example of Mrs. Johnson. Clinical strategies for improving motor control using a reflex model would focus on methods to reduce flexor spasticity, which should enhance normal movement capacity.

Despite the limitations in Sherrington's conclusions, many of his assumptions about how the CNS controls movement have been reinforced and have influenced current clinical practices.

Hierarchical Theory

Many researchers contributed to the view that the nervous system is organized as a hierarchy. Among them, Hughlings Jackson, an English physician, argued that the brain has higher, middle, and lower levels of control, equated with higher association areas, the motor cortex and spinal levels of motor function (8).

Hierarchical control in general has been defined as an organizational structure that is *top down*. That is, each successively higher level exerts control over the level below it, as shown in Figure 1.5. In a strict vertical hierarchy, lines of control do not cross and there is never bottom up control.

In the 1920s, Rudolf Magnus began to explore the function of different reflexes within different parts of the nervous system.

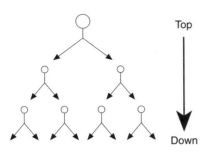

Figure 1.5. The hierarchical control structure is characterized by a top-down structure, where higher centers are always in charge of lower centers.

He found that reflexes controlled by lower levels of the neural hierarchy are only present when cortical centers are damaged. These results were later interpreted to imply that reflexes are part of a hierarchy of motor control, in which higher centers normally inhibit these lower reflex centers (9–10).

Later, Georg Schaltenbrand (11) used the concepts developed by Magnus to explain the development of mobility in children and adults. He described the development of human mobility in terms of the appearance and disappearance of a progression of reflexes. He went on further to say that pathology of the brain may result in the persistence of primitive reflexes. He suggested that a complete understanding of all the reflexes would allow the determination of the neural age of a child or a patient.

In the late 1930s, Stephan Weisz (12) reported on reflex reactions that he felt were the basis for equilibrium in humans. He described the ontogeny of equilibrium reflexes in the normally developing child and proposed a relationship between the maturation of these reflexes and the child's capacity to sit, stand, and walk.

The results of these experiments and observations were drawn together and are often referred to in the clinical literature as a reflex/hierarchical theory of motor control. This reflex/hierarchical theory of motor control combines reflex and hierarchical theories into one. This theory suggests that motor control emerges from reflexes that are nested within hierarchically organized levels of the CNS.

In the 1940s, Arnold Gesell (13, 14) and Myrtle McGraw (15), two well-known developmental researchers, offered detailed descriptions of the maturation of infants. These researchers applied the current scientific thinking about reflex hierarchies of motor control to explain the behaviors they saw in infants. Normal motor development was attributed to increasing corticalization of the CNS resulting in the emergence of higher levels of control over lower level reflexes. This has been referred to as a *neuromaturational theory* of development. An example of this model is illustrated in Figure 1.6. This theory assumes that CNS maturation is the primary agent for change in development. It minimizes the importance of other factors such as musculoskeletal changes during development.

Since Hughlings Jackson's original work, a new concept of *hierarchical* control has evolved. Modern neuroscientists have confirmed the importance of elements of hierarchical organization in motor control. The concept of a strict hierarchy, where higher centers are always in control, has been modified. Current concepts describing hierarchical control within the nervous system recognize the fact that each level of the nervous system can act upon other levels (higher and lower) depending on the task. In addition, the role of reflexes in movement has been modified. Reflexes are not considered the sole determinant of motor control, but only one of many processes important to the generation and control of movement.

LIMITATIONS

One of the limitations of a reflex/hierarchical theory of motor control is that it cannot explain the dominance of reflex behavior in certain situations in normal adults. For example, stepping on a pin results in an immediate withdrawal of the leg. This is an example of a reflex within the lowest level of the hierarchy dominating motor function. It is an ex-

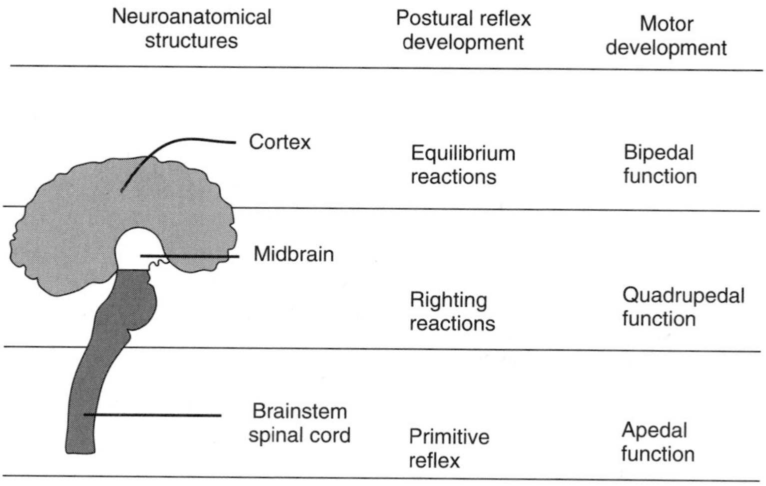

Neuroanatomical structures	Postural reflex development	Motor development
Cortex	Equilibrium reactions	Bipedal function
Midbrain	Righting reactions	Quadrupedal function
Brainstem spinal cord	Primitive reflex	Apedal function

Figure 1.6. Neuromaturational theory of motor control attributes motor development to the maturation of neural processes, including the progressive appearance and disappearance of reflexes.

ample of bottom-up control. Thus, one must be cautious about assumptions that all low-level behaviors are primitive, immature, and nonadaptive, while all higher level (cortical) behaviors are mature, adaptive, and appropriate.

CLINICAL IMPLICATIONS

Abnormalities of reflex organization have been used by many clinicians to explain disordered motor control in the neurological patient. Berta Bobath, an English physical therapist, in her discussions of abnormal postural reflex activity in children with cerebral palsy, states that "the release of motor responses integrated at lower levels from restraining influences of higher centers, especially that of the cortex, leads to abnormal postural reflex activity" (16).

Based on a reflex/hierarchical theory of motor control and development, a number of reflex tests have been developed as part of the clinical assessment of patients with neurological impairments (17). These reflex assessment profiles are used to estimate the level of neural maturation and predict functional ability. In addition, reflex profiles are used to document the presence of persisting and dominating primitive and pathological reflexes believed

to be major deterrents to normal motor control.

A number of treatment approaches have been developed which focus on enhancing or reducing the efficacy of reflexes as an important step in retraining motor control. The goal of treatment is to achieve greater function through the modification of reflex action. One of the difficulties in using a reflex approach to retraining motor control is that successful modification of reflex activity is not always mirrored in improvements in functional skills. Part of the difficulty may lie in the issue of focusing treatment on reactions instead of preparing patients for action.

Motor Programming Theories

More current theories of motor control have expanded our understanding of the CNS. They have moved away from views of the CNS as a mostly reactive system and have begun to explore the physiology of actions rather than the physiology of reactions.

Reflex theories have been useful in explaining certain stereotyped patterns of movement. However, an interesting way of viewing reflexes is to consider that one can remove the stimulus, or the afferent input, and still have a patterned motor response (18). If we remove the motor response from its stimulus, we are left with the concept of a central motor pattern. This concept of a motor pattern is more flexible than the concept of a reflex because it can either be activated by sensory stimuli or by central processes.

A motor program theory of motor control has considerable experimental support. For example, experiments in the early 1960s studied the grasshopper or locust and showed that the timing of the animal's wing beat in flight depended on a rhythmic pattern generator. Even when the sensory nerves were cut, the nervous system by itself could generate the output with no sensory input; however, the wing beat was slowed (20). This suggested that movement is possible in the absence of reflexive action. Sensory input, while not essential in driving movement, has an important function in modulating action. These conclusions were further supported by work examining locomotion in cats (21). The results of these experiments showed that in the cat, spinal neural networks could produce a locomotor rhythm without either sensory inputs or descending patterns from the brain. By changing the intensity of stimulation to the spinal cord, the animal could be made to walk, trot, or gallop. Thus, it was again shown that reflexes do not drive action, but that central pattern generators by themselves can generate such complex movements as the walk, trot, and gallop. Further experiments showed the important modulatory effects of incoming sensory inputs on the central pattern generator (22).

These experiments led to the motor program theory of motor control. This term has been used in a number of ways by different researchers, so care should be taken in determining how the term is being used. The term **motor program** may be used to identify a central pattern generator (CPG), that is, a specific neural circuit like that for generating walking in the cat. In this case the term represents neural connections that are stereotyped and hardwired.

But the term motor program is also used to describe the higher level motor programs that represent actions in more abstract terms.

A significant amount of research in the field of psychology has supported the existence of hierarchically organized motor programs that store the rules for generating movements so that we can perform the tasks with a variety of effector systems.

ACTIVE LEARNING MODULE

You can see this for yourself. Try writing your signature as you normally would on a small piece of paper. Now write it larger, on a blackboard. Now try it with your other hand. While you may be much more proficient with one hand versus the other, you will see elements of your signature that are common to all situations. As shown in Figure 1.7, the rules for writing your name are stored as a motor program at higher levels within the CNS. As a result, neural commands from these higher centers to write your name can be sent to various parts of the body. Yet, elements of the written signature remain constant regardless of the part of the body used to carry out the task (23).

LIMITATIONS

The concept of central pattern generators expanded our understanding of the role of the nervous system in the control of movement. However, we must be careful to realize that the central pattern generator concept has never been intended to replace the concept of the importance of sensory input in controlling movement. It simply expanded our understanding of the flexibility of the nervous system in creating movements, to include its ability to create movements in isolation from feedback.

An important limitation of the motor program concept is that a central motor program cannot be considered to be the sole determinant of action (23). Two identical commands to the elbow flexors, for example, will produce very different movements depending on whether your arm is resting at your side, or if you are holding your arm out in front of you. The forces of gravity will act differently on the limb in the two conditions, and thus

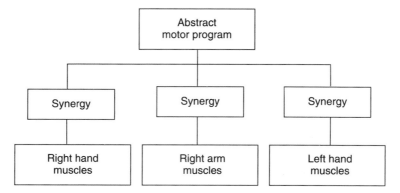

Figure 1.7. Levels of control for motor programs and their output systems. Rules for action are represented at the highest level, in abstract motor programs. Lower levels of the hierarchy contain information essential for effecting action.

modify the movement. In addition, if your muscles are fatigued, similar nervous system commands will give very different results. Thus, the motor program concept does not take into account the fact that the nervous system must take into account both musculoskeletal and environmental variables in achieving movement control.

CLINICAL IMPLICATIONS

Motor program theories of motor control have allowed clinicians to move beyond a reflex explanation for disordered motor control. Explanations for abnormal movement have been expanded to include problems resulting from abnormalities in central pattern generators, or in higher level motor programs.

Mrs. Johnson, our stroke patient, may indeed have flexor spasticity in her arms which may affect her ability to move. However, it will be important to determine what levels of motor programming are involved. If her higher levels of motor programming are not affected, she will be able to continue to use such programs as handwriting, but will find alternate effectors, for example, her unaffected hand, to carry out the tasks. Of course, these less used lower level synergy and muscular systems will have to be trained to carry out these higher level programs.

In patients whose higher levels of motor programming are affected, motor program theory suggests the importance of helping patients relearn the correct rules for action. In addition, treatment should focus on retraining movements important to a functional task, not just on reeducating specific muscles in isolation.

Systems Theory

Even before motor program concepts were developed, another researcher, Nicolai Bernstein (1896–1966), a Russian scientist, was looking at the nervous system and body in a whole new way. Previous neurophysiologists had focused primarily on neural control aspects of movement. Bernstein recognized that you cannot understand the neural control of movement without an understanding of the characteristics of the system you are moving, and the external and internal forces acting on the body.

In describing the characteristics of the *system* being moved, he looked at the whole body as a mechanical system, with mass, and subject to both external forces, like gravity, and internal forces, including both inertial and movement-dependent forces. During the course of any movement the amounts of force acting on the body will change as potential and kinetic energy change. He thus showed that the same central command could result in quite different movements because of the interplay between external forces and variations in the initial conditions (23). For the same reasons, different commands could result in the same movement.

Bernstein also suggested that control of integrated movement was probably distributed throughout many interacting systems working cooperatively to achieve movement. This gave rise to the concept of a *distributed model of motor control.*

How does Bernstein's approach to motor control differ from the reflex, hierarchical, or motor program approaches presented previously? Bernstein asked questions about the organism in a continuously changing situation. He found answers that were different from previous researchers about the nature and cause of movement, since he asked different questions, such as: How does the body as a mechanical system influence the control process? How do the initial conditions affect the properties of the movement?

In describing the body as a mechanical system, Bernstein noted that we have many **degrees of freedom** that need to be controlled. For example, we have many joints, all of which flex or extend and many of which can be rotated as well. This complicates movement control incredibly. He said, "Coordination of movement is the process of mastering the redundant degrees of freedom of the moving organism" (23). In other words, it involves converting the body into a controllable system.

As a solution to the *degrees of freedom problem,* Bernstein hypothesized that hierarchical control exists to simplify the control of the body's multiple degrees of freedom. In this way, the higher levels of the nervous system activate lower levels. The lower levels activate **synergies**, or groups of muscles that are constrained to act together as a unit. We can think of our movement repertoire like sentences made up of many words. The letters within the words are the muscles; the words themselves are the synergies, and the sentences are the actions themselves.

Thus, Bernstein believed that synergies play an important role in solving the degrees of freedom problem. This is achieved by constraining certain muscles to work together as a unit. He hypothesized that though there are few synergies, they make possible almost the whole variety of movements we know. For example, he considered some simple synergies to be the locomotor, postural, and respiratory synergies.

LIMITATIONS

What are the limitations of Bernstein's systems approach? As you can see, it is the broadest of the approaches we have discussed thus far, and since it takes into account not only the contributions of the nervous system to action, but also the contributions of the muscle and skeletal systems, as well as the forces of gravity and inertia, it predicts actual behavior much better than previous theories. However, as it is presented today, it does not focus as heavily on the interaction of the organism with the environment, as do some other theories of motor control.

CLINICAL IMPLICATIONS

The systems theory has a number of implications for therapists. First, it stresses the importance of understanding the body as a mechanical system. Movement is not solely determined by the output of the nervous system, but is the output of the nervous system as filtered through a mechanical system, the body. When working with the patient who has a central nervous system deficit, the therapist must be careful to assess the contribution of impairments in the musculoskeletal system, as well as the neural system, to overall loss of motor control.

In our example of Mrs. Johnson, the long-term loss of mobility in her arm and leg will potentially affect the musculoskeletal system. She may show shortening of the elbow flexors and loss of range of motion at the ankle joint. These musculoskeletal limitations will have a significant effect on her ability to recover motor control.

The systems theory suggests that assessment and treatment must focus not only on the impairments within individual systems contributing to motor control, but the effect of interacting impairments among multiple systems. A good example of this in Mrs. Johnson is the interacting impairments in the musculoskeletal and neuromuscular systems that constrain her ability to move her arm.

Dynamical Action Theory

The dynamical action theory approach to motor control has begun to look at the moving person from a new perspective (24–26). The perspective comes from the broader study of dynamics or synergetics within the physical world, and asks the questions: How do the patterns and organization we see in the world come into being from their orderless constituent parts? And, how do these systems change over time? For example, we have thousands of muscle cells in the heart that work together to make the heart beat. How is this system of thousands of degrees of freedom (each cell we add contributes a new degree of freedom to the system) reduced to one of few degrees of freedom, so that all the cells function as a unit?

This phenomenon, which we see not only in heart muscle, but in the patterns of cloud formations and the patterns of movement of water as it goes from ice to liquid to boiling to evaporation, illustrates the principle of *self-organization*, which is a fundamental dynamical systems principle. It says that when a system of individual parts comes together, its elements behave collectively in an ordered way. There is no need for a "higher" center issuing instructions or commands to achieve coordinated action. This principle applied to motor control suggests that movement emerges as a result of interacting elements, without the need for specific commands, or motor programs within the nervous system.

The dynamical action or *synergetics perspective* also tries to find mathematical descriptions of these self-organizing systems. Critical features that are examined are what are called the *nonlinear properties* of the system (27).

What is nonlinear behavior? It is a situation in which, as one parameter is altered and reaches a critical value, the system goes into a whole new behavior pattern. For example, as an animal walks faster and faster, there is a point at which, suddenly, it shifts into a trot. As the animal continues to move faster, there is a second point at which it shifts into a gallop. This is shown in Figure 1.8.

The dynamical action approach does not seek to explain these shifts in terms of the nervous system circuitry, but instead simply attempts to describe mathematically the function of these systems. This allows the prediction of the ways that a given system will act in different situations. One of the points that proponents of this perspective put forth is that many body movement transitions may be explainable without invoking a specific neural pattern generator to cause the transition. The transitions instead may be due to the oscillatory or pendulum-like properties of the limbs themselves. Thus, the dynamical action perspective has deemphasized the notion of commands from the central nervous system in controlling movement and has sought physical explanations that may contribute to movement characteristics as well (28).

The dynamical action theory has recently been modified to incorporate many of Bernstein's concepts. This has resulted in the blending of these two theories of motor control into a dynamical systems model (24). This model suggests that movement underlying action results from the interaction of both physical and neural components (29).

LIMITATIONS

This approach has added to our understanding of the elements contributing to movement itself, and serves as a reminder that understanding the nervous system in isolation will not allow the prediction of movement. However, a limitation of this model can be the presumption that the nervous system has a fairly unimportant role, and that the relationship between the physical system of the animal and the environment in which it operates primarily determines the animal's be-

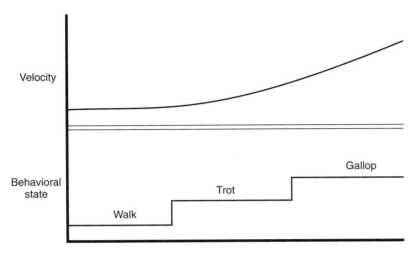

Figure 1.8. A dynamical action model predicts discrete changes in behavior resulting from changes in the linear dynamics of a moving system. For example, as velocity increases linearly, a threshold is reached that results in a change in behavioral state of the moving animal from a walk, to a trot, and a gallop.

havior. The focus of the dynamical action theory is usually at the level of this interface, not at understanding the neural contributions to the system.

CLINICAL IMPLICATIONS

One of the major implications of the dynamical action theory is the view that movement is an emergent property. That is, it emerges from the interaction of multiple elements that self-organize based on certain dynamical properties of the elements themselves. This means that shifts or alterations in movement behavior can often be explained in terms of physical principles rather than necessarily in terms of neural structures.

What are the implications of this for treating motor dyscontrol in patients? If as clinicians we understood more about the physical or dynamical properties of the human body, we could make use of these properties in helping patients to regain motor control. For example, velocity can be an important contributor to the dynamics of movement. Often, patients are asked to move slowly in an effort to move safely. Yet, this approach to retraining fails to take into account the interaction between speed and physical properties of the body, which produce momentum, and

therefore can help a weak patient move with greater ease.

In our example of Mrs. Johnson, moving slowly may not be the best strategy for getting from sit to stand, if weakness is a primary impairment. Instead, teaching her to increase the speed of trunk motion may allow her to generate sufficient momentum to succeed in standing.

Parallel Distributed Processing Theory

The parallel distributed processing (PDP) theory of motor control describes how the nervous system processes information for action. This theory has been used to explain how we acquire new skills, since it makes predictions about the processes used by the nervous system during the development or acquisition of new skills (30).

The PDP theory is consistent with current knowledge in neurophysiology that the nervous system operates both through serial processing, that is, processing information through a single pathway, and through parallel processing, that is, processing information through multiple pathways that process the same information simultaneously in different ways (31).

Figure 1.9. Parallel distributed processing model showing three layers, the input, hidden, and output layers, hypothetically equivalent to sensory, interneuron, and motor units.

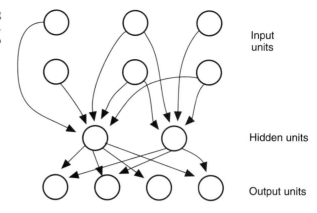

Input units

Hidden units

Output units

Scientists have begun to model neural processing using computer programs. These programs have been developed with sophisticated circuitry similar to brain networks. This is how the modeling is done: Models consist of elements that are hooked together in circuits. Like neuronal synapses, each element can be affected in a positive or negative way by the other elements. Also, like neuronal synaptic transmission, each element can have different magnitudes of either positive or negative effect on the next element. Each element then summates all the incoming positive and negative inputs. These models have been made into layered networks containing input elements, intermediate processing layers called hidden layers, and output elements. This is shown in Figure 1.9. These layers are equivalent to sensory neurons, interneurons, and motor neurons (30).

Just as in the nervous system, the efficiency of performance in this system depends on two factors. The first is the pattern of connections between the layers, and the second is the strength of individual connections. The beauty of this model is that the researcher can determine the most efficient connections to perform a particular function through a technique called *back propagation*. Through the process of back propagation, the most efficient output from the "motor neuron" layer is determined. It starts with a random set of inputs to the system. The system then calculates the difference between the desired and the actual activity of the output unit. The dif-

ference between actual and desired activity is called the *error*. The error is used to modify the connections among those elements that have produced the error.

The process is run over and over, simulating the repetition of a task performed again and again. With this activity, the system self-corrects until it solves the output problem.

The model has correctly predicted processes in both perceptual and action systems. For example, a PDP has been used to simulate the processing of visual stimuli underlying the ability to recognize and identify letters. In addition, the models have been used to predict how we calculate the correct joint angles associated with moving a limb to a particular position in space (31).

PDP is somewhat unique in its emphasis on explaining neural mechanisms associated with motor control. This theory and its related models are of great interest right now because, though they are not exact replicas of the nervous system, they have many of the properties that are also seen in the nervous system. Thus, they may help us understand how the nervous system solves particular movement problems.

LIMITATIONS

This theory is not intended to be an exact replica of the nervous system, and therefore many of its functions, such as back propagation, do not mimic nervous system processing of information during performance and learning.

CLINICAL IMPLICATIONS

The PDP theory is relatively new, and thus its clinical applications are relatively unknown. There are several ways that PDP models could be integrated into clinical practice.

A PDP model could be used to predict how injury within the nervous system affects function. The theory predicts that because of the availability of parallel redundant pathways, the loss of just a few elements will not necessarily affect function. However, the theory might predict that once a certain level or threshold is attained, the loss of additional elements will affect the capacity of the system to function. This concept of a threshold for dysfunction can be seen in many cases of pathology. For example, in Parkinson's disease there is a gradual loss of cells in the basal ganglia. Clinical symptoms may not be apparent initially, until the number of neurons lost reaches a critical threshold.

Redundant pathways suggest the possibility of multiple roads to recovery; thus, the theory could be used to suggest approaches to retraining motor dyscontrol. It suggests that recovery might be best when rehabilitation training is applied to multiple pathways. For example, Mrs. Johnson's rehabilitation program might include both voluntary activation of the gastrocnemius muscle to help improve muscle strength, but also practice, using that muscle in postural and locomotor tasks.

Task-Oriented Theories

In the last 50 years, a tremendous amount of information on the basic structure of the CNS has emerged from neuroscience research. But there is still the recognition that we *know* a lot but *understand* very little. That is, we know much about neural circuitry, but little about how the neurons operate together to achieve function. Peter Greene (32), a theoretical biologist, suggested that what was needed in the field of motor control was a

theory of tasks. By tasks, Greene was referring to the fundamental problems that the CNS was required to solve in order to accomplish motor tasks. According to Greene, an example of a fundamental task inherent in motor control is the degrees of freedom problem described by Bernstein.

According to Greene, a theory of tasks would help neuroscientists find observable behaviors to measure that are relevant to the tasks the brain is called upon to perform. Thus, an understanding of motor control requires more than an understanding of circuits. It requires an understanding of the underlying problems the CNS is required to solve in order to accomplish motor tasks. A task-oriented approach to the study of motor control would provide the basis for a more coherent picture of the motor system. Greene suggests that once the essentials of a task have been organized into a coherent picture, it becomes possible to know less and understand more.

An adaptation of Greene's theory of tasks has been elaborated by Gordon (33) and Horak (34). The task-oriented approach presented by Gordon and Horak, however, defines task from a more functional perspective. That is, what control issues are inherent in the accomplishment of functional tasks in meaningful environments? The task-oriented approach is based on the recognition that the goal of motor control is the control of movement to accomplish a particular task, not the elaboration of movement for the sake of moving alone (except in unusual cases such as dance). The task-oriented approach assumes that control of movement is organized around goal-directed functional behaviors such as walking or talking.

LIMITATIONS

A limitation of a task-oriented theory of motor control is a lack of consistent agreement about what the fundamental tasks of the CNS are. In addition, scientists don't always agree on what the essential elements being controlled within a task are. For example, some scientists studying postural control believe that controlling head position is the essential goal of the postural system. However, other scientists studying postural control believe that controlling center of mass position to achieve body stability is the essential goal of postural control.

CLINICAL IMPLICATIONS

The most significant implication of a task-oriented theory of motor control is the concept that motor retraining needs to focus on essential functional tasks. It suggests the importance of understanding the role of perceptual, cognitive, and action systems in accomplishing these tasks. One of the challenges for clinicians is to analyze essential components of everyday tasks we are called upon to retrain. This requires more than an understanding of the biomechanical features of the task, that is, the motor strategies used to accomplish the task. It also requires understanding the perceptual basis for action, and the cognitive contributions to action.

In our example of Mrs. Johnson, what are the essential tasks that will be retrained during the course of her recovery? How will these tasks be retrained? How much time will the clinician spend on retraining function, as opposed to working on some of the essential elements contributing to function, such as strength and range of motion? How can the clinician ensure that tasks learned in a clinical setting will be retained when Mrs. Johnson finally returns to her own home?

Ecological Theory

In the 1960s, independent of the research in physiology, a psychologist named James Gibson was beginning to explore the way in which our motor systems allow us to interact most effectively with the environment in order to perform goal-oriented behavior (35). His research focused on how we detect information in our environment that is relevant to our actions, and how we use this information to control our movements (see Fig. 1.10).

This view was expanded by the students of Gibson (36, 37) and became known as the

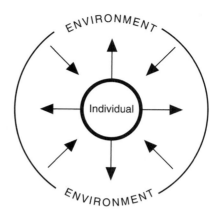

Figure 1.10. Ecological approach stresses the interaction between the individual and the environment. The individual actively explores the environment, which in turn supports the individual's actions.

ecological approach to motor control. It suggests that motor control evolved so that animals could cope with the environment around them, moving in it effectively in order to find food, run away from predators, build shelter, and even play (28). What is new about this approach? It was really the first time that researchers began focusing on how actions are geared to the environment. Actions require perceptual information that is specific to a desired goal-directed action performed within a specific environment. The organization of action is specific to the task and the environment in which the task is being performed.

Whereas many previous researchers had seen the organism as a sensory-motor system, Gibson stressed that it was not sensation per se that was important to the animal, but perception. Specifically, what is needed is the perception of environmental factors important to the task. He stated that perception focuses on detecting information in the environment that will support the actions necessary to achieve the goal. From an ecological perspective, it is important to determine how an organism detects information in the environment that is relevant to action, what form this information takes, and how this information is used to modify and control movement (28).

In summary, the ecological perspective has broadened our understanding of nervous system function from that of a sensory-motor system, reacting to environmental variables, to that of a perception-action system which actively explores the environment to satisfy its own goals.

LIMITATIONS

Although the ecological approach has expanded our knowledge significantly concerning the interaction of the organism and the environment, it has tended to give less emphasis to the organization and function of the nervous system, which led to this interaction. Thus, the research emphasis has shifted from the nervous system to the organism-environment interface.

CLINICAL IMPLICATIONS

A major contribution of this view is in describing the individual as an active explorer of the environment. The active exploration of the task and the environment in which the task is performed allows the individual to develop multiple ways to accomplish a task. Adaptability is important not only in the way we organize movements to accomplish a task, but also in the way we use our senses during action.

An important part of treatment is helping Mrs. Johnson explore the possibilities for achieving a functional task in multiple ways. The ability to develop multiple adaptive solutions to accomplishing a task requires that the patient explore a range of possible ways to accomplish a task, and discover the best solution for them, given the patient's set of limitations. In Mrs. Johnson's case, this ability to actively discover a range of solutions is hampered by a reduced ability to move, inaccurate perceptions, and possible cognitive limitations.

WHICH THEORY OF MOTOR CONTROL IS BEST?

So which motor control theory best suits the current theoretical and practice needs of therapists? Which is the most com-

plete theory of motor control, the one that really predicts the nature and cause of movement and is consistent with our current knowledge of brain anatomy and physiology?

As you no doubt can already see, there is no one theory that has it all. We believe the best theory of motor control is one that combines elements from all of the presented theories. A comprehensive, or integrated, theory recognizes the elements of motor control we do know about and leaves room for the things we don't. Any current theory of motor control is in a sense *unfinished*, since there must always be room to revise and incorporate new information.

Many people have been working to develop an integrated theory of motor control (24, 34, 38–43). In some cases, as theories are modified, new names are applied. As a result, it becomes difficult to distinguish among evolving theories. For example, systems, dynamical, dynamical action, and dynamical action systems are all terms that are often used interchangeably.

In previous articles we (40, 42) have called the theory of motor control on which we base our research and clinical practice a *systems approach*. We have continued to use this name, though our concept of *systems* theory differs from Bernstein's systems theory and has evolved to incorporate many of the concepts proposed by other theories of motor control. In this book we will continue to refer to our theory of motor control as a *systems approach*. This approach argues that it is critical to recognize that movement emerges from an interaction between the individual, the task, and the environment in which the task is being carried out. Thus, movement is not solely the result of muscle-specific motor programs, or stereotyped reflexes, but results from a dynamic interplay between perceptual, cognitive, and action systems.

Action systems are defined here to include both the neuromuscular aspects and the physical or dynamic properties of the musculoskeletal system itself. The organizational properties of the system emerge as a function of the task and the environment in which the task is performed.

This theoretical framework will be used throughout this text, and is the basis for clinical methods for assessing and treating motor dyscontrol in the patient with neurological problems. We have found the theory useful in helping us to generate research questions and hypotheses about the nature and cause of movement.

SUMMARY

1. The study of motor control is the study of the nature and cause of movement. It deals with both stabilizing the body in space, that is, postural and balance control, and with moving the body in space.
2. The specific practices used to assess and treat the patient with motor dyscontrol are determined by underlying assumptions about the nature and cause of movement that come from specific theories of motor control.
3. A theory of motor control is a group of abstract ideas about the nature and cause of movement. Theories provide: (a) a framework for interpreting behavior; (b) a guide for clinical action; (c) new ideas; and (d) working hypotheses for assessment and treatment.
4. Rehabilitation practices reflect the theories, or basic ideas, we have about the cause and nature of function and dysfunction.
5. In this chapter we have reviewed many motor control theories that have an impact on our perspective regarding assessment and treatment, including the reflex theory, hierarchical theory, motor programming theories, systems theory, dynamical action theory, parallel distributed processing theory, task-oriented theories, and ecological theory.
6. In this text we use our systems theory approach as the foundation for many clinical applications. According to this theory, movement arises from the interaction of multiple processes, including (a) perceptual, cognitive, and motor processes within the individual, and (b) interactions between the individual, the task, and the environment.

REFERENCES

1. Rosenbaum D. Human motor control. New York: Academic Press, 1991.
2. Brooks VB. The neural basis of motor control. New York: Oxford University Press, 1990.
3. Shepard K. Theory: criteria, importance and impact. In: Contemporary management of motor control problems: proceedings of the II Step Conference. Alexandria, VA: APTA, 1991:5–10.
4. Rothstein JM, Echternach JL. Hypothesis-oriented algorithm for clinicians: a method for evaluation and treatment planning. Phys Ther 1986;66:1388–1394.
5. Sherrington, C. The integrative action of the nervous system. 2nd ed. New Haven: Yale University Press, 1947.
6. Gallistel, CR. The organization of action: a new synthesis. Hillsdale, NJ: Lawrence Erlbaum, 1980.
7. Taub E, Berman AJ. Movement and learning in the absence of sensory feedback. In: Freedman SJ, ed. The neurophysiology of spatially oriented behavior. Homewood: Dorsey Press, 1968:173–192.
8. Foerster O. The motor cortex in man in the light of Hughlings Jackson's doctrines. In: Payton OD, Hirt S, Newman, R, eds. Scientific bases for neurophysiologic approaches to therapeutic exercise. Philadelphia: FA Davis, 1977:13–18.
9. Magnus R. Animal posture (Croonian lecture). Proc Roy Soc London 1925;98:339.
10. Magnus R. Some results of studies in the physiology of posture. Lancet 1926;2:531–585.
11. Schaltenbrand G. The development of human motility and motor disturbances. Arch Neurol Pyschiatr 1928;20:720–730.
12. Weisz S. Studies in equilibrium reaction. J Nerv Ment Dis 1938;88:150–162.
13. Gesell A, Amatruda CS. Developmental diagnosis. 2nd ed. New York: Paul B. Hoeber, 1947.
14. Gesell A. Behavior patterns of fetal-infant and child. Genetics. Proceedings of the Association for Research in Nervous and Mental Disease 1954;33:114.
15. McGraw M. Neuromuscular maturation of the human infant. New York: Hafner Press, 1945.
16. Bobath B. Abnormal postural reflex activity caused by brain lesions. London: Heinemann, 1965:8.
17. Fiorentino M. Reflex testing methods for

evaluating CNS Development. Springfield, IL: Charles C Thomas, 1963.

19. van Sant AF. Concepts of neural organization and movement. In: Connolly BH, Montgomery PC, eds. Therapeutic exercise in developmental disabilities. Chattanooga, TN: Chattanooga Corp, 1987:1–8.

20. Wilson DM. The central nervous control of flight in a locust. J Exp Biol 1961;38:471–490.

21. Grillner S. Control of locomotion in bipeds, tetrapods and fish. In: Geiger SR, ed. Handbook of physiology, vol 2. Bethesda, MD: American Physiological Society, 1981:1179–1236.

22. Forssberg H, Grillner S, Rossignol S. Phase dependent reflex reversal during walking in chronic spinal cats. Brain Res 1975;85:103–107.

23. Bernstein, N. The coordination and regulation of movement. London: Pergamon Press, 1967.

24. Thelen E, Kelso JAS, Fogel A. Self-organizing systems and infant motor development. Developmental Review 1987;7:39–65.

25. Kamm K, Thelen E, Jensen J. A dynamical systems approach to motor development: In: Rothstein JM, ed. Movement science. Alexandria, VA: APTA Association, 1991: 11–23.

26. Kelso JAS, Tuller B. A dynamical basis for action systems. In: Gazanniga MS, ed. Handbook of cognitive neuroscience. NY: Plenum Press, 1984:321–356.

27. Kugler PN, Turvey MT. Information, natural law and self assembly of rhythmic movement. Hillsdale, NJ: Erlbaum, 1987.

28. Schmidt R. Motor and action perspectives on motor behaviour. In: Meijer OG, Roth K, eds. Complex movement behavior: the motor-action controversy. Amsterdam: Elsevier, 1988:3–44.

29. Crutchfield CA, Heriza CB, Herdman S. Motor control. Morgantown, WV: Stokesville Publishers, in press.

30. Rumelhart DE, McClelland JL, eds. Parallel distributed processing, explorations in the microstructure of cognition, vol 1: Foundations. Cambridge, Mass: MIT Press, 1986.

31. Kandel E, Schwartz JH, Jessell TM, eds. Principles of neuroscience. 3rd ed. New York: Elsevier, 1991:420–439.

32. Green PH. Problems of organization of motor systems. In: Rosen R, Snell FM, eds. Progress in theoretical biology. San Diego: Academic Press, 1972:304–338.

33. Gordon J. Assumptions underlying physical therapy intervention: theoretical and historical perspectives. In: Carr JH, Shepherd RB, Gordon J, et al., eds. Movement sciences: foundations for physical therapy in rehabilitation. Rockville, Md: Aspen Publishers, 1987:1–30.

34. Horak F. Assumptions underlying motor control for neurologic rehabilitation. In: Contemporary management of motor control problems. Proceedings of the II Step Conference. Alexandria, VA: APTA, 1992: 11–28.

35. Gibson, JJ. The senses considered as perceptual systems. Boston: Houghton Mifflin, 1966.

36. Reed ES. An outline of a theory of action systems. Journal of Motor Behavior. 1982;14:98–134.

37. Lee DN. The functions of vision. In: Pick H, Saltzman E, eds. Modes of perceiving and processing information. Hillsdale, NJ: Erlbaum, 1978.

38. Mulder T, Geurts A. Recovery of motor skill following nervous system disorders: a behavioral emphasis. Clinical Neurology. In press.

39. Patla A. The neural control of locomotion. In: Spivack BS, ed. Mobility and gait. In press.

40. Woollacott M, Shumway-Cook A. Changes in posture control across the life span—a systems approach. Phys Ther 1990;70:799–807.

41. Shumway-Cook A. Equilibrium deficits in children. In: Woollacott M, Shumway-Cook A, eds. Development of posture and gait across the life span. Columbia, SC: Univ of SC Press, 1989: 229–252.

42. Woollacott M, Shumway-Cook A, Williams H. The development of posture and balance control. In: Woollacott MH, Shumway-Cook A, eds. Development of posture and gait across the life span. Columbia, SC: Univ of SC Press, 1989:77–96.

43. Horak F, Shumway-Cook A. Clinical implications of postural control research. In: Duncan P, ed. Balance. Alexandria, VA: APTA, 1990.

Chapter 2

MOTOR LEARNING AND RECOVERY OF FUNCTION

INTRODUCTION TO MOTOR LEARNING

Mr. Smith has been receiving therapy for 5 weeks now, following his stroke. He has gradually regained the ability to stand, walk, and feed himself again. What is the cause of Mr. Smith's recovery of motor function? How much is due to "spontaneous recovery"? How much of his recovery may be attributed to therapeutic interventions? How many of his re-acquired motor skills will he be able to retain and use when he leaves the rehabilitation facility and returns home? These questions and issues reflect the importance of motor learning to clinicians involved in retraining the patient with motor control problems.

What Is Motor Learning?

In Chapter 1, we defined the field of motor control as the study of the nature and cause of movement. We define the field of **motor learning** as the study of the acquisition and or modification of movement. While motor control focuses on understanding the control of movement already acquired, motor learning focuses on understanding the acquisition and or modification of movement.

The field of motor learning has traditionally referred to the study of the acquisition or modification of movement in normal subjects. In contrast, **recovery of function** has referred to the re-acquisition of movement skills lost through injury.

While there is nothing inherent in the term motor learning to distinguish it from processes involved in the recovery of movement function, the two are often thought of as separate. This separation between recovery of function and motor learning may be misleading. Issues facing clinicians concerned with helping patients reacquire skills lost as the result of injury are similar to those faced by people in the field of motor learning. Questions common to both include: how can I best structure practice (therapy) to ensure learning? How can I ensure that skills learned in one context transfer to others? Will simplifying a task, that is making it easier to perform, result in more efficient learning?

In this chapter we use the term motor learning to encompass both the acquisition and reacquisition of movement. We will describe various theories of motor learning and recovery of function.

EARLY DEFINITIONS OF MOTOR LEARNING

Learning has been described as the process of acquiring knowledge about the world; motor learning has been described as a set of processes associated with practice or experience leading to relatively permanent changes in the capability for producing skilled action (1). This definition of motor learning reflects four concepts: (1) learning is a process of acquiring the capability for skilled action; (2) learning results from experience or practice; (3) learning cannot be measured directly—instead, it is inferred based on behavior; and (4) learning produces relatively permanent changes in behavior, thus short-term alterations are not thought of as learning (1).

BROADENING THE DEFINITION OF MOTOR LEARNING

In this chapter the definition of motor learning has been expanded to encompass many aspects not traditionally considered part of motor learning.

Motor learning involves more than motor processes. Rather, it involves learning new strategies for sensing as well as moving. Thus, motor learning, like motor control, emerges from a complex of perception-cognition-action processes.

Previous views of motor learning have focused primarily on changes in the individual. But the process of motor learning can be described as the search for a task solution that emerges from an interaction of the individual with the task and the environment. Task solutions are new strategies for perceiving and acting (2).

Similarly, the recovery of function involves the reorganization of both perceptual and action systems in relationship to specific tasks and environments. Thus, one cannot study motor learning or recovery of function outside of the context of how individuals are solving functional tasks in specific environments.

Relating Performance and Learning

Traditionally, the study of motor learning has focused solely on motor outcomes. Earlier views of motor learning did not always distinguish it from performance (3). Changes in performance that resulted from practice were usually thought to reflect changes in learning. However, this view failed to consider that certain practice effects improved performance initially but were not necessarily retained, a condition of learning. This led to the notion that learning could not be evaluated during practice, but rather during specific retention or transfer tests. Thus, learning, defined as a relatively permanent change, has been distinguished from performance, defined as a temporary change in motor behavior seen during practice sessions.

We view the term performance from a slightly different perspective. Performance is behavior observed at any specific moment in time, and not limited to describing behaviors observed during practice sessions. Performance, whether observed during practice sessions or during retention and transfer tasks, is the result of a complex interaction among many variables, one of which is the level of learning. Some other variables that may affect performance include fatigue, anxiety, and motivation. Thus, performance, regardless of when it is measured, is not necessarily a measure of absolute learning. This is because changes in performance can reflect not only changes in learning, but changes in other variables as well.

FORMS OF LEARNING

The recovery of function following injury involves the reacquisition of complex tasks. However, it is difficult to understand the processes involved in learning using the study of complex tasks. Therefore, many researchers have begun by exploring simple forms of learning, with the understanding that these simple forms of learning are the basis for the acquisition of skilled behavior. However, there is very little information about how these simple forms of learning contribute to the acquisition of more complex skills.

We begin by reviewing these simple forms of learning and discussing some of their clinical applications. We then consider theories of motor learning that have been developed to describe the acquisition of skilled behavior and suggest how each might be used to explain the acquisition of the skill such as reaching for a glass of water. At the outset, we provide a review of simple nonassociative forms of learning such as habituation and sensitization.

Nonassociative Forms of Learning

Nonassociative learning occurs when animals are given a single stimulus repeatedly. As a result, the nervous system learns about the characteristics of that stimulus. Habituation and sensitization are two very simple forms of nonassociative learning (4). **Habituation** is a decrease in responsiveness that occurs as a result of repeated exposure to a non-painful stimulus.

Habituation is used in many different ways in the clinical setting. For example, habituation exercises are used to treat dizziness

in patients with certain types of vestibular dysfunction. Patients are asked to repeatedly move in ways that provoke their dizziness. This repetition results in habituation of the dizziness response. Habituation forms the basis of therapy for children who are termed "tactile defensive," that is, who show excessive responsiveness to cutaneous stimulation. Children are repeatedly exposed to gradually increasing levels of cutaneous inputs in an effort to decrease their sensitivity to this stimulus.

Sensitization is an increased responsiveness following a threatening or noxious stimulus (4). For example, if I receive a painful stimulus on the skin, and then a light touch, I will react more strongly than normal to the light touch. After a person has habituated to one stimulus, another painful stimulus can dishabituate the first. That is, sensitization counteracts the effects of habituation.

There are times when increasing a patient's sensitivity to a threatening stimulus is important. For example, increasing a patient's awareness of stimuli indicating a likelihood for impending falls might be an important aspect of balance retraining.

Not all nonassociative forms of learning are simple. Sensory learning, where you form a sensory experience, is an example of nonassociative learning. It is learning that relates to understanding about a stimulus, in this case, the sensory inputs. Helping patients to explore their perceptual space, as it relates to learning a particular skill—like reaching or transferring—would be an example of nonassociative learning.

Associative Forms of Learning

What is *associative learning*? One possible answer is that it involves the association of ideas. For example, if you tell your patients who are having problems walking to try to associate shifting their center of gravity with lifting their leg, you are helping them combine two aspects of a movement into one integrated whole. It is through associative learning that a person learns to predict relationships, either relationships of one stimulus to another (classical conditioning) or the relationship of one's behavior to a consequence (operant conditioning).

It has been suggested that associative learning has evolved to help animals learn to detect causal relationships in the environment (4). Establishing lawful and therefore predictive relationships among events is part of the process of making sense and order of our world. Recognizing key relationships between events is an essential part of the ability to adapt behavior to novel situations (4).

Patients who have suffered an injury that has drastically altered their ability to sense and move about their world have the task of reexploring their body in relationship to their world, in order to determine what new relationships exist between the two.

Pavlov studied how humans and animals learn the association of two stimuli, through the simple form of learning that is now called **classical conditioning**.

CLASSICAL CONDITIONING

Classical conditioning consists of learning to pair two stimuli. During classical conditioning an initially weak stimulus (the conditioned stimulus) becomes highly effective in producing a response when it becomes associated with another stronger stimulus (the unconditioned stimulus). The conditioned stimulus is usually something that initially produces no response (like a bell). In contrast, the unconditioned stimulus (UCS), which could be food, always produces a response. After repeated pairing of the conditioned and the unconditioned stimulus, one begins to see a conditioned response (CR) to the conditioned stimulus (CS). Remember—it originally produced no response (4). This relationship is shown in Figure 2.1.

What the subject is doing in this type of learning is to predict relationships between two stimuli or events that have occurred and to respond accordingly. For example, in a therapy setting, if we repeatedly give patients a verbal cue in conjunction with giving them aid in making a movement, they may even-

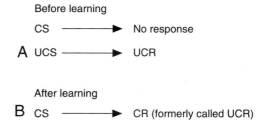

Figure 2.1. The process of classical conditioning is diagrammed showing the relationship between the conditioned stimulus (CS), unconditioned stimulus (UCS), conditioned response (CR), and unconditioned response (UCR) before learning (**A**) and during the course of learning (**B**).

tually begin to make the movement with only the verbal cue.

Thus, as patients gain skills we see them move along the continuum of assistance from hands-on assistance from the therapist, to performing the task with verbal cues, and eventually to performing the action unassisted.

It has recently been shown that we generally learn relationships that are relevant to our survival; it is more difficult to associate biologically meaningless events. These findings underscore an important learning principle: the brain is most likely to perceive and integrate aspects of the environment that are most pertinent. With regard to therapy, learning in patients is most likely to occur in tasks and environments that are relevant and meaningful to them.

OPERANT CONDITIONING

Operant or instrumental conditioning is a second type of associational learning (4). It is basically trial and error learning. During **operant conditioning** we learn to associate a certain response, from among many that we have made, with a consequence. The classic experiments in this area were done with animals who were given food rewards whenever they randomly pressed a lever inside their cages. They soon learned to associate the lever press with the presentation of food, and lever pressing frequency became very high.

The principle of operant conditioning could be stated as follows: behaviors that are rewarded tend to be repeated at the cost of other behaviors. And likewise, behaviors followed by aversive stimuli are not usually repeated. This has been called the *law of effect* (4).

Operant conditioning plays a major role in determining the behaviors shown by patients referred for therapy. For example, the frail elderly person who leaves her home to go shopping and experiences a fall is less likely to repeat that activity again. A decrease in activity results in declining physical functions, which in turn increases the likelihood she will fall. This increased likelihood for falls will reinforce her desire to be inactive, and on it goes, showing the law of effect in action. Therapists may make use of a variety of techniques to assist this patient in regaining her activity level and in reducing her likelihood of falling. One technique is to use the process of desensitization to decrease her anxiety and fear of falling.

Operant conditioning can be an effective tool during clinical intervention. Verbal praise by a therapist for a job well done serves as a reinforcer for some (though not all!) patients. Setting up a therapy session so that a particular movement is rewarded by the successful accomplishment of a task desired by the patient is a powerful example of operant conditioning. Using biofeedback to help a patient learn to control the foot during the swing portion of gait is also an example of operant conditioning.

PROCEDURAL AND DECLARATIVE LEARNING

Some researchers have begun to classify associative learning based on the type of knowledge that is acquired by the learner. Using this type of classification, two types of learning have been identified based on the type and recall of information learned (4).

Procedural learning refers to learning tasks that can be performed automatically without attention or conscious thought, like a habit. Procedural learning develops slowly through repetition of an act over many trials, and is expressed through improved performance of the task that was practiced. Procedural learning does not depend on awareness, attention, or other higher cognitive processes. During motor skill acquisition, repeating a movement continuously under varying circumstances would typically lead to procedural learning. That is, one automatically learns the movement itself, or the rules for moving, called a movement schema.

For example, when teaching a patient to transfer from chair to bed, we often have the patient practice an optimal movement strategy to move from one to the other. To better prepare patients to transfer effectively in a wide variety of situations and contexts, patients learn to move from chairs of differing heights, and at different positions relative to the bed. They thus begin to form the *rules associated with the task of transfer*. The development of rules for transferring will allow them to safely transfer in unfamiliar circumstances. This constant practice and repetition results in efficient procedural learning and effective and safe transfers.

On the other hand, **declarative learning** results in knowledge that can be consciously recalled and thus requires processes such as awareness, attention, and reflection (4). Declarative learning can be expressed in declarative sentences, like: first I button the top button, then the next one. Constant repetition can transform declarative into procedural knowledge. For example, when patients are first relearning a skill, they may verbally describe each movement as they do it. However, with repetition, the movement becomes an automatic motor activity, that is, one that does not require conscious attention and monitoring.

The advantage of declarative learning is that it can be shown in other forms than it was learned. So, for example, expert ski racers, when preparing to race down a slalom hill at 120 miles an hour, rehearse in their minds the race and how they will run it. So, too, figure skaters preparing to perform will often mentally practice the sequences to be skated prior to getting on the ice.

In therapy, when helping patients reacquire skills lost through injury, the emphasis is often on practices leading to procedural learning, learning a movement, rather than on declarative learning. Declarative learning requires the ability to verbally express the process to be performed and is often not possible with patients who have both cognitive and language deficits that impair their ability to recall and express knowledge. Teaching movement skills declaratively would, however, allow patients to rehearse their movements mentally, increasing the amount of practice available to them when physical conditions such as fatigue would normally limit it.

THEORIES RELATED TO SKILLED LEARNING

Just as there are theories of motor control, there are theories of motor learning, that is, a group of abstract ideas about the nature and cause of the acquisition or modification of movement. Theories of motor learning, like theories of motor control, must be based on current knowledge regarding the structure and function of the nervous system. The following section reviews current theories of motor learning. Included in this section is a brief discussion of several theories related to recovery of function, the reacquisition of skills lost through injury.

Adams' Closed-Loop Theory

Adams (5), a researcher in physical education, was the first person to attempt to create a comprehensive theory of motor learning. This theory generated a lot of interest during the 1970s as researchers attempted to determine its applicability to motor skill acquisition.

The most important aspect of the theory is that it is founded on the concept of **closed-loop** processes in motor control. In a closed-loop process sensory feedback is used for the ongoing production of skilled movement. This theory hypothesizes that, in motor learning, sensory feedback from the ongoing movement is compared within the nervous system with the stored memory of the intended movement (6). This internal reference of correctness, which Adams called a **perceptual trace**, is built up over a period of practice.

Adams predicted that the perceptual trace by itself could not lead to the accurate production of skilled movement. He proposed that a second trace, the **memory trace**, is used to select and initiate the movement (1). After movement is initiated by the memory trace, he proposed that the perceptual trace would take over to carry out the movement and detect error.

According to Adams' theory, when learning to pick up a glass, you would gradually develop a perceptual trace for the movement, which would serve as a guide toward your endpoint. The more you practiced the specific movement, the stronger the perceptual trace would become. The accuracy of the movement would be directly proportional to the strength of the perceptual trace.

LIMITATIONS

Adams' closed-loop theory of motor learning has been criticized for several reasons. It has been shown that animals and humans can make movements even when they have no sensory feedback (7–9). In addition, animals are capable of conditioned learning in order to avoid shocks, even after deafferentation (7). Thus, Adams' closed-loop theory could not explain these open-loop movements, that is, movements made in the absence of sensory feedback.

Schmidt's Schema Theory

In the 1970s, in response to many of the limitations of the closed-loop theory of motor learning, Richard Schmidt, another researcher from the field of physical education, proposed a new motor learning theory, which he called the schema theory. It emphasized open-loop control processes and the motor program concept (10). Though the concept of motor programs was considered essential to understanding motor control, no one had yet addressed the question of how motor programs can be learned. As other researchers before him, Schmidt proposed that motor programs do not contain the specifics of movements, but instead contain generalized rules for a specific class of movements. He predicted that when learning a new motor program, the individual learns a generalized set of rules that can be applied to a variety of contexts.

At the heart of this motor learning theory is the concept of **schema**, which has been important in psychology for many years. The term schema originally referred to an abstract representation stored in memory following multiple presentations of a class of objects. For example, after seeing many different types of dogs, it is proposed that we begin to store an abstract set of rules for general dog qualities in our brain, so that whenever we see a new dog, no matter what size, color, or shape, we can identify it as a dog.

Schmidt expanded the concept of schema and applied it to the area of motor control. He proposed that, after an individual makes a movement, four things are stored in memory: (*a*) the initial movement conditions, such as the position of the body and the weight of the object manipulated; (*b*) the parameters used in the generalized motor program; (*c*) the outcome of the movement, in terms of **knowledge of results** (KR); and (*d*) the sensory consequences of the movement, that is, how it felt, looked, and sounded. This information is abstracted and stored in the form of a **recall** (motor) schema and a **recognition** (sensory) schema, as you see in Figure 2.2.

The recall schema is used for the selection of a specific response. When making a given movement, the initial conditions and desired goal of the movement are inputs to the recall schema. Other inputs are the abstract memory of previous response specifications in similar tasks.

The recognition schema is used for the evaluation of the response. In this case the sensory consequences and outcomes of previous movements are coupled with the current initial conditions to create a representation of the expected sensory consequences. This is then compared to the sensory information from the ongoing movement in order to evaluate the efficiency of the response. The recognition schema is primarily used for learning rather than on-line control.

When the movement is over, the error signal is fed back into the schema and the schema is modified as a result of the sensory feedback and KR. Thus, according to this theory, learning consists of the ongoing process of updating the recognition and recall schemas with each movement that is made.

According to schema theory, when learning to reach for a glass, you would optimally practice many variations on the task itself. This would allow you to develop a set of rules for reaching, which you would then apply when reaching for the glass in front of you. The better your rules for reaching, the more optimal would be your strategy for picking up an unfamiliar glass, and the less likely that you would drop the glass or spill the milk.

LIMITATIONS

Is schema theory supported by research? Yes and no. One of the predictions of schema theory is that when practicing a skill, variable forms of practice will produce the most effective schema or motor program. Research to test this prediction has used the following paradigms. Two groups of subjects are trained in a new task, one given constant practice conditions and the other given variable practice conditions. Both groups are then tested on a new, but similar movement. According to schema theory, the second group should show higher level performance than the first, because they have developed a broad set of rules about the task, which should allow them to apply the rules to a new situation. On the other hand, the first group should have developed a very narrow schema with limited rules that would not be easily applicable to new situations.

In studies on normal adults, the support is mixed. Many studies show large effects of variable practice, while some studies show very small effects or no effect at all. However, with regard to studies in children, there has been strong support. For example, 7- and 9-year-old children were trained to toss bean bags over a variable distance or a fixed dis-

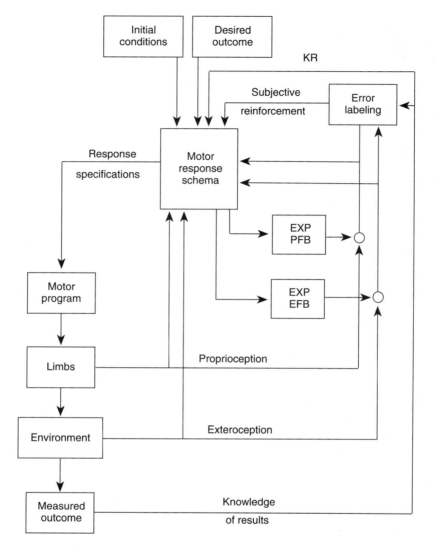

Figure 2.2. Diagram of Schmidt's schema theory, illustrating the critical elements in the acquisition of movement. EXP PFB = expected proprioceptive feedback; EXP EFB = expected exteroceptive feedback. (Adapted from Schmidt RA. A schema theory of discrete motor skill learning. Psychol Rev 1975;82:225–260.)

tance. When asked to throw at a new distance, the variable practice group produced significantly better scores than the fixed practice group (11). Why might there be differences between children and adults in these experiments? It has been suggested that it may be difficult to find experimental tasks at which adults don't already have significant variable practice during normal activities, while children, with much less experience, are more naive subjects (12). Therefore, the experiments may be more valid in children.

Another limitation of the theory is that it lacks specificity. Because of its generalized nature, there are few recognizable mechanisms that can be tested. Thus, it is not clear how schema processing itself interacts with other systems to learn movement and how it aids to control that movement.

Another challenge to the schema theory has been its inability to account for the immediate acquisition of new types of coordination or new forms of movement. For example, researchers have shown that if all of a centipede's limbs except for two pairs are removed, the centipede will immediately produce a quadrupedal gait (13). It has been argued that findings such as these cannot be accounted for by schema theory (2).

Fitts and Posner: Stages of Motor Learning

Fitts and Posner (14), two researchers from the field of psychology, described a theory of motor learning related to the stages that people go through in learning a new skill. They suggest there are three main phases involved in skill learning. In the first stage the learner is concerned with understanding the nature of the task, developing strategies that could be used to carry out the task, and determining how the task should be evaluated. These efforts require a high degree of cognitive activity such as attention. Accordingly, this stage is referred to as the **cognitive stage** of learning.

In this stage the person experiments with a variety of strategies, abandoning those that don't work while keeping those that do. Performance tends to be quite variable, perhaps because many strategies are being sampled for performing the task. However, improvements in performance are also quite large in this first stage, perhaps as a result of selecting the most effective strategy for the task.

The second stage in skill acquisition is described by Fitts and Posner as the **associative stage**. By this time the person has selected the best strategy for the task and now begins to refine the skill. Thus, during this stage there is less variability in performance, and improvement also occurs more slowly. It is proposed that verbal-cognitive aspects of learning are not as important at this stage because the person focuses more on refining a particular pattern rather than on selecting among alternative strategies (1). This stage may last from days to weeks or months, depending on the performer and the intensity of practice. This stage is equivalent to the motor stage described by Adams.

The third stage of skill acquisition has

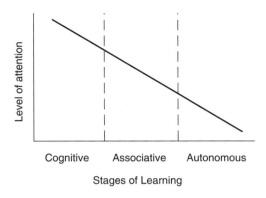

Figure 2.3. The changing attentional demands associated with the three stages of motor skill acquisition outlined by Fitts and Posner.

been described as the **autonomous stage**. Fitts and Posner define this stage by the automaticity of the skill, and the low degree of attention required for its performance, as shown in Figure 2.3. Thus, in this stage the person can begin to devote his or her attention to other aspects of the skill in general, like scanning the environment for obstacles that might impede performance, or one may choose to focus on a secondary task (like talking to a friend while performing the task), or save one's energy, so that one does not become fatigued.

Using this theory of motor learning we would learn to reach for a glass in the following way. Your first experience of using the glass would require a great deal of attention and conscious thought. You might make a lot of errors and spill a lot of water, while you experimented with different movement strategies to accomplish the task. When moving into the second stage, however, the movement toward the glass would be refined and you would use an optimal strategy. At this point the task wouldn't require your full attention. In the third autonomous stage, you would be able to reach for the glass while carrying on a conversation or being engaged in other tasks.

LIMITATIONS

Schmidt (1) notes that very little research has been focused on the autonomous

Figure 2.4. A diagram showing the process proposed by Newell of exploring the sensory and motor workspace (**A**) in order to find optimal solutions to movement tasks (**B**).

Exploration of perceptual and motor workspaces

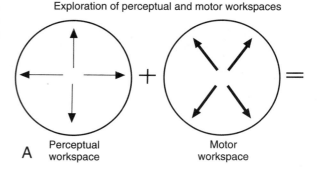

A   Perceptual   Motor
     workspace   workspace

Mapping perceptual-motor workspaces to create optimal solutions

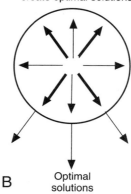

B   Optimal
     solutions

stage of learning, partly because it would take months or years to bring many subjects to this skill level on a laboratory task. Thus, he states that the principles that govern motor learning in this stage are largely unknown.

Newell's Theory of Learning as Exploration

Karl Newell drew heavily from both systems and ecological motor control theories to create a theory of motor skill acquisition based on search strategies (2). In the previous learning theories proposed by Adams and Schmidt, practice produced a cumulative continuous change in behavior due to a gradual buildup of the strength of motor programs. It was proposed that, with practice, a more appropriate representation of action is developed.

In contrast, Newell suggests that motor learning is a process that increases the coor-

dination between perception and action in a way consistent with the task and environmental constraints. What does he mean by this? He proposes that, during practice, there is a search for optimal strategies to solve the task, given the constraints. Part of the search for optimal strategies involves finding the most appropriate perceptual cues and motor responses for the task. Thus, the perception and action systems can be considered to be incorporated or mapped into an optimal task solution.

Critical to the search for optimal strategies is the exploration of the *perceptual-motor workspace*. This process of exploring the sensory and motor workspace in order to find optimal solutions is shown diagrammatically in Figure 2.4. Newell believes that one useful outcome of his theory will be the impetus to identify critical perceptual variables essential to optimal task-relevant solutions. These critical variables will be useful in designing search strategies that produce efficient mapping of perceptual information and movement parameters.

Newell believes that perceptual information has a number of roles in motor learning. In a *prescriptive* role, perceptual information relates to understanding the goal of the task and the movements to be learned. This information has typically been given to learners through demonstrations.

Another role of perceptual information is as *feedback*, both during the movement (concurrent feedback, sometimes called knowledge of performance) and on completion of the movement (knowledge of results). Finally, he proposes that perceptual information can be used to structure the search for a perceptual-motor solution that is appropriate for the demands of the task. Thus, in this approach, motor learning is characterized by optimal task-relevant mapping of perception and action, not by a rule-based representation of action.

In Newell's approach, during the course of learning to reach for a glass, repeated practice with reaching for a variety of glasses that contain a variety of substances within them, results in learning to match the appropriate movement dynamics for the task of reaching. But in addition, we learn to distinguish what characteristics of the task we need to know to organize our actions. Such characteristics as the size of the glass, how slippery the surface is, how full it is, are essential perceptual cues that help us develop optimal movement strategies for grasping any variation of glasses.

Various sensory cues help us to create optimal motor strategies. If a perceptual cue suggests a heavy glass, we grasp with more force. If the glass is full, we modulate our speed and trajectory to accommodate the situation. If we lack preciseness in these sensory cues, we can still create a motor strategy, but it might be less than optimal. That is, the fluid may spill, or the glass may slip. Knowledge about the critical perceptual cues associated with a task is essential in dealing with a new variation of the task. When faced with a novel variant, we actively explore the perceptual

cues to find the information we need to optimally solve the task problem.

This idea of a search of the workspace is similar to the concept of discovery learning, yet discovery learning concepts do not address the best ways for the learner to channel the search through the workspace.

Newell discusses ways to augment skill learning. The first is to help the learner understand the nature of the perceptual motor workspace. The second is to understand the natural search strategies used by performers in exploring space. And the third is that of providing augmented information to facilitate the search.

One central prediction of this theory is that the transfer of motor skills will be dependent on the similarity between the two tasks of the optimal perceptual-motor strategies and relatively independent of the muscles used or the objects manipulated in the task.

In summary, this new approach to motor learning emphasizes skill as a reflection of a dynamic exploratory activity, involved in mapping the perceptual-motor workspace to create optimal strategies for performing a task.

LIMITATIONS

This is a very new theory. One of its major limitations is that it has yet to be applied to specific examples of motor skill acquisition in any systematic way. As a result, it is an untested theory.

FACTORS CONTRIBUTING TO MOTOR LEARNING

Very often therapists ask themselves questions like: Is the type of feedback that I am giving to my patients concerning the quality of their movements really effective? Could I give a different form of feedback that might be better? Should I give feedback with every trial that the patient makes, or would it be better to withhold feedback occasionally and make the patients try to discern by themselves if their movement is accurate or efficient?

What is the best timing for feedback? In the following section we discuss research in motor learning that has attempted to answer these questions. We review the research in relation to the different motor learning factors that are important to consider when retraining patients with motor control problems, including feedback, practice conditions, and variability of practice.

Feedback

We have already discussed the importance of feedback in relation to motor learning. Clearly, some form of feedback is essential for learning to take place. In the following section we describe the types of feedback that are available to the performer, and the contributions of these different types of feedback to motor learning.

The broadest definition of feedback includes all the sensory information that is available as the result of a movement that a person has produced. This is typically called **response-produced feedback** (1). This feedback is usually further divided into two subclasses, that of **intrinsic feedback** and **extrinsic feedback**.

INTRINSIC FEEDBACK

Intrinsic feedback is feedback that comes to the individual simply through the various sensory systems as a result of the normal production of the movement. This includes such things as visual information concerning whether a movement was accurate, as well as somatosensory information concerning the position of the limbs as one was moving (1).

EXTRINSIC FEEDBACK

Extrinsic feedback is information that supplements intrinsic feedback. For example, when you tell a patient that he/she needs to pick up his/her foot higher to clear an object while walking, you are offering extrinsic feedback.

Extrinsic feedback can be given *concur-* *rently* with the task and in addition, at the end of the task, in which case it is called *terminal feedback*. An example of concurrent feedback would be *verbal* or manual guidance to the hand of a patient learning to reach for objects. An example of terminal feedback would be telling a patient after a first unsuccessful attempt to rise from a chair, to push harder the next time, using the arms to create more force to stand up (1).

KNOWLEDGE OF RESULTS

Knowledge of results (KR) is one important form of extrinsic feedback. It has been defined as terminal feedback about the *outcome* of the movement, in terms of the movement's goal (1). This is in contrast to **knowledge of performance** (KP), which is feedback relating to the movement pattern used to achieve the goal.

Research has been performed to determine the types of feedback that are the best to give a subject. Almost all of the research that has been performed involves studying the efficacy of different types of knowledge of results. Typically, research has shown that knowledge of results is an important learning variable, that is, it is important for learning motor tasks (15). However, there are certain types of tasks where intrinsic feedback (for example, visual or kinaesthetic) is sufficient to provide most error information, and KR has only minimal effects. For example, in learning tracking tasks KR only minimally improves the performance and learning of a subject (1).

It has also been shown that KR is a performance variable, that is, it has temporary effects on the ability of the subject to perform a task. This may be due to motivational or alerting effects on the performer, as well as guidance effects (that is, it tells the subject how to perform the task better in the next trial).

When should KR be given for optimal results? Should it be given right after a movement? What delay is best before the next movement is made, to ensure maximum learning efficiency? Should KR be given after every movement? These are important questions for the therapist who wants to optimize the learning or relearning of motor skills in patients with motor disorders.

Experiments attempting to determine the optimum KR delay interval have found very little effect of KR delay on motor learning efficacy. The same is true of the post-KR delay interval. There may be a slight reduction in learning if the KR delay is very short, but any effects are very small. However, it has been shown that it is good not to fill the KR-delay interval with other movements, since these appear to interfere with the learning of the target movements. Research on the effects of filling the post-KR delay interval with extraneous activities is less clear. Apparently, this interval is not as important as the KR-delay interval for the integration of KR information. It has also been recommended that the *intertrial interval* should not be excessively short, but the literature in this area shows conflicting results (1, 16) concerning the effects of different lengths of intertrial intervals on learning.

What happens to learning efficacy if KR is not given every trial? For example, if you ask a patient to practice a reaching movement and only give the patient feedback on the accuracy of the movement every five or 10 trials, what do you think might happen? One might assume that decreasing the amount of KR given would have a detrimental effect on learning. However, experiments in this area have shown surprising results.

Experimenters compared the performance of (*a*) subjects who had KR feedback on every trial; (*b*) subjects who had *summary KR*, that is KR for each of the trials only at the end of an entire block of 20 trials; and (*c*) subjects who had both types of feedback. It was found that at the end of the acquisition trials, performance was best if KR was given after every trial (groups 1 and 3 were far better than group 2). However, when performance was then compared for the groups on transfer tests, where no KR was given at any time, the group that was originally the least accurate, the summary KR only group (group 2), was now the most accurate (17).

These results suggest that summary KR is the best feedback, but if this were so, group 3 should have been as good as group 2, and this was not the case. It has thus been concluded that immediate KR is detrimental to learning, because it provides too much information, and allows the subject to rely on the information too strongly (1).

What is the best number of trials to complete before giving KR? This appears to vary depending on the task. For very simple movement timing tasks, in which KR was given after one trial, five trials, 10 trials, or 15 trials, the performance on acquisition trials was best for the most frequent feedback, but when a transfer test was given, the performance was best for the 15-trial summary group. In a more complex task, where a pattern of moving lights had to be intercepted by an arm movement (like intercepting a ball with a bat), the most effective summary length for learning was five trials, and anything more or less was less efficient (1).

How precise must KR be in order to be most effective? The answer varies for adults vs. children. For adults, quantitative KR appears to be best, with the more precise KR giving more accurate performance, up to a point, beyond which there is no further improvement. For adults, units of measure (for example, inches, centimeters, feet, miles) do not seem to be important, with nonsense units even being effective. However, in children, unfamiliar units or very precise KR can be confusing and degrade learning (1, 18).

Practice Conditions

We have already discussed the importance of KR to learning. A second variable that is also very important is practice. Typically, the more practice you can give a patient, the more the patient learns, with other things being equal. Thus, in creating a therapy session, the number of practice attempts should be maximized. But what about fatigue? How should the therapist schedule practice periods vs. rest periods? Research to answer these questions is summarized in the following sections.

MASSED AND DISTRIBUTED PRACTICE

To answer these questions researchers have performed experiments comparing two types of practice sessions: massed and distributed. **Massed practice** is defined as a session in which the amount of practice time in a trial is greater than the amount of rest between trials. This may lead to fatigue in some tasks. **Distributed practice** is defined as a session in which the amount of rest between trials equals or is greater than the amount of time for a trial (1). For continuous tasks, massed practice has been proven to decrease performance markedly while it is present, but affects learning only slightly when learning is measured on a transfer task in distributed conditions. In this case fatigue may mask the original learning effects during massed practice, but they become apparent on the transfer tasks. For discrete tasks, the research results are not as clear, and appear to depend considerably on the task (1).

Keep in mind that in the therapy setting a risk of injury due to fatigue will increase during massed practice for tasks that may be somewhat dangerous for the patient, such as tasks in which a fall could result. In this case, it is best not to overly fatigue the patient and risk injury.

VARIABLE PRACTICE

As we mentioned when discussing Schmidt's schema theory, generalizability of practice is considered a very important variable in motor learning. In general, research has shown that variable practice increases the adaptability of learning. For example, in one experiment one group of subjects practiced a timing task (they had to press a button when a moving pattern of lights arrived at a particular point) at variable speeds of 5, 7, 9, and 11 miles/hr, while a second group (constant practice) practiced at only one of those speeds. Then, all subjects performed a transfer test, in which they performed at a novel light speed outside their previous range of experience. The absolute errors were smaller for the

variable than for the constant practice group (19). Thus, in general, variable practice appears to allow a person to perform significantly better on novel variations of the task.

CONTEXTUAL INTERFERENCE

Surprisingly, it has also been found that factors that make performing a task more difficult initially very often make learning more effective in the long run. These types of factors have been called *context effects* (1). For example, if you were to ask a person to practice five different tasks in random order, vs. blocking the trials for each task into individual groups, you might presume that it would be easier to learn each task in a blocked design. However, this is not the case. While performance is better during the acquisition phase, when tested on a transfer task, performance is actually better in the randomly ordered conditions.

It has been concluded that the critical factor in improving learning is that the subject has to do something different on consecutive trials (1). What are the implications of these results? Clearly, traditional methods for retraining by practicing one skill repeatedly are probably not the most effective. On the contrary, encouraging the patient to practice a number of tasks in random order would probably be more successful for long-term retention (1).

WHOLE VS. PART TRAINING

One approach to retraining function is to break the task down into interim steps, helping the patient to master each step prior to learning the entire task. This has been called task analysis and is defined as the process of identifying the components of a skill or movement and then ordering them into a sequence. How are the components of a task defined? They are defined in relationship to the goals of the task. So, for example, a task analysis approach to retraining mobility would be to break down the locomotor pattern into naturally occurring components such as step initiation, stability during stance, or push-off to achieve progression. During mobility retraining, the patient would practice each of these components in isolation, before combining them into the whole gait pattern. But each of these components must be practiced within the overall context of gait. For example, having a patient practice hip extension while prone will not necessarily increase the patient's ability to achieve the goal of stance stability, even though both require hip extension. Thus part-task training can be an effective way to retrain some tasks, if the task itself can be naturally divided into units that reflect the inherent goals of the task (20, 21).

TRANSFER

A critical issue in rehabilitation is how training transfers, either to a new task, or to a new environment. For example, will learning a task in a clinical environment transfer to a home environment? Or does practicing standing balance transfer to a dynamic balance task such as walking around the house?

What determines how well a task learned in one condition will transfer to another? Researchers have determined that the amount of transfer depends on the similarity between the two tasks or the two environments (22, 23). A critical aspect in both appears to be whether the neural processing demands in the two situations are similar. For example, training a patient to maintain standing balance in a well-controlled environment, such as on a firm, flat surface, in a well-lit clinic, will not necessarily enable the patient to balance in a home environment that contains thick carpets, uneven surfaces, and visual distractions. The more closely the demands in the practice environment resemble those in the actual environment, the better the transfer (20, 21).

MENTAL PRACTICE

It has been shown that mentally practicing a skill (the act of performing the skill in one's imagination, without any action involved) can produce large positive effects on the performance of the task. For example, Rawlings et al. (24) taught subjects a **rotary pursuit task**. On the first day, all subjects practiced 25 trials. On days 2–9, one group of subjects continued with physical practice, while a second group performed only mental practice, and a third group was given no practice. On day 10, all subjects were retested, and the mental practice group had improved almost as much as the physical practice group, while the no-practice group showed little improvement.

Why is this the case? One hypothesis is that the neural circuits underlying the motor programs for the movements are actually triggered during mental practice, and the subject either does not activate the final muscle response at all, or activates responses at very low levels which do not produce movement. In Chapter 3, we discussed experiments showing that one part of the brain, the supplementary motor cortex, is activated during mental practice.

GUIDANCE

One technique often used in therapy is guidance, that is, the learner is physically guided through the task to be learned. Research has again explored the efficiency of this form of learning vs. other forms of learning that involve trial and error discovery procedures. In one set of experiments (1), various forms of physical guidance were used in teaching a complex elbow movement task. When performance was measured on a no-guidance transfer test, physical guidance was no more effective than simply practicing the task under unguided conditions. In other experiments (25), practice under unguided conditions was found less effective for acquisition of the skill, but was more effective for later retention and transfer. This is similar to the results just cited, which showed that conditions that made the performance acquisition more difficult enhanced performance in transfer tests.

This doesn't mean that we should never use guidance in teaching skills, but it implies that if guidance is used, it should be used only at the outset of teaching a task, to acquaint the performer with the characteristics of the task to be learned.

RECOVERY OF FUNCTION

Concepts Related to Recovery of Function

To understand concepts related to recovery of function it is necessary first to define terms such as function and recovery.

FUNCTION

Function is defined here as the complex activity of the whole organism that is directed at performing a behavioral task (26). Optimal function is characterized by behaviors that are efficient in accomplishing a task goal in a relevant environment.

RECOVERY

The term **recovery** has a number of different meanings pertaining to regaining function that has been lost following an injury. A stringent definition of recovery requires achieving the functional goal in the same way it was performed premorbidly, that is, using the same processes utilized prior to the injury (27). Less stringent definitions define recovery as the ability to achieve task goals using effective and efficient means, but not necessarily those used premorbidly (28).

RECOVERY VS. COMPENSATION

Is recovery the same or different from compensation? **Compensation** is defined as behavioral substitution, that is, alternative behavioral strategies are adopted to complete a task. Recovery is achieving function through original processes, while compensation is achieving function through alternative processes. Thus function returns, but not in its identical premorbid form.

A question of concern to many therapists is: Should therapy be directed at recovery of function or compensation? The response to this question has changed over the years as our knowledge about the plasticity and malleability of the adult CNS has changed (29). For many years, the adult mammalian CNS was characterized as both rigid and unaltera-ble. Upon maturation, function was localized to various parts of the CNS. Research at the time suggested that regeneration and reorganization was not possible within the adult CNS. This view of the CNS naturally led to therapy directed at compensation, since recovery in the strict sense of the word was not possible. More recent research in the field of neuroscience has begun to show that the adult CNS has great plasticity and retains an incredible capacity for reorganization. Studies on neural mechanisms underlying recovery of function are covered in Chapter 4 of this text.

SPARING OF FUNCTION

When a function is not lost, despite a brain injury, it is referred to as a **spared function** (26). For example, when language develops normally in children who have suffered brain damage early in life, retained language function is said to be spared.

STAGES OF RECOVERY

Stages of recovery from neural injury have been described by several authors. Stages of recovery are based on the assumption that the process of recovery can be broken down into discrete stages. Classically, recovery is divided into spontaneous recovery and forced recovery. Forced recovery is recovery obtained through specific interventions designed to impact neural mechanisms (30).

The presumption is that different neural mechanisms underlie these relatively discrete stages of recovery. Chapter 4 describes how research on neural mechanisms might contribute to various stages of recovery.

Factors Contributing to Recovery of Function

Jean Held (31), a physical therapist who has written extensively on the neural basis for recovery of function, summarizes a number of factors that affect the outcome of damage to the nervous system as well as the extent of subsequent recovery.

EFFECT OF AGE ON RECOVERY

Dr. Held notes that the age of the individual at the time of the lesion affects recovery of function, but in a complex manner. Early views on age-related effects on recovery of brain function proposed that injury during infancy caused fewer deficits than damage in the adult years. For example, in the 1940s, Kennard (32, 33) performed experiments in which she removed the motor cortex of infant vs. adult monkeys and found that infants were able to feed, climb, walk, and grasp objects, while adults were not. In humans, this effect has been noted in language function, where damage to the dominant hemisphere shows little or no effect on speech in infants, but causes different degrees of aphasia in adults.

However, as we understand more about the function of different brain areas, researchers are concluding that not all areas show the same capacity for regeneration. For example, injury to some areas of the brain shows similar deficits whether it occurs in the infant or adult, while damage to other areas may show little effect in infancy, yet problems develop later with further maturation.

Why is this? It has been hypothesized that if an area is mature, injury will cause similar damage in infants and adults. But, if another area that is functionally related is not yet mature, it may assume the function of the injured area. In addition, if an immature area is damaged and no other area assumes its function, no problems may be seen in infancy, but in later years, deficits may become apparent.

In addition, when children have brain injuries in the speech areas, there is probably loss of other functions to spare the function of speech. Researchers have found that the IQ's of children with spared speech following early brain injury were consistently lower than those of children who had a brain injury when they were older (34). This implies that when a function is spared, a crowding effect may occur, and thus it occurs at the cost of compromising another behavior (26).

QUALITY OF THE LESION AND RECOVERY

Held (31) notes that there are a number of characteristics of lesions that affect the extent of recovery from injury. For example, a small lesion has a greater chance of recovery, as long as a functional area hasn't been entirely removed. In addition, slowly developing lesions appear to cause less functional loss than lesions that happen quickly. For example, case studies have shown that a person who functioned well until near death, upon autopsy, had a large lesion in the brain tissue. This phenomenon has been explored experimentally, by making serial lesions in animals, in which the animal is allowed to recover between lesions (26). If a single large lesion is made in the motor cortex (Brodmann's areas 4 & 6), animals become immobilized, where similar lesions produced serially over a period of time allow the animal to walk, feed, and right itself with no difficulty (35).

EFFECT OF EXPERIENCE ON RECOVERY

Held (31) notes that studies in which rats were raised in enriched environments show many resultant changes in the brain morphology and biochemistry, including increased brain weight, dendritic branching, and enzyme activity. As a result of these findings, researchers wondered if this enrichment would improve responses to brain injury. Experiments showed that preinjury environmental enrichment protects animals against certain deficits after brain lesions. For example, two sets of rats received lesions of the cortex, one group with preoperative enrichment and a control group. After surgery, the enriched animals made fewer mistakes during maze learning, and in fact performed better than control animals without brain damage.

In a second study by Held et al. (36) the effect of pre- and postoperative enrichment was compared for a locomotor task following removal of sensorimotor cortex. They found that preoperatively enriched rats were no different from enriched sham-lesioned controls on both behavioral and fine-grained movement analysis. The group that was only postoperatively enriched was mildly impaired in locomotor skills, but recovered more quickly than the lesioned controls, though they never regained full locomotor function. Thus, postoperative enrichment is effective, but doesn't allow the same extent of recovery as preoperative enrichment.

Held suggests that enriched subjects may have developed functional neural circuitry that is more varied than that of restricted subjects, and this could provide them with a greater ability to reorganize the nervous system after a lesion, or simply to use alternate pathways to perform a task.

EFFECT OF TRAINING ON RECOVERY

According to Held, training is a different form of exposure to enriched environments in that activities used are specific rather than generalized. Ogden and Franz (37) performed an interesting study in which they produced hemiplegia in monkeys by making lesions in the motor cortex. They then gave four types of postoperative training: (*a*) no treatment, (*b*) general massage of the involved arm, (*c*) restraint of the noninvolved limb, and (*d*) restraint of the noninvolved limb coupled with stimulation of the involved limb to move, along with forced active movement of the animal. The last condition was the only one to show recovery, and in this condition it occurred within 3 weeks.

A second study by Black et al. (38) examined recovery from a motor cortex forelimb area lesion. They initiated training immediately after surgery or at 4 months, with training lasting 6 months. They found that training of the involved hand alone, or training of the involved and normal hand together, was more effective than training the normal hand alone. When training was delayed, recovery was worse than when it was initiated immediately following the lesion.

Held concludes that recovery is affected by the state of the system at the time of a lesion, and that training after the lesion improves recovery best when it occurs immedi-ately after the lesion and is specific to the involved limb.

CLINICAL OVERVIEW

By now it should be clear that the field of rehabilitation has much in common with the field of motor learning, defined as the study of the acquisition of movement. More accurately, therapists involved in treating the adult neurological patient are concerned with issues related to motor relearning, or the reacquisition of movement. The pediatric patient who is born with a CNS deficit, or experiences injury early in life, faces the task of acquisition of movement in the face of unknown musculoskeletal and neural constraints. In either case, the therapist is concerned with structuring therapy in ways to maximize acquisition and/or recovery of function.

Remember Mr. Smith from the beginning of this chapter? Mr. Smith had been receiving therapy for 5 weeks and had recovered much of his ability to function. We wanted to know more about why this happened. What is the cause of Mr. Smith's recovery of motor function? How much of his recovery may be attributed to therapeutic interventions? How many of his reacquired motor skills will he be able to retain and use when he leaves the rehabilitation facility and returns home?

Mr. Smith's reacquisition of function cannot be attributed to any one factor. Some of Mr. Smith's functional return will be due to recovery, that is, regaining original control of original mechanisms; some will be due to compensatory processes. In addition, age, premorbid function, site and size of lesion, and the effect of interventions all interact to determine the degree of function regained.

Mr. Smith has had excellent therapy as well! Mr. Smith has been involved in carefully organized therapy sessions that have contributed to his reacquisition of task-relevant behaviors. Both associative and nonassociative forms of learning may have played a role in his recovery. Habituation was used to decrease complaints of dizziness associated with inner ear problems.

Trial and error learning (operant conditioning) was used to help him discover optimal solutions to many functional tasks. His therapist carefully structured his environment so that optimal strategies were reinforced. For example, biofeedback was used to help him develop better foot control during locomotion.

Functionally relevant tasks were practiced under wide-ranging conditions. Under optimal conditions, this would lead to procedural learning, ensuring that Mr. Smith would be able to transfer many of his newly gained skills to his home environment. Practicing tasks under varied conditions was aimed at the development of rule-governed action or schemas. Recognizing the importance of developing optimal perceptual and motor strategies, his therapist structured his therapy sessions so that Mr. Smith explored the perceptual environment. This was designed to facilitate the optimal mapping of perceptual and motor strategies for achieving functional goals. Finally, therapy was directed at helping Mr. Smith repeatedly solve the sensory-motor problems inherent in various functional tasks, rather than teaching him to repeat a single solution.

or the relationship of one's behavior to a consequence (operant conditioning).

6. Classical conditioning consists of learning to pair two stimuli. During operant conditioning we learn to associate a certain response, from among many that we have made, with a consequence.

7. Procedural learning refers to learning tasks that can be performed automatically without attention or conscious thought, like a habit.

8. Declarative learning results in knowledge that can be consciously recalled, and thus requires processes such as awareness, attention, and reflection.

9. Different theories of motor control include Adams' closed loop theory of motor control, Schmidt's schema theory, Fitts' and Posner's theory on the stages of motor learning, and Newell's theory of learning as exploration.

10. Classical recovery is divided into spontaneous recovery and forced recovery, that is, recovery obtained through specific interventions designed to impact neural mechanisms.

11. Experiments show that preinjury environmental enrichment protects animals against certain deficits after brain lesions.

12. Training after the lesion improves recovery best when it occurs immediately after the lesion and when it is specific to the involved limb.

SUMMARY

1. Motor learning, like motor control, emerges from a complex set of processes including perception, cognition, and action.

2. Motor learning results from an interaction of the individual with the task and environment.

3. Nonassociative learning occurs when an organism is given a single stimulus repeatedly. As a result, the nervous system learns about the characteristics of that stimulus.

4. Habituation and sensitization are two very simple forms of nonassociative learning. Habituation is a decrease in responsiveness that occurs as a result of repeated exposure to a nonpainful stimulus. Sensitization is an increased responsiveness following a threatening or noxious stimulus.

5. In associative learning a person learns to predict relationships, either relationships of one stimulus to another (classical conditioning)

REFERENCES

1. Schmidt RA. Motor control and learning. 2nd ed. Champaign, IL: Human Kinetics, 1988.

2. Newell KM. Motor skill acquisition. Annu Rev Psychol 1991;42:213–237.

3. Schmidt RA. Motor learning principles for physical therapy. In: Contemporary management of motor control problems. Proceedings of the II Step Conference. Alexandria, VA: APTA, 1992:49–62.

4. Kupfermann I. Learning and memory. In: Kandel ER, Schwartz JH, Jessell TM, eds. Principles of neuroscience. 3rd ed. New York: Elsevier, 1991:997–1008.

5. Adams JA. A closed-loop theory of motor learning. J Motor Behav 1971;3:111–150.

6. Ivry R. Representational issues in motor learning: phenomena and theory. In: Keele S, Heuer H, eds. Handbook of perception and

action: motor skills. New York: Academic Press, in press.

7. Taub E, Berman AJ. Movement and learning in the absence of sensory feedback. In: Freedman SJ, ed. The neuropsychology of spatially oriented behavior. Homewood, IL: Dorsey Press, 1968.

8. Rothwell JC, Traub MM, Day BL, Obeso JA, Marsden CD. Manual motor performance in deafferented man. Brain 1982;105:515–542.

9. Fentress JC. Development of grooming in mice with amputated forelimbs. Science 1973;179:704.

10. Schmidt RA. A schema theory of discrete motor skill learning. Psychol Rev 1975;82:225–260.

11. Kerr R, Booth B. Skill acquisition in elementary school children and schema theory. In: Landers DM, Christina RW, eds. Psychology of motor behavior and sport, vol. 2. Champaign, IL: Human Kinetics, 1977.

12. Shapiro DC, Schmidt RA. The schema theory: recent evidence and developmental implications. In: Kelso FAS, Clark JE, eds. The development of movement control and coordination. New York: John Wiley & Sons, 1982:113–173.

13. Kugler PN, Kelso JAS, Turvey MT. On the concept of coordinative structures as dissipative structures: I. Theoretical line. In: Stelmach GE, Requin J, eds. Tutorials in motor behavior. Amsterdam: North-Holland, 1980:3–37.

14. Fitts PM, Posner MI. Human performance. Belmont, CA: Brooks/Cole, 1967.

15. Bilodeau EA, Bilodeau IM, Schumsky DA. Some effects of introducing and withdrawing knowledge of results early and late in practice. J Exper Psych 1959;58:142–144.

16. Salmoni AW, Schmidt RA, Walter CB. Knowledge of results and motor learning: a review and critical reappraisal. Psychol Bull 1984;95:355–386.

17. Lavery JJ. Retention of simple motor skills as a function of type of knowledge of results. Can J Psych 1962;16:300–311.

18. Newell KM, Kennedy JA. Knowledge of results and children's motor learning. Dev Psych 1978;14:531–536.

19. Catalano JF, Kleiner BM. Distant transfer and practice variability. Percept Mot Skills 1984; 58:851–856.

20. Winstein CJ. Designing practice for motor learning: clinical implications. Contemporary

management of motor control problems. Proceedings of the II Step Conference. Alexandria, VA: APTA, 1991.

21. Schmidt RA. Motor learning principles for physical therapy. Contemporary management of motor control problems. Proceedings of the II Step Conference. Alexandria, VA: APTA, 1991.

22. Schmidt RA, Young DE. Augmented kinematic information feedback for skill learning: a new research paradigm. J Mot Behav 1987.

23. Lee TD. Transfer-appropriate processing: a framework for conceptualizing practice effects in motor learning. In: Meijer OG, Roth K, eds. Complex movement behavior: the motor-action controversy. Amsterdam: North Holland, 1988.

24. Rawlings EI, Rawlings IL, Chen CS, Yilk MD. The facilitating effects of mental rehearsal in the acquisition of rotary pursuit tracking. Psychonomic Science 1972;26:71–73.

25. Singer RN. Motor learning and human performance. 3rd ed. New York: Macmillan, 1980.

26. Craik RL. Recovery processes: maximizing function. In: Contemporary management of motor control problems. Proceedings of the II Step Conference. Alexandria, VA: APTA, 1992:165–173.

27. Almli RB, Finger S. Toward a definition of recovery of function. In: Le Vere TE, Almli RB, Stein DG, eds. Brain injury and recovery: theoretical and controversial issues. New York: Plenum, 1988:1–4.

28. Slavin MD, Laurence S, Stein DG. Another look at vicariation. In: Le Vere TE, Almli RB, Stein DG, eds. Brain injury and recovery: theoretical and controversial issues. New York: Plenum, 1988:165–179.

29. Gordon J. Assumptions underlying physical therapy intervention: theoretical and historical perspectives. In: Carr JH, Shepherd, RB, Gordon J et al., eds. Movement sciences: foundations for physical therapy in rehabilitation. Rockville, MD: Aspen Systems, 1987:1–30.

30. Bach-y-Rita P, Balliet R. Recovery from stroke. In: Duncan P, Badke MB, eds. Stroke rehabilitation: the recovery of motor control. Chicago: Year Book Medical Publishers, 1987:79–107.

31. Held JM. Recovery of function after brain damage: theoretical implications for thera-

peutic intervention. In: Carr JH, Shepherd, RB, Gordon J, et al., eds. Movement sciences: foundations for physical therapy in rehabilitation. Rockville, MD: Aspen Systems, 1987:155–177.

32. Kennard MA. Relation of age to motor impairment in man and in sub-human primates. Arch Neurol Psychiatry 1940;44:377–398.

33. Kennard MA. Cortical reorganization of motor function: studies on a series of monkeys of various ages from infancy to maturity. Arch Neurol Psychiatr 1942;48:27–240.

34. Woods BT. The restricted effects of right hemispheric lesions after age one: Wechsler test data. Neuropsychologia 1980;18:65–70.

35. Travis AM, Woolsey CN. Motor performance of monkeys after bilateral partial and total cerebral decortication. Am J Phys Med 1956; 35:273–310.

36. Held JM, Gordon F, Gentile AM. Environmental influences on locomotor recovery following cortical lesions in rats. Behav Neurosci 1985;99:678–690.

37. Ogden R, Franz SI. On cerebral motor control: the recovery from experimentally produced hemiplegia. Psychobiology 1917; 1:33–49.

38. Black P, Markowitz RS, Cianci SN. Recovery of motor function after lesions in motor cortex of monkeys. Ciba Found Symp 1975; 34:65–83.

Chapter 3

PHYSIOLOGY OF MOTOR CONTROL

INTRODUCTION AND OVERVIEW

Motor Control Theories and Physiology

As we mentioned in Chapter 1, theories of motor control are not simply a collection of concepts regarding the nature and cause of movement. They must take into consideration current research findings about the structure and function of the nervous system. Remember that motor control is about the nature and cause of movement. It arises from the interaction of both perceptual and action systems, with cognition affecting both systems at many different levels. Within each of these systems are many levels of processing, which are illustrated in Figure 3.1. For example, perception can be thought of as progressing through various processing stages. Each stage reflects specific brain structures that process sensory information at different levels, from initial stages of sensory processing to increasingly abstract levels of interpretation and integration in higher levels of the brain.

Recent neuroscience research suggests that movement control is achieved through

45

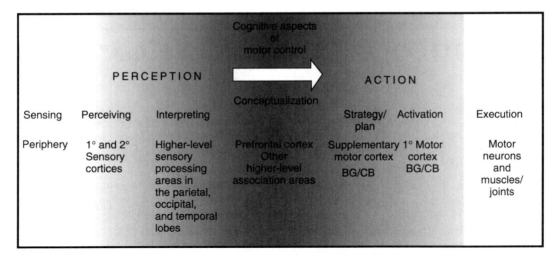

Figure 3.1. Model of the interaction between perceptual, action and cognitive processes involved in motor control. BG = basal ganglia; CB = cerebellum.

the cooperative effort of many brain structures, which are organized both hierarchically and in parallel. This means that a signal may be processed in two ways. A signal may be processed **hierarchically**, within ascending levels of the central nervous system (CNS). In addition, the same signal may be processed simultaneously among many different brain structures, showing **parallel distributed processing.** Hierarchical processing, in conjunction with distributed processing, occurs in both the perceptual and action systems of movement control.

When we talk about "hierarchical" processing in this chapter, we are describing a system in which higher levels of the brain are concerned with issues of abstraction of information. For example, within the perceptual system, hierarchical processing means that higher brain centers *integrate* inputs from many senses, and *interpret* incoming sensory information. On the action side of movement control, higher levels of brain function form motor *plans* and *strategies* for action. Thus, higher levels might select the specific response to accomplish a particular task. Lower levels of processing would then carry out the detailed monitoring and regulation of the response execution, making it appropriate for the context in which it is carried out.

In parallel distributed processing, the same signal is processed simultaneously among many different brain structures, though for different purposes. For example, the cerebellum and the basal ganglia process higher level motor information simultaneously, before sending it back to the motor cortex for action.

This chapter reviews the processes underlying the production of human movement. The first section of this chapter presents an overview of the major components of the CNS and the structure and function of a neuron, the basic unit of the CNS. The remaining sections of this chapter discuss in more detail the neural anatomy (the basic circuits), and the physiology (the function) of the systems involved in the production and control of movement. The chapter follows the neural anatomy and physiology of movement control from perception into action, recognizing that it is often difficult to distinguish where one ends and the other begins.

Overview of Brain Function

Brain function underlying motor control is typically divided into multiple processing levels, including the spinal cord, the brainstem, the cerebellum, the diencephalon, and the cerebral hemispheres, including the cerebral cortex and basal ganglia (1, 2).

SPINAL CORD

At the lowest level of the perception-action hierarchy is the spinal cord, and the sensory receptors and muscles that it innervates. The circuitry of the spinal cord is involved in the initial reception and processing of somatosensory information (from the muscles, joints, and skin) contributing to the control of posture and movement. At the level of spinal cord processing, we can expect to see a fairly simple relationship between the sensory input and motor output. At the spinal cord level, we see the organization of reflexes, the most stereotyped responses to sensory stimuli, and the basic flexion and extension patterns of the muscles involved in leg movements, such as kicking and locomotion (1).

Sherrington called the motor neurons of the spinal cord the "final common pathway," since they are the last processing level before muscle activation occurs. Figure 3.2A shows the anatomist's view of the nervous system with the spinal cord positioned caudally. Figure 3.2B shows an abstract model of the nervous system with the spinal cord positioned at the bottom of the hierarchy, with its many parallel pathways. In this view, the sensory receptors are represented by input arrows and the muscles by output arrows.

BRAINSTEM

The spinal cord extends rostrally to join the next neural processing level, the brainstem. The brainstem contains important nuclei involved in postural control and locomotion, including the vestibular nuclei, the red nucleus, and the reticular nuclei. The brainstem receives somatosensory input from the skin and muscles of the head, as well as sensory input from the vestibular and visual systems. In addition, nuclei in the brainstem control the output to the neck, face, and eyes, and are critical to the function of hearing and taste. In fact, all the descending motor pathways except the corticospinal tract originate in the brainstem. Finally, the reticular formation, which regulates our arousal and awareness, is also found within the brainstem (1).

The anatomist's view of the brainstem (Fig. 3.2A) shows divisions from caudal to rostral into the medulla, pons, and midbrain, while the abstract model (Fig. 3.2B) shows its input connections from the spinal cord and higher centers (the cerebellum and motor cortex) and its motor pathways back to the spinal cord.

CEREBELLUM

The cerebellum lies behind the brainstem and is connected to it by tracts called "peduncles" (Fig. 3.2A). As you can see from Figure 3.2B, the cerebellum receives inputs from the spinal cord (giving it feedback about movements) and from the cerebral cortex (giving it information on the planning of movements), and it has outputs to the brainstem. The cerebellum has many important functions in motor control. One is to adjust our motor responses by comparing the intended output with sensory signals, and then to update the movement commands if they deviate from the intended trajectory. The cerebellum also modulates the force and range of our movements and is involved in motor learning.

DIENCEPHALON

As we move rostrally in the brain, we next find the diencephalon, which contains the thalamus (Fig. 3.2A). The thalamus processes most of the information coming to the cortex from the many parallel input pathways (from the spinal cord, cerebellum, and brainstem) (Fig. 3.2B). These pathways stay segregated during the thalamic processing, and during the subsequent output to the different parts of the cortex (1).

CEREBRAL HEMISPHERES (CEREBRAL CORTEX AND BASAL GANGLIA)

As we move higher, we find the cerebral hemispheres, which include the cerebral cor-

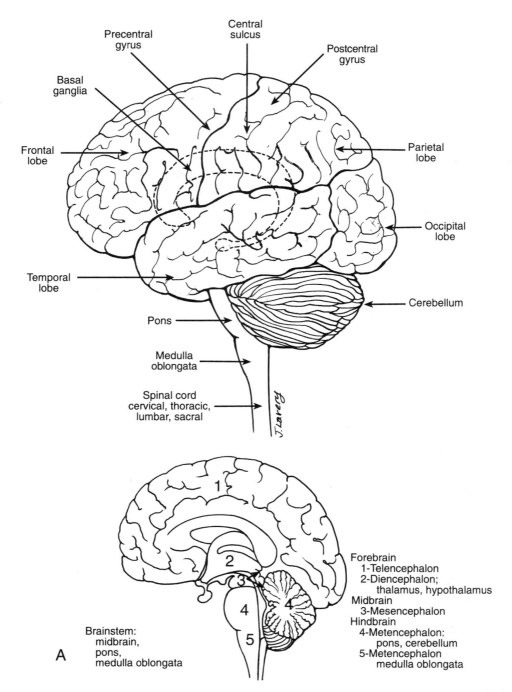

Figure 3.2.   **A**, Illustration of the nervous system from an anatomist's view. **B**, An abstract model of the nervous system. (Adapted from Kandel E, Schwartz JH, Jessell TM, eds. Principles of neuroscience. 3rd ed. NY: Elsevier; 1991:8.)

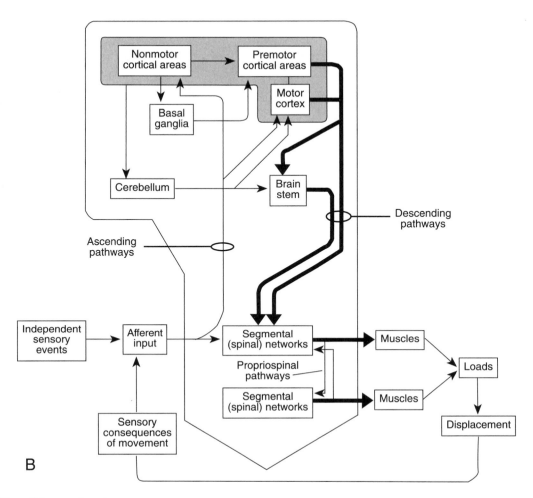

Figure 3.2.—*continued*

tex and basal ganglia. Lying at the base of the cerebral cortex, the basal ganglia (Fig. 3.2) receive input from most areas of the cerebral cortex, and send their output back to the motor cortex, via the thalamus. Some of the functions of the basal ganglia involve higher-order, cognitive aspects of motor control, such as the planning of motor strategies (1).

The cerebral cortex (Fig. 3.2A) is often considered the highest level of the motor control hierarchy. The parietal and premotor areas, along with other parts of the nervous system, are involved in identifying targets in space, choosing a course of action, and programming movements. The premotor areas send outputs mainly to the motor cortex, which sends its commands on to the brainstem and spinal cord via the corticospinal tract and the corticobulbar system (Fig. 3.2A).

In light of these various subsystems involved in motor control, clearly, the nervous system is organized both hierarchically and "in parallel." Thus, the highest levels of control not only affect the next levels down, they also can act independently on the spinal motor neurons. This combination of parallel and hierarchical control allows a certain overlap of functions, so that one system is able to take over from another when environmental or task conditions require it. This also allows a certain amount of recovery from traumatic injury, by the use of alternative pathways.

To better understand the function of the different levels of the nervous system, let's examine a specific action and walk through the pathways of the nervous system that contribute to its planning and execution. For example, perhaps you're thirsty and want to pour some milk from the milk carton in front of you into a glass. Sensory inputs come in from the periphery to tell you what is happening around you, where you are in space, and where your joints are relative to each other: they give you a map of your body in space. Higher centers in the cortex make a plan to act on this information in relation to the goal: reaching for the carton of milk.

From your sensory map, you make a movement plan (using, possibly, the parietal lobes and premotor cortex). You're going to reach over the box of corn flakes in front of you. This plan is sent to the motor cortex, and muscle groups are specified. The plan is also sent to the cerebellum and basal ganglia, and they modify it to refine the movement. The cerebellum sends an update of the movement output plan to the motor cortex and brainstem. Descending pathways from the motor cortex and brainstem then activate spinal cord networks, spinal motor neurons activate the muscles, and you reach for the milk. If the milk carton is full, when you thought it was almost empty, spinal reflex pathways will compensate for the extra weight that you didn't expect and activate more motor neurons. Then, the sensory consequences of your reach will be evaluated, and the cerebellum will update the movement—in this case, to accommodate a heavier milk carton.

Neuron—Basic Unit of the CNS

The lowest level in the hierarchy is the single neuron in the spinal cord. How does it function? What is its structure? To explore more fully the ways that neurons communicate between the levels of the hierarchy of the nervous system, we need to review some of the simple properties of the neuron, including the resting potential, the action potential, and synaptic transmission.

Remember that the neuron, when it is at rest, always has a negative electrical charge or potential on the inside of the cell, with respect to the outside. Thus, when physiologists record from a neuron intracellularly with an electrode, they discover that the inside of the cell has a **resting potential** of about −70 mv with respect to the outside (Fig. 3.3). This electrical potential is caused by an unequal concentration of chemical ions on the inside vs. the outside of the cell. Thus, K^+ ions are high on the inside of the cell and Na^+ ions are high on the outside of the cell, and an electrical pump within the cell membrane keeps the ions in their appropriate concentrations. When the neuron is at rest, K^+ channels are open and keep the neuron at this negative potential (2–4).

When a neuron is excited, one sees a series of dramatic jumps in voltage across the cell membrane. These are the **action potentials**, nerve impulses, or spikes. They don't go to zero voltage, but to +30 mv (as shown in Fig. 3.3). That is, the inside of the neuron becomes positive. Action potentials are also about 1 msec in duration and quickly repolarize. The height of the action potential is always about the same: −70 + 30 mv = ca. 100 mv.

How does the neuron communicate this information to the next cell in line? It does this through the process of **synaptic transmission**. A cleft 200Å wide separates neurons. Each action potential in a neuron releases a small amount of transmitter substance. It diffuses across the cleft and attaches to receptors on the next cell, which open up channels in the membrane and depolarize the cell. One action potential makes only a small depolarization, called an **excitatory postsynaptic potential**, the EPSP. The EPSP normally dies away after 3 to 4 msec, and as a result, the next cell is not activated (2).

But if the first cell fires enough action potentials, there is a series of EPSPs, and they continue to build up depolarization to the threshold voltage for the action potential in the next neuron. This is called **summation**. There are two kinds of summation, temporal and spatial, and these are illustrated in Figure 3.3. **Temporal summation** results in depolarization because of synaptic potentials that occur close together in time. **Spatial sum-**

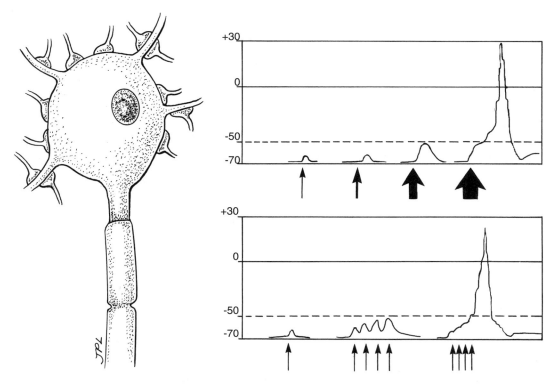

Figure 3.3. A schematic drawing illustrating important aspects of neuron physiology including the resting potential (RP) of −70 mv and changes during an action potential, and the spatial (*top*) and temporal (*bottom*) summation properties of a neuron.

mation produces depolarization because of the action of multiple cells synapsing on the postsynaptic neuron. Spatial summation is really an example of parallel distributed processing, since multiple pathways are affecting the same neuron (2).

The effectiveness of a given synapse changes with experience. For example, if a given neuron is activated over a short period of time, it may show **synaptic facilitation**, in which it releases more transmitter and therefore more easily depolarizes the next cell. Alternatively, a cell may also show **defacilitation**, or **habituation**. In this case, the cell is depleted of transmitter, and thus is less effective in influencing the next cell. Many mechanisms can cause synaptic facilitation or habituation in different parts of the nervous system. Increased use of a given pathway can result in synaptic facilitation. However, in a different pathway, increased use could result in defacilitation or habituation. Variations in the coding within the neuron's internal chem-

istry and the stimuli activating the neuron will determine how it will respond to these signals in one mode or another (3).

With this overview of the essential elements of the nervous system, we can now turn our attention to the heart of this chapter, an in-depth discussion of the sensory-motor processes underlying motor control.

SENSORY/PERCEPTUAL SYSTEMS

What is the role of sensation in the production and control of movement? In the chapter on motor control theories, there were divergent views about the importance of sensory input in motor control. Current neuroscience research suggests that sensory information plays many different roles in the control of movement.

Sensory inputs serve as the stimuli for reflexive movement organized at the spinal cord level of the nervous system. In addition, sensory information has a vital role in modulating the output of movement that results from the activity of pattern generators in the spinal cord. An example of this type of movement might be locomotor output from pattern generators in the spinal cord. Likewise, at the spinal cord level, sensory information can modulate movement that results from commands originating in higher centers of the nervous system. The reason that sensation can modulate all these types of movement is that sensory receptors converge on the motor neurons, considered the final common pathway. But another role of sensory information in movement control is accomplished via ascending pathways, which contribute to the control of movement in much more complex ways.

Somatosensory System

The somatosensory system, from the lowest to the highest level of the CNS hierarchy, going from the reception of signals in the periphery to the integration and interpretation of those signals relative to other sensory systems, is described in this section. Pay close attention to how hierarchical and parallel distributed processing contribute to the analysis of somatosensory signals.

PERIPHERAL RECEPTORS

Muscle Spindle

Most muscle spindles are located in the muscle belly of skeletal muscles. They consist of specialized muscle fibers, called **intrafusal fibers**, surrounded by a connective tissue capsule (extrafusal fibers are the regular muscle fibers). In humans, the muscles with the highest spindle density (spindles per muscle) are the extraocular, hand, and neck muscles. Is it surprising that neck muscles have such a high spindle density? This is because we use these muscles in eye-head coordination as we reach for objects and move about in the environment (5).

Intrafusal muscle fibers are much smaller than extrafusal fibers. There are two types: *nuclear bag* and *nuclear chain fibers*.

The bag fiber is thicker than the chain fiber, and projects beyond the capsule, attaching to the connective tissue surrounding the extrafusal fiber fascicle. The chain fibers attach to the spindle capsule or to the bag fiber (Fig. 3.4A). Each fiber type can be divided into equatorial, juxtaequatorial, and polar regions. The nuclear bag fiber has many spherical nuclei at the equatorial region, and gives a slow twitch contraction, while the nuclear chain fiber has a single row of nuclei, and gives a fast twitch contraction. The equatorial region is very elastic, like a balloon full of water.

The muscle spindle sends fibers into the nervous system via afferent fibers, and it is controlled by the CNS via efferent fibers. Let's consider the afferent endings. The muscle spindle sends information to the nervous system via two kinds of afferent fibers, the *group Ia* and the *group II afferents*. The Ia fiber sensory endings wrap around the equatorial region, while the group II endings are on the juxtaequatorial region. The Ia afferents go to both bag and chain fibers, while the group II afferents go to mainly to the chain fibers (Fig. 3.4A) (2, 5).

Both bag and chain muscle fibers are innervated by **γ-motor neurons**. The cell bodies of the γ-motor neurons are inside the ventral horn of the spinal cord, intermingled with the **α-motor neurons**, innervating the extrafusal fibers. The γ-motor neuron endings are at the polar, striated region of the bag and the chain muscle fibers, as shown in Figure 3.4A. There are two types of γ-fibers: (*a*) the γ-dynamic, innervating the bag fiber, and (*b*) the γ-static, innervating the chain fiber.

Passive muscle stretch causes stretch of the equator of intrafusal fibers. The equator of the bag fiber is easily stretched, because it is so elastic, while the chain fiber equator stretches less rapidly because it is stiffer, with less nuclei. Remember, the Ia's are on the equator of the bag and chain fibers; thus, they have a low threshold to stretch and will follow changes in length easily. This means that the Ia afferents code the rate of stretch (a dynamic response) and the length of the muscle at the end of stretch (static response) (5).

The group II afferents end on the jux-

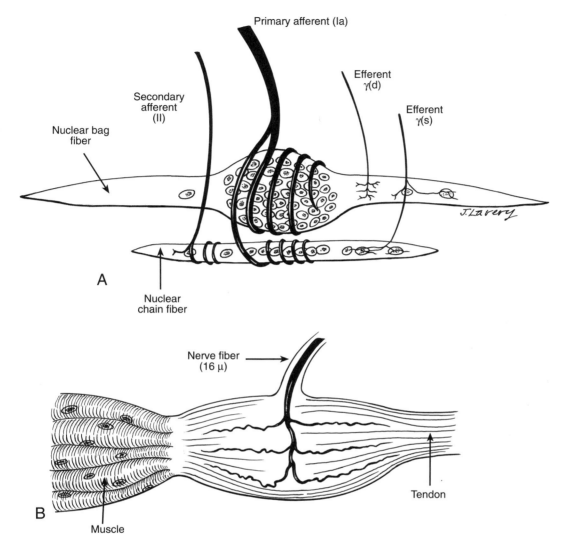

Figure 3.4. Anatomy of the muscle receptors: muscle spindle and Golgi tendon organ. **A,** The contents of the muscle spindle showing the nuclear bag and chain fibers. **B,** The spindle-shaped Golgi tendon organ, located at the muscle-tendon junction and connected to 15 to 20 muscle fibers.

taequatorial region of the chain fiber. This is a stiffer region, and as a result, the group II afferents have a higher threshold than do the Ia's. The group II afferents code only muscle length and have no dynamic response. Static responses are linearly correlated with the length of the muscle. Thus, the Ia afferents respond well to slight tendon taps, sinusoidal stretches, and even vibration of the muscle tendon, while group II afferents do not respond to these stimuli (5).

How is information from the muscle spindle utilized during motor control? Muscle spindle information is employed at many levels of the CNS hierarchy. At the lowest level, it is involved in reflex activation of muscles. However, as the information ascends the CNS hierarchy, it is used in increasingly complex and abstract ways. For example, it may contribute to our perception of our sense of effort. In, addition, it is carried over different pathways to different parts of the brain, in this way contributing to the parallel distributed nature of brain processing.

Stretch reflex loop. When a muscle is stretched, it stretches the muscle spindle, exciting the Ia afferents. They have excitatory monosynaptic connections to the α motor neurons, which activate their own muscle and synergistic muscles. They also excite Ia inhibitory interneurons, which then inhibit the α motor neurons to the antagonist muscles. For example, if the gastrocnemius muscle is stretched, the muscle spindle Ia afferents in the muscle are excited, and, in turn, excite the α motor neurons of the gastrocnemius, which cause it to contract. The Ia afferent also excites the Ia inhibitory interneuron, which inhibits motor neurons to the antagonist muscle, the tibialis anterior, so that, if this muscle was contracting, it now relaxes. The group II afferents also excite their own muscle, but disynaptically (2, 5).

What is the purpose of γ fiber activity, and when are these fibers active? Whenever there is a voluntary contraction, there is α-γ coactivation. Without this coactivation, spindle afferents would be silent during muscle contraction. With it, the nuclear bag and chain fibers contract as well as the regular extrafusal fibers of the muscle, and thus the polar region of the muscle spindle can't go slack. Because of this coactivation, if there is unexpected stretch during the contraction, the group Ia and II afferents will be able to sense it, and compensate.

Golgi Tendon Organs

Golgi tendon organs (GTOs) are spindle-shaped and located at the muscle-tendon junction (Fig. 3.4*B*). They connect to 15 to 20 muscle fibers. Afferent information from the GTO is carried to the nervous system via the Ib afferent fibers. Unlike the muscle spindles, they have no efferent connections, and thus are not subject to CNS modulation.

This is how GTOs function. The GTO is sensitive to tension changes that result from either stretch or contraction of the muscle. The GTO responds to as little as 2 to 25 g force. The GTO reflex is an inhibitory disynaptic reflex, inhibiting its own muscle and exciting its antagonist.

Researchers used to think that the GTO was only active in response to large amounts of tension. So they hypothesized that the role of the GTO was to protect the muscle from injury. Current research has shown that these receptors constantly monitor muscle tension and are very sensitive to even small amounts of tension changes caused by muscle contraction. A newly hypothesized function of the GTO is that it modulates muscle output in response to fatigue. Thus, when muscle tension is reduced due to fatigue, the GTO output is reduced, lowering its inhibitory effect on its own muscle (2, 5).

It has also been shown that the GTOs of the extensor muscles of the leg are active during the stance phase of locomotion and act to excite the extensor muscles and inhibit the flexor muscles until the GTO is unloaded (6). This is exactly the opposite of what would be expected from the reflex when it is activated when the animal is in a passive state. Thus, the reflex appears to have different properties under different task conditions.

Researchers have hypothesized that the function of the muscle spindles and GTOs together may be that of muscle stiffness regulation. Muscle stiffness may be defined as the force/unit length of a muscle. This is exactly what the GTO and muscle spindle are reciprocally controlling: Force (GTO)/unit length (muscle spindle) (5).

Joint Receptors

How do joint receptors work and what is their function? There are a number of different types of receptors within the joint itself, including Ruffini-type endings or spray endings, paciniform endings, ligament receptors, and free nerve endings. They are located in different portions of the joint capsule. Morphologically, they share the same characteristics as many of the other receptors found in the nervous system. For example, the ligament receptors are almost identical to GTOs, while the paciniform endings are identical to pacinian corpuscles in the skin.

Joint function has many intriguing aspects. The joint receptor information is used at several levels of the hierarchy of sensory processing. Some researchers have found that joint receptors appear to be sensitive only to extreme joint angles (7). Because of this, the joint receptors may provide a danger signal about extreme joint motion.

Other researchers have reported that many individual joint receptors respond to a limited range of joint motion. This phenomenon has been called *range fractionation*, with multiple receptors being activated in overlapping ranges. Afferent information from joint receptors ascends to the cerebral cortex and contributes to our perception of our position in space. The CNS determines joint position by monitoring which receptors are activated at the same time, and this allows the determination of exact joint position.

Cutaneous Receptors

There are also several types of cutaneous receptors: (*a*) mechanoreceptors, including pacinian corpuscles, Merkel's discs, Meissner's corpuscles, Ruffini endings, and lanceolate endings around hair follicles, detecting mechanical stimuli; (*b*) thermoreceptors, detecting temperature changes; and (*c*) nociceptors, detecting potential damage to the skin. The number of receptors within the sensitive areas of the skin, such as the tips of the fingers, is very high, on the order of 2500 per square centimeter (8).

Information from the cutaneous system is also used in hierarchical processing in several different ways. At lower levels of the CNS hierarchy, cutaneous information gives rise to reflex movements. Information from the cutaneous system also ascends and provides information concerning body position essential for orientation within the immediate environment.

The nervous system uses cutaneous information for reflex responses in various ways, depending on the extent and type of cutaneous input. A light diffuse stimulus to the bottom of the foot tends to produce extension in the limb, as for example, when you touch the pad of a cat's foot lightly, it will extend it. This is called the placing reaction, and it is found in human infants as well. In contrast, a sharp focal stimulus tends to produce withdrawal, or flexion, even when it is applied to exactly the same area of the foot. This is called the flexor withdrawal reflex, and it is used to protect us from injury. The typical pattern of response in the cutaneous reflex is ipsilateral flexion, and contralateral extension, which allows you to support your weight on the opposite limb (mediated by group III and IV afferents).

It is important to remember that even though we consider reflexes to be stereotyped, they are modulated by higher centers, depending on the task and the context. Remember our example of the flexor reflex, which typically causes withdrawal of a limb from a noxious stimulus. However, if there is more at stake than not hurting yourself, such as saving the life of your child, the CNS inhibits the activation of this reflex movement in favor of actions more appropriate to the situation.

ROLE OF SOMATOSENSATION AT THE SPINAL CORD LEVEL

Information from cutaneous, muscle, and joint receptors modifies the output of circuits at the spinal cord level that control such basic activities as locomotion. In the late 1960s, Grillner performed experiments in which he cut the dorsal roots to the cat spinal cord to eliminate sensory feedback from the periphery (9). He stimulated the spinal cord and was able to activate the neural pattern generator for locomotor patterns. He found that low rates of repetitive stimulation gave rise to a walk, higher rates to a trot, and then a gallop. This suggests that complex movements, such as locomotion, can be generated at the spinal cord level without supraspinal influences or inputs from the periphery.

If we don't need sensory information to generate complex movement, does that mean there is no role for sensory information in its execution? No. Hans Forssberg and his colleagues have shown that sensory information

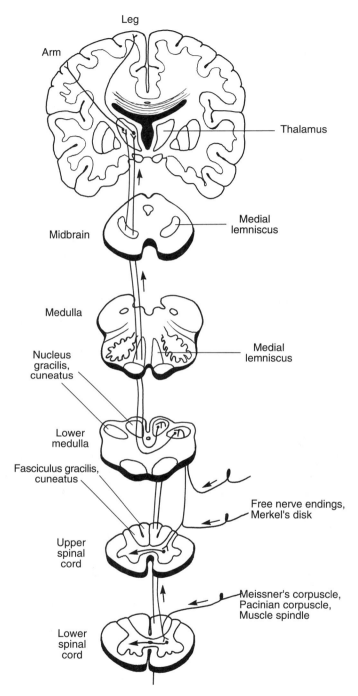

Figure 3.5. Ascending sensory systems: the dorsal-column pathway containing information from touch and pressure receptors.

modulates locomotor output in a very elegant way (10). When he brushed the paw of a spinalized cat with a stick during the swing phase of walking, it caused the paw to flex more strongly and get out of the way of the stick. But during stance, the very same stimulation caused stronger extension, in order to push off more quickly and avoid the stick in this way. Thus, he found that the same cutaneous input could modulate the step cycle in different functional ways, depending on the context in which it was used.

ASCENDING PATHWAYS

Information from the trunk and limbs is also carried to the sensory cortex and cerebellum. Two systems ascend to the cerebral cortex: the dorsal column-medial lemniscal (DC-ML) system and the anterolateral system. (Systems that ascend to the cerebellum are discussed later in the chapter.) These are shown in Figures 3.5 and 3.6. They are examples of parallel ascending systems. Each relays information about somewhat different functions, but there is some redundancy between the two pathways. What is the advantage of parallel systems? They give extra subtlety and richness to perception, by using multiple modes of processing information. They also give a measure of insurance of continued function in case of injury (2, 11).

Dorsal Column-Medial Lemniscal System

The *dorsal columns* are formed mainly by dorsal root neurons. These are thus first-order neurons. The majority of the fibers branch on entering the spinal cord, synapsing on interneurons and motor neurons to modulate spinal activity, and send branches to ascend in the dorsal column pathway toward the brain. What are the functions of the dorsal column neurons? They send information on muscle, tendon, and joint sensibility up to the somatosensory cortex and other higher brain centers. There is an interesting exception, however. Leg proprioceptors have their own private pathway to the brainstem, the lateral column. They join the dorsal column pathway

in the brainstem. The D-C pathway also contains information from touch and pressure receptors, and codes especially for discriminative fine touch. This pathway is shown in Figure 3.5 (11).

Where does this information go, and how is it processed? The pathways synapse at multiple levels in the nervous system, including the medulla, where second-order neurons become the *medial lemniscal* pathway and cross over to the thalamus, synapsing with third-order neurons, which proceed to the somatosensory cortex. Every level of the hierarchy has the ability to modulate the information coming into it from below. Through synaptic excitation and inhibition, higher centers have the ability to shut off or enhance ascending information. This allows higher centers to selectively tune (up or down) the information coming from lower centers.

As the neurons ascend through each level to the brain, the information from the receptors is increasingly processed to allow meaningful interpretation of the information. This is done by selectively enlarging the receptive field of each successive neuron.

Anterolateral System

The second ascending system, shown in Figure 3.6, is the *anterolateral* (AL) system. It consists of the spinothalamic, spinoreticular, and spinomesencephalic tracts. These fibers cross over upon entering the spinal cord and then ascend to brainstem centers. The anterolateral system has a dual function. First, it transmits information on crude touch and pressure, and thus contributes in a minor way to touch and limb proprioception. It also plays a major role in relaying information related to thermal and nociception to higher brain centers. All levels of the sensory processing hierarchy act on the AL system in the same manner as for the DC-ML system (11).

There is a redundancy of information in both tracts. A lesion in one tract doesn't cause complete loss of discrimination in any of these senses. However, a lesion in both tracts causes severe loss. Hemisection of the spinal cord

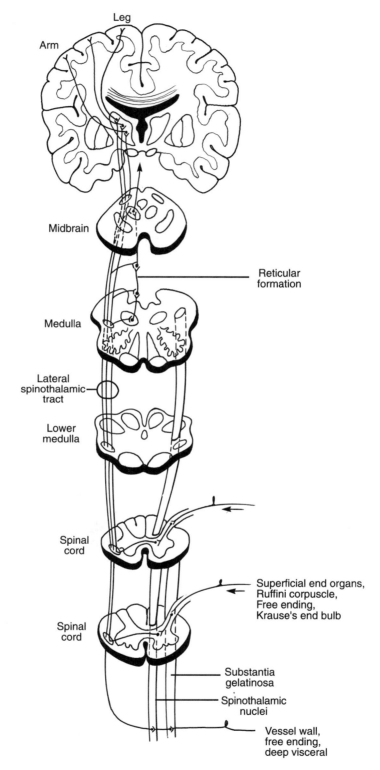

Figure 3.6.   Ascending sensory systems: the anterolateral system, containing information on pain and temperature.

(caused by a serious accident, for example) would cause tactile sensation and proprioception in the arms to be lost on the ipsilateral side (fibers haven't crossed yet), while pain and temperature sensation would be lost on the contralateral side (fibers have already crossed upon entering the spinal cord) (11).

THALAMUS

Information from both the ascending somatosensory tracts, like information from virtually all sensory systems, goes through the *thalamus*. This is a major processing center of the brain, and a lesion in this area will cause severe sensory (and motor) problems.

SOMATOSENSORY CORTEX

The *somatosensory* cortex is a major processing area for all the somatosensory modalities, and marks the beginning of conscious awareness of somatosensation. Somatosensory cortex is divided into two major areas: *primary somatosensory cortex* (SI) (also called Brodmann's area 1, 2, 3a, and 3b); and *secondary somatosensory cortex* (SII) (Fig. 3.7A). In SI, kinesthetic and touch information from the contralateral side of the body is organized in a somatotopic manner and spans four cytoarchitectural areas, Brodmann's areas 1, 2, 3a, and 3b (11).

It is in this area that we begin to see cross-modality processing. That means that joint receptors, muscle spindles, and cutaneous information are now integrated to give us information about movement in a given body area. This information is laid on top of a map of the entire body, which is distorted to reflect the relative weight given sensory information from certain areas, as you see in Figure 3.7B. For example, the throat, mouth, and hands are heavily represented because we need more detailed information to support the movements that are executed by these structures. This is the beginning of the spatial processing that is essential to the coordination of movements in space. Coordinated movement requires information about the position of the body relative to your environment and the position of one body segment relative to another (11, 12).

Contrast sensitivity is very important to movement control, since it allows the detection of the shape and edges of objects. The somatosensory cortex processes incoming information to increase contrast sensitivity so that we can more easily identify and discriminate between different objects through touch. How does it do this? It has been shown that the receptive fields of the somatosensory neurons have an excitatory center and inhibitory surround. This inhibitory surround aids in two-point discrimination through *lateral inhibition*.

How does lateral inhibition work? The cell that is excited inhibits the cells next to it, thus enhancing contrast between excited and nonexcited regions of the body. The receptors don't have lateral inhibition. But it comes in at the level of the dorsal columns, and at each subsequent step in the relay. In fact, humans have a sufficiently sensitive somatosensory system to perceive the activation of a single tactile receptor in the hand (11, 12).

There are also special cells within the somatosensory cortex that respond best to moving stimuli and are directionally sensitive. One does not find this feature in the dorsal columns, nor in the thalamus. These higher level processing cells also have larger receptive fields than the typical cells in SS, often encompassing a number of fingers. These cells appear to respond preferentially when neighboring fingers are stimulated. This could indicate their participation in such functions as the grasp of objects.

It has recently been found that the receptive fields of neurons in the somatosensory cortex are not fixed in size. Both injury and experience can change their dimensions considerably. The implications of these studies are considered in the motor learning sections of this book (8).

Somatosensory cortex also has descending connections to the thalamus, dorsal column nucleus, and the spinal cord, and thus has the ability to modulate ascending information coming through these structures.

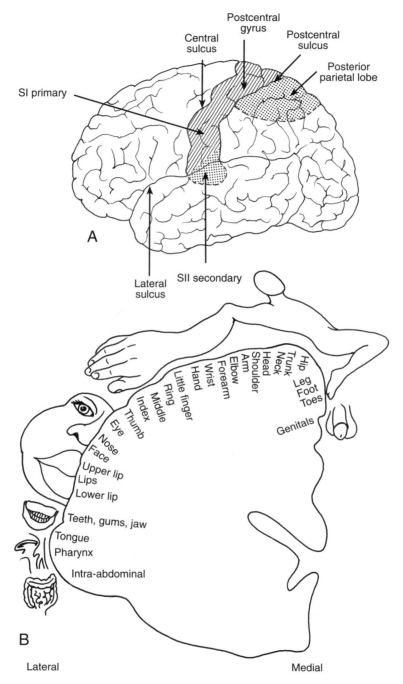

Figure 3.7. Somatosensory cortex and association areas. **A,** Located in the parietal lobe, the somatosensory cortex contains three major divisions: the primary (SI), secondary (SII), and the posterior parietal cortex. **B,** Sensory homunculus showing the somatic sensory projections from the body surface. (Adapted from Kandel E, Schwartz JH, Jessell TM, eds. Principles of neuroscience. 3rd ed. NY: Elsevier, 1991:368, 372.)

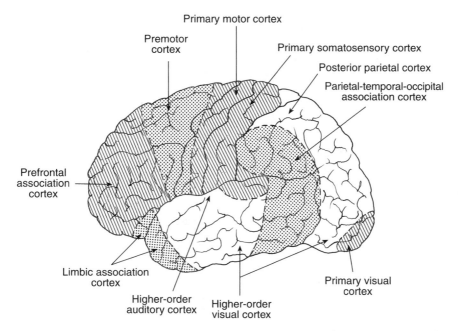

Figure 3.8. Schematic drawing showing the locations of primary sensory areas, higher-level sensory association areas, and higher-level cognitive (abstract) association cortices. (Adapted from Kandel E, Schwartz JH, Jessell TM, eds. Principles of neuroscience. 3rd ed. NY: Elsevier, 1991:825.)

ASSOCIATION CORTICES

It is in the many association cortices that we begin to see the transition from perception to action. It is here too that we see the interplay between cognitive and perceptual processing. The association cortices, found in parietal, temporal, and occipital lobes, include centers for higher level sensory processing and higher level abstract cognitive processing. The locations of these various areas are shown in Figure 3.8.

Within the parietal, temporal, and occipital cortices are association areas, which are hypothesized to link information from several senses. Area 5 of the parietal cortex is a thin strip posterior to the postcentral gyrus. After intermodality processing has taken place within area SI, outputs are sent to area 5, which integrates information between body parts. Area 5 connects to area 7 of the parietal lobe. Area 7 also receives processed visual information. Thus, area 7 probably combines eye-limb processing in most visually triggered or guided activities.

Lesions in areas 5 or 7 in either humans or other animals cause problems with the learning of skills that use information regarding the position of the body in space. In addition, certain cells in these areas appear to be activated during visually guided movements, with their activity becoming more intense when the animal attends to the movement. These findings support the hypothesis that the parietal lobe participates in processes involving attention to the position of and manipulation of objects in space (13).

These experimental results are further supported by observations of patients with damage to the parietal lobes. Their deficits include problems with body image and perception of spatial relations, which may be very important in both postural control and voluntary movements. Clearly, lesions to this area don't simply reduce the ability to perceive information coming in from one part of the body; in addition, they can affect the ability to interpret this information.

For example, people with lesions in the right angular gyrus (the nondominant hemisphere), just behind area 7, show complete neglect of the contralateral side of body, objects, and drawings. This is called **agnosia** or the inability to recognize. When their own arm or leg is passively moved into their visual field, they may claim that it isn't theirs. In certain cases, patients may be totally unaware of the hemiplegia that accompanies the lesion and may thus desire to leave the hospital early since they are unaware that they have any problem (13). Many of these same patients show problems when asked to copy drawn figures. They may draw objects in which one-half of it is missing. This is called *constructional apraxia*. Larger lesions may cause the inability to operate and orient in space or the inability to perform complex sequential tasks.

When right-handed patients have lesions in the left angular gyrus (the dominant hemisphere), they show such symptoms as confusion between left and right, difficulty in naming their fingers, though they can sense touch, and difficulty in writing, though their motor and sensory functions are normal for the hands. Alternatively, when patients have lesions to both sides of these areas, they often have problems attending to visual stimuli, in using vision to grasp an object, and in making voluntary eye movements to a point in space (13).

We have just taken one sensory system, the somatosensory system, from the lowest to the highest level of the CNS hierarchy, going from the reception of signals in the periphery to the integration and interpretation of those signals relative to other sensory systems. We have also looked at how hierarchical and parallel distributed processing have contributed to the analysis of these signals. We are now going to look at a second sensory system, the visual system, in the same way.

Visual System

Vision serves motor control in a number of ways. Vision allows us to identify objects in space, and to determine their movement. When vision plays this role, it is considered an exteroceptive sense. But vision also gives us information about where our body is in space, about the relation of one body part to an-

other, and the motion of our body. When vision plays this role, it is referred to as visual-proprioception, which means that it gives us information not only about the environment, but about our own body. Later chapters show how vision plays a key role in the control of posture, locomotion, and manipulatory function. In the following sections, we consider the anatomy and physiology of the visual system to show how it supports these roles in motor control.

PERIPHERAL VISUAL SYSTEM

Photoreceptors

Let's first look at an overall view of the eye. The eye is a great instrument, designed to focus the image of the world on the retina with great precision. As illustrated in Figure 3.9, light enters the eye through the cornea and is focused by the cornea and lens on the retina at the back of the eye. An interesting feature of the retina is that light must travel through all the layers of the eye and the neural layers of the retina before it hits the photoreceptors, which are at the back of the retina, facing away from the light source. Luckily, these layers are nearly transparent.

There are two types of photoreceptor cells: the *rods* and the *cones*. The cones are functional for vision in normal daylight and are responsible for color vision. The rods are responsible for vision at night when the amount of light is very low and too weak to activate the cones. Right at the fovea, the rest of the layers are pushed aside so the cones can receive the light in its clearest form. The blind spot (where the optic nerve leaves the retina) has no photoreceptors, and therefore we are blind in this one part of the retina. Except for the fovea, there are 20 times more rods than cones in the retina. However, cones are more important than rods for normal vision, because their loss causes legal blindness, while total loss of rods causes only night blindness (14).

Remember that sensory differentiation is a key aspect of sensory processing that supports motor control. To accomplish this, the

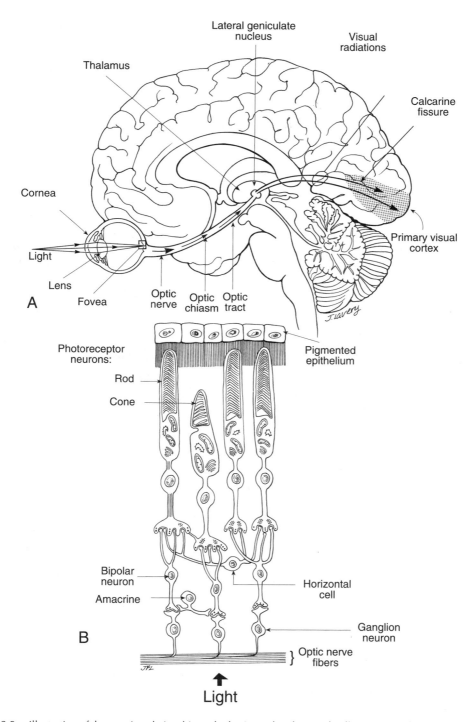

Figure 3.9. Illustration of the eye, its relationship to the horizontal and vertical cells (insert), and the visual pathways from the retina to the thalamus, midbrain, and area 17 of the cerebral cortex. (Adapted from Kandel E, Schwartz JH, Jessell TM, eds. Principles of neuroscience. 3rd ed. NY: Elsevier, 1991:401, 415, 423.)

visual system has to identify objects and determine if they are moving. So how are *object identification* and *motion sense* accomplished in the visual system? There are two separate pathways to process them. We will follow these pathways from the retina all the way up to the visual cortex. In addition, *contrast sensitivity* is used in both pathways to accomplish the goal of object identification and motion sense. Contrast sensitivity enhances the edges of objects, giving us greater precision in perception. As in the somatosensory system, all three processes are used extensively in the visual system. This processing begins in the retina. So let's first look at the cells of the retina, so that we can understand how they work together to process information (14).

Vertical Cells

In addition to the rods and cones, the retina contains *bipolar* cells and *ganglion cells*, which you might consider "vertical" cells, since they connect in series to one another but have no lateral connections (Fig. 3.9). For example, the rods and cones make direct synaptic contact with bipolar cells. The bipolar cells in turn connect to the ganglion cells. And the ganglion cells then relay visual information to the CNS, by sending axons to the lateral geniculate nucleus and superior colliculus as well as to brainstem nuclei (14–15).

Horizontal Cells

There is another class of neurons in the retina, which we are calling "horizontal" cells. These neurons modulate the flow of information within the retina by connecting the "vertical" cells together laterally. These are called the *horizontal* and *amacrine* cells. The horizontal cells mediate interactions between the receptors and bipolar cells, while the amacrine cells mediate interactions between bipolar and ganglion cells. The horizontal cells and amacrine cells are critical for achieving contrast sensitivity. Though it may appear that there are complex interconnections between the receptor cells and other neurons before the final output of the ganglion cells is

reached, the pathways and functions of the different classes of cells are straightforward.

Let's first look at the bipolar cell pathway. There are two types of pathways that involve bipolar cells, a "direct" pathway and a "lateral" pathway. In the direct pathway, a cone, for example, makes a direct connection with a bipolar cell, which makes a direct connection with a ganglion cell. In the lateral pathway, activity of cones is transmitted to the ganglion cells lateral to them through horizontal cells or amacrine cells. If you look at Figure 3.9, you will see these organizational possibilities (14, 15).

In the direct pathway, cones (or rods) connect directly to bipolar cells with either "on-center" or "off-center" receptive fields. The **receptive field** of a cell is the specific area of the retina to which the cell is sensitive, when that part of the retina is illuminated. The receptive field can be either excitatory or inhibitory, increasing or decreasing the cell's membrane potential. The receptive fields of bipolar cells (and ganglion cells) is circular. At the center of the retina, the receptive fields are small, while in the periphery, receptive fields are large. The term "on-center" means that the cell has an excitatory central portion of the receptive field, with an inhibitory surrounding area. "Off-center" refers to the opposite case of an inhibitory center and excitatory surround (15).

How do the cells take on their antagonistic surround characteristics? It appears that horizontal cells in the surround area of the bipolar cell receptive field (RF) make connections onto cones in the center of the field. When light shines on the periphery of the receptive field, the horizontal cells inhibit the cones adjacent to them.

Each type of bipolar cell then synapses with a corresponding type of ganglion cell: on-center and off-center, and makes excitatory connections with that ganglion cell (14, 15).

On-center cells give very few action potentials in the dark, and are activated when their RF is illuminated. When the periphery of their RF is illuminated, it inhibits the effect of stimulating the center. Off-center ganglion cells likewise show inhibition when light is applied to the center of their RF, and they fire at the fastest rate just after the light is turned off. They also are activated if light is applied only to the periphery of their RF.

Ganglion cells are also influenced by the activity of amacrine cells. Many of the amacrine cells function in a similar manner to horizontal cells, transmitting inhibitory inputs from nearby bipolar cells to the ganglion cell, increasing contrast sensitivity.

These two types of pathways (on- and off-center) for processing retinal information are two examples of *parallel distributed processing* of similar information within the nervous system. We talked about a similar *center-surround inhibition* in cutaneous receptor receptive fields. What is the purpose of this type of inhibition? It appears to be very important in detecting contrasts between objects, rather than the absolute intensity of light produced or reflected by an object. This inhibition allows us to detect edges of objects very easily. It is very important in locomotion, when we are walking down stairs and need to see the edge of the step. It is also important in manipulatory function in being able to determine the exact shape of an object for grasping.

The ganglion cells send their axons, via the optic nerve, to three different regions in the brain, the lateral geniculate nucleus, the pretectum, and the superior colliculus (16) (Fig. 3.9).

CENTRAL VISUAL PATHWAYS

Lateral Geniculate Nucleus

To understand what part of the retina and visual field are represented in these different areas of the brain, let's first discuss the configuration of the visual fields and hemiretina. The left half of the visual field projects on the nasal (medial—next to the nose) half of the retina of the left eye and the temporal (lateral) half of the retina of the right eye. The right visual field projects on the nasal half of the retina of the right eye and the temporal half of the retina of the left eye (16).

Thus, the optic nerves from the left and right eyes leave the retina at the optic disc, in the back. They travel to the optic chiasm where the nerves from each eye come together, and axons from the nasal side of the eyes cross, while those from the temporal side do not cross. At this point, the optic nerve becomes the optic tract. Because of this resorting of the optic nerves, the left optic tract has a map of the right visual field. This is similar to what we found for the somatosensory system, in which information from the opposite side of the body was represented in the thalamus and cortex.

One of the targets of cells in the optic tract is the lateral geniculate nucleus (LGN) of the thalamus. The lateral geniculate nucleus has six layers of cells, which map the contralateral visual field. The ganglion cells from different areas project onto specific points in the LGN, but just as we find for somatosensory maps of the body, certain areas are represented much more strongly than others. The fovea of the retina, which we use for high acuity vision, is represented to a far greater degree than the peripheral area. Each layer of the LGN gets input from only one eye. The first two layers (most ventral) are called the *magnocellular* (large cells) layers, and layers four through six are called the *parvocellular* (small cells) layers. The projection cells of each layer send axons to the visual cortex (16).

The receptive fields of neurons in the LGN are very similar to those found in the ganglion cells of the retina. There are separate on-center and off-center receptive field pathways. The magnocellular layers appear to be involved in the analysis of movement of the visual image, and the coarse details of an object, while the parvocellular layers function in color vision and a more detailed structural analysis. Thus, magnocellular layers will be more important in motor functions like balance control, where movement of the visual field gives us information about our body sway, and in reaching for moving objects. The parvocellular layers will be more important in the final phases of reaching for an object, when we need to grasp it accurately.

Superior Colliculus

Ganglion cell axons in the optic tract also terminate in the *superior colliculus* (in addition to indirect visual inputs coming from the visual cortex). It has been hypothesized that the superior colliculus maps the visual space around us in terms of not only visual, but also auditory and somatosensory cues. The three sensory maps in the superior colliculus are different from those seen in the sensory cortex. Body areas here are not mapped in terms of density of receptor cells in a particular area, but in terms of their relationship to the retina. Areas close to the retina (the nose) are given more representation than areas far away (the hand). For any part of the body, the visual, auditory, and somatosensory maps are aligned, in the different layers of the colliculus (16).

In addition to these three maps, located in the upper and middle of the seven layers of the colliculus, there is a motor map in the deeper layers of the colliculus. Through these output neurons, the colliculus controls saccadic eye movements that cause the eye to move toward a specific stimulus. The superior colliculus then sends outputs to (*a*) regions of the brainstem that control eye movements, (*b*) the tectospinal tract, mediating the reflex control of the neck and head, and (*c*) the tectopontine tract, which projects to the cerebellum, for further processing of eye-head control (16).

Pretectal region

Ganglion cells also terminate in the *pretectal* region. The pretectal region is an important visual reflex center involved in pupillary eye reflexes, in which the pupil constricts in response to light shining on the retina.

PRIMARY VISUAL CORTEX

From the LGN, axons project to the *visual cortex* (also called striate cortex) to Brodmann's area 17, which is in the occipital lobe (Fig. 3.9). The inputs from the two eyes alternate throughout the striate cortex, producing what are called *ocular dominance columns*.

Output cells from primary visual cortex then project to Brodmann's area 18. From area 18, neurons project to the medial temporal cortex (area 19), the inferotemporal cortex (areas 20, 21), and the posterior parietal cortex (area 7). In addition, outputs go to the superior colliculus and also project back to the LGN (feedback control). The primary visual cortex contains a map of the retina with topographic mapping. There are six additional representations of the retina in the occipital lobe alone (16).

The receptive fields of cells in the visual cortex are not circular anymore, but linear: the light must be in the shape of a line, a bar, or an edge to excite them. These cells are classified as *simple* or *complex* cells. Simple cells respond to bars, with an excitatory center and an inhibitory surround, or vice versa. They also have a specific axis of orientation, for which the bar is most effective in exciting the cell. All axes of orientation for all parts of the retina are represented in the visual cortex. Results of experiments by Hubel and Wiesel (18) suggest that this bar-shaped receptive field is created from many geniculate neurons with partially overlapping circular receptive fields in one line, converging onto a simple cortical cell. It has been suggested that complex cells have convergent input from many simple cells. Thus, their receptive fields are larger than simple cells, and have a critical axis of orientation. For many complex cells, the most useful stimulus is movement across the field.

The visual cortex is divided into columns, with each column consisting of cells with one axis of orientation, and neighboring columns receiving input from the left vs. the right eye. Hubel and Wiesel used the name *hypercolumn* to describe a set of columns from one part of the retina, including all orientation angles for the two eyes (17).

HIGHER-ORDER VISUAL CORTEX

Central visual processing pathways continue on to include cells in the primary visual cortex, located in the occipital lobe, and cells in the higher-order visual cortices, located in the temporal and parietal cortex as well. These areas are shown in Figure 3.9. Higher order-cortices are involved in the integration of so-matosensory and visual information underly-ing spatial orientation, an essential part of all actions. This interaction between visual and somatosensory inputs within higher-order as-sociation cortices was previously discussed in the somatosensory section of this chapter.

It has been suggested that the cells within the visual pathways contribute to a *hi-erarchy* within the visual system, with each level of the hierarchy increasing the visual ab-straction (19). In addition, there are *parallel pathways* through which this information is processed. These pathways involve the mag-nocellular layers (processing movement and coarse detail—processing the "where") and parvocellular layers (processing fine detail and color—processing the "what") of the lateral geniculate nucleus (20).

There is interesting clinical evidence to support the existence of these parallel pro-cessing pathways. A perceptual deficit called "movement agnosia" occurs after damage to the medial temporal (MT) area or the medial superior temporal (MST) regions of the cor-tex. Patients show a specific loss of motion perception without any other perceptual problems. Other patients with damage to Brodmann's areas 18 or 37 lose only color vision, but can still identify form (achroma-topsia). Still other patients lose the ability to identify forms (with damage to areas 18, 20, 21) (20).

How do we sense motion? The mag-nocellular pathway continues to area MT and MST and the visual motor area of the parietal lobe. In MT, the activity in the neurons is re-lated to the velocity and movement direction of objects. This information is then further processed in MST for visual perception, pur-suit eye movements, and guiding the move-ments of the body through space.

How do we take the information pro-cessed by these parallel pathways and organize it into a perceptual whole? This process by which the brain recombines information pro-cessed in its different regions is called the "binding problem." The recombination of

this information appears to require attention, which may be mediated by subcortical struc-tures such as the superior colliculus, as well as cortical areas, such as the posterior parietal and prefrontal cortex. It has been hypothe-sized that the CNS takes information related to color, size, distance, and orientation and organizes it into a "master map" of the image (21). Our attentional systems allow us to fo-cus on one small part of the master map as we identify objects or move through space.

Vestibular System

The vestibular system is sensitive to two types of information: the position of the head in space and sudden changes in the direction of movement of the head. Although we aren't consciously aware of vestibular sensation, as we are of the other senses, vestibular inputs are important for the coordination of many motor responses and help to stabilize the eyes and to maintain postural stability during stance and walking. Abnormalities within the vestibular system result in sensations such as dizziness or unsteadiness, which do reach our awareness, as well as problems with focusing our eyes and in keeping our balance.

Like other sensory systems, the vestib-ular system can be divided into two parts, a peripheral and a central component. The pe-ripheral component consists of the sensory re-ceptors and 8th cranial nerve, while the cen-tral part consists of the four vestibular nuclei as well as the ascending and descending tracts.

PERIPHERAL RECEPTORS

Let's first look at the anatomy of the vestibular system (Fig. 3.10). The vestibular system is part of the *membranous labyrinth* of the inner ear. The other part of the labyrinth is the *cochlea*, which is concerned with hear-ing. The membranous labyrinth consists of a continuous series of tubes and sacs located in the temporal bone of the skull. The membra-nous labyrinth is surrounded by a fluid called the *perilymph*, and filled with a fluid called the *endolymph*. The endolymph has a density greater than water, giving it inertial charac-

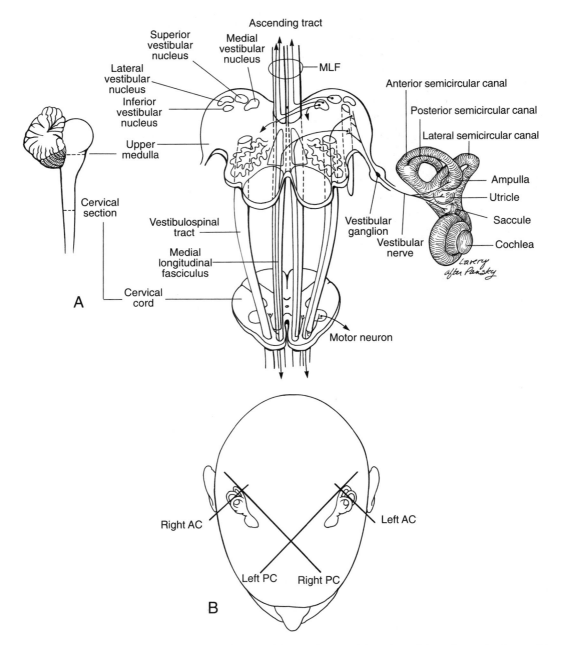

Figure 3.10.   Vestibular system. **A**, Schematic drawing of the membranous labyrinth (otoliths and semicircular canals) and the central connections of the vestibular system. Shown are the ascending vestibular inputs to the oculomotor complex, important for stabilizing gaze, and the descending vestibulospinal system, important for posture and balance. **B**, Location of the paired semicircular canals within the temporal bone of the skull. AC = anterior canal; PC = posterior canal.

teristics, which are important to the way the vestibular system functions.

The vestibular portion of the labyrinth includes five receptors: three *semicircular canals*, the *utricle*, and the *saccule*.

Semicircular Canals

The semicircular canals function as angular accelerometers. They lie at right angles to each other, and are named the anterior, posterior, and horizontal canals on either side of the head (Fig. 3.10). At least one pair is affected by any given angular acceleration of the head or body. The sensory endings of the semicircular canals are in the enlarged end of each canal, which is called the *ampulla*, near its junction with the utricle. Each ampulla has an *ampullary crest*, which contain the vestibular hair cells. The hair cells project upward into the *cupula* (Latin for small inverted cup), made of gelatinous material, and extending to the top of the ampulla, preventing movement of the endolymph past the cupula. The hair cells are the vestibular receptors, and are innervated by bipolar sensory neurons, which are part of the 8th nerve. Their cell bodies are located in the vestibular ganglion (22, 23).

How do the semicircular canals signal head motion to the nervous system? When the head starts to rotate, the fluid in the canals doesn't move initially, due to its inertial characteristics. As a result, the cupula, along with its hair cells, bends in the opposite direction to head movement. When head motion stops, the cupula and hair cells are deflected in the opposite direction, that is, the direction in which the head had been moving.

When the hair cells bend, they cause a change in the firing frequency of the nerve, depending on which way the hair cells are bent. For each hair cell, there is a *kinocilium* (the tallest tuft) and 40 to 70 *stereocilia*, which increase in length as they get closer to the kinocilium. Bending the hair cell toward the kinocilium causes a depolarization of the hair cell and an increase in firing rate of the bipolar cells of the 8th nerve, and bending away causes hyperpolarization and a decrease in firing rate of bipolar cells. At rest, the hair

cells fire at 100 Hz, so they have a wide range of frequencies for modulation. Thus, changes in firing frequency of the neurons either up or down are possible because of this tonic resting discharge, which occurs in the absence of head motion (22, 23).

Because canals on each side of the head are approximately parallel to one another, they work together in a reciprocal fashion. The two horizontal canals work together, while each anterior canal is paired with a posterior canal on the opposite side of the head. When head motion occurs in a plane specific to a pair of canals, one canal will be excited, while its paired opposite canal will be hyperpolarized.

Thus, angular motion of the head, either horizontal or vertical, results in either an increase or decrease in hair cell activity, which produces a parallel change in the frequency of neuronal activity in paired canals. Receptors in the semicircular canal are very sensitive: they respond to angular accelerations of $.1°/sec^2$, but do not respond to steady-state motion of the head. During prolonged motion of the head, the cupula returns to its resting position, and firing frequency in the neurons returns to its steady state.

Utricle and Saccule

The utricle and saccule provide information about body position with reference to the force of gravity and linear acceleration or movement of the head in a straight line. On the wall of these structures is a thickening where the epithelium contains hair cells. This area is called the *macula* (Latin for spot), and is where the receptor cells are located. The hair cells project tufts or processes up into a gelatinous membrane: the *otolith organ* (Greek, from "lithos"—stone). The otolith organ has many calcium carbonate crystals called *otoconia*, or otoliths (22).

The macula of the utricle lies in the horizontal plane when the head is held horizontally, so the otoliths rests upon it. But if the head is tilted, or accelerates, the hair cells are bent by the movement of the gelatinous mass. The macula of the saccule lies in the vertical plane when the head is positioned normally, so it responds selectively to vertically directed linear forces. As in the semicircular canals, hair cells in the otoliths respond to bending in a directional manner.

CENTRAL CONNECTIONS

Vestibular Nuclei

Neurons from both the otoliths and the semicircular canals go through the 8th nerve, and have their cell bodies in the vestibular ganglion (Scarpa's ganglion). The axons then enter the brain in the pons, and most go to the floor of the medulla, where the vestibular nuclei are located. There are four nuclei in the complex: the *lateral vestibular nucleus* (Deiters'), the *medial vestibular nucleus*, the *superior vestibular nucleus*, and the *inferior*, or *descending vestibular nucleus*. A certain portion of the vestibular neurons go from the sensory receptors to the cerebellum, the reticular formation, the thalamus, and the cerebral cortex. The central connections of the vestibular system are pictured in Figure 3.10.

The lateral vestibular nucleus receives input from the utricle, semicircular canals, cerebellum, and spinal cord. The output contributes to vestibulo-ocular tracts and to the lateral vestibulospinal tract, which activates antigravity muscles in the neck, trunk, and limbs.

Inputs to the medial and superior nuclei are from the semicircular canals. The outputs of the medial nucleus are to the medial vestibulospinal tract (MVST), with connections to the cervical spinal cord, controlling the neck muscles. Information in the MVST plays an important role in coordinating interactions between head and eye movements. In addition, neurons from the medial and superior nuclei ascend to motor nuclei of the eye muscles, and aid in stabilizing gaze during head motions.

The inputs to the inferior vestibular nucleus include neurons from the semicircular canals, utricle, saccule, and cerebellar vermis, while the outputs are part of the vestibulospinal tract and vestibuloreticular tracts.

Ascending information from the vestibular system to the oculomotor complex is responsible for the *vestibulo-oculomotor reflex*, which rotates the eyes opposite to head movement, allowing the gaze to remain steady on an image even when the head is moving (22, 23).

Vestibular nystagmus is the rapid alternating movement of the eyes in response to continued rotation of the body. One can create vestibular nystagmus in a subject by rotating the person seated on a stool to the left: when the acceleration first begins, the eyes go slowly to the right, to keep the eyes on a single point in space. When the eyes reach the end of the orbit, they "reset" by moving rapidly to the left; then they move again slowly to the right.

This alternating slow movement of the eyes in the direction opposite head movement, and rapid resetting of the eyes in the direction of head movement, is called nystagmus. It is a normal consequence of acceleration of the head. However, when nystagmus occurs without head movement it is usually an indication of dysfunction in the peripheral or central nervous system.

Postrotatory nystagmus is a reversal in the direction of nystagmus, and occurs when a person who is spinning stops abruptly. Postrotatory nystagmus has been used clinically to evaluate the function of the vestibular system (24).

The vestibular apparatus has both static and dynamic functions. The dynamic functions are controlled mainly by the semicircular canals, allowing us to sense head rotation and angular accelerations, and allowing the control of the eyes through the vestibulo-ocular reflexes. The static functions are controlled by the utricle and saccule, allowing us to monitor absolute position of the head in space, and are important in posture. (The utricle and saccule also detect linear acceleration, a dynamic function.)

ACTION SYSTEMS

The action system includes areas of the nervous system such as motor cortex, cerebellum, and basal ganglia, which perform processing essential to the coordination of movement.

Remember our example presented in the beginning of this chapter. You're thirsty and want to pour some milk from the milk carton in front of you into a glass. We've already seen how sensory structures help you form the map of your body in space and locate the milk carton relative to your arm. Now you need to generate the movement that will allow you to pick up the carton and pour the milk. You will need a plan to move, you will need to specify specific muscles (both timing and force), and you will need a way to modify and refine the movement. So let's look at the structures that allow you to do that.

Motor Cortex

The *motor cortex* is situated in the frontal lobe and consists of a number of different processing areas, including the *primary motor cortex* (MI) the *supplementary motor area* (SM), (occasionally called MII), and the *premotor cortex* (Fig. 3.11A). These areas interact with sensory processing areas in the parietal lobe and also with basal ganglia and cerebellar areas to identify where we want to move, to plan the movement, and finally, to execute our actions (25).

All three of these areas have their own somatotopic maps of the body, so that if different regions are stimulated, different muscles and body parts move. The primary motor cortex (Brodmann's area 4) contains a very complex map of the body. There is often a one-to-one correspondence between cells stimulated and the activation of individual α motor neurons in the spinal cord. In contrast to a one-to-one activation pattern typical of neurons in the primary motor cortex, stimulation of neurons in the premotor and supplementary motor areas (Brodmann's area 6) typically activates multiple muscles at multiple joints, giving coordinated actions.

The motor map, or motor homunculus (shown in Fig. 3.11B), is similar to the sensory map in the way it distorts the representations of the body. In both cases, the areas that require the most detailed control (the mouth, throat, and hand), allowing finely graded movements, are most highly represented (26).

Inputs to the motor areas come from the basal ganglia, the cerebellum, and from sensory areas, including the periphery (via the thalamus), SI, and sensory association areas in the parietal lobe. Interestingly, MI neurons receive sensory inputs from their own muscles and also from the skin above the muscles. It has been suggested that this transcortical pathway might be used in parallel with the spinal reflex pathway to give additional force output in the muscles when an unexpected load is encountered during a movement (27). This pathway has also been hypothesized to be an important proprioceptive pathway functioning in postural control (25).

CORTICOSPINAL TRACT

Outputs from the motor cortex contribute to the corticospinal tract (also called the pyramidal tract) and often make excitatory monosynaptic connections onto α motor neurons, in addition to polysynaptic connections to γ motor neurons, which control muscle spindle length. In addition to their monosynaptic connections, corticospinal neurons make many polysynaptic connections through interneurons within the spinal cord.

The corticospinal tract includes neurons from primary motor cortex (about 50%), supplementary motor cortex, premotor areas, and even somatosensory cortex (Fig. 3.12). The fibers descend ipsilaterally from the cortex through the internal capsule, the midbrain, and the medulla. In the medulla, the fibers concentrate to form "pyramids" and near the junction of the medulla and the spinal cord, most (90%) cross to form the lateral corticospinal tract. The remaining 10% continue uncrossed to form the anterior corticospinal tract. The majority of the anterior corticospinal neurons cross just before they terminate in the ventral horn of the spinal cord. Most axons enter the ventral horn and terminate in the intermediate and ventral areas on interneurons and motor neurons.

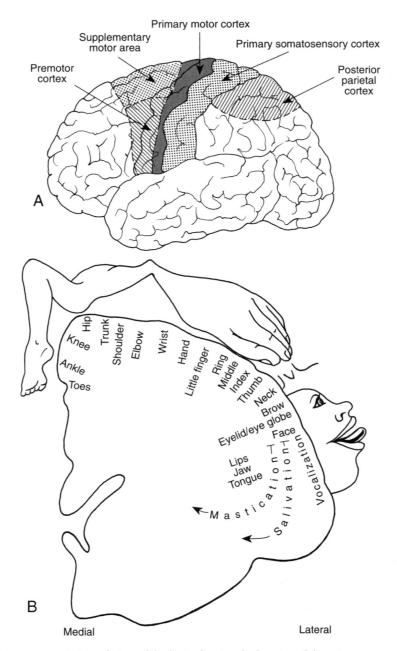

Figure 3.11. Motor cortex. **A**, Lateral view of the brain showing the location of the primary motor cortex, supplementary motor area, and premotor cortex. **B**, Motor homunculus. (Adapted from Kandel E, Schwartz JH, Jessell TM, eds. Principles of neuroscience. 3rd ed. NY: Elsevier, 1991:610, 613.)

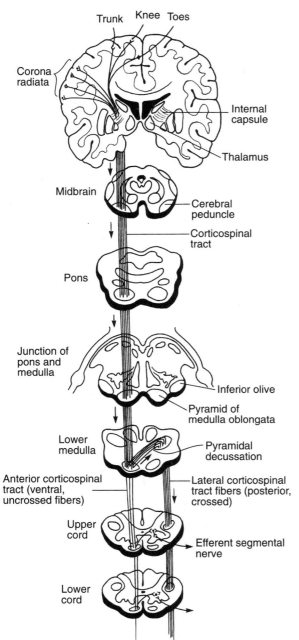

Figure 3.12.   Pyramidal or (corticospinal) tract.

FUNCTION

Motor Cortex

What is the specific function of motor cortex in movement control? Evarts (28) recorded the activity of corticospinal neurons in monkeys while they made wrist flexion and extension movements. He found that the firing rate of the corticospinal neurons codes (a) the force used to move a limb, and (b) in some cases, the rate of change of force. Thus, both absolute force and the speed of a movement are controlled by the primary motor cortex.

Now, think about a typical movement that we make—reaching for the carton of milk, for example. How does the motor cortex encode the execution of such a complex movement? Researchers performed experiments in which a monkey made arm movements to many different targets around a central starting point (29). They found that there were specific movement directions where each neuron was activated maximally, yet each responded for a wide range of movement directions. To explain how movements could be finely controlled when neurons are so broadly tuned, these researchers suggested that actions are controlled by a population of neurons. The activity of each of the neurons can be represented as a vector, whose length represents the degree of activity in any direction. The sum of the vectors of all of the neurons would then predict the movement direction and amplitude.

If this is the case, does it mean that whenever we make a movement, for example, with our ankle, the exact same neurons are activated in the primary motor cortex? No. It has been shown that specific neurons in the cortex, activated when we pick up an object, may remain totally silent when we make a similar movement such as a gesture in anger. This is a very important point to understand because it implies that there are many parallel motor pathways for carrying out an action sequence, just as there are parallel pathways for sensory processing. Thus, simply by training a patient in one situation, we can't automatically assume that the training will transfer to all other activities requiring the same set of muscles (25).

Supplementary and Premotor Cortex

What are the functions of the supplementary and premotor areas? Roland and his colleagues (30) performed some interesting experiments with humans, which have begun to clarify their functions. He asked subjects to perform tasks ranging from very simple to complex movements, and while they were making the movements, he assessed the amount of cerebral blood flow in different areas of the brain. (To measure blood flow, one

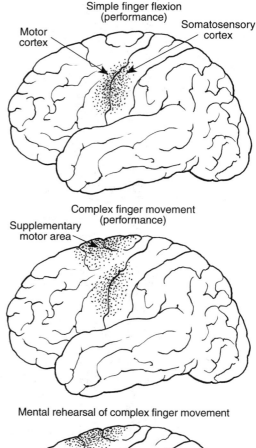

Figure 3.13. Changes in blood flow during different motor behaviors indicating the areas of the motor cortex involved in the behavior. (Adapted from Roland PE, Larsen B, Lassen NA, Skinhof E. Supplementary motor area and other cortical areas in organization of voluntary movements in man. J Neurophysiol 1980;43:118–136.)

injects short-lived radioactive tracer into the blood, then measures the radioactivity in different brain areas with detectors on the scalp.)

As shown in Figure 3.13, when subjects were asked to perform a simple task (simple repetitive movements of the index finger or pressing a spring between the thumb and index finger), the blood flow increase was only in the motor and sensory cortex. In contrast, when they were asked to perform a complex task (a sequence of movements involving all four fingers, touching the thumb in different orders), subjects showed a blood flow increase in the supplementary motor area, bilaterally, and in the primary motor and sensory areas. Finally, when they were asked to rehearse the task, but not perform it, the blood flow increase was only in the supplementary motor area, not the primary sensory or motor cortex. Roland concluded that the supplementary area is active when a sequence of simple ballistic movements is planned. Thus, it participates in the assembly of the central motor program or forms a motor subroutine.

These experiments were performed by the subjects in intrapersonal space (moving one body part in relation to another, where only a body reference system is needed). Moving the limbs in extrapersonal space requires a different reference system, which is three-dimensional, and fixed by points in the environment. For example, picking up a milk carton from a table requires this framework.

Since these two types of movements are different, one might expect the cerebral organization to be different. To test this, Roland had the subjects perform a new movement. They were asked to make a spiraling movement in the air or move their fingers (using no vision) over a grid according to specific cues (maze test). At that point, the superior parietal region was active along with the other regions. So this region must be necessary for the planning of voluntary movements in extrapersonal space.

Roland noted that the premotor area was activated only when a new motor program was established, or alternatively when a previously learned program was modulated.

Therefore, the premotor area probably has a role in motor learning (30).

Higher-Level Association Areas

ASSOCIATION AREAS OF THE FRONTAL REGION

The association areas of the frontal regions (areas rostral to Brodmann's area 6) are important for motor planning and other cognitive behaviors. For example, these areas probably integrate sensory information and then select the appropriate motor response from the many possible responses (31).

The prefrontal cortex can be divided into the principal sulcus and the prefrontal convexities (refer back to Fig. 3.8). Experiments have indicated that the neurons of the principal sulcus are involved in the strategic planning of higher motor functions. For example, experiments on monkeys in which this area was lesioned showed that they had difficulty with performing spatial tasks in which information had to be stored in working memory in order to guide future action. In other experiments, neurons in this area were shown to be active as soon as a cue was presented and to remain active throughout a delay period, when the cue wasn't present, but the monkey had to keep the cue in working memory, before performing the task (13).

This area is densely interconnected with the posterior parietal areas. The prefrontal and parietal areas are hypothesized to work closely together in spatial tasks that require attention.

By contrast, lesions in the prefrontal convexity cause problems in performing any kind of delayed response task. Animals with these lesions have problems with tasks where they have to inhibit certain motor responses at specific moments. Lesions in adjacent areas cause problems with a monkey's ability to select from a variety of motor responses when given different sensory cues (13).

Lesions in other prefrontal regions cause patients to have difficulty with changing strategies when they are asked to. Even when they are shown their errors, they fail to correct them.

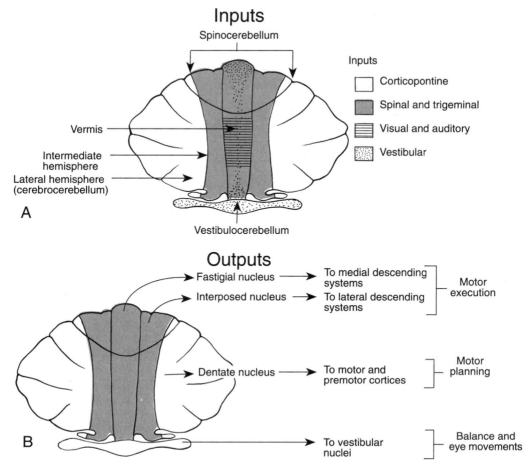

Figure 3.14. A schematic drawing showing the basic anatomy of the cerebellum, including **A**, its inputs, and **B**, its outputs. (Adapted from Ghez C. The cerebellum. In: Kandel E, Schwartz JH, Jessell TM, eds. Principles of neuroscience. 3rd ed. NY: Elsevier, 1991:633.)

Cerebellum

The cerebellum is considered one of three important brain areas contributing to coordination of movement, in addition to the motor cortex and the basal ganglia complex. Yet, despite its important role in the coordination of movement, the cerebellum doesn't play a primary role in either sensory or motor function. If the cerebellum is destroyed, we don't lose sensation or become paralyzed. However, lesions of the cerebellum do produce devastating changes in our ability to perform movements, from the very simple to the most elegant. The cerebellum receives afferent information from almost every sensory

system, consistent with its role as a regulator of motor output (32, 33).

How does the cerebellum adjust the output of the motor systems? Its function is related to its neuronal circuitry. Through this circuitry and its input and output connections, it appears to act as a comparator, a system that compensates for errors by comparing intention with performance.

The cerebellum's input and output connections are vital to its role as error detector, and are summarized in Figure 3.14. Its inputs (Fig. 3.14A) include information from other modules of the brain related to the programming and execution of movements. This information is often referred to as "efference copy" or "corollary discharge" when it comes from the primary motor cortex, since it is hypothesized to be a direct copy of the motor cortex output to the spinal cord. The cerebellum also receives sensory feedback information (reafference) from the receptors about the movements as they are being made. After processing this information, outputs (Fig. 3.14*B*) from the cerebellum go to the motor cortex and other systems within the brainstem to refine the movement.

ANATOMY OF THE CEREBELLUM

An understanding of the anatomy of the cerebellum is helpful in explaining its function. The cerebellum consists of an outer layer of gray matter (the cortex), internal white matter (input and output fibers), and three pairs of *deep nuclei*: the *fastigial nucleus*, the *interposed nucleus*, and the *dentate nucleus*. All the inputs to the cerebellum go first to one of these three deep cerebellar nuclei and then proceed to the cortex. All the outputs of the cerebellum go back to the deep nuclei, before going on to the cerebral cortex or the brainstem (32, 33).

The cerebellum can be divided into three zones, phylogenetically (refer back to Fig. 3.14). The oldest zone corresponds to the *flocculonodular lobe*. It is functionally related to the vestibular system. The phylogenetically more recent areas to develop are the *vermis* and *intermediate* part of the hemispheres and the *lateral hemispheres*, respectively. These three parts of the cerebellum have distinct functions and input output connections.

Flocculonodular Lobe

The flocculonodular lobe receives inputs from both the visual system and the vestibular system, and its outputs return to the vestibular nuclei. It functions in the control of the axial muscles that are used in equilibrium control. If a patient experiences dysfunction in this system, one observes an ataxic gait, wide-based stance and nystagmus.

Vermis and Intermediate Hemispheres

The vermis and intermediate hemispheres receive proprioceptive and cutaneous inputs from the spinal cord (via the spinocerebellar tracts) in addition to visual, vestibular, and auditory information. Researchers used to think that there were two maps of the complete body in the cerebellum, but now it has been shown that the maps are much more complex and can be divided into many smaller maps. This has been called *fractured somatotopy*. These smaller maps appear to be related to functional activities: thus, in the rat, the mouth and paw receptive fields are positioned closely together, possibly to contribute to the control of grooming behavior. Inputs to this part of the cerebellum go through the fastigial nucleus (vermis) and interposed nucleus (intermediate lobes) (34).

There are four spinocerebellar tracts that relay information from the spinal cord to the cerebellum. Two tracts relay information from the arms and the neck, and two relay information from the trunk and legs. Inputs are also from the spino-olivo-cerebellar tract, through the inferior olivary nucleus (climbing fibers). These latter inputs are important in learning and are discussed later.

What are the output pathways of this part of the cerebellum? The outputs go to the (*a*) brainstem reticular formation, (*b*) vestibular nuclei, (*c*) thalamus and motor cortex, and (*d*) red nucleus in the midbrain.

What are the functions of the vermis and intermediate lobes? First, they appear to function in the control of the actual execution of movement: they correct for deviations from an intended movement through comparing feedback from the spinal cord with the intended motor command. They also modulate muscle tone. This occurs through the continuous output of excitatory activity from the fastigial and interpositus nucleus, which modulates the activity of the γ-motor neurons to the muscle spindles. When there are lesions in these nuclei, there is a significant drop in muscle tone (hypotonia) (32).

Lateral Hemispheres

The last part of the cerebellum and the newest phylogenetically is the lateral zone of the cerebellar hemispheres (Fig. 3.14). It receives inputs from the pontine nuclei in the brainstem that relay information from wide areas of the cerebral cortex (sensory, motor, premotor, and posterior parietal). Its outputs are to the thalamus, motor, and premotor cortex.

What is the function of the lateral hemispheres? This part of the cerebellum functions in the preparation of movement, whereas the intermediate lobes function in movement execution and fine-tuning of ongoing movement via feedback information. It appears that the lateral hemispheres of the cerebellum participate in programming the motor cortex for the execution of movement. The cerebellar pathways are one of many parallel pathways affecting the motor cortex. The others probably include the supplementary and premotor areas.

The lateral hemispheres also appear to function in the coordination of ongoing movements. It has been shown that cooling parts of the cerebellum disturbs the timing of agonist and antagonist muscle responses during rapid movements (35). The antagonist activity becomes delayed, giving a hypermetric or "overshooting" movement. As corrections are attempted in cerebellar patients, one sees unintended movements in the opposite direction, giving intention tremor.

In addition, the lateral cerebellum may contribute to a more general timing function that affects perception as well as action. Patients with cerebellar lesions often make timing errors during movement. Those with lateral hemisphere lesions show errors in timing related to perceptual abilities, which researchers think may be related to problems with a central clock-like mechanism (36). In contrast, patients with intermediate lobe lesions make errors related to movement execution (36).

Finally, many parts of the cerebellum, including the lateral cerebellum, seem to be important in motor learning. The unique cellular circuitry of the cerebellum has been shown to be perfect for the long-term modification of motor responses. Experiments have shown that as animals learn a new task, the climbing fiber, a type of neuron that detects movement error, alters the effectiveness of the synapse of a second fiber, the granule cell parallel fiber, onto the main output cells of the cerebellum, the Purkinje cells (37).

This type of cerebellar learning also occurs in vestibulo-ocular reflex circuitry, which includes cerebellar pathways. This reflex keeps the eyes fixed on an object when the head turns. In experiments in which humans wore prismatic lenses that reversed the image on the eye, the gain of the vestibulo-ocular reflex was altered over time. This modification of the reflex did not occur in patients with cerebellar lesions (38).

Basal Ganglia

The basal ganglia complex consists of a set of nuclei at the base of the cerebral cortex, including the *putamen, caudate nucleus, globus pallidus, subthalamic nucleus,* and *substantia nigra.* Basal means "at the base," or in other words, "just below the cortex." As with patients with cerebellar lesions, patients with basal ganglia damage are not paralyzed, but have problems with the coordination of movement. Advancement in our understanding of basal ganglia function first came from clinicians, especially from James Parkinson, who in 1817 first described Parkinson's disease as "the shaking palsy" (39).

The basal ganglia were once believed to be part of the extrapyramidal motor system, which was believed to act in parallel with the pyramidal system (the cortico-spinal tract) in movement control. Thus, clinicians defined pyramidal problems as relating to spasticity and paralysis, while extrapyramidal problems were defined as involuntary movements and rigidity. As we have seen in this chapter, this distinction is no longer valid since many other brain systems also control movement. In addition, the pyramidal and extrapyramidal systems are not independent, but work together in controlling movements.

ANATOMY OF THE BASAL GANGLIA

The major connections of the basal ganglia are summarized in Figure 3.15, including the major afferent (3.15*A*), central (3.15*B*), and efferent (3.15*C*) connections. The main input nuclei of the basal ganglia complex are the caudate and the putamen. The caudate and the putamen develop from the same structure and are often discussed as a single unit, the *striatum*. Their primary inputs are from widespread areas of the neocortex, including sensory, motor, and association areas (39, 40).

The globus pallidus has two segments, internal and external, and is situated next to the putamen, while the substantia nigra is situated a little more caudally, in the midbrain. The internal segment of the globus pallidus and the substantia nigra are the major output areas of the basal ganglia. Their outputs terminate in the prefrontal and premotor cortex areas, by way of the thalamus. The final nucleus, the subthalamic nucleus, is situated just below the thalamus.

The connections within the basal ganglia complex are as follows: Cells in both the caudate and putamen terminate in the globus pallidus and the substantia nigra in a somatotopic manner, as seen for other pathways in the brain. Cells from the external segment of the globus pallidus terminate in the subthalamic nucleus, while the subthalamic nucleus projects to the globus pallidus and substantia nigra. Other inputs to the subthalamic nucleus include direct inputs from the motor and premotor cortex.

ROLE OF THE BASAL GANGLIA

The basal ganglia and cerebellum have many similarities in the way they interact with the rest of the elements of the motor system. But what are their differences? First, their input connections are different. The cerebellum receives input only from the sensory and motor areas of the cerebral cortex. It also receives somatosensory information directly from the spinal cord. However, the basal ganglia complex is the termination site for tracts from the entire cerebral cortex, but not the spinal cord (39).

Their outputs also influence different parts of the motor system. The basal ganglia complex sends its outputs to the prefrontal and premotor cortex areas, involved in higher level processing of movement, while the cerebellar output goes back to the motor cortex, and also to the spinal cord via brainstem pathways. This suggests that the cerebellum is more directly involved in the on-line control of movement (correcting errors), while the basal ganglia function may be more complex, including functions related to the planning and control of more complex motor behavior.

The basal ganglia may play a role in selectively activating some movements as they suppress others (39, 40). Diseases of the basal ganglia typically produce involuntary movements (dyskinesia), poverty and slowness of movement, and disorders of muscle tone and postural reflexes. Parkinson's disease symptoms include resting tremor, increased muscle tone or rigidity, slowness in the initiation of movement (akinesia) as well as in the execution of movement (bradykinesia). The site of the lesion is in the dopaminergic pathway from the substantia nigra to the striatum. The tremor and rigidity may be due to loss of inhibitory influences within the basal ganglia. Huntington's disease characteristics include chorea and dementia. Symptoms appear to be caused by loss of cholinergic neurons and GABA-ergic neurons in the striatum (39, 40).

This concludes our review of the physiological basis for motor control. In this chapter we have tried to show you the substrates for movement. This has involved a review of the perception and action systems, and the higher-level cognitive processes that play a part in their elaboration. We have tried to show the importance of both the hierarchical and distributed nature of these systems. The presentation of the perception and action systems separately is somewhat misleading. In real life, as movements are generated to accomplish tasks in varied environments, the boundaries between perception, action, and cognition are blurred.

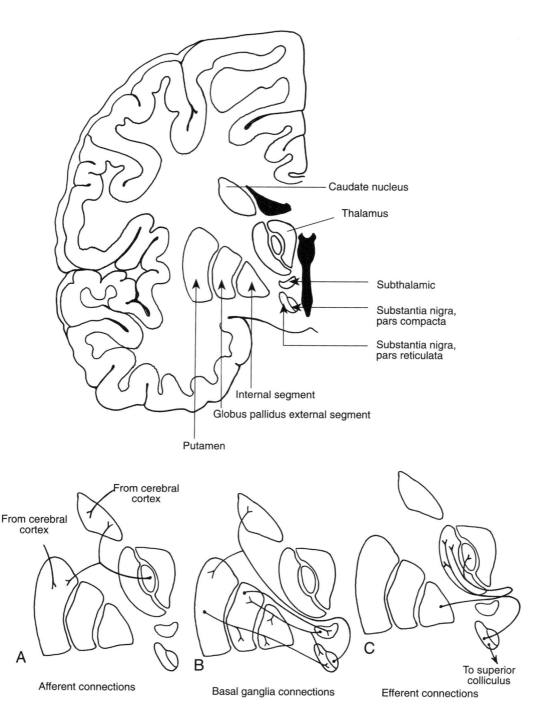

Figure 3.15.   Illustration summarizing **A**, the major afferent, **B**, the central, and **C**, the efferent connections of the basal ganglia. (Adapted from Cote L, Crutcher MD. The basal ganglia. In: Kandel E, Schwartz JH, Jessell TM, eds. Principles of neuroscience. 3rd ed. NY: Elsevier, 1991:649.)

SUMMARY

1. Movement control is achieved through the cooperative effort of many brain structures, which are organized both hierarchically and in parallel.
2. Sensory inputs perform many functions in the control of movement. They (a) serve as the stimuli for reflexive movement organized at the spinal cord level of the nervous system; (b) modulate the output of movement that results from the activity of pattern generators in the spinal cord; (c) modulate commands that originate in higher centers of the nervous system; and (d) contribute to the perception and control of movement through ascending pathways in much more complex ways.
3. In the somatosensory system, muscle spindles, Golgi tendon organs, joint receptors, and cutaneous receptors contribute to spinal reflex control, modulate spinal pattern generator output, modulate descending commands, and contribute to perception and control of movement through ascending pathways.
4. Vision (a) allows us to identify objects in space, and to determine their movement (exteroceptive sensation) and (b) gives us information about where our body is in space, about the relation of one body part to another, and the motion of our body (visual-proprioception).
5. The vestibular system is sensitive to two types of information: the position of the head in space and sudden changes in the direction of movement of the head.
6. As sensory information ascends to higher levels of processing, every level of the hierarchy has the ability to modulate the information coming into it from below, allowing higher centers to selectively tune (up or down) the information coming from lower centers.
7. Information from sensory receptors is increasingly processed as it ascends the neural hierarchy, enabling meaningful interpretation of the information. This is done by selectively enlarging the receptive field of each successively higher neuron.
8. The somatosensory and visual systems process incoming information to increase contrast sensitivity so that we can more easily identify and discriminate between different objects. This is done through lateral inhibition, in which the cell that is excited inhibits the cells next to it, thus enhancing contrast between excited and nonexcited regions of the body or visual field.
9. There are also special cells within the SS and visual systems that respond best to moving stimuli and are directionally sensitive.
10. In the association cortices, we begin to see the transition from perception to action. The parietal lobe participates in processes involving attention to the position of and manipulation of objects in space.
11. The action system includes areas of the nervous system such as motor cortex, cerebellum, and basal ganglia.
12. The motor cortex interacts with sensory processing areas in the parietal lobe and with basal ganglia and cerebellar areas to identify where we want to move, to plan the movement, and finally, to execute our actions.
13. The cerebellum appears to act as a comparator, a system that compensates for errors by comparing intention with performance. In addition, it modulates muscle tone, participates in the programming of the motor cortex for the execution of movement, contributes to the timing of movement, and to motor learning.
14. Basal ganglia function is related to the planning and control of complex motor behavior. In addition, it may play a role in selectively activating some movements and suppressing others.

REFERENCES

1. Kandel E. Brain and behavior. In: Kandel E, Schwartz JH, Jessell TM, eds. Principles of neuroscience. 3rd ed. NY: Elsevier, 1991:5–17.
2. Patton HD, Fuchs A, Hille B, Scher A, Steiner R. Textbook of physiology, vol 1. 21st ed. Philadelphia: WB Saunders, 1989.
3. Koester J. Passive membrane properties of the neuron. In: Kandel E, Schwartz JH, Jessell TM, eds. Principles of neuroscience. 3rd ed. NY: Elsevier, 1991:95–103.
4. Kandel ER. Cellular basis of behavior: an introduction to behavioral neurobiology. San Francisco: Freeman, 1976.
5. Gordon J, Ghez C. Muscle receptors and spinal reflexes: the stretch reflex. In: Kandel E,

Schwartz JH, Jessell TM, eds. Principles of neuroscience. 3rd ed. NY: Elsevier, 1991:564–580.

6. Pearson KG, Ramirez JM, Jiang W. Entrainment of the locomotor rhythm by group Ib afferents from ankle extensor muscles in spinal cats. Exp Brain Res 1992;90:557–566.

7. Burgess PR, Clark FJ. Characteristics of knee-joint receptors in the cat. J Physiol (Lond) 1969;203:317–325.

8. Kandel E, Jessell TM. Touch. In: Kandel E, Schwartz JH, Jessell TM, eds. Principles of neuroscience. 3rd ed. NY: Elsevier, 1991:367–384.

9. Grillner S, Wallen P. Central pattern generators for locomotion, with special reference to vertebrates. Annu Rev Neurosci 1985; 8:233–261.

10. Forssberg H, Grillner S, Rossignol S. Phasic gain control of reflexes from the dorsum of the paw during spinal locomotion. Brain Res 1977;132:121–139.

11. Martin JH, Jessell TM. Anatomy of the somatic sensory system. In: Kandel E, Schwartz JH, Jessell TM, eds. Principles of neuroscience. 3rd ed. NY: Elsevier, 1991:353–366.

12. Martin J. Coding and processing of sensory information. In: Kandel E, Schwartz JH, Jessell TM, eds. Principles of neuroscience. 3rd ed. NY: Elsevier, 1991:329–340.

13. Kupfermann I. Localization of higher cognitive and affective functions: the association cortices. In: Kandel E, Schwartz JH, Jessell TM, eds. Principles of neuroscience. 3rd ed. NY: Elsevier, 1991:823–838.

14. Tessier-Lavigne M. Phototransduction and information processing in the retina. In: Kandel E, Schwartz JH, Jessell TM, eds. Principles of neuroscience. 3rd ed. NY: Elsevier, 1991:400–417.

15. Dowling JE. The retina: an approachable part of the brain. Cambridge, MA: Belknap Press, 1987.

16. Mason C, Kandel ER. Central visual pathways. In: Kandel E, Schwartz JH, Jessell TM, eds. Principles of neuroscience. 3rd ed. NY: Elsevier, 1991:420–439.

17. Hubel DH, Wiesel TN. Receptive fields of single neurones in the cat's striate cortex. J Physiol (Lond) 1959;148:574–591.

18. Hubel DH, Wiesel TN. Receptive fields, binocular interaction and functional architecture in the cat's visual cortex. J Physiol (Lond) 1962;160:106–154.

19. Hubel DH. Eye, brain and vision. NY: Scientific American Library, 1988.

20. Kandel ER. Perception of motion, depth and form. In: Kandel E, Schwartz JH, Jessell TM, eds. Principles of neuroscience. 3rd ed. NY: Elsevier, 1991:440–466.

21. Treisman A. Features and objects: the fourteenth Bartlett memorial lecture. J Exp Psychol 1988;40A:201–237.

22. Kelly JP. The sense of balance. In: Kandel E, Schwartz JH, Jessell TM, eds. Principles of neuroscience. 3rd ed. NY: Elsevier, 1991:500–511.

23. Baloh RW: Dizziness, hearing loss and tinnutus: the essentials of neurotology. Philadelphia: FA Davis, 1984.

24. Ayres J. Sensory integration and learning disorders. Los Angeles: Western Psychological Services; 1972.

25. Ghez C. Voluntary movement. In: Kandel E, Schwartz JH, Jessell TM, eds. Principles of neuroscience. 3rd ed. NY: Elsevier, 1991:609–625.

26. Penfield W, Rasmussen T. The cerebral cortex of man: a clinical study of localization of function. NY: Macmillan, 1950.

27. Conrad B, Matsunami K, Meyer-Lohmann J, Wiesendanger M, Brooks VB. Cortical load compensation during voluntary elbow movements. Brain Res 1974;71:507–514.

28. Evarts EV. Relation of pyramidal tract activity to force exerted during voluntary movement. J Neurophysiol 1968;31:14–27.

29. Georgopoulos AP, Kalaska JF, Caminiti R, Massey JT. On the relations between the direction of two-dimensional arm movements and cell discharge in primate motor cortex. J Neurosci 1982;2:1527–1537.

30. Roland PE, Larsen B, Lassen NA, Skinhof E. Supplementary motor area and other cortical areas in organization of voluntary movements in man. J Neurophysiol 1980;43: 118–136.

31. Fuster JM. The prefrontal cortex: anatomy, physiology and neuropsychology of the frontal lobe. 2nd ed. NY: Raven Press. 1989.

32. Ghez C. The cerebellum. In: Kandel E, Schwartz JH, Jessell TM, eds. Principles of neuroscience. 3rd ed. NY: Elsevier, 1991:627–646.

33. Ito M. The cerebellum and neural control. New York: Raven Press, 1984.

34. Shambes GM, Gibson JM, Welker W. Frac-

tured somatotopy in granule cell tactile areas of rat cerebellar hemispheres revealed by micromapping. Brain Behav Evol 1978;15:94–140.

35. Brooks VB, Thatch WT. Cerebellar control of posture and movement. In: Brooks VB, ed. Handbook of physiology, section 1: nervous system, vol 2, Motor control, part 2. Bethesda, MD: American Physiological Society, 1981:877–946.

36. Ivry RB, Keele SW. Timing functions of the cerebellum. J Cogn Neurosci 1989;1:136–152.

37. Gilbert PFC, Thach WT. Purkinje cell activity during motor learning. Brain Res 1977;128:309–328.

38. Gonshor A, Melvill Hones G. Short-term adaptive changes in the human vestibulo-ocular reflex arc. J Physiol (Lond) 1976;256:361–379.

39. Cote L, Crutcher MD. The basal ganglia. In: Kandel E, Schwartz JH, Jessell TM, eds. Principles of neuroscience. 3rd ed. NY: Elsevier, 1991:647–659.

40. Alexander GE, Crutcher MD. Functional architecture of basal ganglia circuits: neural substrates of parallel processing. Trends Neurosci 1990;13:266–271.

Chapter 4

PHYSIOLOGICAL BASIS OF MOTOR LEARNING AND RECOVERY OF FUNCTION

INTRODUCTION

In Chapter 2 we defined *learning* as the process of acquiring knowledge about the world, and *motor learning* as the process of the acquisition and/or modification of movement. We also mentioned that, just as motor control must be seen in light of the interaction between the individual, the task, and the environment, this also applies to motor learning.

In this chapter we extend our knowledge of the physiological basis of motor control to include motor learning. This chapter demonstrates that the physiological basis for motor learning, like motor control, is distributed among many brain structures and processing levels, rather than being localized to a particular learning site of the brain. Likewise, it illustrates that the physiological basis for the recovery of function is similar to learning, in that recovery involves processes occurring throughout the nervous system and not just at the lesioned site. These processes have many common properties with those occurring during learning.

This chapter focuses on the physiological basis of motor learning and recovery of function, showing the similarities and differences between these important functions. The material in this chapter builds on material presented in the chapter on the physiological basis of motor control. Since we assume that the reader has a basic familiarity with the concepts presented in Chapter 3, these concepts will not be reviewed again in this chapter.

Integral to a discussion on the physiological basis of motor learning are issues related to the physiological basis for memory. A fundamental question addressed in this chapter is: how does learning change the structure and function of neurons in the brain? Of equal concern is the question: what changes in the structure and function of neurons underlie the recovery of function following injury? We also explore whether physiological plasticity associated with recovery of function is the same or different from that involved with learning. Previous views have typically held that recovery and learning are different, but physiological studies suggest that they are

85

similar in that many of the same neural mechanisms underlie both types of change.

Defining Neural Plasticity

We define **plasticity** as the ability to show modification. Throughout this book we use the term plasticity as it relates to neural modifiability. Plasticity, or neural modifiability, may be seen as a continuum from short-term functional changes to long-term structural changes. *Short-term functional plasticity* refers to changes in the efficiency or strength of synaptic connections. In contrast, *structural plasticity* refers to changes in the organization and numbers of connections among neurons.

Similarly, learning can be seen as a continuum of short-term to long-term changes in the capability to produce skilled actions. The gradual shift from short-term to long-term learning reflects a move along the continuum of neural modifiability, as increased synaptic efficiency gradually gives way to structural changes, which are the underpinning of long-term modification of behavior. This relationship is shown in Figure 4.1.

Learning and Memory

Learning is defined as the acquisition of knowledge or ability; memory is the retention and storage of that knowledge or ability (1). Learning reflects the *process* by which we acquire knowledge; memory is the *product* of that process. Memory is often divided into short- and long-term storage. **Short-term memory** refers to *working* memory, which has a limited capacity for information and lasts for only a few moments. Short-term memory reflects a momentary attention to something, such as when we remember a phone number only long enough to dial it and then it's gone.

Long-term memory is intimately related to the process of learning. Long-term memory can also be seen as a continuum. Initial stages of long-term memory formation would reflect functional changes in the efficiency of synapses. Later stages of memory formation reflect structural changes in synaptic connections. These memories are less subject to disruption.

Localization of Learning and Memory

Are learning and memory localized in a specific brain structure? It appears that they are not. In fact, learning can occur in all parts of the brain. Learning and the storage of that learning, memory, appear to involve both parallel and hierarchical processing within the CNS. Even for relatively simple learning tasks,

Figure 4.1. A diagram showing the gradual shift from short-term to long-term learning is reflected in a move along the continuum of neural modifiability. Short-term changes, associated with an increased synaptic efficiency, persist and gradually give way to structural changes, the underpinning of long-term learning.

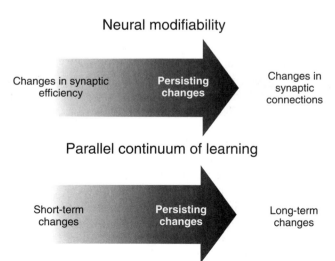

Neural modifiability

Changes in synaptic efficiency   Persisting changes   Changes in synaptic connections

Parallel continuum of learning

Short-term changes   Persisting changes   Long-term changes multiple parallel channels of information are used. In addition, the information can be stored in many different areas of the brain.

Apparently, mechanisms underlying learning and memory are the same whether the learning is occurring in fairly simple circuits, or involves very complex circuits incorporating many aspects of the CNS hierarchy. Thus, current neuronal models of memory suggest that a memory consists of a pattern of changes in synaptic connections among networks of neurons distributed throughout the brain (1).

This chapter describes the continuum of plasticity within the nervous system which represents learning, and specifically, motor learning. The processes underlying learning in the nervous system, as well as those that underlie recovery of function, are described. Once understood, principles of plasticity related to learning and recovery of function can be derived. Then, in later chapters, these principles are applied to therapy settings.

HOW DOES LEARNING CHANGE THE STRUCTURE AND FUNCTION OF NEURONS WITHIN THE BRAIN?

Many factors potentially modify synaptic connections. During development, synaptic connectivity develops under the control of genetic and developmental processes. These connections are fine-tuned during various critical periods of development due to interacting environmental and genetic factors. We are concerned in this chapter with *activity-dependent* modifications of synaptic connections, that is, both the *transient* and *long-term modulation* of synapses resulting from experience. Learning alters our capability for acting by changing both the effectiveness and anatomic connections of neural pathways. We discuss modifications of synaptic connections at both the cellular level and at the level of whole networks of neurons.

Physiological Basis of Nonassociative Forms of Learning

Remember that in *nonassociative* forms of learning, the person is learning about properties of a stimulus that is repeated. The learned suppression of a response to a non-noxious stimulus is called *habituation*. In contrast, an increased response to one stimulus that is consistently preceded by a noxious stimulus is called *sensitization*. Keep in mind that nonassociative forms of learning can be short-term or long-lasting. What are the neural mechanisms underlying these simple forms of learning, and do the same neural mechanisms underlie both short- and long-term changes?

HABITUATION

Habituation was first studied by Sherrington, who found that the flexion reflex habituated with many stimulus repetitions. More recent research examining habituation in relatively simple networks of neurons in invertebrate animals has shown that habituation is related to a decrease in synaptic activity between sensory neurons and their connections to interneurons and motor neurons (2, 3).

During habituation, there is a reduction in the amplitude of synaptic potentials (a decreased excitatory postsynaptic potential [EPSP]) produced by the sensory neuron on the interneuron and motor neuron. This short-term change in EPSP amplitude during habituation is illustrated in Figure 4.2A. During initial stages of learning, the decreased size of the EPSP may last for only several minutes. With continued presentation of the stimulus, persisting changes in synaptic efficacy occur, representing longer-term memory for habituation.

During the course of learning, continued presentation of the stimulus results in structural changes in the sensory cells themselves. Structural changes include a decrease in the number of synaptic connections between the sensory neuron and interneurons

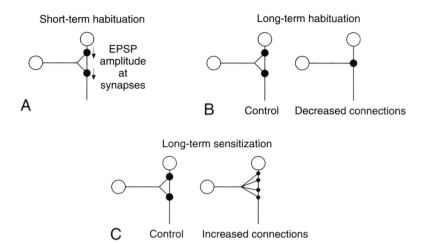

Figure 4.2. Neuronal modifications underlying short- and long-term nonassociative learning. **A,** Short-term habituation results from a decrease in EPSP amplitude at the synapse between the sensory and motor neuron. **B,** Long-term habituation results in a decrease in numbers of connections. **C,** Long-term sensitization results in an increase in numbers of connections. (Adapted from Kandel ER. Cellular mechanisms of learning and the biological basis of individuality. In: Kandel ER, Schwartz JH, Jessell TM, eds. Principles of neuroscience. 3rd ed. New York: Elsevier, 1991:1009–1031.)

and motor neurons, shown diagrammatically in Figure 4.2B. In addition, the number of active transmitting zones within existing connections decreases. As a result of these structural changes, habituation persists over weeks and months, representing long-term memory for habituation. Thus, the process of habituation does not involve specific *memory* storage neurons found in specialized parts of the CNS. Rather, memory (retention of habituation) results from a change in the neurons that are normal components of the response pathway.

How might this research apply to treatment strategies used by therapists in the clinic? As we mentioned earlier, habituation exercises are given to patients who have certain types of inner ear disorders resulting in complaints of dizziness when they move their head in certain ways (4). When patients begin therapy, they may experience an initial decline in the intensity of their dizziness symptoms during the course of one session of exercise. But the next day, dizziness is back at the same level. Gradually, over days and weeks of practicing the exercises, the patient begins to see that decreases in dizziness persist across sessions (4).

Kandel's research suggests that initially

with exercise there is a temporary decrease in the synaptic effectiveness of certain vestibular neurons and their connections, due to a decrease in the size of the EPSPs. With continued exercise, changes in synaptic effectiveness become more permanent. In addition, structural changes, including a reduction in the number of vestibular neuron synapses connecting to interneurons, occurs. With the advent of structural changes, the decline in dizziness in response to the repeated head movement persists, allowing the patient to discontinue the exercise without reexperiencing symptoms of dizziness. It is possible that if exercises are discontinued too soon, before structural changes have occurred in the sensory connections, dizziness symptoms will recur due to the loss of habituation.

SENSITIZATION

As we mentioned in Chapter 2, sensitization is caused by a strengthening of responses to potentially injurious stimuli. Sensitization may also be short- or long-term, and it may involve the exact set of synapses that show habituation. However, the mechanisms involved in sensitization are a little more complex than those involved in habituation. One way that sensitization may occur is by prolonging the action potential through changes in potassium conductance. This allows more transmitter to be released from the terminals, giving an increased EPSP. It also appears to improve the *mobilization* of transmitter, making it more available for release (2).

Sensitization, like habituation, can be short- or long-term. Mechanisms for long-term memory of sensitization involve the same cells as short-term memory, but now reflect structural changes in these cells (3, 5). Kandel (6) has shown that in invertebrates short-term sensitization involves changes in preexisting protein structures, while long-term sensitization involves the synthesis of new protein. This synthesis of new protein at the synapse implies that long-term sensitization involves changes that are genetically influenced.

This genetic influence also encompasses the growth of new synaptic connections, as illustrated in Figure 4.2C. Animals who showed long-term sensitization were found to have twice as many synaptic terminals as untrained animals, increased dendrites in the postsynaptic cells, and an increase in numbers of active zones at synaptic terminals, from 40 to 65% (7).

In summary, the research on habituation and sensitization suggests that short-term and long-term memory may not be separate categories, but may be part of a single graded memory function. With sensitization, as with habituation, long-term and short-term memory involve changes at the same synapses. While short-term changes reflect relatively temporary changes in synaptic effectiveness, structural changes are the hallmark of long-term memory (2).

Neural Plasticity and Associative Learning

Remember that during *associative learning* a person learns to predict relationships, either relationships of one stimulus to another (*classical conditioning*), or the relationship of one's behavior to a consequence

(*operant conditioning*). Through associative learning we learn to form key relationships that help us adapt our actions to the environment.

Researchers examining the physiological basis for associative learning have found that it can take place through simple changes in synaptic efficiency without requiring complex learning networks. Associative learning, whether short-term or long-term, utilizes common cellular processes. Initially, when two neurons fire at the same time (that is, in association), there is a modification of existing proteins within these two neurons that produces a change in synaptic efficiency. Long-term association results in the synthesis of new proteins and the subsequent formation of new synaptic connections between the neurons.

CLASSICAL CONDITIONING

During classical conditioning, an initially weak stimulus (the conditioned stimulus) becomes highly effective in producing a response when it becomes associated with another stronger stimulus (the unconditioned stimulus). It is similar to, though more complex than, sensitization. In fact, it may be that classical conditioning is simply an extension of the processes involved in sensitization.

Remember that in classical conditioning, timing is critical. When conditioned and unconditioned stimuli converge on the same neurons, facilitation occurs if the conditioned stimulus causes action potentials in the neurons just before the unconditioned stimulus arrives. This is because action potentials allow Ca^+ to move into the presynaptic neuron and this Ca^+ activates special modulatory transmitters involved in classical conditioning. If the activity occurs after the unconditioned stimulus, Ca^+ is not released at the right time and the stimulus has no effect (2, 8).

OPERANT CONDITIONING

Although operant conditioning and classical conditioning may seem like two different processes, in fact, the laws that govern the two are similar, indicating that the same neural mechanisms may control them. In each type of conditioning, learning involves the development of predictive relationships. In classical conditioning, a specific stimulus predicts a specific response. In operant conditioning, we learn to predict the outcome of specific behaviors. However, the same cellular mechanisms that underlie classical conditioning are also responsible for operant conditioning.

DECLARATIVE LEARNING

Remember that associative learning can also be thought of in terms of the type of knowledge acquired. *Procedural learning* refers to learning tasks that can be performed automatically without attention or conscious thought. In contrast, *declarative learning* requires conscious processes such as awareness and attention, and results in knowledge that can be expressed consciously. Procedural learning is expressed through improved performance of the task learned, while declarative learning can be expressed in a form other than that in which it was learned.

Consistent with the two types of associative learning described, scientists believe that the circuits involved in the storage of these two types of learning are different. Procedural memory involves primarily cerebellar circuitry, while declarative memory involves temporal lobe circuitry (1).

Wilder Penfield, a neurosurgeon, was one of the first researchers to understand the important role of the temporal lobes in memory function. While performing temporal lobe surgery in patients with epilepsy, he stimulated the temporal lobes of the conscious patients, in order to determine the location of the diseased vs. normal tissue. The patients experienced memories from the past as if they were happening again. For example, one patient heard music from an event long ago, and saw the situation and felt the emotions that surrounded the singing of that music, with everything happening in real time (9).

In humans, lesions in the temporal lobe of the cortex and the hippocampus may interfere with the laying down of declarative memory. A few patients have been studied after having the hippocampus and related temporal lobe areas removed due to epilepsy. After surgery, the patients were no longer able to acquire long-term declarative memories, though they remembered old memories. Their short-term memory was normal, but if their attention was distracted from an item held in short-term memory, they forgot it completely. However, skill learning was unaffected in these patients. They would often learn a complex task but be unable to remember the procedures that made up the task or the events surrounding learning the task (10).

This work suggests that the temporal lobes and hippocampus may be important to the establishment of memory, but are not a part of the memory storage area.

The hippocampus, which is a subcortical structure, and part of the temporal lobe circuitry, is critical for declarative learning. Research has shown evidence of plastic changes in hippocampal neurons similar to those found in neural circuits of simpler animals when learning takes place.

Researchers have shown that pathways in the hippocampus show a facilitation that has been called **long-term potentiation (LTP)**, which is similar to the mechanisms causing sensitization (2, 11). For example, in one region of the hippocampus LTP occurs when a weak and an excitatory input arrive at the same region of a neuron's dendrite. The weak input will be enhanced if it is activated in association with the strong one. This process is shown in Figure 4.3. LTP appears to require the simultaneous firing of both pre- and postsynaptic cells. After this occurs, LTP is maintained through an increase in presynaptic transmitter release.

Long-term potentiation has been found in many areas of the brain, in addition to the hippocampus, and it has been shown that it is involved in *spatial memory* (2). For example, Morris et al. (12) performed an experiment in which rats swam a water maze to find a platform under the water. The water was made opaque in order to block the use of vision in finding the target. The rats were released in different parts of the maze and were required to use spatial cues related to the position of

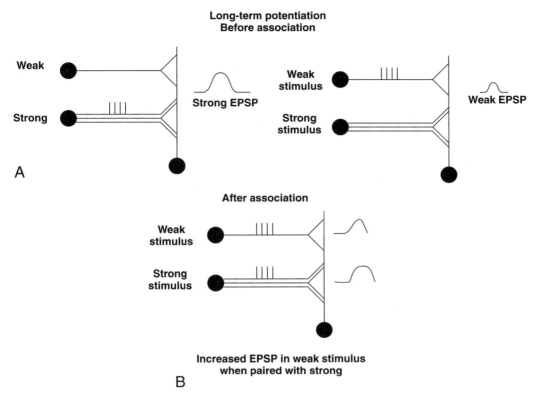

Figure 4.3. Schematic of the cellular basis for long-term potentiation. **A,** Prior to pairing with a strong stimulus, the weak stimulus produces only a weak EPSP. **B,** After association, there is an increased EPSP produced by the weak stimulus when paired with the strong. (Adapted from Kandel ER. Cellular mechanisms of learning and the biological basis of individuality. In: Kandel ER, Schwartz JH, Jessell TM, eds. Principles of neuroscience. 3rd ed. New York: Elsevier, 1991:1009–1031.)

the walls to find the target. They also performed a nonspatial task where the platform was above the water and the rat could simply use visual cues to swim to the target.

These experimenters showed that blocking special receptors in hippocampal neurons caused the rats to fail to learn the spatial version of the task. This finding suggests that certain hippocampal neurons are involved in spatial learning through LTP.

PROCEDURAL LEARNING

Procedural learning appears to involve the cerebellum.

The unique cellular circuitry of the cerebellum has been shown to be perfect for the long-term modification of motor responses. You will recall that the cerebellum has two

types of input fibers, the climbing fibers and the mossy fibers, and one type of output fiber, the Purkinje cells. Climbing fiber input to the Purkinje cells typically signals error and is important in the correction of ongoing movements. In contrast, mossy fiber input to the Purkinje cells provides kinesthetic information about ongoing movements, important in the control of those movements. Figure 4.4 reviews the relationship of these fibers.

It has been shown that the climbing fiber inputs signaling error to the Purkinje cells may increase or decrease the strength of mossy fiber synapses onto the same Purkinje cells. This produces a long-term change in Purkinje cell output, which contributes to motor learning.

Gilbert and Thach (13) examined the role of the cerebellum in motor learning dur-

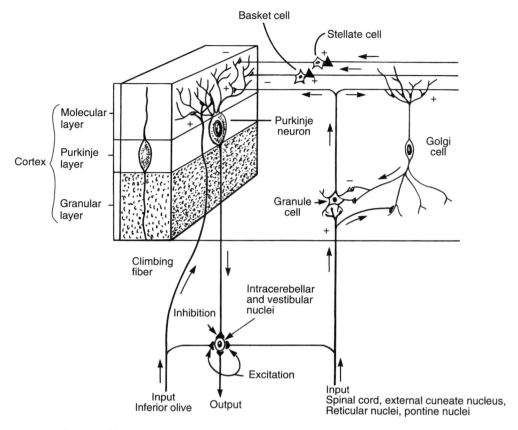

Figure 4.4.   A diagram of the cerebellum showing the relationship between mossy and climbing fiber input important to learning.

ing experiments in which monkeys were trained to return a handle to a central position whenever it was moved to the left or right. During the sessions, they recorded the activity of Purkinje neurons in the arm area of the anterior lobe of the cerebellum. Once the task was learned and repeatedly performed in the same way, the arm movement was accompanied by predictable changes occurring primarily in mossy fiber inputs reporting the kinesthetics of the movement, with an occasional climbing fiber input.

Then the experimenters modified the task, requiring the monkeys to use more force to return the handle to the original position. At first the animal wasn't able to return the handle in one simple movement. But gradually, the animal learned to respond correctly. On the first few trials of the new task, there

was a sudden increase in activity in the climbing fibers, signaling the error.

This increase in climbing fiber activity was associated with a reduction in the efficiency of the mossy fiber connections to the Purkinje cells. The reduction in Purkinje cell output then was associated with an increase in force generation, allowing the monkey to now successfully complete the task. Thus, it appears that changes in synaptic efficiency between these neurons in the cerebellum are an important link in the modification of movements through procedural learning.

This type of cerebellar learning may also occur in the vestibulo-ocular reflex circuitry, which includes cerebellar pathways. This reflex keeps the eyes fixed on an object when the head turns. In experiments in which humans wore prismatic lenses that reversed the image on the eye, the vestibulo-ocular reflex was reversed over time. This modification of the reflex did not occur with cerebellar lesions (14).

PERCEPTUAL LEARNING

Perceptual learning, or the formation of sensory memories, is actually a form of non-associative learning (1). It is a more complex form of nonassociative learning than either habituation or sensitization, so it is presented separately. How does perceptual learning actually occur? For example, when you are first introduced to a new skill, and see someone perform it, you are often able to remember the essence of the skill after only one exposure. One hypothesis is that, in the process of viewing a new scene, the brain stores a coded representation of it in our visual cortex, and that we recognize that stimulus when this visual representation is reactivated by the same scene at a later time.

Experiments on monkeys by Mishkin et al. (15) support this hypothesis and indicate that these coded representations of visual stimuli are stored in higher-order sensory association areas of the visual cortex. How does this representation get stored? When we see a unique scene, this new set of visual stimuli is coded by parallel neural circuits in the visual cortex, coding for size, color, texture, and shape of the stimulus. These circuits are in such places as Brodmann's areas, 18, 20, 21, and 37 of higher visual cortex. These parallel pathways converge on a single set of inferior temporal cortex neurons, and they, in turn, stimulate a reverberating circuit that includes neurons in a cortico-limbo-thalamo-cortico pathway (including neurons in the amygdala, hippocampus, thalamus, returning to the visual cortex). This circuit serves as a spontaneous rehearsal mechanism that serves to strengthen the connections that were part of the first activation of the circuit.

When the neurons are later reactivated, the pathway can be considered the stored representation of that scene. This visual memory will also interact with other memories that were laid down at the same time, such as sensory memories, emotional memories, spatial memories, or motor memories. Thus, the first pathway can arouse the other pathways or be aroused by them through reciprocal connections between these different parts of the cortex.

PLASTICITY AND RECOVERY OF FUNCTION

In the early part of this century, Ramon y Cajal performed experiments which suggested that growth was not possible in neurons in the adult mammalian CNS. This led to a view of the CNS as a static structure with rigid and unalterable connections (16). This view persisted until the late 1960s and 1970s, when researchers began to discover growth and reorganization of neurons in the adult CNS after injury. Much of this early work showed that cells which lost their normal input as a consequence of injury could receive new connections (17). These early studies have contributed to more current views of the CNS as a structure capable of dynamic changes in parallel pathways throughout distributed sites.

Continued research examining the reorganization of neuronal circuits following injury has shown that the CNS has amazing capacities for reorganization following injury, and that this reorganization of neuronal circuits has functional consequences (17). How much can the CNS reorganize following injury? Can postinjury reorganizational processes be manipulated to facilitate CNS reorganization? These and other questions have critical importance for basic scientists and clinicians involved in the rehabilitation of brain-injured patients.

Injury to the CNS can affect neuronal function through direct damage to the neurons themselves. In addition, disruption of neuronal function can occur as the result of indirect effects of injuries that impair cerebral blood flow, control of the cerebrospinal fluid, or cerebral metabolism. As shown in Figure 4.5, whether the trauma occurs through a direct or indirect mechanism, the effect on neuronal function can include (*a*) interrupting

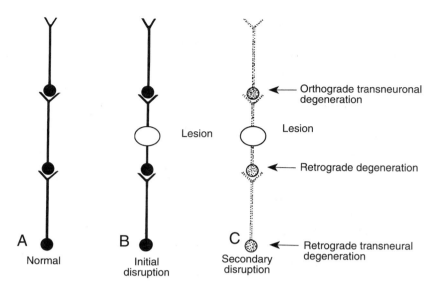

Figure 4.5. Schematic showing the secondary neuronal disruption that occurs as part of the cascade of events following neural injury. **A**, Normal neuronal function. **B**, Interruption of axonal projections from injured area. **C**, Secondary neuronal disruption.

axonal projections from areas injured (Fig. 4.5*B*); (*b*) denervation of the population of neurons innervated by the injured neurons (Fig. 4.5*C*); and (*c*) removing some neurons entirely (Fig. 4.5*C*) (17).

Aside from the loss of neurons damaged at the site of injury, the consequences of synaptic loss from these neurons produces a cascading degeneration along neuronal pathways, increasing the extent of neuronal disruption with time (17).

Cellular Responses to Injury

The following sections review some of the events occurring within the nervous system following injury. These events may contribute to and limit recovery of function.

NEURONAL SHOCK

One of the first events following nervous system injury is **neuronal shock** or *diaschisis* (18, 19). This includes the short-term loss of function in neuronal pathways at a distance from the lesion itself. Such a situation could arise with the loss of the normal neuronal activation of the intact areas. If the intact areas recover to some extent from the loss

of input from the injured area, the symptoms caused by the disruption of input will be reduced.

SYNAPTIC EFFECTIVENESS

Neurons directly affected by the lesion will show loss of synaptic effectiveness. Craik (19) notes that edema at the site of neuronal injury may lead to a compression of axons and physiological blocking of neuronal conduction. Reduction of the edema would then restore a portion of the functional loss.

This process is shown in Figure 4.6.

DENERVATION SUPERSENSITIVITY

Denervation supersensitivity can occur when neurons show a loss of input from another brain region. In this case, the postsynaptic membrane of a neuron becomes hyperactive to a released transmitter substance. For example, Parkinson's disease causes a loss of dopamine producing neurons in the substantia nigra of the basal ganglia. In response to this disease-induced denervation, their postsynaptic target neurons in the striatum become hypersensitive to the dopamine that is released by the remaining substantia nigra neurons.

SILENT SYNAPSES

Recruitment of previously silent synapses also occurs during recovery of function. This suggests that structural synapses are present in many areas of the brain that may not normally be functional due to competition within neuronal pathways. However, experiential factors or lesions may lead to their being unmasked when they are released from these previous effects.

REGENERATIVE AND REACTIVE SYNAPTOGENESIS

Regenerative synaptogenesis occurs when injured axons begin sprouting. **Reactive synaptogenesis**, called collateral sprouting, may occur when neighboring normal axons sprout to innervate synaptic sites that were previously activated by the injured axon. Examples of regenerative and reactive synaptogenesis are shown in Figure 4.7 (18, 19).

Global Aspects of Plasticity

With this understanding of some of the responses of neurons to injury, we might ask how this contributes to more global aspects of plasticity within the nervous system. For example, how modifiable are the sensory-motor maps of our brain?

Research on the development of the visual system has shown that the visual cortex is highly modifiable by experience during certain critical periods shortly after birth. Is this modifiability also possible in other sensory and motor systems, and is it possible to change these systems in the adult as well as early in the developmental process? The answers to these questions are YES!

In Chapter 3, we talked about the primary somatosensory cortex areas 1, 2, 3a, and 3b, each having a separate sensory map of the body. Research (20) has shown that these maps of the somatosensory cortex vary from

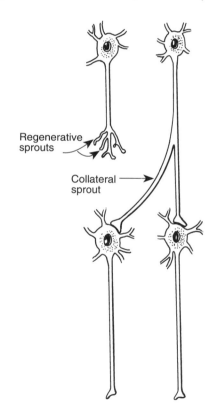

Figure 4.7. Examples of regenerative and reactive synaptogenesis in related neurons following injury. (Adapted from Held JM. Recovery of function after brain damage: theoretical implications for therapeutic intervention. In: Carr JH, Shepherd RB, Gordon F, et al., eds. Movement sciences: foundations for physical therapy in rehabilitation. Rockville, MD: Aspen Systems, 1987:155–177.)

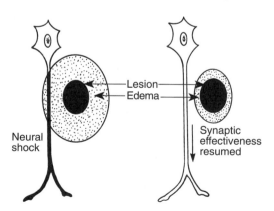

Figure 4.6. Diagram of recovery of synaptic effectiveness due to the resolution of edema, allowing nerve conduction to resume. (Adapted from Craik RL. Recovery processes: maximizing function. In: Contemporary management of motor control problems. Proceedings of the II Step Conference. Alexandria, VA: APTA, 1992:165–173.)

individual to individual according to past experience.

What have researchers learned about how these maps change during recovery of function? When the median nerve (which innervates the cutaneous regions of the monkey's hand) of the monkey is severed, one might expect that its corresponding parts of the somatosensory cortex would become silent, since there would be no input coming into them. But when experiments were performed to test the mapping of the cortex after surgery, it was found that neighboring maps had expanded their receptive fields to cover much of the denervated region. These representations increased even further in the weeks following denervation (21, 22).

Other research by Mortimer Mishkin and his colleagues (23) has shown that somatosensory cortex area II (SII) is also very plastic. These researchers removed all of the inputs for the hand representation coming into SII and noted that the area was initially unresponsive. However, within 2 months, the area was again responsive and occupied by the inputs from the foot. This reorganization involved over half of the SII representation.

Additional studies (20) have shown that the somatotopic maps in normal animals show extensive differences between individuals. But how do we know whether these differences are due to inherited genetic differences or to experience? To test for this, Merzenich and coworkers (24) performed an experiment in which monkeys were able to reach for food by using a strategy that involved use of their middle fingers only. After considerable experience with this task, the monkeys' cortical map showed an area for the middle fingers that was significantly larger than normal. This reorganization in somatosensory cortex resulting from training is shown in Figure 4.8.

It has also been shown that these changes occur at other levels of the nervous system besides the cerebral cortex. The dorsal column nuclei, which are the first synaptic juncture within the somatosensory system, also show reorganization after peripheral lesions (25).

What mechanisms contribute to the changes in receptive fields as a result of lesions

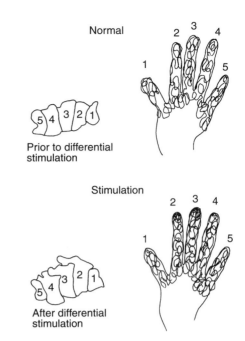

Figure 4.8. Training causes an expansion of cortical representation (Adapted from Jenkins WM, Merzenich MM, Och MT, Allard T, Guic-Robles E. Functional reorganization of primary somatosensory cortex in adult owl monkeys after behaviorally controlled tactile stimulation. J Neurophysiol 1990;63:82–104.)

or learning? The mechanisms involved appear to be very similar to those that we have previously discussed in relation to associative learning. In further experiments with monkeys, Merzenich and his colleagues connected two fingers of the monkey together, so that these fingers would always be used together in the monkey's actions (26). This means that the inputs from the two areas would always be highly correlated in the cortex. This changed the mapping of area 3b in the somatosensory cortex, eliminating the sharp boundaries between the maps of these two fingers. Thus, the normal sharp boundaries between different parts of the body within our sensory and motor maps may depend significantly on the activity of these areas.

What do these studies tell us? They suggest that we have multiple pathways innervating any given part of the sensory or motor cortex, with only the dominant pathway showing functional activity. However, when a lesion occurs in one pathway, the less dominant pathway may immediately show functional connections. This leads us to the conclusion that cortical maps are very dynamic. Even in adults there appears to be use-dependent competition among neurons for synaptic connections. So when one area becomes inactive, a neighboring area can take over its former targets and put them to functional use.

These experiments also suggest that our sensory and motor maps in the cortex are constantly changing in accordance with the amount to which they are activated by peripheral inputs. Since each one of us has been brought up in a different environment and has practiced very different types of motor skills, the maps of each of our brains are unique and constantly changing as a result of these experiences.

How can we apply this information to therapy? First, it means that whenever a patient experiences a neural lesion, the cortical maps show both (*a*) immediate reorganization, due to the unmasking of previously nonfunctional synaptic connections from neighboring areas, and (*b*) a longer-term change, where neighboring inputs to the areas take over the parts of the map that were previously occupied by damaged or destroyed cells.

Second, it tells us that experience is very important in shaping cortical maps. Thus, if we leave patients without rehabilitation training for many weeks or months, their brains will show changes in organization, reflecting disuse, which will be most detrimental to these patients. However, the good news is that training appears to make a difference no matter when it is given, since the brain continues to be plastic throughout our lives.

SUMMARY

The research on the neurophysiological basis for learning, memory, and recovery of function covered in this chapter suggests the following important principles:

1. The brain is incredibly plastic, and has great capacity to change; this includes not just the immature brain but the mature adult brain.
2. The most important way in which the environment changes behavior in humans is through learning.
3. CNS structural changes occur because of the interaction between both genetic and experiential factors.
4. A key factor in experience is the concept of *active competition*, and this may be summed up in the phrase "the squeaky wheel gets the oil," or in this case, it gets the new synaptic connections. This concept is applicable from simple circuits to complex neural pathways.
5. Research suggests that short-term and long-term memory may not be separate categories, but may be part of a single graded memory function, involving the same synapses.
6. Short-term changes reflect relatively temporary changes in synaptic effectiveness; structural changes are the hallmark of long-term memory.
7. Scientists believe that the circuits involved in the storage of procedural and declarative learning are different, with procedural memory involving cerebellar circuitry and declarative memory involving temporal lobe circuitry.

REFERENCES

1. Kupfermann I. Learning and Memory. In: Kandel ER, Schwartz JH, Jessell TM, eds. Principles of neuroscience. 3rd ed. New York: Elsevier, 1991:997–1008.
2. Kandel ER. Cellular mechanisms of learning and the biological basis of individuality. In: Kandel ER, Schwartz JH, Jessell TM, eds. Principles of neuroscience. 3rd ed, New York: Elsevier, 1991:1009–1031.
3. Kandel ER, Schwarz JH. Molecular biology of learning: modulation of transmitter release. Science 1982;218:433–443.
4. Shumway-Cook A, Horak FB. Rehabilitation strategies for patients with vestibular deficits. Neurol Clin 1990;8:441–457.
5. Sweatt JD, Kandel ER. Persistent and transcriptionally-dependent increase in protein phosphorylation in long-term facilitation of Aplysia sensory neurons. Nature 1989; 339:51–54.
6. Kandel ER. Genes, nerve cells, and the remembrance of things past. J Neuropsychiatry 1989;1:103–125.
7. Bailey CH, Chen M. Morphological basis of long-term habituation and sensitization in Aplysia. Science 1983;220:91–93.
8. Abrams TW, Kandel ER. Is contiguity detection in classical conditioning a system or a cellular property? Learning in Aplysia suggests a

possible molecular site. Trends Neurosci 1988;11:128–135.

9. Penfield W. Functional localization in temporal and deep Sylvian areas. Res Publ Assoc Res Nerv Ment Dis 1958;36:210–226.

10. Milner B. Amnesia following operation on the temporal lobes. In: Whitty CWM, Zangwill OL, eds. Amnesia. London: Butterworths, 1966:109–133.

11. Bliss TVP, Lomo T. Long-lasting potentiation of synaptic transmission in the dentate area of the anaesthetized rabbit following stimulation of the perforant path. J Physiol (Lond) 1973;232:331–356.

12. Morris RGM, Anderson E, Lynch GS, Baudry M. Selective impairment of learning and blockage of long-term potentiation by an N-methyl-D-aspartate receptor antagonist, AP5. Nature 1986;319:774–776.

13. Gilbert PFC, Thach WT. Purkinje cell activity during motor learning. Brain Res 1977;70:1–18.

14. Melville-Jones G, Mandl G. Neurobionomics of adaptive plasticity: integrating sensorimotor function with environmental demands. In: Desmedt JE, ed. Motor control mechanisms in health and disease. Adv Neurol 1983;39:1047–1071.

15. Mishkin MH, Malamut B, Bachevalier J. Memories and habits: two neural systems. In: McGaugh JL, Lynch G, Weinberger NM, eds. The neurobiology of learning and memory. New York: Guilford Press, 1984:65–77.

16. Gordon J. Assumptions underlying physical therapy intervention: theoretical and historical perspectives. In: Carr JH, Shepherd RB, Gordon F, et al., eds. Movement sciences: foundations for physical therapy in rehabilitation. Rockville, MD: Aspen Systems, 1987:1–30.

17. Steward O. Reorganization of neuronal connections following CNS trauma: principles and experimental paradigms. J Neurotrauma 1989;6:99–151.

18. Held JM. Recovery of function after brain damage: theoretical implications for therapeutic intervention. In: Carr JH, Shepherd, RB, Gordon F, et al., eds. Movement sciences: foundations for physical therapy in rehabilitation. Rockville, MD: Aspen Systems, 1987:155–177.

19. Craik RL. Recovery processes: maximizing function. In: Contemporary management of motor control problems. Proceedings of the II Step Conference. Alexandria, VA: APTA, 1992:165–173.

20. Merzenich MM. Sources of intraspecies and interspecies cortical map variability in mammals: conclusions and hypotheses. In: Cohen MJ, Strumwassser F, eds. Comparative neurology: modes of communication in the nervous system. New York: John Wiley & Sons, 1985:105–116.

21. Merzenich MM, Kaas JH, Wall J, Nelson RJ, Sur M, Felleman D. Topographic reorganization of somatosensory cortical areas 3B and 1 in adult monkeys following restricted deafferentation. Neuroscience 1983;8:33–55.

22. Merzenich MM, Kaas JH, Wall JT, Sur M, Nelson RJ, Felleman DJ. Progression of change following median nerve section in the cortical representation of the hand in areas 3b and 1 in adult owl and squirrel monkeys. Neuroscience 1983;10:639–665.

23. Pons TP, Garraghty PE, Mishkin M. Lesion-induced plasticity in the second somatosensory cortex of adult macaques. Proc Natl Acad Sci USA 1988;85:5279–5281.

24. Jenkins, WM, Merzenich MM, Och MT, Allard T, Guic-Robles E. Functional reorganization of primary somatosensory cortex in adult owl monkeys after behaviorally controlled tactile stimulation. J Neurophysiol 1990;63:82–104.

25. Wall PD, Egger MD. Formation of new connections in adult rat brains after partial deafferentation. Nature 1971;232:542–545.

26. Clark SA, Allard T, Jenkins WM, Merzenich MM. Receptive fields in the body-surface map in adult cortex defined by temporally correlated inputs. Nature 1988;332:444–445.

Chapter 5

A CONCEPTUAL FRAMEWORK FOR CLINICAL PRACTICE

INTRODUCTION

Clinicians responsible for retraining movement in the patient with neurological impairments are faced with an overwhelming number of decisions. What is the most appropriate way to assess my patient? How much time should be spent on documenting functional ability versus evaluating underlying problems leading to dysfunction? What criteria should I use in deciding what the priority problems are? How do I establish goals that are realistic and meaningful? What should be treated? What is the best approach to treatment and the most effective way to structure my therapy sessions? What are the most ap-

propriate outcomes for evaluating the effects of my treatment?

These questions reflect the critical need for a conceptual framework for clinical practice. A **conceptual framework** is a logical structure that helps the clinician organize clinical practices related to assessment and treatment into a cohesive and comprehensive plan. It provides the clinician with guidelines for how to proceed through the clinical intervention process.

Clinical practices related to retraining the patient with motor control problems are changing in response to a number of factors, including new views on the physiological basis of motor control. As new models of motor

99

control evolve, clinical practices are modified to reflect current concepts in how the brain controls movement. Thus, a conceptual framework for structuring clinical practice is dynamic, changing in response to new scientific theories about motor control.

The purpose of this chapter is threefold: (*a*) to consider elements that contribute to a comprehensive conceptual framework for clinical practice; (*b*) to discuss the changing face of clinical practice and its relationship to underlying theories of motor control; and (*c*) to describe a conceptual framework for retraining the patient with movement disorders, which we call a task-oriented approach. A task-oriented approach is used in later chapters as the framework for retraining posture, mobility, and upper extremity control in the patient with a neurological deficit (1).

CONCEPTUAL FRAMEWORK FOR CLINICAL INTERVENTION

Again, a conceptual framework for clinical practice provides a structure for clinical intervention. It guides the clinician through the intervention process, unifying clinical practices related to assessment and treatment. We propose that there are four key concepts or elements that contribute to a comprehensive conceptual framework for clinical practice. These include:

1. The **clinical decision-making process**, which is a procedure for gathering information essential to developing a plan of care consistent with the problems and needs of the patient;
2. A **hypothesis-oriented clinical practice**, which provides the means to systematically test assumptions about the nature and cause of motor control problems;
3. A **model of disablement**, which imposes an order on the effects of disease and enables the clinician to develop a hierarchical list of problems towards which treatment can be directed; and
4. A **theory of motor control** from which

assumptions about the cause and nature of normal and abnormal movement are derived.

These assumptions guide the clinician in making decisions about key elements to assess and treat when retraining the patient with a movement disorder.

The following sections describe each of these important components in detail.

Clinical Decision-Making Process

Mrs. Claire Stern has been referred for therapy with a history of recurrent falls. She is 72 years old, and lives alone in an assisted living retirement center. She walks with a cane, and while she used to be fairly active, walking a half-mile every day with her neighbor, since her last two falls, she is reluctant to leave her apartment. She is becoming less and less active, is having increasing difficulty in getting around her retirement home, and is referred for therapy. She is referred for balance and mobility retraining, to reduce the likelihood of falling again.

Mr. George Johnson is a 68-year-old man who was diagnosed with Parkinson's disease approximately 15 years ago. He lives in his own home with his wife, who is in relatively good health. He is spending more and more time sitting, and his balance and walking have become increasingly worse as has his ability to assist in his own transfers. His wife is finding it increasingly difficult to assist him during transfers. They are referred for therapy to try to improve Mr. Johnson's mobility skills, in particular, to improve his independence in transfer abilities.

Sam Churchill is an 18-year-old with a recent history of a motor vehicle accident in which he suffered a closed head injury. Primary pathology was to the cerebellum. In addition, Sam has significant cognitive impairments, including attention and memory problems. He is unable to stand and walk independently due to severe ataxia, and is dependent in most of his activities of daily living (ADL) due to dysmetria and dyscoordination. He spent 4 weeks in coma, but with the return of consciousness has been admitted to the unit to begin rehabilitation.

Sara is a 3-year-old child who was born with cerebral palsy, and has moderate spastic hemiplegia. She has been in an early intervention program since she was 4 months old. She has recently moved into a new area, and is referred for a continuation of her therapy to improve posture, mobility, and upper extremity skills.

This diverse group of patients is typical of those referred for retraining motor control problems affecting their ability to move and carry out activities of daily life. Can the same approach used to assess motor control in an elderly man with Parkinson's disease be appropriate for an 18-year-old head-injured patient? Can the same approach to retraining posture and mobility problems in a 72-year-old elderly faller be used to habilitate mobility in a 3-year-old child with cerebral palsy?

As you will see, the answer to these questions is yes. Despite the diversity of these patients, the clinical decision-making process used to gather information and design an intervention program is similar for all patients. While each patient's motor control problems and therapeutic solutions may be different, the process used to identify problems and establish a plan of care will be consistent across patients.

Clinical decision making is the process of gathering information essential to developing a plan of care consistent with the problems and needs of the patient (2, 3). The clinical decision-making process involves (*a*) assessment of the patient, (*b*) analysis and interpretation of the assessment data, (*c*) development of short- and long-term goals, (*d*) development of an appropriate treatment plan to achieve these goals, (*e*) carrying out the treatment plan, and (*f*) reassessment of the patient and treatment outcome.

The purpose of clinical decision making is to establish a scientifically sound and cost-effective plan of care geared to the problems and needs of each individual patient. The first step in establishing a plan of care is assessment. A good definition of **assessment** is the systematic acquisition of information that is relevant and meaningful in providing the clinician with a comprehensive picture of the patient's abilities and problems. Planning an effective treatment program requires that the clinician identify the patient's functional problems, and determine the underlying cause(s).

The process of identifying problems and their underlying cause(s) is not always easy. Most CNS pathology affects multiple systems, resulting in a diverse set of impairments. This means that functional problems in the patient with a neurological deficit are often associated with many possible causes. How does a therapist establish a link between impairment and functional disability? Which impairments are critical to loss of function? Which impairments should be treated and in what order? What is the most efficacious approach to treatment? Hypothesis-driven clinical practice can assist the clinician in answering some of these questions (4).

Hypothesis-Oriented Clinical Practice

What is a hypothesis and how do we use it in the clinic? A **hypothesis** can be defined as a proposal to explain certain facts. In clinical practice, it can be considered one possible explanation about the cause or causes of a patient's problem (4, 5). To a great extent, the hypotheses generated reflect the theories a clinician has about the cause and nature of function and dysfunction in patients with neurological disease (6). As noted in Chapter 1, there are many theories of motor control that present varying views on the nature and cause of movement. As a result, there can be many different hypotheses about the underlying cause(s) of motor control problems in the patient with neurological dysfunction.

Clarifying functional movement problems requires the clinician to (*a*) generate several alternative hypotheses about the potential cause(s); (*b*) determine the crucial test(s) and their expected outcomes, which would rule out one or more of the hypotheses; (*c*) carry out the tests; and (*d*) continue the process of generating and testing hypotheses, refining one's understanding of the cause(s) of the problem (5).

The generation and testing of hypoth-

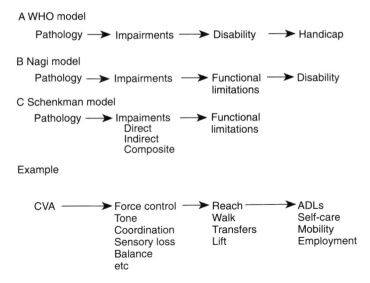

A WHO model

Pathology → Impairments → Disability → Handicap

B Nagi model

Pathology → Impairments → Functional → Disability
limitations

C Schenkman model

Pathology → Impaiments → Functional
Direct   limitations
Indirect
Composite

Example

CVA → Force control → Reach → ADLs
Tone   Walk   Self-care
Coordination   Transfers   Mobility
Sensory loss   Lift   Employment
Balance
etc

Figure 5.1. Models of disablement. Illustrated are three models of disablement. **A,** The WHO. **B,** The Nagi. **C,** The Schenkman. The effects of a cerebral vascular accident (CVA) at the various levels are also described.

eses are an important part of clinical practice. However, there is a difference between hypothesis testing in a research laboratory versus in a clinic. In the laboratory, it is often possible to set up a carefully controlled experiment that will test the hypotheses. The outcome is a *clean result*, that is, a result that accepts one hypothesis and rejects the alternative hypothesis. In contrast, in the clinic, we are often unable to get a clean result. Clinical tests are often not sensitive and specific enough to clearly differentiate between two hypotheses. Rather, they indicate the likelihood for the origin of the problem. Despite the limitations of clinical tests, the generation, testing, and revision of alternative hypotheses are important in the clinical decision-making process.

Models of Disablement

While the clinical decision making-process suggests how to proceed, it does not shed light on what to assess. A different approach is needed to answer the questions: What shall I assess? Toward what goals should I direct my treatment? In what order should problems be tackled? A model of disablement suggests a framework for structuring the effects of disease on the individual. It suggests a hierar-

chical system for categorizing patient problems and can be used as a framework for organizing and interpreting assessment data, and developing a comprehensive plan for treatment (7). Three models are reviewed in this chapter.

WORLD HEALTH ORGANIZATION MODEL

The International Classification of Impairments, Disabilities and Handicaps is a model of disablement developed by the World Health Organization (WHO) (8). The WHO model categorizes problems according to four levels of analysis: pathology, impairment, disability, and handicap. This model is shown in Figure 5.1*A*.

The first level, the *pathology* level of analysis, represents a description of the disease or injury process at the organ level. The second level, *impairment*, includes psychological, physiological, or anatomical problems related to structure or function, such as decreased strength or range of motion (ROM), or the presence of spastic hemiplegia. The third level, *disability*, represents a disturbance in task-oriented or functional behaviors, such as walking, climbing, transferring, lifting, reaching, or maintaining a posture. Finally, the fourth level, *handicap*, is defined with respect to the society and family network of the patient. Categories of handicap include physical dependence and mobility, occupation, social integration, and economic self-sufficiency. The degree of handicap is not usually established by one professional, but rather through the comprehensive assessment of the patient by a team of professionals.

NAGI MODEL

The Nagi model, shown in Figure 5.1*B*, also contains four levels of dysfunction (9–11). The first two levels, *pathology* and *impairment*, are consistent with the WHO terminology. The remaining two levels are conceptually similar to the WHO model, but the terminology is different. In the Nagi model, the next level of dysfunction following impairment is *functional limitation* (comparable to the *disability* level in the WHO model). Functional limitations describe a patient's problems with reference to functional tasks. At the top of the disablement hierarchy is the disability level of dysfunction, which reflects the inability of the individuals to carry out their roles in society. This is roughly equivalent to the handicapped level in the WHO model. Many clinicians prefer the Nagi model because of the growing pressure in society to discontinue the use of the term "handicapped" (10).

SCHENKMAN MODEL

Margaret Schenkman, a physical therapist, has also suggested a model of disablement to be used as the basis for a multisystem evaluation and treatment of individuals with neurological impairments (12). Her model, shown in Figure 5.1*C*, is composed of three levels: pathophysiology, impairments, and disabilities. Similar to the previous models, impairments refer to abnormalities within specific organs and systems which constrain a patient's ability to function normally, for example, spasticity, weakness, or loss of joint mobility. Disability refers to functional restrictions, for example, problems with gait, bed mobility, or transfers.

Schenkman further divides impairments into those that are the direct effect of pathophysiology, those that result indirectly from pathology, and those that are the composite effects of both direct and indirect impairments. It is important to differentiate between direct, or primary, impairments and indirect, or secondary, impairments. Secondary impairments develop as a result of the primary impairments, not the pathology itself. For example, in the patient with UMN disease, musculoskeletal contractures can develop secondary to weakness and immobility (primary impairments). However, secondary impairments can often be prevented with appropriate treatment.

CLINICAL IMPLICATIONS

How do models of disablement assist the clinician in formulating a clinical plan for intervention? Figure 5.1*D* illustrates how these three models would potentially describe the effects of a cerebral vascular accident (CVA) at the various levels. Clinicians are primarily involved in identifying and documenting the effects of pathology at both the impairment and disability levels (10, 12). During assessment, clinicians identify and document limitations in the patient's functional capacity, for example, the ability to walk, transfer, reach for, and manipulate objects. In addition, clinicians determine and document the sensory, motor, and cognitive impairments that constrain functional abilities. These impairments can be the direct result of a neurological lesion, for example, weakness, or the indirect effect of another impairment, such as contractures in the weak and immobile patient.

Theories of Motor Control

The fourth element that contributes to a comprehensive conceptual framework for clinical practice is a theory of motor control. Theories of motor control have led to the development of clinical practices, which then apply assumptions from these theories to improving the control of movement. Thus, the approach a clinician chooses when assessing and treating a patient with movement disorders is based in part on both implicit and explicit assumptions associated with an underlying theory of motor control (1, 13–15).

PARALLEL DEVELOPMENT OF CLINICAL PRACTICE AND SCIENTIFIC THEORY

Much has been written recently about the influence of changing scientific theories on the treatment of patients with movement disorders. Several excellent articles discuss in detail the parallel development between scientific theory and clinical practice (1, 13–15).

Neuroscience researchers identify the scientific basis for movement and movement disorders, but it is up to the clinician to develop the applications of this research (13). Thus, scientific theory provides a framework that allows the integration of practical ideas into a coherent treatment philosophy. As we mentioned in Chapter 1, a theory is not right or wrong in an absolute sense, but judged to be more or less useful in solving the problems presented by patients with movement dysfunction (1, 13).

Just as scientific assumptions about the important elements that control movement are changing, so too, clinical practices related to the assessment and treatment of the patient with a neurological deficit are changing. New assumptions regarding the nature and cause of movement are replacing old assumptions. Clinical practice evolves in parallel with scientific theory, as clinicians assimilate changes in scientific theory and apply them to practice. Let's explore the evolution of clinical practice in light of changing theories of motor control in more detail.

NEUROLOGICAL REHABILITATION: REFLEX-BASED NEUROFACILITATION APPROACHES

In the late 1950s and early 1960s, the so-called neurofacilitation approaches were

developed, resulting in a dramatic change in clinical treatment of the patient with neurological impairments (1, 13). For the most part, these approaches still dominate the way clinicians assess and treat the patient with neurological deficits.

Neurofacilitation approaches include the Bobath Approach, developed by Karl and Berta Bobath (16–18), the Rood Approach, developed by Margaret Rood (19–20), Brunnstrom's approach, developed by Signe Brunnstrom (21), Proprioceptive Neuromuscular Facilitation (PNF), developed by Kabat and Knott and expanded by Voss (22), and Sensory Integration Therapy, developed by Jean Ayres (23–25). These approaches were based largely on assumptions drawn from both the reflex and hierarchical theories of motor control (1, 13, 15).

Prior to the development of the neurofacilitation approaches, therapy for the patient with neurological dysfunction was largely directed at changing function at the level of the muscle itself. This has been referred to as a *muscle re-education* approach to treatment (1, 13). While the muscle re-education approach was effective in treating movement disorders resulting from polio, it had less impact on altering movement patterns in patients with upper motor neuron lesions. Thus, the neurofacilitation techniques were developed in response to clinicians' dissatisfaction with previous modes of treatment, and a desire to develop approaches that were more effective in solving the movement problems of the patient with neurological dysfunction (13).

Clinicians working with patients with UMN lesions began to direct clinical efforts towards modifying the CNS itself (13). Neurofacilitation approaches focused on retraining motor control through techniques designed to facilitate and/or inhibit different movement patterns. Facilitation refers to treatment techniques that increase the patient's ability to move in ways judged to be appropriate by the clinician. Inhibitory techniques decrease the patient's use of movement patterns considered abnormal.

Underlying Assumptions

NORMAL MOTOR CONTROL

Neurofacilitation approaches are largely associated with both the reflex and hierarchical theories of motor control (1, 13, 15). Thus, clinical practices have been developed based on assumptions regarding the nature and cause of normal motor control, abnormal motor control, and the recovery of function (1, 13; see also Chapter 1 of this text).

For example, it is assumed that reflexes are the basis for motor control. This approach suggest that normal movement probably results from a chaining of reflexes that are organized hierarchically within the CNS. Thus, control of movement is *top-down*. Normal movement requires that the highest level of the CNS, the cortex, be in control of both intermediate (brainstem) and lower (spinal cord) levels of the CNS. This means that the process of normal development, sometimes called corticalization, is characterized by the emergence of behaviors organized at sequentially higher and higher levels in the CNS. A great emphasis is placed on the understanding that incoming sensory information stimulates, and thus drives, a normal movement pattern (1).

ABNORMAL MOTOR CONTROL

Explanations regarding the physiological basis for abnormal motor control from a reflex and hierarchical perspective largely suggest that a disruption of normal reflex mechanisms underlies abnormal movement control. It is assumed that lesions at the highest cortical levels of the CNS cause release of abnormal reflexes organized at lower levels within the CNS. The release of these lower level reflexes constrains the patient's ability to move normally. Another prevalent assumption is that abnormal or atypical patterns of movement seen in the patient with UMN lesions are the direct result of the lesion itself, as opposed to considering some behaviors as developing either secondary to the lesion or in response to the lesion, that is, compensa-

tory to the lesion (13). Thus, it is predicted that in the child with UMN lesions the process of increasing corticalization is disrupted, and as a result, motor control is dominated by primitive patterns of movement organized at lower levels of the CNS. In addition, in the adult with acquired UMN lesions, damage to higher levels of the CNS probably results in a release of lower centers from higher center control. Likewise, primitive and pathological behaviors organized at these levels re-emerge to dominate, preventing normal patterns of movement from occurring (1, 14, 15).

RECOVERY OF FUNCTION AND REACQUISITION OF SKILL

A central assumption concerning the recovery of function in the patient with a UMN lesion is that recovery of normal motor control cannot occur unless higher centers of the CNS once again regain control over lower centers. According to this approach, recovery of function in a sense recapitulates development, with higher centers gradually regaining their dominance over lower centers of the CNS.

Two key assumptions are that (*a*) functional skills will automatically return once abnormal movement patterns are inhibited and normal movement patterns facilitated; and (*b*) repetition of these normal movement patterns will automatically transfer to functional tasks.

Clinical Implications

What are some of the clinical implications of these assumptions? First, assessment of motor control should focus on identifying the presence or absence of normal and abnormal reflexes controlling movement. Also, treatment should be directed at modifying the reflexes that control movement. The importance of sensory input for stimulating normal motor output suggests a treatment focus of modifying the CNS through sensory stimulation (1, 13). A hierarchical theory suggests that one goal of therapy is to regain independent control of movement by higher centers of the CNS. Thus, treatment is geared towards helping the patient regain normal patterns of movement as a way of facilitating functional recovery.

Limitations

More recently, questions have been raised about the assumptions related to neurofacilitation models (13–15). Dissatisfaction with neurofacilitation approaches is reflected in a growing number of questions regarding their underlying assumptions, including: Can inhibition of abnormal reflexes alone produce more normal patterns of movement? Will this carry over to improved function? Are the atypical movement patterns seen in patients with neurological impairments the result of the abnormal CNS, or compensatory to the problem? Is it appropriate to train a patient to use a particular pattern of movement when the hallmark of normal function is variability of movement strategies?

Changing Practices

The neurofacilitation approaches still dominate the way clinicians assess and treat the patient with UMN lesions. However, just as scientific theory about the nature and cause of movement has changed in the past 30 years, so too, many of the neurofacilitation approaches have changed their approach to practice. Currently, within the neurofacilitation approaches, there is a greater emphasis on explicitly training function, and less emphasis on inhibiting reflexes and retraining normal patterns of movement. In addition, there is more consideration of motor learning principles when developing treatment plans. The boundaries between approaches are less distinct as each approach integrates new concepts related to motor control into its theoretical base.

Systems-Based Task-Oriented Approach

One of the newer approaches to retraining is the task-oriented approach to clinical intervention, which is based on a systems theory of motor control. As we mentioned in Chapter 1, a task-oriented approach to retraining is a term used to describe a newer neurological rehabilitation approach that is evolving in parallel with new theories of motor control (1). Others have referred to these new clinical methods as a *motor control approach* (13). In the past, we have referred to this new clinical approach as a *systems approach* (14–15, 26). However, it has recently been suggested that separate names be given to each to distinguish between clinical treatment approaches and their theoretical bases (1).

Underlying Assumptions

NORMAL CONTROL OF MOVEMENT

Some underlying assumptions that guide a task-oriented approach to retraining follow. First, normal movement emerges as an interaction among many different systems, each contributing different aspects of control. In addition, movement is organized around a behavioral goal; thus, multiple systems are organized according to the inherent requirements of the task being performed. These assumptions suggest that when retraining movement control, it is essential to work on identifiable functional tasks, rather than on movement patterns for movement's sake alone.

Another key assumption in this approach is the recognition that organization of the various elements contributing to movement is also determined by various aspects of the environment. This means that strategies for moving and sensing emerge from an interaction of the individual with the environment to accomplish a functional task. Thus, both functional goals and environmental constraints play an essential role in determining movement.

Finally, the role of sensation in normal movement is not limited to a stimulus-response reflex mode. Instead, sensation is hypothesized to contribute to predictive and adaptive control of movement as well.

ABNORMAL MOTOR CONTROL

From a systems perspective, abnormal motor control results from impairments within one or more of the systems controlling movement. In addition, movements observed in the patient with a UMN lesion represent behavior that emerges from the best mix of the systems remaining to participate. This means that what is observed is not just the result of the lesion itself, but the efforts of the remaining systems to compensate for the loss and still be functional. However, the compensatory strategies developed by patients are not always optimal. Thus, a goal in treatment may be to improve the efficiency of compensatory strategies used to perform functional tasks.

RECOVERY OF FUNCTION AND THE REACQUISITION OF SKILL

A systems perspective suggests that patients learn by actively attempting to solve the problems inherent to a functional task, rather than repetitively practicing normal patterns of movement. Adaptation to changes in the environmental context is a critical part of recovery of function. In this context, patients are helped to learn a variety of ways to solve the task goal rather than a single muscle activation pattern.

TASK-ORIENTED CONCEPTUAL FRAMEWORK FOR CLINICAL INTERVENTION

In the beginning of this chapter, we discussed the importance of a comprehensive conceptual framework for guiding clinical practice. We suggested there were four key elements in a comprehensive conceptual framework including: the clinical decision-making process, hypothesis-oriented practice, models of disablement, and a theory of motor control. We have just discussed the assumptions underlying a task-oriented approach to retraining, based on a systems theory of motor control. We now incorporate our task-ori-

ented approach into a complete conceptual framework which includes these other elements.

Using the clinical decision-making process, we can identify the steps to follow during the course of clinical intervention, including assessment, identification of problems and goals, and the establishment of a treatment plan to achieve those goals. The two levels of analysis from Schenkman's model help us to identify problems that are commonly assessed and treated by physical and occupational therapists: impairments and functional disability. In addition, we add a third level of analysis that focuses on identifying the strategies patients use to perform functional tasks despite their impairments. This represents an intermediate level of analysis, between functional disability and underlying impairments.

Finally, we draw on a systems theory of motor control to generate hypotheses about the potential causes of functional movement disorders and their treatment. We will continue to refer to this framework as a task-oriented approach. The remaining section of this book discusses in more detail the essential elements of assessment and treatment based on a task-oriented approach. In later chapters, we will show the specific application of this approach to retraining posture, mobility, and uppper extremity function in the patient with neurological dysfunction.

Assessment

We begin with assessment, the first step in the clinical decision-making process. A task-oriented assessment evaluates motor behavior at three levels: (*a*) objective measurement of functional skills, (*b*) a description of the strategies used to accomplish functional skills, and (*c*) quantification of the underlying sensory, motor, and cognitive impairments that constrain performance (27–29).

Since there is no single test that allows one to collect information at all levels, clinicians are required to assemble a battery of tests, enabling them to document problems at all three levels of analysis. This concept is illustrated in Figure 5.2, which examines the

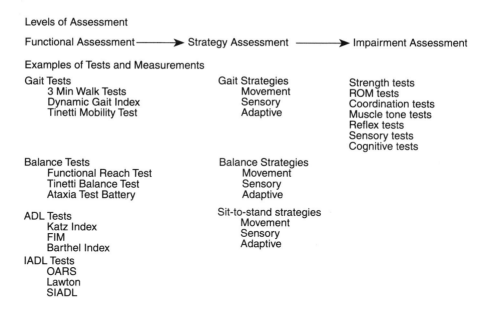

Figure 5.2.   A conceptualization of the relationship between the three levels of testing within a task-oriented model, and the types of tests a clinician could choose from within each of these levels.

three levels of testing within a task-oriented model, and the types of tests a clinician could choose from within each of these levels. The figure is not intended to present a comprehensive list of all tests and measurements available within each level, but presents the concept itself.

PERFORMANCE-BASED FUNCTIONAL ASSESSMENT

Assessment tools that focus on measuring the first level of performance, functional abilities, are called **performance-based functional measures**. These tests allow the clinician to document a patient's level of independence in carrying out daily life activities and are an important part of justifying ongoing therapy to the patient, the patient's family, and third-party insurers.

There are a number of different approaches to assessing functional behavior. For example, standardized assessment tools have been developed to test Activities of Daily Living (ADL), or Instrumental Activities of Daily Living (IADL). ADL scales test the patients' ability to care for themselves including: bathing, dressing, toileting, feeding, mobility, and continence. Examples of ADL scales include

the Katz Index (30); Functional Independence Measure (FIM) (31); and the Barthel Index (32).

IADL scales assess activities in which the person interacts with the environment, including: telephone usage, traveling, shopping, preparing meals, housework, and finances. An example is the Scale for Instrumental Activities of Daily Living (IADL) (33).

Some assessment scales limit their focus to specific tasks such as balance, mobility, or upper extremity control. Examples of these types of assessment tools include: the Tinetti Test of Balance and Mobility (34), the Ataxia Test Battery (35), or the Erhardt Test of Manipulatory Skills (36). These tests have been developed to provide clinicians with a clearer picture of the patient's functional skills related to a limited set of tasks the clinician will be directly involved in retraining. These task-specific tests will be covered in later chapters, which discuss retraining posture, mobility, and upper extremity functions.

A number of assessment tools have been developed to assess functional limitations and underlying impairments in specific patient populations. The most prevalent of this type of tool relates to assessing function following stroke. Examples of these include the Motor Assessment Scale for Stroke Patients (37), the Fugl-Meyer Test (38), or the Motor Assessment in Hemiplegia by Signe Brunnstrom (39). Several scales have been developed to evaluate the severity of symptoms associated with Parkinson's disease, including the Unified Rating Scale for Parkinsonism (40) and the Schwab Classification of Parkinson Progression (41).

A General Taxonomy of Movement Tasks

Ann Gentile, a motor control scientist from Columbia University in New York, has proposed a comprehensive approach to categorizing functional movement tasks (corresponding to a level 1 analysis) based on the goals of the task and the environmental context in which the action takes place (29, 42). She points out that different tasks have inherently different requirements with respect to the environment and thus make different demands on sensory, motor, and cognitive processes. These requirements can be used to classify tasks into a hierarchy according to the demands of the task.

How does a classification of functional movement tasks help in the assessment and treatment of movement disorders in the pa-

tient with a neurological disorder? The classification of functional movement tasks into distinct categories provides an inherent order or structure to tasks that involve the performer, the task, and the environment.

Gentile's classification of movement tasks, shown in Table 5.1, represents a hierarchy of tasks that could form the basis for an assessment profile, as well as a progression for retraining motor control in the patient with a neurological disorder. Tasks that have minimal variation and relatively fixed environmental features are considered simple closed tasks. Closed tasks require fixed and habitual patterns of movement, and therefore have fairly limited information processing and attentional demands. In contrast, open tasks vary greatly from trial to trial, have changing environmental features, and as a result, have large information processing and attentional demands. Movements used to perform open tasks are constantly changing, adapting to changing task and environmental demands.

One limitation of Gentile's classification scheme of movement tasks is that, while it represents an interesting theoretical framework for assessing and retraining motor control, a formal application of this framework to retraining the patient with movement disorders has not yet been proposed.

Table 5.1. Gentile's Taxonomy of Movement Tasks[a]

| Environmental Context | Body Stability | | Body Transport | |
	No Manipulation	Manipulation	No Manipulation	Manipulation
Stationary No intertrial variability	Closed Body stability	Closed Body stability plus manipulation	Closed Body transport	Closed Body transport plus manipulation
Stationary Intertrial variability	Variable Motionless Body stability	Variable Motionless Body stability plus manipulation	Variable Motionless Body stability	Variable Motionless Body stability plus manipulation
Motion No intertrial variability	Consistent Motion Body stability	Consistent Motion Body stability plus manipulation	Consistent Motion Body transport	Consistent Motion Body transport plus manipulation
Intertrial variability	Open Body stability	Open Body stability plus manipulation	Open Body transport	Open Body transport plus manipulation

[a]From Gentile A. Skill acquisition: action, movement, and neuromotor processes. In: Carr J, Shepherd R, Gordon J, et al., eds. Movement science: foundations for physical therapy in rehabilitation. Rockville, MD: Aspen Systems, 1987:115.

Limitations of Functional Tests

There are a number of limitations inherent in functional performance-based testing. Performance-based measures will not necessarily provide information as to *why* the patient is dependent in performing functional skills. As a result, functional tests will not allow the therapist to test hypotheses about the cause of motor dysfunction. Therefore, performance-based functional tests will not tell the clinician what to treat, since treatment strategies are often directed at underlying sensorimotor impairments constraining function.

Performance-based measures assess performance quantitatively rather than qualitatively. That is, they evaluate the degree to which a patient can carry out a task, but not *how* they perform the task. To understand how a patient is performing a task, we need to focus on a strategy level of analysis. Another limitation of functional performance-based tests is that they examine performance in one instant in time, under a fairly limited set of circumstances. Results from a functional-based assessment do not always predict performance in less than ideal situations. For example, because a patient can walk safely and independently with a cane in the clinic does not necessarily mean the patient can (or will) walk safely and independently in a cluttered, poorly lit home environment.

STRATEGY ASSESSMENT

The second level of assessment of motor control examines the strategies used to accomplish functional tasks. The term **strategy** is not limited to the evaluation of the movement pattern used to accomplish a task, but includes how the person organizes sensory and perceptual information necessary to performing a task and how this changes under various conditions.

Why is it important for clinicians to examine the strategies a patient uses when performing a functional task? One answer is that the strategies used to perform a task largely determine the level of performance. According to Welford (43), a psychologist from England, performance depends on four different factors. The first relates to the demands of the task and the person's desire for particular standards of achievement. The second relates to the capacities, both mental and physical, that a person brings to the task. The third is the strategies that the person uses to meet the demands of the task, while the fourth is the ability to choose the most efficient strategy for a given task.

Note that two of the four factors relate to strategies, emphasizing their importance in determining our level of performance. Thus, the strategies we use relate the demands of the task to our capacity to perform the task. If we choose poor strategies, and the task is difficult, we may reach the limits of our capacities well before we have met the demands of the task. In contrast, inefficient strategies may still be effective in carrying out simple, less demanding tasks. As capacity to perform a task declines either because of age or disease, we may be unable to meet the demands of a task, unless we use alternative strategies to maintain performance.

For example, as a young adult you rise quickly out of a chair without the need to use your arms. You rely on the ability to generate momentum using movements of your trunk to rise from the sitting position. As you age, strength may slowly decline without affecting your ability to use this strategy for getting up. But at some threshold, the loss of strength no longer allows you to get up using your once effective momentum strategy. Instead, you begin to use your arms to get up, thereby maintaining the functional ability to rise from a chair, albeit with a new strategy.

Thus, in the individual with a neurological deficit, maintaining functional performance depends on the capacity of the individual to meet the demands of the task in a particular environment. When impairments limit the capacity to use well-learned strategies, the patient must learn new ways to accomplish functional tasks despite these limitations.

Limitations

Clinicians are hampered in their ability to assess sensory, motor, and cognitive strategies used to perform daily tasks because assessment tools to evaluate these strategies are just being developed. There is only limited information defining sensory, motor, and cognitive strategies in neurologically intact subjects. In addition, we know very little about how compensatory strategies develop as a result of neurological impairments.

Researchers have begun to quantify movement strategies used in functional tasks such as gait, stance postural control, and other mobility skills such as moving from sit to stand, supine to prone, and supine to stance. Clinical tools to assess movement strategies have grown out of these analyses. An example is the use of observational gait analysis to define the movement strategies used during ambulation.

IMPAIRMENT ASSESSMENT

Finally, the third level of assessment focuses on identifying the impairmentsthat potentially constrain functional movement skills. This requires an evaluation of the sensory, motor, and cognitive systems contributing to movement control. Assessment of the motor system includes an evaluation of both the neuromuscular and musculoskeletal systems. Since perception is essential to action, assessment of motor control requires the assessment of sensory and perceptual abilities in the control of movement. Since task-specific movement is performed within the context of intent and motivation, cognitive aspects of motor control including mental status, attention, motivation, and emotional considerations must be assessed.

Impairments that affect motor control can be either direct or indirect effects of the neural lesion (12). In addition, as first described by Hughlings Jackson, upper motor neuron disease (UMN) can result in both positive and negative signs or impairments (44). Positive signs refer to the emergence of behaviors that are not normally present and constrain motor function. Examples of positive signs include the presence of increased muscle tone, or involuntary movements such as tremors. Negative signs refer to the absence of behaviors normally present. An example of negative signs associated with UMN disease would be weakness, or sensory loss.

INTEGRATING HYPOTHESIS TESTING INTO ASSESSMENT

Earlier, we described the importance of hypothesis testing in clarifying the cause(s) of functional movement problems. We suggested it required the clinician to generate and test several alternative hypotheses about the potential cause(s), and continue this process until a clear understanding of the cause(s) of the problem emerge (5).

For example, a patient with hemiplegia is referred for balance retraining because of recurrent falls. During the course of your evaluation, you observe that when standing, the patient tends to fall primarily in the backward direction. Your knowledge of normal postural control suggests the importance of the ankle muscles during the recovery of stance balance. You generate three hypotheses that could explain why the patient is falling backwards: (*a*) weak anterior tibialis muscle, (*b*) shortened gastrocnemius, (*c*) a problem coordinating the anterior tibialis muscle within a postural response synergy. What clinical tests can be used to distinguish among these hypotheses? Strength testing indicates the patient is weak but able to voluntarily generate force, thus weakening support for the first hypothesis. Range of motion tests suggest normal passive range of motion at the ankle, weakening support for the second hypothesis. In response to the Nudge Test (a brief displacement in the backwards direction), the patient does not dorsiflex the foot of the hemiplegic leg. The inability to dorsiflex the foot, even though the capacity to generate force voluntarily is present, suggests support for the third hypothesis. If it were available, surface electromyography could be used to investigate further whether the anterior tibialis is activated as part of a postural synergy responding to backwards instability.

How much confidence can we have that our clinical tests have given us a *clean result*, that is a result that clearly supports one hypothesis and rejects the others? A clean result depends on clinical tests that are valid ways to differentiate between underlying problems. Sometimes this is not the case. For example, in the case presented above, passive range of motion tests may not be a valid way of predicting the active range of a muscle during dynamic activities. In addition, manual muscle testing may not be a valid way to test strength in the patient with upper motor neuron disease.

Despite the limitations of clinical tests, the generation, testing, and revision of alternative hypotheses is an important part of the clinical decision-making process. Hypothesis generation assists the clinician in determining the relationship between functional limitations and underlying impairments. We treat those impairments that relate directly to functional limitations and reach within the scope of treatments available to us (4).

In summary, a task-oriented approach to assessment is directed at answering the following questions:

1. To what degree can the patient perform functional tasks?
2. What strategies does the patient use to perform the tasks, and can he/she adapt strategies to changing task conditions?
3. What are the sensory, motor, and cognitive impairments that constrain how the patient performs the task, and can these impairments be changed through intervention?
4. Is the patient performing optimally given the current set of impairments, or can therapy improve the strategies being used to accomplish functional tasks despite the impairments?

Making the Transition from Assessment to Treatment

The next three steps in the clinical decision-making process, analysis and interpretation of the assessment data, development of short- and long-term goals, and development of an appropriate treatment plan, establish the link between assessment and treatment.

INTERPRETING ASSESSMENT DATA

Interpreting the data collected during the assessment process is no easy task. A number of important issues arise when analyzing assessment information. For example, by what criteria do we determine *normalcy*? Most often, assessment is carried out to distinguish normal motor behavior from abnormal behavior, and to determine the most appropriate approach to retraining motor dyscontrol and regaining functional independence. This requires that we have some criteria for determining what "normal" means.

Clinicians are hampered in their ability to discriminate normal from abnormal because there are no standards by which to judge normal movement function. Determining normal performance is often based on our visual observations and assumption that if the person is using a typical strategy for moving, he/she is normal. Alternatively, the patient using an atypical strategy is considered abnormal and in need of therapy. However, an important aspect of assessing motor control is determining whether the patient is using an optimal strategy (albeit atypical) given the constellation of sensory, motor, and cognitive problems involved.

Once all three levels of assessment are completed, the clinician can translate these assessment data into a list of patient problems categorized according to functional disability, problems associated with task-specific strategies, and underlying sensory, motor, and cognitive impairments. From a comprehensive list, the therapist and patient identify the most difficult problems, which will become the focus for initial intervention strategies. Thus, a list of short- and long-term treatment goals are established and a specific treatment plan is formulated for each of the problems identified.

SETTING TREATMENT GOALS

Establishing a reasonable and rational plan of treatment requires setting appropriate short- and long-term goals that are consistent with the patients' needs and desires, and within their capacity to attain.

Long-Term Goals

Generally, long-term goals define the patient's expected level of performance at the end of the treatment process. Long-term goals are often expressed in terms of functional outcomes, such as (*a*) amount of independence, (*b*) supervision, or level of assistance required to carry out a task, or (*c*) in relationship to the equipment or environmental adaption needed to perform the task. An example of a long-term goal is: the patient will be able to walk 350 ft using an ankle foot orthosis with quad cane in 3 minutes with no loss of balance; or, the patient will need minimal supervision in all dressing activities.

Short-Term Goals

Short-term goals are goals that are expected to be achieved in a reasonably short period of time, for example, one month. Short-term goals are often defined with respect to expected changes at the impairment level. For example, the patient will gain 15° of knee flexion, or the patient will increase quadriceps strength as indicated by an increased number of standing squats from four to eight. Alternatively, short-term goals may be derived from long-term goals, which are broken down into interim steps. For example, the patient will walk 10 feet with minimum assistance. Thus, treatment strategies geared to attaining short-term goals can focus on resolution of impairments and/or achieving interim steps of functional tasks.

Clinical Implications—Treatment

The remaining steps in the clinical problem-solving process involve establishing a comprehensive plan of care, carrying it out, and evaluating its effectiveness in achieving the short- and long-term goals.

A task-oriented approach to establishing a comprehensive plan of care includes treatment strategies designed to achieve the following goals derived from the three levels of assessment:

1. Resolve or prevent impairments;
2. Develop effective task-specific strategies; and
3. Retrain functional goal-oriented tasks.

A critical aspect of retraining functional skills is helping the patient learn to adapt task-specific strategies to changing environmental contexts.

These goals are not approached sequentially, that is in a set order, but rather in parallel. Thus, a clinician may utilize techniques designed to focus on one or more of the aforementioned goals within the same therapy session. For example, when retraining mobility in a patient who has had a stroke, the clinician may have the patient work on (*a*) strengthening exercises to remediate weakness (impairment), (*b*) improving weightbearing on the involved leg, to produce a more symmetrical gait pattern (strategy), (*c*) practicing level walking (functional task) and walking on slightly uneven surfaces or around obstacles (adaptation).

RETRAINING STRATEGIES: RECOVERY VS. COMPENSATION

A question that frequently arises during the course of rehabilitating the patient with a UMN lesion is how much emphasis should be placed on promoting recovery of *normal* strategies versus teaching *compensatory* strategies for performing a task? Recovery of normal strategies for function is defined as the returning capability of the individual to perform a task using mechanisms previously used. Compensatory strategies are atypical approaches to meeting the sensory and motor requirements of the task using alternative mechanisms not typically used.

When to facilitate normal strategies versus teach compensatory strategies is not easy to determine and will vary from patient to patient. Often, the guideline used to determine when compensatory strategies should be taught is *time*. That is, in the acute patient, emphasis is on recovery of normal function, while in the chronic patient, the emphasis shifts to maximizing function through compensatory strategies.

We have found it helpful in the decision-making process to consider the nature of the impairments themselves. Compensatory strategies will be needed in the case of permanent, unchanging impairments, regardless of whether the patient is acute or chronic. An example would be teaching a patient with a permanent loss of vestibular function to rely on alternative vision and somatosensory cues for maintaining balance during functional tasks. Alternatively, if impairments are temporary and changeable (either through natural recovery or in response to therapy), the emphasis would be on remediating impairments and recovery of normal strategies for action.

A problem arises when it is not known whether impairments will resolve. For example, in the acute CVA patient with flaccidity, it is often not possible to predict whether the patient will remain flaccid or regain control over affected extremities. In this case, the clinician may revert to a time-based decision-making process, working towards recovery of normal strategies in the acute patient, and switching to a compensatory focus in the chronic patient.

We will be discussing treatment strategies in greater depth in later chapters focusing on retraining posture, mobility, and upper extremity function.

SUMMARY

1. A comprehensive conceptual framework for clinical practice is built upon four key elements: (a) the clinical decision-making process that establishes the steps for intervention; (b) hypothesis-oriented practice, which provides a process for testing assumptions regarding the nature and cause of motor control problems; (c) a model of disablement that imposes a hierarchical order on the effects of disease on the individual; and (d) a theory of motor control that suggests essential elements to assess and treat.

2. The clinical decision-making process involves: (a) assessment of the patient, (b) anal-

ysis and interpretation of the assessment data, (c) development of short- and long-term goals, (d) development of an appropriate treatment plan to achieve these goals, (e) carrying out the treatment plan, and (f) reassessment of the patient and assessment of treatment outcome.

3. During the course of clinical intervention, the clinician will be required to generate multiple hypotheses, proposing possible explanations regarding the problem and its cause(s), and must investigate these hypotheses through observation, tests, and measurement.

4. A model of disablement provides a hierarchical system for categorizing patient problems that can be used as a framework for organizing and interpreting assessment data.

5. Clinical practices evolve in parallel with scientific theory, as clinicians assimilate changes in scientific theory and apply them to practice. Neurofacilitation approaches to treatment were developed in parallel with the reflex and hierarchical theories of motor control. New approaches to treatment are being developed in response to changing theories of motor control.

6. A task-oriented approach to clinical intervention is based on a systems theory of motor control. Crucial to this approach is the assumption that movement emerges as an interaction among many different systems that are organized around a behavioral goal and various aspects of the environment.

7. A task-oriented assessment evaluates behavior at three levels including (a) objective measurement of functional skills; (b) a description of the strategies used to accomplish functional skills; and (c) quantification of the underlying sensory, motor, and cognitive impairments that constrain performance.

8. A task-oriented approach to treatment focuses on (a) resolving or preventing impairments, (b) developing effective task-specific strategies, and (c) retraining functional goal-oriented tasks.

9. A critical aspect of retraining functional skills is helping the patient learn to adapt task-specific strategies to changing environmental contexts.

REFERENCES

1. Horak F. Assumptions underlying motor control for neurologic rehabilitation. In: Contemporary management of motor con-

trol problems. Proceedings of the II Step Conference. Alexandria, VA: APTA, 1991:11–27.

2. O'Sullivan S. Clinical decision making: planning effective treatments. In: O'Sullivan S, Schmitz T, eds. Physical rehabilitation: assessment and treatment. 2nd ed. Philadephia: FA Davis, 1988:1–7.

3. Wolf S. Summation: identification of principles underlying clinical decisions. In: Wolf S, ed. Clinical decision making in physical therapy. Philadelphia: FA Davis, 1985:379–384.

4. Rothstein J, Echternach JL. Hypothesis-oriented algorithm for clinicians: a method for evaluation and treatment planning. Phys Ther 1986;66:1388–1394.

5. Platt JR. Strong inference. Science 1964; 146:347–352.

6. Sheperd K. Theory: criteria, importance, and impact. In: Contemporary management of motor control problems. Proceedings of the II STEP Conference. Alexandria, VA: APTA, 1991:5–10.

7. Campbell S. Framework for the measurement of neurologic impairment and disability. In: Contemporary management of motor control problems. Proceedings of the II Step Conference. Alexandria, VA: APTA, 1991:143–153.

8. International classification of impairment, disabilities and handicaps: a manual of classification relating to the consequences of disease. Geneva, Switzerland: World Health Organization, 1980.

9. Nagi SZ. Some conceptual issues in disability and rehabilitation. In: Sussman MD, ed. Sociology and rehabilitation. Washington, DC: Am Sociological Assoc, 1965:100–113.

10. Jette AM. Diagnosis and classification by physical therapists: a special communication. Phys Ther 1989;69:967–969.

11. Guccione AA. Physical therapy diagnosis and the relationship between impairments and function. Phys Ther 1991;71:499–504.

12. Schenkman M, Butler RB. A model for multisystem evaluation, interpretation, and treatment of individuals with neurologic dysfunction. Phys Ther 1989;69:538–547.

13. Gordon J. Assumptions underlying physical therapy intervention: theoretical and historical perspectives. In: Carr J, Shepherd R, Gordon J, et al., eds. Movement science: foundations for physical therapy rehabilitation. Rockville, MD: Aspen Systems, 1987.

14. Woollacott M, Shumway-Cook A. Changes in posture control across the life span: a systems approach. Phys Ther 1990;70:799–807.

15. Horak F, Shumway-Cook A. Clinical implications of postural control research. In: P Duncan, ed. Balance. Alexandria, VA: APTA, 1990:105–111.

16. Bobath B, Bobath K. Motor development in different types of cerebral palsy. London: Heinemann, 1976.

17. Bobath K, Bobath B. The neurodevelopmental treatment. In: Scrutton D, ed. Management of the motor disorders of cerebral palsy. Clin Dev Med No 90. London: Heinemann, 1984:6–18.

18. Mayston M. The Bobath concept: evolution and application. In: Forssberg H, Hirschfeld H, eds. Movement disorders in children. Med Sport Sci Basel: Karger, 1992.

19. Stockmyer S. An interpretation of the approach of Rood to the treatment of neuromuscular dysfunction. Am J Phys Med 1967; 46:950–955.

20. Minor MA. Proprioceptive neuromuscular facilitation and the approach of Rood. In: Contemporary management of motor control problems. Proceedings from the II Step Conference. Alexandria, VA: APTA, 1992:137–139.

21. Brunnstrom S. Movement therapy in hemiplegia. New York: Harper & Row; 1970.

22. Voss D, Ionta M, Myers B. Proprioceptive neuromuscular facilitation: patterns and techniques. 3rd ed. New York: Harper & Row; 1985.

23. Ayres J. Sensory integration and learning disorders. Los Angeles: Western Psychological Services; 1972.

24. Montgomery P. Neurodevelopmental treatment and sensory integrative theory. Contemporary management of motor control problems. Proceedings from II Step. Alexandria VA: APTA, 1991.

25. Fisher A, Bundy AC. Sensory integration theory. In: Forssberg H, Hirschfeld H, eds. Movement disorders in children. Basel: Karger, 1992:16–20.

26. Shumway-Cook A, Horak FB. Balance rehabilitation in the neurological patient. Seattle: NERA, 1992.

27. Shumway-Cook A. Retraining balance and mobility: the integration of research into clin-

ical practice. Presentation at the APTA Annual Meeting, Cincinnati; 1993.

28. Woollacott M, Shumway-Cook A. Clinical and research methodology for the study of posture and balance. In: Sudarsky L, ed. Gait disorders of aging: mechanisms, falls and therapy. In press.

29. Gentile, A. The nature of skill acquisition: therapeutic implications for children with movement disorders. In: Forssberg H, Hirschfeld H, eds. Movement disorders in children. Basel: Karger, 1992:31–40.

30. Katz S, Downs TD, Cash HR, Grotz RC. Progress in development of the index of ADL. Gerontologist 1970:20–30.

31. Keith RA, Granger CV, Hamilton BB, Sherwin FS. The functional independence measure: a new tool for rehabilitation. In: Eisentberg MG, Grzesiak RC, eds. Advances in clinical rehabilitation, vol 1. New York: Springer Verlag, 1987:6–18.

32. Mahoney RI, Barthel DW. Functional evaluation: the Barthel Index. Maryland State Medical Journal 1965;14:61–65.

33. Lawton MP. The functional assessment of elderly people. J Am Geriatr Soc 1971;19:465–481.

34. Tinetti ME. Performance oriented assessment of mobility problems in elderly patients. J Am Geriatr Soc 1986;34:119–126.

35. Fregly AR, Graybeil A. An ataxia test battery not requiring rails. Aerospace Medicine 1968:277–282.

36. Erhardt RP. Developmental hand dysfunction: theory, assessment, treatment. Laurel, MD: Ramsco Publishing Co., 1982.

37. Carr J, Shepherd R. Motor relearning programme for stroke. Rockville, MD: Aspen Systems, 1985.

38. Fugl-Myer AR, Jaasko L, Leyman I, et al. The post-stroke hemiplegic patient: a method for evaluation of physical performance. Scand J Rehabil Med 1975;7:13–31.

39. Brunnstrom S. Motor testing procedures in hemiplegia: based on sequential recovery stages. Phys Ther 1966;46:357–375.

40. Hoehn MM, Yahr MD. Parkinsonism: onset, progression and mortality. Neurology 1967; 17:433–450.

41. Schwab RS. Progression and prognosis in Parkinson's disease. J Nerv Ment Dis 1960; 130:556–572.

42. Gentile A. Skill acquisition: action movement, and neuromotor processes. In: Carr J, Shepherd R, Gordon J, et al., eds. Movement science: foundations for physical therapy in rehabilitation. Rockville, MD: Aspen Systems, 1987.

43. Welford AT. Motor skills and aging. In: Mortimer J, Pirozzolo FJ, Maletta G, eds. The aging motor system. New York: Praeger, 1982:152–187.

44. Foerster, O. The motor cortex in man in the light of Hughlings Jackson's doctrines. In: Payton OD, Hirt S, Newman R, eds. Scientific bases for neurophysiologic approaches to therapeutic exercise. Philadelphia: FA Davis, 1977:13–18.

Section II

POSTURE/BALANCE

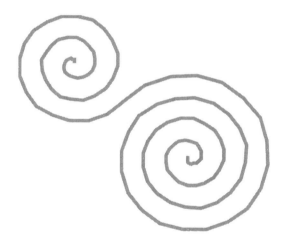

Chapter 6

CONTROL OF POSTURE AND BALANCE

INTRODUCTION

Picture yourself getting out of the car at the airport, in a hurry to catch your flight. You pick up your suitcase and run towards the terminal building. On the way, you misjudge the height of the curb, trip, but recovering, go into the terminal and check your bags. You get on the moving walkways that take you to your gate, moving quickly to avoid running into other people. Finally, you board the plane and sink gratefully into your seat.

The many tasks involved in getting from your car to your seat on the plane place heavy demands on the systems that control posture and balance. In examining some of these tasks you can see that posture and balance involve not just the ability to recover from instability, but also the ability to anticipate and move in ways that will help you avoid instability.

While few clinicians would argue the importance of posture and balance to independence in activities such as sitting, standing, and walking, there is no universal defi-

nition of posture and balance, nor agreement on the neural mechanisms underlying the control of these functions.

Over the last several decades, research into posture and balance control and their disorders has shifted and broadened. The very definitions of posture and balance have changed, as has our understanding of the underlying neural mechanisms. In rehabilitation science, there are at least two different conceptual theories to describe the neural control of posture and balance: the reflex/hierarchical theory and the systems theory (1–3).

A reflex/hierarchical theory suggests that posture and balance result from hierarchically organized reflex responses triggered by independent sensory systems. According to this theory, during development there is a progressive shift from the dominance of primitive spinal reflexes to higher levels of postural reactions, until *mature* cortical responses dominate. This theory of balance control will be presented in more detail in the next chapter.

119

This chapter discusses normal posture and balance control from a systems perspective. Sitting and standing postural control are described as well. Posture related to mobility, however, is covered in the next section of the book.

As noted in Chapter 1, the systems approach suggests that action emerges from an interaction of the individual with the task and the environment (Fig. 6.1). The systems approach implies that the ability to control our body's position in space emerges from a complex interaction of musculoskeletal and neural systems, collectively referred to as the postural control system.

Defining the Task of Postural Control

To understand postural behavior in the individual, we must understand the *task* of postural control, and examine the effect of the environment on the task of posture.

The task of **postural control** involves controlling the body's position in space for the dual purposes of stability and orientation. **Postural orientation** is defined as the ability to maintain an appropriate relationship between the body segments, and between the body and the environment for a task (4). For most functional tasks, we maintain a vertical

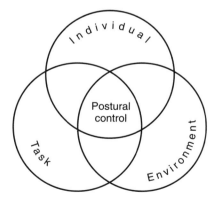

Figure 6.1. Postural actions emerge from an interaction of the individual, the task with its inherent postural demands, and the environmental constraints on postural actions.

orientation of the body. In the process of establishing a vertical orientation, we use multiple sensory references, including gravity (the vestibular system), the support surface (somatosensory system), and the relationship of our body to objects in our environment (visual system).

Postural stability is defined as the ability to maintain the position of the body, and specifically, the center of body mass (COM), within specific boundaries of space, referred to as stability limits. **Stability limits** are boundaries of an area of space in which the body can maintain its position without changing the base of support. Stability limits are not fixed boundaries, but change according to the task, the individual's biomechanics, and various aspects of the environment. The term *stability* is used in this text interchangeably with *balance* or *equilibrium*. Stability involves establishing an equilibrium between destabilizing and stabilizing forces (5).

Stability and orientation represent two distinct goals of the postural control system (6, 7). Some tasks place importance on maintaining an appropriate orientation at the expense of stability. The successful blocking of a goal in soccer, or catching a flyball in baseball, requires that the player always remain oriented with respect to the ball, sometimes falling to the ground in an effort to block a goal, or to catch a ball. Thus, while postural control is a requirement that most tasks have in common, stability and orientation demands change with each task (8).

Defining Systems for Postural Control

Postural control for stability and orientation requires (*a*) the integration of sensory information to assess the position and motion of the body in space, and (*b*) the ability to generate forces for controlling body position. Thus, postural control requires a complex interaction of musculoskeletal and neural systems, as shown in Figure 6.2.

Musculoskeletal components include such things as joint range of motion, spinal

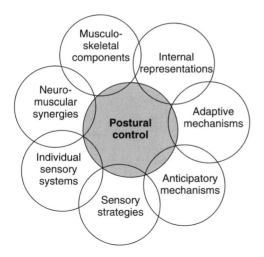

Figure 6.2. Conceptual model representing systems contributing to postural control.

flexibility, muscle properties, and biomechanical relationships among linked body segments.

Neural components essential to postural control encompass (*a*) motor processes, including neuromuscular response synergies; (*b*) sensory processes, including the visual, vestibular, and somatosensory systems; (*c*) sensory strategies that organize these multiple inputs; (*d*) internal representations important for the mapping of sensation to action; and (*e*) higher level processes essential for adaptive and anticipatory aspects of postural control.

In this book we refer to higher level neural processes as cognitive influences on postural control. It is very important to understand, however, that the term cognitive as it is used here does not mean conscious control. Higher level cognitive aspects of postural control are the basis for adaptive and anticipatory aspects of postural control. **Adaptive postural control** involves modifying sensory and motor systems in response to changing task and environmental demands. Anticipatory aspects of postural control pretune sensory and motor systems for postural demands based on previous experience and learning. Other aspects of cognition that affect postural control include such processes as attention, motivation, and intent (6).

Thus, in a systems approach, postural control results from a complex interaction among many bodily systems that work cooperatively to control the body's position in space. The specific organization of postural systems is determined both by the functional task and the environment in which it is being performed.

Postural Requirements Vary with Functional Task

The ability to control our body's position in space is fundamental to everything we do! All tasks have postural requirements. That is, every task has an orientation component and a stability component. However, the stability and orientation requirements will vary with the task and the environment.

The task of sitting in a chair and reading has an orientation requirement of keeping the head and gaze stable and fixed on the reading material. The arms and hands maintain an appropriate task-specific orientation that allows the book to be held in the appropriate position in relationship to the head and eyes. The stability requirements of this task are lenient. Since the contact of the body with the chair back and seat provides a fairly large base of support, the primary requirement is controlling the unsupported mass of the head with respect to the mass of the trunk.

In contrast, the task of standing and reading a book has roughly the same orientation requirements with respect to the head, eyes, arms, and book, but the stability requirements are considerably more stringent. This task requires that the center of mass be kept within a much smaller base of support defined by the two feet.

Finally, a person standing on a moving bus has to constantly regain stability which is threatened by the constant motion of the bus. The task of stability is more rigorous, reflecting the changing and unpredictable nature of the task. In this case, the task demands vary from moment to moment, requiring constant adaptation of the postural system.

Thus, you can see that while these tasks

demand postural control, the specific orientation and stability requirements vary according to the task and the environment. Because of this, the sensory and motor strategies used to accomplish postural control must adapt to varying task and environmental demands (6).

STANCE POSTURAL CONTROL

How do the sensory and motor systems work together to control stance? The task of stance postural control has stringent stability demands, requiring that the center of body mass (COM) be kept within stability limits, defined principally by the length of the feet and the distance between them (5).

Stance postural control is usually associated with the maintenance of a vertical orientation, though this is not an invariant requirement of the task. That is, one could maintain a standing position but be bent over, looking at something on the ground, or alternatively, stand with the head extended, looking at a bird. In both instances, one can vary the configuration of body parts to accomplish these two standing tasks, but the stability requirements do not vary. If the center of body mass is not kept within the support base of the feet, a fall will occur, unless the base of support is changed by taking a step.

Over the past decade, sensory and motor strategies for controlling stance posture have been widely studied. What do we mean by strategies for postural control? A strategy is a plan for action, an approach to organizing individual elements within a system into a collective structure. Postural **motor strategies** refer to the organization of movements appropriate for controlling the body's position in space. **Sensory strategies** organize sensory information from visual, somatosensory, and vestibular systems for postural control. Finally, **sensorimotor strategies** reflect the rules for coordinating sensory and motor aspects of postural control (6).

Research in stance postural control has focused primarily on examining strategies for controlling forward and backward sway. Why?

ACTIVE LEARNING MODULE

You can determine this for yourself. Try standing up with your feet shoulder distance apart. First notice: are you standing perfectly still, or do you move very slightly? In which direction do you feel yourself swaying most? Try leaning forward and backwards as far as you can without taking a step. Does your body move the same way as when you only lean forward or backward a little? What muscles do you feel working to keep you balanced when you sway a little? What muscles work when you sway further? What happens when you lean so far forward that your center of mass moves outside the base of support of your feet?

As you have already discovered, no one stands absolutely still; instead, the body sways in small amounts, mostly in the forward and backward direction. This is why researchers have concentrated on understanding how normal adults maintain stability in the sagittal plane.

Now we can explore the underlying control mechanisms in depth, beginning with the motor mechanisms underlying postural control. In our discussion of motor mechanisms important to postural control, we first consider the role of muscle tone and postural tone in controlling small oscillations of the body during quiet stance. Then we review motor strategies and underlying muscle synergies that help us to recover stability when our balance is threatened.

Motor Mechanisms for Postural Control

Postural control requires the generation, scaling, and coordination of forces that produce movements effective in controlling the body's position in space. How does the nervous system organize the motor system to ensure postural control during quiet stance? How does the organization change when stability is threatened?

MOTOR CONTROL OF QUIET STANCE

What are the behavioral characteristics of quiet stance, and what is it that allows us to remain upright during quiet stance or sitting? Quiet stance is characterized by small amounts of spontaneous postural sway. A number of factors contribute to our stability in this situation. First, body alignment can minimize the effect of gravitational forces, which tend to pull us off center. Second, muscle tone keeps the body from collapsing in response to the pull of gravity. Three main factors contribute to our background muscle tone during quiet stance: (*a*) the intrinsic stiffness of the muscles themselves, (*b*) the background muscle tone, which exists normally in all muscles because of neural contributions, and (*c*) postural tone, the activation of antigravity muscles during quiet stance. Let's look at these factors (9–12).

Alignment

How does alignment contribute to postural stability? In a perfectly aligned posture, shown in Figure 6.3, the vertical line of gravity falls in the midline between (*a*) the mastoid process; (*b*) a point just in front of the shoulder joints, (*c*) the hip joints (or just behind), (*d*) a point just in front of the center of the knee joints, and (*e*) a point just in front of the ankle joints (10). The ideal alignment

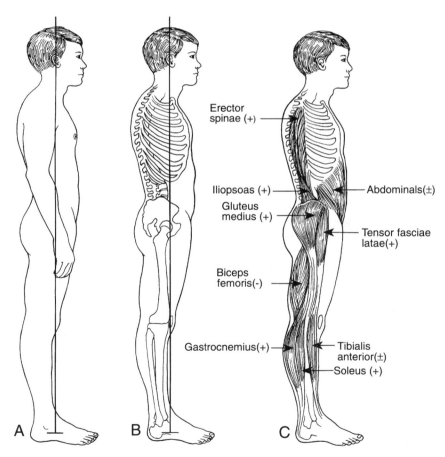

Figure 6.3. Diagrammatic illustration of (**A** and **B**) the ideal alignment in stance, requiring minimal muscular effort to sustain the vertical position, and **C**, the muscles that are tonically active during the control of quiet stance. (Adapted from Kendell FP, McCreary EK. Muscles: testing and function. 3rd ed. Baltimore: Williams & Wilkins, 1983:280.)

TECHNOLOGY BOX 1

ELECTROMYOGRAPHY is a technique used for measuring the activity of muscles through electrodes placed on the surface of the skin, over the muscle to be recorded, or in the muscle itself. The output signal from the electrode (the electromyogram or EMG) describes the output to the muscular system from the motor neuron pool. It provides the clinician with information about (*a*) the identity of the muscles that are active during a movement, (*b*) the timing and relative intensity of muscle contraction, and (*c*) whether antagonistic or synergistic muscle activity is occurring. Surface electrodes are most often used; however the ability of these electrodes to differentiate between the activity of neighboring muscles is not very effective.

The amplitude of the EMG signal is often interpreted as a rough measure of tension generated in the muscle. However, caution must be used when interpreting EMG amplitude measurements. There are many variables that can affect the amplitude of EMG signals, including how rapidly the muscle is changing length, resistance associated with cutaneous tissue and subcutaneous fat, and location of the electrode. Thus, generally, it is not accurate to compare absolute amplitudes of EMG activity of a muscle across subjects, or within the same subject across different days. Researchers who utilize EMG amplitude data to compare temporal and spatial patterns of muscle activity across subjects or within a subject on different days generally convert absolute amplitude measures to relative measures. For example, one can determine the ratio between the response amplitude and the amplitude of a maximum voluntary contraction of that muscle. Or, the ratio between agonist and antagonist muscles at a joint can be determined. Likewise, the ratio of synergistic muscles can be found. One can then examine how this ratio changes as a function of changing task or environmental conditions (61, 62).

TECHNOLOGY BOX 2

KINEMATIC ANALYSIS is the description of the characteristics of an object's movement, including linear and angular displacements, velocities, and accelerations. Displacement data are usually gathered from the measurement of the position of markers placed over anatomic landmarks and reported relative to either an anatomic coordinate system, that is, relative joint angle, or to an external spatial reference system.

There are various ways to measure the kinematics of body movement. Goniometers, or electrical potentiometers, can be attached to measure a joint angle where a change in joint angle produces a proportional change in voltage.

Accelerometers are usually force transducers that measure the reaction forces associated with acceleration of a body segment. The mass of the body is accelerated against a force transducer, producing a signal voltage proportional to the acceleration. Finally, imaging measurement techniques, including cinematography, video, or optoelectric systems, can be used to measure body movement. Optoelectric systems require the subject to wear special infrared lights or reflective markers on each anatomic landmark, which are recorded by one or more cameras. The location of the light, or marker, is expressed in terms of x and y coordinates in a two-dimensional system, or x, y and z coordinates in a three-dimensional system. Output from these systems is expressed as changes in segment displacements, joint angles, velocities, or accelerations, and the data can be used to create a reconstruction of the body's movement in space (61, 62).

TECHNOLOGY BOX 3

KINETIC ANALYSIS refers to the analysis of the forces that cause movement, including both internal and external forces. Internal forces come from muscle activity, ligaments, or from friction in the muscles and joints; external forces come from the ground or external loads. Kinetic analysis gives us insight into the forces contributing to movement. Force-measuring devices or force transducers are used to measure force, with output signals that are proportional to the applied force.

Force plates measure ground reaction forces, which are the forces under the area of the foot, from which center of pressure data are calculated. The term center of gravity (CG) of the body is not the same as the center of pressure (CP). The CG of the body is the net location of the center of mass in the vertical direction. CP is the location of the vertical ground reaction force on the forceplate and is equal and opposite to all the downward acting forces (61, 62).

in stance allows the body to be maintained in equilibrium with the least expenditure of internal energy.

Before we continue reviewing the research concerning the control of posture and movement, be sure to review the information contained in the adjacent boxes, which discuss techniques for movement analysis at different levels of control, including electromyography, kinematics, and kinetics.

Muscle Tone

What is muscle tone, and how does it help us to keep our balance? **Muscle tone** refers to the force with which a muscle resists being lengthened, that is, its stiffness (10). Muscle tone is often tested clinically by passively extending and flexing a relaxed patient's limbs and feeling the resistance offered by the muscles. Both non-neural and neural mechanisms contribute to muscle tone or stiffness.

A certain level of muscle tone is present in a normal, conscious, and relaxed person. However, in the relaxed state no electrical activity is recorded in normal human skeletal muscle using EMGs. This has led researchers to argue that non-neural contributions to muscle tone are the result of small amounts of free calcium in the muscle fiber, which cause a low level of continuous recycling of cross-bridges (13).

There are also neural contributions to muscle tone or stiffness, associated with the activation of the stretch reflex, which resists lengthening of the muscle. Changes in muscle length are sensed by the muscle spindles. This afferent information is sent to the motor neurons, which alter their firing to achieve the needed force to change the muscle length to the desired value. In this way, the stretch reflex loop acts continuously to keep the muscle length at a set value. For a more detailed review of the role of the muscle spindle, review Chapter 3.

The role of the stretch reflex as a contributor to normal muscle tone is fairly clear. The role of stretch reflexes in controlling upright stance posture, however, is not. According to one theory, stretch reflexes play a feedback role during the maintenance of posture. Thus, this theory suggests that, as we sway back and forth while standing, the ankle muscles are stretched, activating the stretch reflex. This results in a reflex shortening of the muscle, and subsequent control of forward and backward sway.

While some authors suggest that the stretch reflex is critical for maintaining posture, others have questioned the role of the stretch reflex in the control of quiet stance. Reports that the gain of the stretch reflex is quite low during stance has led some researchers to question its relevance to controlling sway (14).

Postural Tone

We have explained the mechanisms contributing to the generation of tone in individual muscles, when a person is in a relaxed state. This background level of activity changes in certain anti-gravity postural muscles when we stand upright, thus counteracting the force of gravity. This increased level of activity in anti-gravity muscles is referred to as **postural tone**. What are the factors that contribute to postural tone?

A number of factors influence postural tone. Evidence from experiments showing that lesions of the dorsal (sensory) roots of the spinal cord reduced postural tone, indicates that postural tone is influenced by inputs coming in from the somatosensory system (15). In addition, it has long been known that activation of cutaneous inputs on the soles of the feet causes a placing reaction, which results in an automatic extension of the foot toward the support surface, thus increasing postural tone in extensor muscles. Somatosensory inputs from the neck activated by changes in head orientation can also influence the distribution of postural tone in the trunk and limbs (15). These have been referred to as the tonic neck reflexes, and are discussed further in the next chapter on postural development (9).

Inputs from the visual and vestibular systems also influence postural tone. Vestibular inputs, activated by a change in head orientation, alter the distribution of postural tone in the neck and limbs, and have been referred to as the vestibulocollic and vestibulospinal reflexes (15–17).

Often, these reflex contributions to posture control are highly emphasized in the clinical literature. However, it is important to remember that there are many influences on postural control in a normal, intact, functioning individual (16). It is possible that in the neurologically impaired individual, who has lost varying amounts of nonreflex influences, reflex pathways take a more commanding role in the control of posture.

In the clinical literature, much emphasis is placed on the concept of postural tone as a major mechanism in supporting the body against gravity. In particular, many clinicians have suggested that postural tone in the trunk segment is the key element for control of normal postural stability in the erect position (12, 18, 19). How consistent is this assumption with EMG studies that have examined the muscles active in quiet stance?

Researchers have found that many muscles in the body are tonically active during quiet stance (10). Some of these muscles are shown in Figure 6.3*C*, and include (*a*) the soleus and gastrocnemius, since the line of gravity falls slightly in front of the knee and ankle; (*b*) the tibialis anterior, when the body sways in the backward direction; (*c*) the gluteus medius and tensor fasciae latae but not the gluteus maximus; (*d*) the iliopsoas, which prevents hyperextension of the hips, but not the hamstrings and quadriceps; and (*e*) the thoracic erector spinae in the trunk (along with intermittent activation of the abdominals), because the line of gravity falls in front of the spinal column.

These studies suggest that muscles throughout the body, not just those limited to the trunk, are tonically active to maintain the body in a narrowly confined vertical position during quiet stance. Once the center of mass moves outside the narrow range defined by the *ideal alignment*, more muscular effort is required to recover a stable position. In this situation, compensatory postural strategies are used to return the center of gravity to a stable position within the base of support.

MOTOR STRATEGIES DURING PERTURBED STANCE

Many research labs, including Lewis Nashner's lab from the United States and the labs of Dichgans, Dietz, and Allum in Europe, have studied the organization of movement strategies used to recover stability in response to brief displacements of the supporting surface, using a variety of moving platforms such as the one shown in Figure 6.4 (20–22). In addition, characteristic patterns of muscle activity, called muscle synergies, which are associated with postural movement strategies,

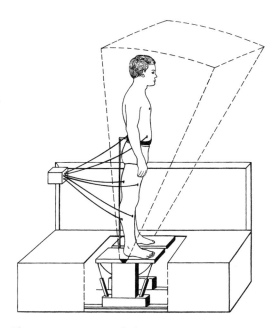

Figure 6.4. Moving platform posturography used to study postural control. (Adapted from Woollacott MH, Shumway-Cook A, Nashner LM. Aging and posture control: changes in sensory organization and muscular coordination. Int J Aging Hum Dev 1986;22:332.)

have been described (23–25). These movement patterns are referred to as the ankle, hip, and suspensory/or stepping strategies, and are illustrated in Figure 6.5.

These postural movement strategies are used in both a feedback and feedforward (anticipatory) manner to maintain equilibrium in a number of circumstances. Here are some examples of such situations:

1. In response to external disturbances to equilibrium, such as when the support surface moves;
2. To prevent a disturbance to the system, for example, prior to a voluntary movement that is potentially destabilizing;
3. During gait and in response to unexpected disruptions to the gait cycle; and
4. During volitional center of mass movements in stance.

Nashner and his colleagues (23–25) have explored the muscle patterns that un-

derlie movement strategies for balance. Results from postural control research in neurologically intact young adults suggest the nervous system combines independent, though related muscles, into units called **muscle synergies**. A **synergy** is defined as the functional coupling of groups of muscles such that they are constrained to act together as a unit; this simplifies the control demands on the CNS. It is important to keep in mind that while muscle synergies are important, they are only one of many motor mechanisms that affect outputs for postural control (23–25).

What are some of the muscle synergies underlying movement strategies critical for stance postural control? How do scientists know whether these neuromuscular responses are due to neural programs (that is, synergies) or if they are the result of independent stretch of the individual muscles at mechanically coupled joints?

Ankle Strategy

The ankle strategy and its related muscle synergy were among the first patterns for controlling upright sway to be identified. The ankle strategy restores the COM to a position of stability through body movement centered primarily about the ankle joints. Figure 6.6*A* shows the typical synergistic muscle activity and body movements associated with corrections for loss of balance in the forward direction. In this case, motion of the platform in the backward direction causes the subject to sway forward. Muscle activity begins at about 90 to 100 msec after perturbation onset in the gastrocnemius, followed by activation of the hamstrings 20 to 30 msec later, and finally by the activation of the paraspinal muscles (23).

Activation of the gastrocnemius produces a plantarflexion torque that slows, then reverses, the body's forward motion. Activation of the hamstrings and paraspinal muscles maintains the hip and knees in an extended position. Without the synergistic activation of the hamstrings and paraspinal muscles, the indirect effect of the gastrocnemius ankle torque on proximal body segments would re-

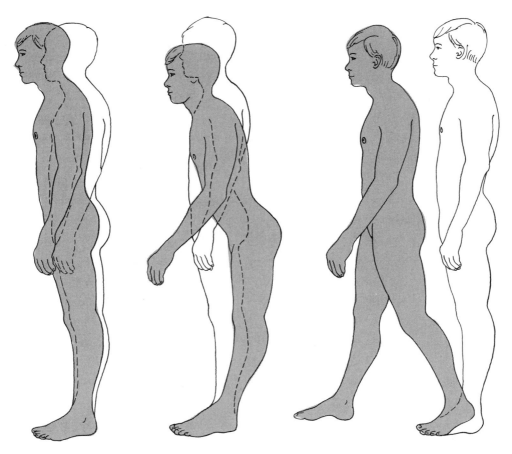

Figure 6.5.   Three postural movement strategies used by normal adults for controlling upright sway. (From Shumway-Cook A, Horak F. Vestibular rehabilitation: an exercise approach to managing symptoms of vestibular dysfunction. Seminars in Hearing 1989;10:199.)

sult in forward motion of the trunk mass relative to the lower extremities.

Figure 6.6*B* shows the synergistic muscle activity and body motions used when reestablishing stability in response to backwards instability. Muscle activity begins in the distal muscle, the anterior tibialis, followed by activation of the quadriceps and abdominal muscles.

How do scientists know that the ankle, knee, and hip muscles are part of a neuromuscular synergy, instead of being activated in response to stretch of each individual joint? Some of the first experiments in postural control (23, 24) provide some evidence for synergistic organization of muscles.

In these early experiments the platform was rotated in a *toes-up* or *toes-down* direction. In a toes-up rotation, the platform motion

provides stretch to the gastrocnemius muscle and dorsiflexion of the ankle, but these inputs are not associated with movements at the mechanically coupled knee and hip. The neuromuscular response that occurs in response to toes-up platform rotation includes activation of muscles at the ankle, knee, and hip joints, despite the fact that motion has occurred only at the ankle joint. Evidence from these experiments supports the hypothesis of a neurally programmed muscle synergy (20, 23, 24), including knee and hip muscles on the same side of the body as the stretched ankle muscle.

Since these responses are destabilizing, in order to regain balance, muscles on the opposite side of the body are activated. These responses have been hypothesized to be activated in response to visual and vestibular inputs (21) and are sometimes referred to as M3

ANKLE STRATEGY

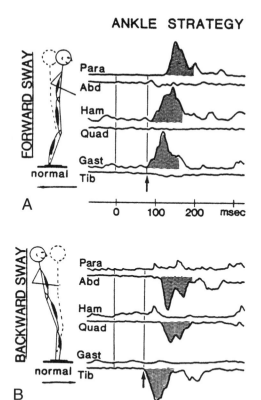

Figure 6.6. Muscle synergy and body motions associated with ankle strategy for controlling **A**, forward sway and **B**, backward sway. (From Horak F, Nashner L. Central programming of postural movements: adaptation to altered support surface configurations. J Neurophysiol 1986;55:1372.)

responses, as opposed to an M1 response, that is, a monosynaptic stretch reflex, and the longer latency stretch responses, which have been called M2 responses (22).

The ankle movement strategy described earlier appears to be used most commonly in situations in which the perturbation to equilibrium is small and the support surface is firm. Use of the ankle strategy requires intact range of motion and strength in the ankles. What happens if the perturbation to balance is large, or if we are in a situation where we are unable to generate force using ankle joint muscles?

Hip Strategy

Scientists have identified another strategy for controlling body sway, the hip move-

ment strategy (25). This strategy controls motion of the COM by producing large and rapid motion at the hip joints with antiphase rotations of the ankles (refer back to Fig. 6.5).

Figure 6.7*A* shows the typical synergistic muscle activity associated with a hip strategy. Motion of the platform in the backward direction again causes the subject to sway forward. As shown in Figure 6.7*A*, the muscles that typically respond to forward sway when a subject is standing on a narrow beam are different from the muscles that become activated in response to forward sway while standing on a flat surface. Muscle activity begins at about 90 to 100 msec after perturbation onset in the abdominal muscles, followed by activation of the quadriceps (25). Figure 6.7*B* shows the muscle pattern and body motions associated with the hip strategy correcting for backward sway.

HIP STRATEGY

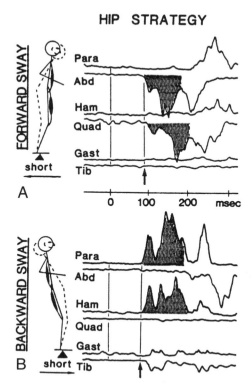

Figure 6.7. Muscle synergy and body motions associated with the hip strategy for controlling **A**, forward sway and **B**, backward sway. (From Horak F, Nashner L. Central programming of postural movements: adaptation to altered support surface configurations. J Neurophysiol 1986;55:1372.)

Horak and Nashner suggest that the hip strategy is used to restore equilibrium in response to larger, faster perturbations, or when the support surface is compliant, or smaller than the feet, for example, when standing on a beam (25).

Stepping Strategy

When a postural perturbation is strong enough to displace the COM outside the base of support of the feet, a step or hop (the stepping strategy) is used to bring the support base back into alignment under the COM (refer back to Fig 6.5) (6, 26).

While the aforementioned strategies and their associated muscular synergies are presented as discrete entities, researchers have shown that most neurologically intact individuals use various mixtures of these strategies when controlling forward and backward sway in the standing position (25).

ADAPTING MOTOR STRATEGIES

Studies have shown that normal subjects can shift relatively quickly from one postural movement strategy to another (25). For example, when asked to stand on the narrow beam, most subjects shifted from an ankle to a hip strategy within five to 15 trials, and when returned to a normal support surface, they shifted back to an ankle strategy, within six trials. During the transition from one strategy to the next, subjects used complex movement strategies that were combinations of the pure strategies.

Scientists theorize that the CNS may represent the different movement strategies with respect to the boundaries in space in which they can be safely used. That is, the CNS appears to map the relationship between body movements in space and the motor strategies used to control those movements (27). These conceptual boundaries are shown in Figure 6.8. Boundaries may be dynamic, shifting in response to the demands of the task and environment. For example, boundaries for using hip, ankle, and stepping strategies when standing on a firm, flat surface (refer to Fig. 6.8A) may be different from those used

when standing on a narrow beam (Fig. 6.8B) (27).

This information is interesting, but is it true that we modify the amplitude of postural responses only when they are inappropriate to the task? In fact, no. Recent research has shown that we are constantly modulating the amplitudes of our postural responses, even when they are appropriate. For example, Woollacott and colleagues examined the responses of adults to repeated translational platform movements, and found that with repeated exposure to the movements, the subjects swayed less and showed smaller amplitude postural responses (28). Thus, with repeated exposure to a given postural task, subjects refine their response characteristics to optimize response efficiency.

How do we modify our postural strategies to accommodate multiple task goals? For example, if we are trying to stand on a moving bus while carrying a cup of coffee, do we use a different strategy from when we are trying to read a book? To answer this question, researchers asked adults to stand on a moveable platform while either keeping their arms at a fixed angle, as if they were reading

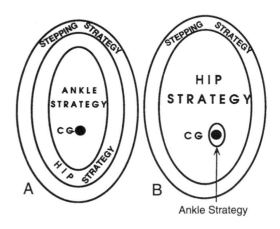

Figure 6.8. Changes in boundaries for motor strategies used to control sway change as a function of the support surface. Mapping the relationship between body movements in space and the motor strategies used to control those movements while standing **A**, on a firm flat surface vs. **B**, crosswise on a narrow beam. (From Horak FB. Effects of neurological disorders on postural movement strategies in the elderly. In: Vellas B, Toupet M, Rubenstein L, Albarede JL, Christen Y, eds. Falls, balance and gait disorders in the elderly. Paris: Elsevier, 1992:147.)

a book, or keeping their finger at a fixed point in space, as if they were trying to keep a glass of water from spilling (29, 30). They found that people continued to use the ankle strategy during both tasks, but changed the coupling of the arm to the trunk in order to perform the additional upper extremity task.

To learn more about postural sway strategies in other directions, MacPherson performed experiments in which she perturbed cats in 16 different directions, around a 360° continuum (31). Despite the fact that cats were perturbed in 16 different directions, they responded with force vectors in only two directions. In addition, while some muscles appeared to be functionally coupled into synergies, others appeared to be controlled independently and used to fine-tune the synergies.

How does this work with cats relate to human postural control experiments? Until recently, human postural research stressed the importance of a limited number of muscle synergies that are the basis for postural control. The work with cats suggests that some muscles within the synergy may be tightly coupled, but other muscle activity may be highly modifiable. Thus, the CNS may combine muscles in more ways than was originally thought. However, the way in which forces are applied may be very limited. This would change the emphasis in postural control from a limited number of muscle synergies, to a limited number of force strategies.

There is some support for this hypothesis in humans from postural experiments examining muscle responses used to control sway in various directions in young adults (32). The experimenters found stereotypical muscle response synergies when sway was forward or backwards, but the responses were much more variable in other directions. As perturbation direction was changed, activation of the recorded muscles varied continuously as a function of perturbation direction.

In summary, we know that the ability to generate and apply forces in a coordinated way to control the body's position in space is an essential part of postural control. We know the CNS must activate synergistic muscles at mechanically related joints to ensure that forces generated at one joint for balance control do not produce instability elsewhere in the body. We believe the CNS internally represents the body's position in space with reference to behavioral strategies that are effective in controlling that movement; however, it is not clear whether these behavioral strategies are internally represented as muscle synergies, movement strategies, or force strategies.

Sensory Mechanisms Related to Posture

Effective postural control requires more than the ability to generate and apply forces for controlling the body's position in space. In order to know *when and how* to apply restoring forces, the CNS must have an accurate picture of *where* the body is in space, and whether it is stationary or in motion. How does the CNS accomplish this?

SENSES CONTRIBUTING TO POSTURE CONTROL

The CNS must organize information from sensory receptors throughout the body before it can determine the body's position in space. Normally, peripheral inputs from visual, somatosensory (proprioceptive, cutaneous, and joint receptors), and vestibular systems are available to detect the body's position and movement in space with respect to gravity and the environment. Each sense provides the CNS with specific information about position and motion of the body; thus, each sense provides a different *frame of reference* for postural control (33, 34).

What information does each of the senses provide for postural control? Is one sense more important than others? Does the CNS use all three senses all the time? If not, how does the CNS decide which sense to use?

Visual Inputs

Visual inputs report information regarding the position and motion of the head with respect to surrounding objects. Visual inputs provide a reference for verticality, since many things that surround us, like windows and doors, are aligned vertically. In addition, the visual system reports motion of the head, since as your head moves forward, surrounding objects move in the opposite direction. Visual inputs include both peripheral visual information, as well as foveal information, though there is some evidence to suggest that a peripheral (or a large visual field) stimulus is more important for controlling posture (35).

Visual inputs are an important source of information for postural control, but are they absolutely necessary? No, since most of us can keep our balance when we close our eyes, or are in a dark room. In addition, visual inputs are not always an accurate source of orientation information about *self-motion*. If you are sitting in your car at a stop light and the car next to you moves, what do you do? You quickly put your foot on the brake. In this situation, visual inputs signal *motion*, which the brain initially interprets as self-motion; in other words, *my car is rolling*. The brain therefore sends out signals to the motor neurons of the leg and foot, so you step on the brake and *stop* the motion.

Thus, visual information may be misinterpreted by the brain. The visual system has difficulty distinguishing between object motion, referred to as exocentric motion, and self-motion, referred to as egocentric motion.

Somatosensory Inputs

The somatosensory system provides the CNS with position and motion information about the body's position in space with reference to supporting surfaces. In addition, somatosensory inputs throughout the body report information about the relationship of body segments to one another. Somatosensory receptors include joint and muscle proprioceptors, cutaneous, and pressure receptors.

Under normal circumstances, when standing on a firm, flat surface, somatosensory receptors provide information about the position and movement of your body with respect to a horizontal surface. However, if you

are standing on a surface that is moving relative to you, for example, a boat, or on a surface that is not horizontal, like a ramp, then it is not appropriate to establish a vertical orientation with reference to the surface. In these situations, inputs reporting the body's position with respect to the surface become less helpful in establishing a vertical orientation.

Vestibular Inputs

Information from the vestibular system is also a powerful source of orientation information. The vestibular system provides the CNS with information about the position and movement of the head with respect to gravity and inertial forces, providing a *gravito-inertial* frame of reference for postural control.

The vestibular system has two types of receptors that sense different aspects of head position and motion. The semicircular canals (SCC) sense angular acceleration of the head. The SCC are particularly sensitive to fast head movements such as those occurring during gait or during imbalance, e.g., slips, trips, or stumbles (7).

The otoliths signal linear position and acceleration. Since gravity is detected in relation to our linear position or movement in space, the otoliths are an important source of information about head position with respect to gravity. The otoliths mostly respond to slow head movements, such as those that occur during postural sway. Thus, the vestibular system reports position and motion of the head, and is important in distinguishing between exocentric and egocentric motion (7).

It is also interesting to note that vestibular signals alone cannot provide the CNS with a *true picture* of how the body is moving in space. For example, the CNS cannot distinguish between a simple head nod (movement of the head relative to a stable trunk) and a forward bend (movement of the head in conjunction with a moving trunk) using vestibular inputs alone (7).

How does the CNS organize this sensory information for postural control? Postural demands during quiet stance, often referred to as static balance control, are different from those during perturbations to stance or during locomotion, which require more dynamic forms of control. Therefore, it is likely that information is organized differently for these tasks.

SENSORY STRATEGIES DURING QUIET STANCE

Somatosensory inputs from all parts of the body contribute to balance control during quiet stance. Studies by the French scientist Roll and his colleagues used minivibrators to excite eye, neck, and ankle muscles (36), and explored the contributions of proprioceptive inputs from these muscles to posture control during quiet stance. They found that vibration to the eye muscles of a standing subject with eyes closed produced body sway, with sway direction depending on the muscle vibrated. Body sway also was produced by vibration to the sternocleidomastoid muscles of the neck or the soleus muscles of the leg. When these muscles were vibrated simultaneously, the effects were additive, with no clear domination of one proprioceptive influence over another. This suggests that proprioception from all parts of the body plays an important role in the maintenance of quiet stance body posture.

Early studies examining the effect of vision on quiet stance examined the amplitude of sway with eyes open vs. eyes closed, and found that there was a significant increase in sway in normal subjects with eyes closed. Thus, it was concluded that vision actively contributes to balance control during quiet stance. The ratio of body sway during eyes open and closed conditions has been referred to as the Romberg quotient (37).

Do we use visual cues in a different manner depending on whether we are standing quietly or responding to an unexpected threat to balance? The answer appears to be yes. Several researchers have studied sensitivity to continuous vs. transient visual motion cues in people of different ages (38–41).

The first experiments of this type were performed by David Lee and his colleagues from Edinburgh, Scotland, using a novel paradigm in which subjects stood in a room that had a fixed floor, but with walls and a ceiling that could be moved forward or backward, creating the illusion of sway in the opposite direction (38). The moving room can be used to create slow oscillations, simulating visual cues during quiet stance sway, or an abrupt perturbation to the visual field, simulating an unexpected loss of balance.

If very small continuous room oscillations are used, neurologically intact adults begin to sway with the room's oscillations, thus showing that visual inputs have an important influence on postural control of adults during quiet stance (38).

Other studies have given adults slow, continuous platform oscillations (simulating quiet stance) vs. fast, transient platform perturbations (creating loss of stability). The results from these studies indicate that visual, vestibular, and somatosensory inputs all influence balance control in normal adults during slow oscillations similar to quiet stance. In contrast, somatosensory inputs appear to dominate postural control in response to transient surface perturbations (42).

What can we conclude from all of these studies? They suggest that all three senses contribute to postural control during quiet stance.

SENSORY STRATEGIES DURING PERTURBED STANCE

How do visual, vestibular, and somatosensory inputs contribute to postural control during recovery from a transient perturbation to balance? Let's look at some of the research examining this question.

Moving rooms, as we just described, have also been used to examine the contribution of visual inputs to recovery from transient perturbations. When abrupt room movements are made, young children (1-year-olds) compensate for this illusory loss of balance with motor responses designed to restore the vertical position. However, since there is no actual body sway, only the illusion of sway, motor responses have a destabilizing effect, causing the infants to stagger or fall in the direction of the room movement (38, 43). This indicates that vision may be a dominant input in compensating for transient perturbations in infants first learning to stand.

Interestingly, older children and adults typically do not show large sway responses to these movements, indicating that in adults, vision does not appear to play an important role in compensating for transient perturbations.

Muscle response latencies to visual cues signaling sway are quite slow, on the order of 200 msec, in contrast to the somatosensory responses that are activated in response to support surface translations (80 to 100 msec) (24, 44). Because somatosensory responses to support surface translations appear to be much faster than those triggered by vision, researchers have suggested that the nervous system preferentially relies on somatosensory inputs for controlling body sway when imbalance is caused by rapid displacements of the supporting surface.

What is the relative contribution of the vestibular system to postural responses to support surface perturbations? Experiments by Dietz and his colleagues indicate that the contribution of the vestibular system is much smaller than that of somatosensory inputs (44). In these experiments, the onset latency and amplitude of muscle responses were compared for two different types of perturbations of stance: (*a*) the support surface was moved forward or backward, stimulating somatosensory inputs; and (*b*) a forward or backward displacement of a load (2 kg) attached to the head was given, stimulating the vestibular system (the response was absent in patients with vestibular deficits). For comparable accelerations, muscle responses to vestibular signals were about 10 times smaller than the somatosensory responses induced by the displacement of the feet. This suggests that vestibular inputs play only a minor role in recovery of postural control when the support surface is displaced horizontally.

However, under certain conditions, vestibular and visual inputs are important in controlling responses to transient perturbations. For example, when the support surface is rotated toes-upward, stretching and activating

the gastrocnemius muscle, this response is destabilizing, pulling the body backward. Allum, a researcher from Switzerland, has shown that the subsequent compensatory response in the tibialis anterior muscle, used to restore balance, is activated by the visual and vestibular systems when the eyes are open. When the eyes are closed, it is primarily (80%) activated by the vestibular semicircular canals (21).

These studies, examining postural control in response to transient horizontal perturbations to stance, suggest that neurologically intact adults tend to rely on somatosensory inputs, in contrast to young children, who may rely more heavily on visual inputs.

Regardless of the task, no one sense by itself can provide the CNS with accurate information regarding the position and motion of the body in space in all circumstances. The ability of the nervous system to adapt its use of sensory information under changing task and environmental conditions is discussed in the next section.

ADAPTING SENSES FOR POSTURAL CONTROL

We live in a constantly changing environment. Adapting how we use the senses for postural control is a critical aspect of maintaining stability in a wide variety of environments, and has been studied by several researchers.

One approach to investigating how the CNS adapts multiple sensory inputs for postural control was developed by Nashner and coworkers. This approach uses a moving platform with a moving visual surround (20, 45). A simplified version of Nashner's protocol was developed by Shumway-Cook and Horak (46) to examine the role of sensory interaction in balance.

In Nashner's protocol, body sway is measured while the subject stands quietly under six different conditions that alter the availability and accuracy of visual and somatosensory inputs for postural orientation. In conditions 1–3, the subject stands on a normal surface with eyes open (1), eyes closed (2) or the visual surround moving with body sway

(3). Conditions 4–6 are identical to 1–3 except that the support surface now rotates with body sway as well. These conditions are shown in Figure 6.9. Differences in the amount of body sway in the different conditions are used to determine a subject's ability to adapt sensory information for postural control.

Many studies have examined the performance of normal subjects when sensory inputs for postural control are varied (45, 47, 48). Generally, these studies have shown that adults and children over the age of 7 easily maintain balance under all six conditions.

Average differences in body sway across the six sensory conditions within a large group of neurologically intact adults are shown in Figure 6.10. Adults sway the least in the conditions where support surface orientation inputs are accurately reporting the body's position in space relative to the surface regardless of the availability and accuracy of visual inputs (Conditions 1, 2, and 3). When support surface information is no longer available as an accurate source of orientation information, adults begin to sway more. The greatest amount of sway is seen in conditions 5 and 6, in which only one accurate set of inputs, the vestibular inputs, is available to mediate postural control (48).

This research suggests a number of things about how the CNS organizes and adapts sensory information for postural control. It supports the concept of hierarchical weighting of sensory inputs for posture based on their relative accuracy in reporting the body's position and movements in space.

In environments where a sense is not providing optimal or accurate information regarding the body's position, the *weight* given to that sense as a source of orientation is reduced, while the weight of other more accurate senses is increased. Because of the redundancy of senses available for orientation and the ability of the CNS to modify the relative importance of any one sense for postural control, individuals are able to maintain stability in a variety of environments.

In summary, postural control includes organizing multiple sensory inputs into sensory strategies for orientation. This process appears to involve the hierarchical ordering of sensory frames of reference, thereby ensuring that the most appropriate sense is selected for the environment and the task. Sensory strategies, that is, the relative weight given to a sense, vary as a function of age, task, and environment. It appears that under normal conditions, the nervous system may *weight* the importance of somatosensory information for postural control more heavily than vision/vestibular inputs.

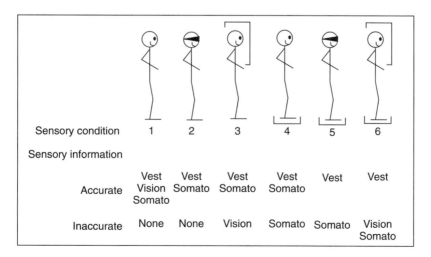

Figure 6.9. The six sensory conditions used to experimentally test how people adapt the senses to changing sensory conditions during the maintenance of stance posture. (Adapted from Horak F, Shumway-Cook A, Black FO. Are vestibular deficits responsible for developmental disorders in children. Insights into Otolaryngology 1988;3:2.)

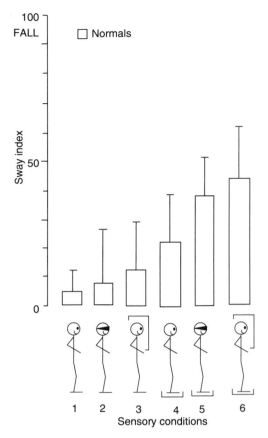

Figure 6.10. Body sway in the six sensory conditions used to test sensory adaptation during stance postural control. (Adapted from Woollacott MH, Shumway-Cook A, Nashner L. Aging and posture control: changes in sensory organization and muscular coordination. Int J Aging Hum Dev 1986;23:108.)

Adaptation to Rotational Support Surface Perturbations

Researchers have performed other types of experiments to explore postural adaptation. Rotational platform movements have been used to study the adaptation of postural responses to different conditions (20, 49, 50). For example, *toes-down* rotational platform movements cause stretch to the tibialis anterior muscles, activating the T-Q-A synergy, but when the synergy is first activated in this situation, it is inappropriate and serves to pull the subject more forward in the direction of the platform rotation. Studies indicate that subjects adapt the responses by attenuating

the response amplitude over a series of approximately 10 trials. It has thus been hypothesized that when subjects receive inaccurate sensory information from one sense (in this case, ankle joint inputs), they are able to compare that information to the other available sensory systems and then readjust the weighting of their sensory inputs driving postural responses, to shift to the remaining, accurate inputs.

Adapting Senses When Learning a New Task

Thus far, we have talked about reweighting sensory information in environments when it is not appropriate to use a particular sense for postural control. Similar reweighting of the senses appears to occur during the process of learning new motor skills. Lee and Lishman (38) found an increased weighting of visual inputs when adults were just learning a task. As the task became more automatic, there appeared to be a decrease in the relative importance of visual inputs for postural control and an increased weighting given to somatosensory inputs.

It has been suggested that adults recovering from a neurological lesion also rely predominantly on vision during the early part of the recovery process. As motor skills, including postural control, are regained, patients become less reliant on vision, and are more able to use somatosensory inputs (51).

Sensorimotor Adaptation

Up to this point in the chapter, we have presented sensory and motor aspects of postural control separately, but postural control is truly a *sensorimotor* task, requiring the coordination of sensory information with motor aspects of postural control. How we move influences how we sense, and in turn, how we sense affects how we move.

Researchers have found an important difference in how the senses are used depending on the type of movement strategy being used to restore stability. Effective use of the ankle strategy appears to depend on intact sensation from somatosensory inputs that report the body's position in space relative to the surface (52). In contrast, vestibular inputs are critical for executing the hip strategy (7). Thus, apparently, there is a relative change in weighting a particular sense, depending on how we move. These experiments emphasize the importance of adaptation in the postural system. To maintain orientation and stability in a wide range of tasks and environments, we are constantly called upon to modify how we sense and move. This capacity to adapt is a critical aspect of normal postural control and is heavily dependent upon experience and learning.

Anticipatory Postural Control

Did you ever pick up a box expecting it to be heavy and find it to be light? The fact that you lifted the box higher than you expected shows that your CNS preprogrammed force based on anticipation of what the task required. Based on previous experience with lifting other boxes of similar and different shapes and weights, the CNS forms a representation of what sensory and motor actions are needed to accomplish this task. It pretunes these systems for the task. Our mistakes are evidence that the CNS uses anticipatory processes in controlling action.

In the 1960s, scientists in Russia first began to explore the way we use posture in an anticipatory manner to steady the execution of our skilled movements. In a paper published in 1967 (53), Belen'kii, Gurfinkel, and Paltsev noted that when a standing adult is asked to raise the arm, both postural (leg and trunk) and prime mover (arm) muscles were activated. They observed that the postural muscle activation patterns could be divided into two parts. The first part was a preparatory phase, in which postural muscles were activated more than 50 msec in advance of the prime mover muscles, to compensate in advance for the destabilizing effects of the movement. The second part was a compensatory phase, in which the postural muscles were again activated after the prime movers, in a feedback manner, to additionally stabilize

the body. They found that the sequence of postural muscles activated, and thus the manner of preparing for the movement, was specific to the task.

After it was discovered that postural responses involved in feedback control of posture were organized into distinct synergies (23), an important question was raised: Are the synergies used in feedback postural control the same synergies that are used in anticipatory posture control? To answer this question, Cordo and Nashner (54) performed experiments in which they asked standing subjects to forcefully push or pull on a handle, in a reaction-time task. They found that the same postural response synergies used in standing balance control were activated in an anticipatory fashion before the arm movements. For example, when a person is asked to pull on a handle, first the gastrocnemius, hamstrings, and trunk extensors are activated, and then the prime mover, the biceps of the arm.

One feature of postural adjustments associated with movement is their adaptability to the conditions of the task. In the aforementioned experiment (54), when the subjects leaned forward against a horizontal bar at chest height, the leg postural adjustments were reduced or disappeared. Thus, there is an immediate preselection of the postural muscles as a function of their ability to contribute appropriate support.

Though we usually think of anticipatory adjustments in terms of activating postural muscles in advance of a skilled movement, we also use anticipation in scaling the amplitude of postural adjustments depending on the size or amplitude of the perturbation we expect.

Horak et al. (55) examined the influence of prior experience and central set on the characteristics of postural adjustments by giving subjects platform perturbations under the following conditions: (a) serial vs. random conditions, (b) expected vs. unexpected conditions, and (c) practiced vs. unpracticed conditions. They found that expectation played a large factor in modulating the amplitude of postural responses. For example, subjects overresponded when they expected a larger perturbation than they received, and under-responded when they expected a smaller one.

Practice also caused a reduction in postural response magnitude and in the amplitude of antagonist muscle responses. However, central set did not affect EMG onset latencies. The authors noted that when different perturbations were presented in random order, all scaling disappeared. Evidently, scaling of postural responses is based on our anticipation of what is needed in a given situation.

It is important to realize that anticipatory postural adjustments are not isolated to tasks we perform while standing.

⊚ ACTIVE LEARNING MODULE

For example, right now, you can test this with a partner. First, take a heavy book in one hand, and ask your partner to lift it off that hand. What did the hand holding the book do? Was it steady? Or did it move upward as the book was lifted off? Now, put the book back on your hand, and lift it off with your other hand. What happened now? Was it steady? What you may have noticed is that you are able to use anticipatory postural adjustments when you are lifting the book out of your own hand, so that your hand does not involuntarily move upward, while you cannot use these adjustments when someone else is lifting the same book from your hand.

Scientists from France and Switzerland, Hugon, Massion, and Wiesendanger (56), first made this discovery in experiments in which they measured the EMGs of the biceps of both the left and right arms during a modification of the task just mentioned. In this case, either the subject or the experimenter lifted a 1 kg weight from the subject's forearm (Fig. 6.11). They found that in the active unloading of the arm by the subject, there was preparatory biceps muscle inhibition to keep the arm from moving upward when it was unloaded. The anticipatory reduction in the biceps EMG of the arm holding the load is time-locked with the onset of the activation of the biceps of the lifting arm. This reduction was not observed in the *passive* unloading condition.

How are these anticipatory postural adjustments associated with movements centrally organized? Animal experiments have been performed

by Massion and his colleagues to look at this question in more detail (57). They trained animals to perform a leg-lifting task that required the animal to simultaneously activate postural muscles in the other three legs when they lifted the prime mover leg. They found that they could also directly stimulate the motor cortex or the red nucleus in the area of the forelimb flexors and produce the leg-lifting movement. When they did this, the movement was always accompanied by a postural adjustment in the other limbs, initiated in a feedforward manner. They hypothesized that the postural adjustments are organized at the bulbospinal level, and that the pyramidal tract activates these pathways as it sends descending commands to the prime mover. Massion suggests that, while the basic mechanisms for postural adjustments could be organized at this level, they appear to be modulated by several other parts of the nervous system, including the cerebellum.

SEATED POSTURAL CONTROL

The maintenance of postural control in the seated position has not been studied to the extent of stance postural control. However, many scientists believe that concepts important for stance postural control will be shown to be equally valid for understanding the control of seated posture.

A recent study was performed to compare the postural responses elicited by platform translations vs. rotations of subjects seated with the legs extended forward (58). The authors noted that forward platform movements, causing the body to sway backward, elicited well-organized, consistent responses in the quadriceps, abdominal and neck flexor muscles at 63 ± 12 msec, 74 ± 21 msec, and 77 ± 10 msec, respectively. Similar responses were elicited by legs-up rotations. However, in response to backward platform perturbations, causing forward sway, smaller and more variable responses were elicited in the trunk and neck extensor muscles. These differences reflect the asymmetry of the stability limits during sitting.

The authors suggest that the postural control system sets a threshold for activation of postural responses according to an internal representation of the body, including the re-

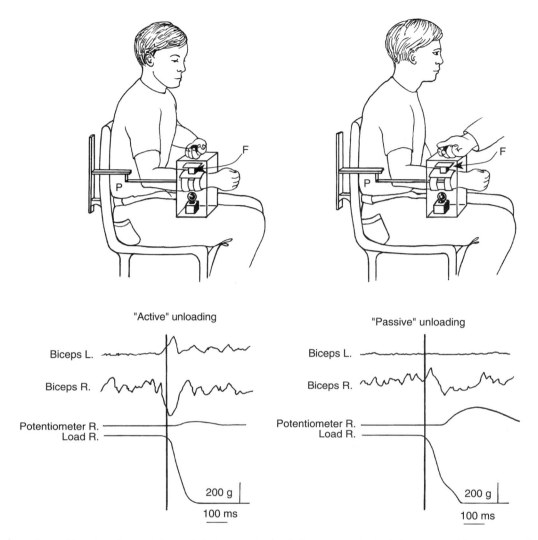

Figure 6.11. Experiments examining anticipatory postural activity associated with lifting a weight from a subject's arm. (Adapted from Hugon M, Massion J, Wiesendanger M. Anticipatory postural changes induced by active unloading and comparison with passive unloading in man. Pflugers Arch 1982;393:292–296.)

lationship between the center of gravity and the support surface. Since the rotational and translational perturbations caused very different head movements, but very similar muscle response patterns, the authors conclude that somatosensory inputs from the backward rotation of the pelvis trigger the postural response synergies in sitting.

Experiments have also been performed to examine the characteristics of anticipatory postural adjustments used in reaching for an object while sitting (59). Researchers found

that increased reach distance and decreased support were associated with earlier, larger postural adjustments. It has also been shown that leg muscles are consistently active during anticipatory postural adjustments in advance of voluntary reaching while sitting (60).

SUMMARY

1. The task of postural control involves controlling the body's position in space for (a) stability, defined as controlling the center of

body mass within the base of support, and (b) orientation, defined as the ability to maintain an appropriate relationship between the body segments, and between the body and the environment for a task.

2. A number of factors contribute to postural control during quiet stance (so-called static balance), including (a) body alignment, which minimizes the effect of gravitational forces, (b) muscle tone, and (c) postural tone, which keeps the body from collapsing in response to the pull of gravity.

3. When quiet stance is perturbed, the recovery of stability requires movement strategies that are effective in controlling the center of mass relative to the base of support.

4. Movement patterns used to recover stance balance from sagittal plane instability are referred to as ankle, hip, and suspensory/or stepping strategies. Normal subjects can shift relatively quickly from one postural movement strategy to another.

5. The CNS activates synergistic muscles at mechanically related joints, possibly to ensure that forces generated at one joint for balance control do not produce instability elsewhere in the body.

6. Inputs from visual, somatosensory (proprioceptive, cutaneous, and joint receptors), and vestibular systems are important sources of information about the body's position and movement in space with respect to gravity and the environment. Each sense provides the CNS with a different kind of information about position and motion of the body; thus, each sense provides a different *frame of reference* for postural control.

7. In adults, all three senses contribute to postural control during quiet stance; in contrast, in response to transient perturbations, adults tend to rely on somatosensory inputs, while young children rely more heavily on visual inputs.

8. Because of the redundancy of senses available for orientation and the ability of the CNS to modify the importance of any one sense for postural control, individuals are able to maintain stability in a variety of environments.

9. Postural adjustments are also activated before voluntary movements to minimize potential disturbances to balance that the movement may cause. This is called anticipatory postural control.

10. The maintenance of postural control in the seated position has not been studied in depth. However, many scientists believe that concepts important for stance postural control will be shown to be equally valid for the control of seated posture.

REFERENCES

1. Shumway-Cook A. Equilibrium deficits in children. In: Woollacott M, Shumway-Cook A, eds. Development of posture and gait across the life span. Columbia, SC: University of South Carolina Press, 1989:229–252.

2. Woollacott M, Shumway-Cook A. Changes in posture control across the life span: a systems approach. Phys Ther 1990;70:799–807.

3. Horak F, Shumway-Cook A. Clinical implications of postural control research. In: Duncan P, ed. Balance: proceedings of the APTA Forum. Alexandria, VA: APTA, 1990:105–111.

4. Shumway-Cook A, Horak F. Balance rehabilitation in the neurologic patient: course syllabus. Seattle: NERA, 1992.

5. McCollum G, Leen T. The form and exploration of mechanical stability limits in erect stance. Journal of Motor Behavior 1989; 21:225–238.

6. Shumway-Cook A, Horak F. Vestibular rehabilitation: an exercise approach to managing symptoms of vestibular dysfunction. Seminars in Hearing 1989;10:196.

7. Horak F, Shupert C. The role of the vestibular system in postural control. In: Herdman S, ed. Vestibular rehabilitation. New York: FA Davis, 1994:22–46.

8. Shumway-Cook A, McCollum G. Assessment and treatment of balance disorders in the neurologic patient. In: Montgomery T, Connolly B, eds. Motor control and physical therapy: theoretical framework and practical applications. Chattanooga, TN: Chattanooga Corp. 1990:123–138.

9. Roberts TDM. Neurophysiology of postural mechanisms. London: Butterworths, 1979.

10. Basmajian JV, DeLuca C. Muscles alive. 5th ed. Baltimore: Williams & Wilkins, 1985.

11. Kendall FP, McCreary EK. Muscles: testing and function. 3rd ed. Baltimore: Williams & Wilkins, 1983.

12. Schenkman M, Butler RB. "Automatic Postural Tone" in posture, movement, and func-

tion. Forum on physical therapy issues related to cerebrovascular accident. Alexandria, VA: APTA, 1992:16–21.

13. Hoyle G. Muscles and their neural control. NY: John Wiley & Sons, 1983.

14. Gurfinkel VS, Lipshits MI, Popov KE. Is the stretch reflex the main mechanism in the system of regulation of the vertical posture of man? Biophysics 1974;19:761–766.

15. Ghez C. Posture. In: Kandel ER, Schwartz JH, Jessell TM, eds. Principles of neural science. 3rd ed. NY: Elsevier, 1991:596–607.

16. Anderson ME, Binder MD. Spinal and supraspinal control of movement and posture. In: Patton HD, Fuchs AF, Hille B, Scher AM, Steiner R. Textbook of physiology, vol. 1: Excitable cells and neurophysiology. Philadelphia: WB Saunders, 1989:563–581.

17. Massion J, Woollacott M. Normal balance and postural control. In: Bronstein AM, Brandt T, Woollacott M. Clinical aspects of balance and gait disorders. London: Edward Arnold. In press.

18. Bobath B. Adult hemiplegia: evaluation and treatment. London: Heinemann, 1978.

19. Davies PM. Steps to follow. New York: Springer-Verlag, 1985.

20. Nashner L. Adapting reflexes controlling the human posture. Exp Brain Res 1976;26:59–72.

21. Allum JHJ, Pfaltz CR. Visual and vestibular contributions to pitch sway stabilization in the ankle muscles of normals and patients with bilateral peripheral vestibular deficits. Exp Brain Res 1985;58:82–94.

22. Diener HC, Dichgans J, Bruzek W, Selinka H. Stabilization of human posture during induced oscillations of the body. Exp Brain Res 1982;45:126–132.

23. Nashner LM. Fixed patterns of rapid postural responses among leg muscles during stance. Exp Brain Res 1977;30:13–24.

24. Nashner L, Woollacott M. The organization of rapid postural adjustments of standing humans: an experimental-conceptual model. In: Talbott RE, Humphrey DR, eds. Posture and movement. NY: Raven Press, 1979:243–257.

25. Horak F, Nashner L. Central programming of postural movements: adaptation to altered support surface configurations. J Neurophysiol 1986;55:1369–1381.

26. Nashner LM. Sensory, neuromuscular, and biomechanical contributions to human balance. In: Duncan P, ed. Balance: Proceedings of the APTA Forum. Alexandria, VA: APTA, 1989:5–12.

27. Horak F, Shupert C, Mirka A. Components of postural dyscontrol in the elderly: a review. Neurobiol Aging 1989;10:727–745.

28. Woollacott M, Roseblad B, Hofsten von C. Relation between muscle response onset and body segmental movements during postural perturbations in humans. Exp Brain Res 1988;72:593–604.

29. Sveistrup H, Massion J, Moore S, Hu MH, Woollacott MH. Are there differences in postural support strategies for simple balance tasks vs. tasks requiring precise hand stabilization? Neuroscience Abstracts 1991; 17:1388.

30. Moore S, Sveistrup H, Massion M, Hu M-H, Woollacott MH. Postural control strategies for simultaneous control tasks. In: Woollacott M, Horak F, eds. Posture and gait: control mechanisms. Eugene, OR: Univ. of Oregon Press, 1992:218–221.

31. MacPherson J. The neural organization of postural control—do muscle synergies exist? In: Amblard B, Berthoz A, Clarac F, eds. Posture and gait: development, adaptation and modulation. Amsterdam: Elsevier, 1988: 381–390.

32. Moore SP, Rushmer DS, Windus SL, Nashner LM. Human automatic postural responses: responses to horizontal perturbations of stance in multiple directions. Exp Brain Res 1988;73:648–658.

33. Hirschfeld H. On the integration of posture, locomotion and voluntary movement in humans: normal and impaired development. Dissertation. Karolinska Institute, Stockholm, Sweden, 1992.

34. Gurfinkel VS, Levick Yu S. Perceptual and automatic aspects of the postural body scheme. In: Paillard J, ed. Brain and space. NY: Oxford Science Publishers, 1991.

35. Paillard J. Cognitive versus sensorimotor encoding of spatial information. In: Ellen P, Thinus-Blanc C, eds. Cognitive processes and spatial orientation in animal and man. Dordrecht: Martinus Nijhoff Publishers BV, 1987:43–77.

36. Roll, JP, Roll R. From eye to foot: a proprioceptive chain involved in postural control. In: Amblard B, Berthoz A, Clarac F, eds. Posture and gait: development, adaptation and modulation. Amsterdam: Elsevier, 1988:155–164.

37. Romberg MH. Manual of nervous diseases of man. London: Sydenham Society, 1853:395–401.

38. Lee DN, Lishman R. Visual proprioceptive control of stance. Journal of Human Movement Studies 1975;1:87–95.

39. Butterworth G, Hicks L. Visual proprioception and postural stability in infancy: a developmental study. Perception 1977;6: 255–262.

40. Butterworth G, Pope M. Origine et fonction de la proprioception visuelle chez le enfant. In: de Schonen S, ed. Le developpement dans la premiere annee. Paris: Presses Universitaires de France, 1983:107–128.

41. Brandt T, Wenzel D, Dichgans J. Die Entwicklung der visuellen Stabilisation des aufrechten standes bein kind: Ein refezeichen in der kinderneurologie (Visual stabilization of free stance in infants: a sign of maturity). Arch Psychiat Nervenkr 1976;223:1–13.

42. Diener HC, Dichgans J, Guschlbauer B, Bacher M. Role of visual and static vestibular influences on dynamic posture control. Human Neurobiology 1986;5:105–113.

43. Lee DN, Aronson E. Visual proprioceptive control of standing in human infants. Perceptual Psychophysiology 1974;15:529–532.

44. Dietz M, Trippel M, Horstmann GA. Significance of proprioceptive and vestibulo-spinal reflexes in the control of stance and gait. In: Patla AE, ed. Adaptability of human gait. Elsevier:Amsterdam, 1991:37–52.

45. Nashner LM. Adaptation of human movement to altered environments. Trends in Neuroscience 1982;358-61.

46. Shumway-Cook A, Horak F. Assessing the influence of sensory interaction on balance. Phys Ther 1986;66:1548–1550.

47. Woollacott MH, Shumway-Cook A, Nashner L. Aging and posture control: changes in sensory organization and muscular coordination. Int J Aging Hum Dev 1986;23:97–114.

48. Peterka RJ, Black FO. Age related changes in human posture control: sensory organization tests. J Vest Res 1990;1:73–85.

49. Keshner E, Allum J. Plasticity in pitch sway stabilization: Normal habituation and compensation for peripheral vestibular deficits. In: Bles W, Brandt T, eds. Disorders of posture and gait. New York: Elsevier, 1986:289–314.

50. Hansen PD, Woollacott MH, Debu B. Postural responses to changing task conditions. Exp Brain Res 1988;73:627–636.

51. Mulder T, Berndt H, Pauwels J, Nienhuis B. Sensorimotor adaptability in the elderly and disabled. In: Stelmach G, Homberg V, eds. Sensori-motor impairment in the elderly. Dordrecht: Kluwer, 1993.

52. Horak F, Diener H, Nashner L. Postural strategies associated with somatosensory and vestibular loss. Exp Brain Res 1991;82:167–177.

53. Belen'kii VY, Gurfinkel VS, Paltsev YI. Elements of control of voluntary movements. Biofizika 1967;12:135–141.

54. Cordo P, Nashner L. Properties of postural adjustments associated with rapid arm movements. J Neurophysiol 1982;47:287–302.

55. Horak F, Diener HC, Nashner LM. Influence of central set on human postural responses. J Neurophysiol 1989;62:841–853.

56. Hugon M, Massion J, Wiesendanger M. Anticipatory postural changes induced by active unloading and comparison with passive unloading in man. Pflugers Arch 1982; 393:292–296.

57. Massion J. Role of motor cortex in postural adjustments associated with movement. In: Asanuma H, Wilson VJ, eds. Integration in the nervous system. Tokyo-New York: Igaku-Shoin, 1979:239–260.

58. Forssberg H, Hirschfeld H. Postural adjustments in sitting humans following external perturbations: muscle activity and kinematics. Exp Brain Res 1994;97:515–527.

59. Moore S, Brunt D, Nesbitt ML, Juarez T. Investigation of evidence for anticipatory postural adjustments in seated subjects who performed a reaching task. Phys Ther 1992; 72:335–343.

60. Shepherd RB, Crosbie J, Squires T. The contribution of the ipsilateral leg to postural adjustments during fast voluntary reaching in sitting. Abstract of International Society for Biomechanics, 14th Congress 1993, Paris.

61. Gronley JK, Perry J. Gait analysis techniques: Rancho Los Amigos Hospital gait laboratory. Phys Ther 1984;64:1831–1837.

62. Winter DA. Biomechanics and motor control of human movement. New York: John Wiley & Sons, 1990.

Chapter 7

DEVELOPMENT OF POSTURAL CONTROL

INTRODUCTION

During the early years of life, the child develops an incredible repertoire of skills, including crawling, independent walking and running, climbing, eye-hand coordination, and the manipulation of objects in a variety of ways. The emergence of all of these skills requires the development of postural activity to support the primary movement.

To understand the emergence of mobility and manipulatory skills in children, therapists need to understand the postural substrate for these skills. Similarly, understanding the best therapeutic approach for a child with difficulties in walking or reaching skills requires the knowledge of any limitations in their postural abilities. Understanding the basis for postural control, then, is the first step in determining the best therapeutic approach for improving related skills.

This chapter discusses the research on the development of postural control and how it contributes to the emergence of stability and mobility skills. Later chapters consider the implications of this research when assessing postural control.

Postural Control and Development

Let's first look at some of the evidence showing that postural control is a critical part of motor development. Research on early development has shown that the simultaneous development of the postural, locomotor, and manipulative systems is essential to the emergence and refinement of skills in all these areas. In the neonate, when the chaotic movements of the head that regularly disturb the infant's seated balance are stabilized, movements and behaviors normally seen in more mature infants emerge (1). For example, as shown in Figure 7.1, the newborn may begin

143

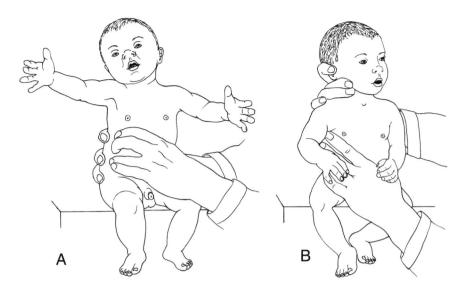

Figure 7.1.   Stabilizing the head in a neonate can produce dramatic changes in behavior. **A,** Uncontrolled movements of the head produce a Moro response. **B,** External support to the child's head and trunk result in more mature behaviors including attending to people and objects, and even reaching. (Adapted from Amiel-Tison C, Grenier A. Neurological evaluation of the human infant. New York: Masson, 1980:81.)

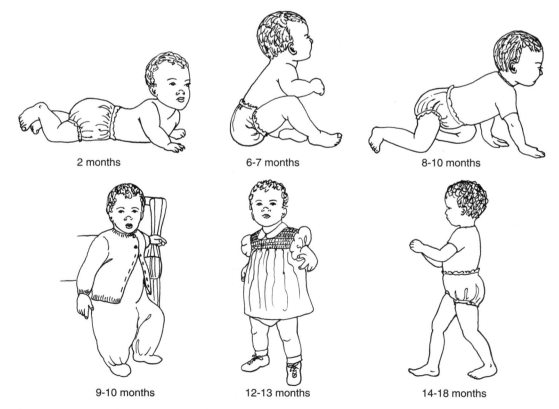

Figure 7.2.   Motor milestones that emerge with the development of postural control. (Adapted from Shumway-Cook A, Woollacott M. Theoretical issues in assessing postural control. In: Wilhelm I, ed. Physical therapy assessment in early infancy. NY: Churchill Livingstone, 1993:163.)

to attend to the examiner, reach for objects, and maintain his arms at his sides, with the fingers open, suggesting inhibition of the grasp and Moro reflexes.

These results support the concept that an immature postural system is a limiting factor or a *constraint* on the emergence of other behaviors such as coordinated arm and hand movements, as well as the inhibition of reflexes. It has also been suggested that delayed or abnormal development of the postural system may also constrain a child's ability to develop independence in mobility and manipulatory skills.

Motor Milestones and Emerging Postural Control

The development of postural control has been traditionally associated with a predictable sequence of motor behaviors referred to as *motor milestones*. Some of the major motor milestones in development are shown in Figure 7.2. They include crawling, sitting, creeping, pull-to-stand, independent stance, and walking. The sequence and timing of the emergence of these motor milestones has been well described by several developmental researchers.

In 1946, Arnold Gesell, a pediatrician, described the emergence of general patterns of behavior in the first few years of life. He noted the general direction of behavioral development as moving from head to foot, and from proximal to distal within segments. Thus, he formulated the *law of developmental direction* (2).

In addition, Gesell portrayed development as a spiralling hierarchy. He suggested that the development of skilled behavior does not follow a strict linear sequence, always advancing, constantly improving with time and maturity. Instead, Gesell believed that development is much more dynamic in nature and seems to be characterized by alternating advancement and regression in ability to perform skills.

Gesell gave the example of children learning to crawl and then creep. Initially, in learning to crawl, the child uses a primarily symmetrical arm pattern, eventually switching to a more complex alternating arm pattern as the skill of crawling is perfected. When the child first begins to creep, there is a return to the symmetrical arm pattern. Eventually, as creeping becomes perfected, the emergence of an alternating arm pattern occurs.

Thus, as children progress to each new stage in the development of a skill, they may appear to regress to an earlier form of the behavior as new, more mature and adaptive, versions of these skills emerge.

Most of the traditional assessment scales created to evaluate the emergence of motor behaviors use developmental norms established by McGraw (3) and Gesell. Using these scales, the therapist evaluates the performance of the infant or child on functional skills that require postural control. These skills include sitting, standing, walking unsupported, reaching forward, and moving from sitting to standing position. Evaluations follow normal development and are used to identify children at risk for developmental problems.

THEORIES OF DEVELOPING POSTURAL CONTROL

What is the basis for the development of postural control underlying this predictable sequence of motor behaviors? Several theories of child development try to relate neural structure and behavior in developing infants. Classic theories of child development place great importance on a reflex substrate for the emergence of mature human behavior patterns. This means that in the normal child the emergence of posture and movement control is dependent on the appearance and subsequent integration of reflexes. According to these theories, the appearance and disappearance of these reflexes reflect the increasing maturity of cortical structures that inhibit and integrate reflexes controlled at lower levels within the CNS into more functional postural and voluntary motor responses (refer to Fig. 1.6 in Chapter 1). This classic theory has been referred to as a reflex/hierarchy theory (4, 5).

Alternatively, more recent theories of motor control, such as the systems, ecological, and dynamic theories, have suggested that posture control emerges from a complex interaction of musculoskeletal and neural systems collectively referred to as the postural control system. The organization of elements within the postural control system is determined both by the task and the environment. Systems theory does not deny the existence of reflexes, but considers them as only one of many influences on the control of posture and movement.

Let's briefly review the reflexes that have been associated with the emergence of postural control.

Reflex-Hierarchical Theory of Postural Control

Postural reflexes were studied in the early part of this century by investigators such as Magnus (6), DeKleijn (7), Rademaker (8), and Schaltenbrand (9). In this early work, researchers selectively lesioned different parts of the CNS and examined an animal's capacity to orient. Magnus and associates took the animal down to what they referred to as the *zero condition*, a condition in which no postural reflex activity could be elicited. Subsequent animals underwent selective lesions, leaving systematically greater and greater amounts of the CNS intact. In this way, Magnus identified individually and collectively all the reflexes that worked cooperatively to maintain postural orientation in various types of animals.

Postural reflexes in animals were classified by Magnus as local static reactions, segmental static reactions, general static reactions, and righting reactions. **Local static reactions** stiffen the animal's limb for support of body weight against gravity. **Segmental static reactions** involve more than one body segment, and include the flexor withdrawal reflex, and the crossed extensor reflex. **General static reactions**, called *attitudinal reflexes*, involve changes in position of the whole body in response to changes in head position. Finally, Magnus described a series of five **righting reactions**, which allowed the animal to assume or resume a species specific orientation of the body with respect to its environment.

POSTURAL REFLEXES IN HUMAN DEVELOPMENT

Examination of reflexes has become an essential part of the study of motor development. Many researchers have tried to document accurately the time frame for appearance and disappearance of these reflexes in normal children, with widely varying results. There is little agreement on the presence and time course of these reflexes, or on the significance of these reflexes to normal and abnormal development (10).

Figure 7.3 summarizes the results from a number of studies examining the presence

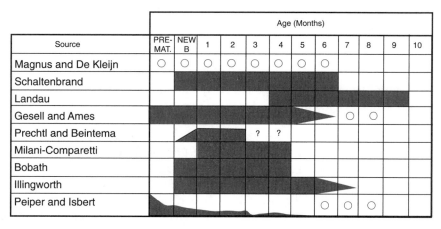

Figure 7.3. A summary of various studies that examined the presence and time-course of the asymmetric tonic neck reflex in normal development. O = reflex not present. (Adapted from Capute AJ, Accardo PJ, Vining EPG, et al. Primitive reflex profile. Baltimore: University Park Press, 1978:36.)

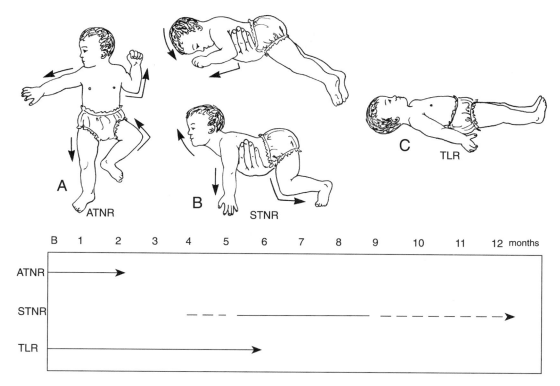

Figure 7.4.   The attitudinal reflexes. **A**, The ATNR reflex produces extension in the *face* arm, and flexion in the *skull* arm when the head is turned. **B**, The STNR reflex results in extension in the upper extremities and flexion in the lower extremities when the head is extended. **C**, The tonic labyrinthine reflex produces an increase in extensor tone when the body is supine, and flexion when prone. Also shown is the time-course for these reflexes. (Adapted from Barnes MR, Crutchfield CA, Heriza CB. The neurophysiological basis of patient treatment. Morgantown, W VA:Stokesville Publishing, 1978:222.)

and time course of the asymmetric tonic neck reflex in normal development. This chart shows obvious disagreement over whether the reflex is present in infancy, and regarding the time course for its appearance and disappearance.

Attitudinal Reflexes

According to the reflex theory of postural control, tonic attitudinal reflexes produce persisting changes in body posture, which result from a change in head position. These reflexes are not obligatory in normal children, but have been reported in children with various types of neural pathology. These reflexes include (*a*) the **asymmetric tonic neck reflex** (ATNR) (Fig. 7.4*A*), (*b*) the **symmetric tonic neck reflex** (STRR) (Fig. 7.4*B*),

and (*c*) the **tonic labyrinthine reflex** (TLR) (Fig. 7.4*C*) (11).

Righting Reactions

According to a reflex-hierarchical model, the interaction of five righting reactions produces orientation of the head in space, and orientation of the body in relationship to the head and ground. Righting reactions are considered automatic reactions that enable a person to assume the normal standing position and maintain stability when changing positions (12).

The three righting reactions that orient the head in space include (*a*) the **optical righting reaction** (Fig. 7.5*A*), which contributes to the reflex orientation of the head using visual inputs; (*b*) the **labyrinthine**

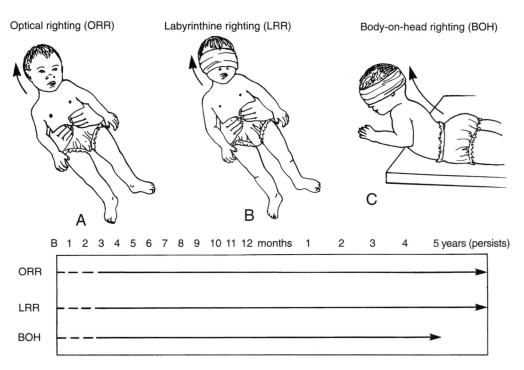

Figure 7.5.   The righting reactions that orient the head. **A,** The optical righting reaction orients the head to vision. **B,** The labyrinthine righting reaction orients the head in response to vestibular signals. **C,** The body-on-head righting reaction uses tactile and neck proprioceptive information to orient the head. Also shown is the time-course for these reflexes. (Adapted from Barnes MR, Crutchfield CA, Heriza CB. The neurophysiological basis of patient treatment. Morgantown, W VA:Stokesville Publishing, 1978:222.)

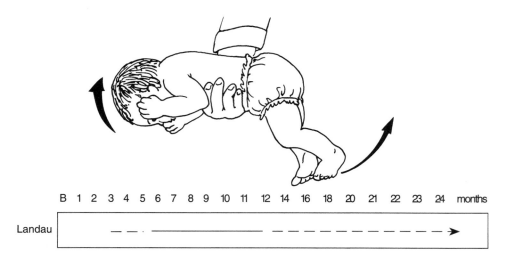

Figure 7.6.   Shown is the Landau reaction and its time-course during development, which combines the effects of all three head-righting reactions. (Adapted from Barnes MR, Crutchfield CA, Heriza CB. The neurophysiological basis of patient treatment. Morgantown, W VA:Stokesville Publishing, 1978:222.)

righting reaction (Fig. 7.5*B*), which orients the head to an upright vertical position in response to vestibular signals (9, 13, 14); and (*c*) the **body-on-head righting reaction** (Fig. 7.5*C*), which orients the head in response to proprioceptive and tactile signals from the body in contact with a supporting surface. The **Landau reaction,** shown in Figure 7.6, combines the effects of all three head-righting reactions (9, 15).

Two reflexes interact to keep the body oriented with respect to the head and the surface. The **neck-on-body righting reaction,** shown in Figure 7.7*A*, orients the body in response to cervical afferents, which report changes in the position of the head and neck. Two forms of this reflex have been reported: an immature form, resulting in log rolling, which is present at birth, and a mature form producing segmental rotation of the body (16). The **body-on-body righting reaction,** shown in Figure 7.7*B*, keeps the body oriented with respect to the ground, regardless of the position of the head.

Balance and Protective Reactions

According to reflex-hierarchical theory, balance control emerges in association with a sequentially organized series of equilibrium reactions. Balance reactions are often separated into three categories. The **tilting reactions**, shown in Figure 7.8 *A–C*, are used for controlling the center of gravity in response to a tilting surface. **Postural fixation reactions**, shown in Figure 7.9*A–C*, are used to recover from forces applied to the other parts of the body (17). **Parachute or protective responses** protect the body from injury during a fall and are shown in Figure 7.10*A–C* (12).

Table 7.1 summarizes the *postural reflex mechanism* purported to underlie the emergence of postural and balance control in children.

Many investigators have suggested that emerging balance reactions are necessary precursors to the acquisition of associated developmental milestones; however, perfection of

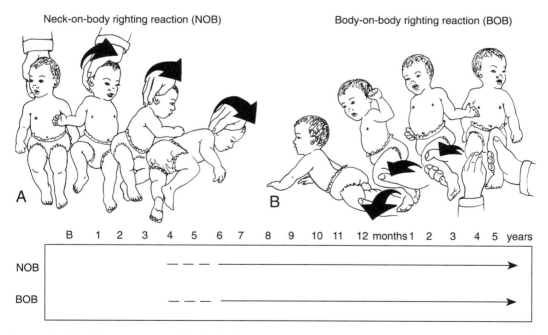

Figure 7.7. The righting reactions of the body. Shown are the mature form of **A**, the neck-on-body (NOB) righting reaction and **B**, the body-on-body (BOB), and their time-course for emergence. (Adapted from Barnes MR, Crutchfield CA, Heriza CB. The neurophysiological basis of patient treatment. Morgantown, W VA: Stokesville Publishing, 1978:222.)

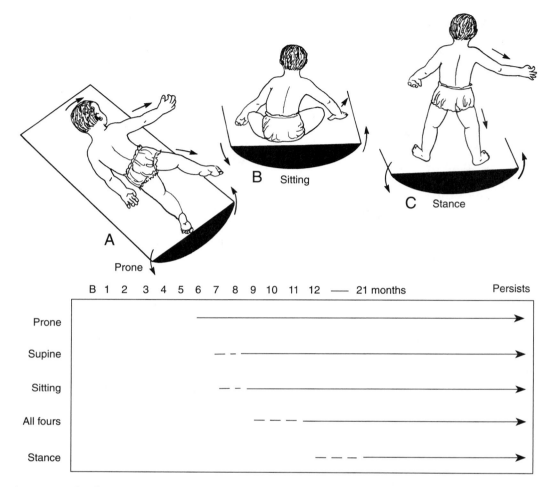

Figure 7.8. The tilting reactions. Tilting responses are purported to emerge first in **A**, prone, then supine (not shown), then **B**, sitting, then emerge in all fours (not shown) and finally **C**, standing. Also shown is the time-course for these reflexes. (Adapted from Barnes MR, Crutchfield CA, Heriza CB. The neurophysiological basis of patient treatment. Morgantown, W VA:Stokesville Publishing, 1978:222.)

the tilting reaction does not occur until the child has moved onto the next developmental milestone (18–20).

ROLE OF REFLEXES IN DEVELOPMENT

What is the role of reflexes in motor development? Scientists do not know for sure; as a result, the role of reflexes in motor control is controversial. Many theorists believe that reflexes form the substrate for normal motor control. For example, it has been suggested that the *asymmetric tonic neck reflex* is part of the developmental process of eye-hand coor-

dination since movement of the head (and eyes) brings the hand within view (21, 22). However, another study showed no relationship between reaching behavior and the presence or absence of this reflex in a 2- to 4-month-old group of infants (23). Various researchers have intimated that the asymmetric tonic neck reflex contributes to movements in adults since there is facilitation of extension in the extremities when the head is rotated (24–27).

The neck-on-body and body-on-body righting reactions are reported to be the basis for rolling in infants. An immature form of rolling at 4 months of age is purported to be

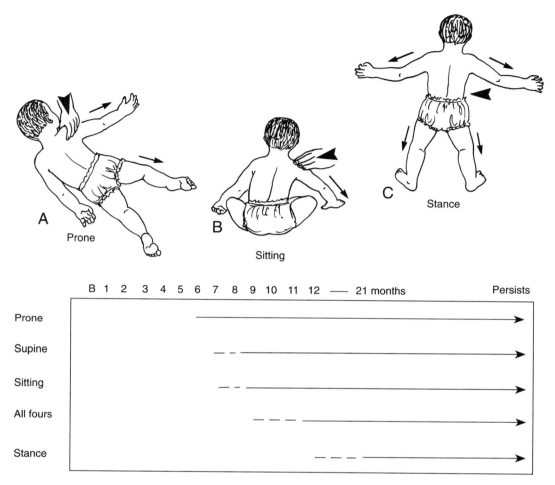

Figure 7.9. The postural fixation reactions. Fixation reactions stabilize the body in response to destabilizing forces applied to the body from anywhere but the supporting surface, and emerge in parallel to the tilting reactions. Shown are reactions in **A**, prone, **B**, sitting, and **C**, stance. Also shown is the time-course for these reflexes. (Adapted from Barnes MR, Crutchfield CA, Heriza CB. The neurophysiological basis of patient treatment. Morgantown, W VA: Stokesville Publishing, 1978:222.)

predictive of CNS pathology, including cerebral palsy (28) and developmental delay (29). The role of these reflexes in more mature rolling patterns has recently been questioned (30).

Clearly, there is considerable uncertainty about the contribution of reflex testing in clarifying the basis for normal and abnormal development in children.

New Models of Development

Many of the newer theories of motor control presented in Chapter 1 have associ-ated theories of motor development. These newer theories are consistent in suggesting that development involves much more than the maturation of reflexes within the CNS. Development is a complex process, with new behaviors and skills emerging from an inter-action of the child (and its maturing nervous and musculoskeletal system) with the environment.

With this framework, the emergence of postural control is likewise ascribed to com-plex interactions between neural and muscu-loskeletal systems. These include (please refer back to Fig. 6.2):

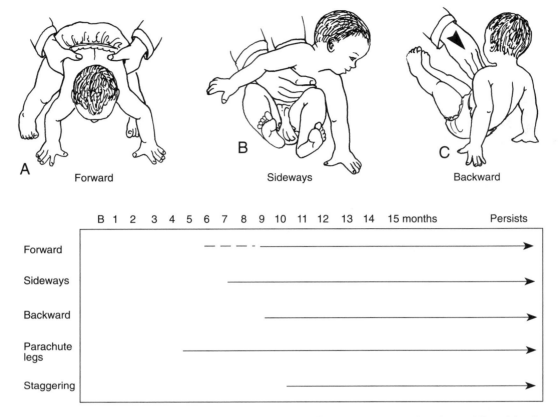

Figure 7.10. The protective reactions. These reactions protect the body from injury resulting from a fall, and develop first **A**, in the forward direction, then **B**, sideways, and **C**, backwards. Also shown is the time-course for these reflexes. (Adapted from Barnes MR, Crutchfield CA, Heriza CB. The neurophysiological basis of patient treatment. Morgantown, W VA:Stokesville Publishing, 1978:222.)

1. Changes in the musculoskeletal system, including development of muscle strength and changes in relative mass of the different body segments;
2. Development or construction of the co-ordinative structures or neuromuscular response synergies used in maintaining balance;
3. Development of individual sensory systems including somatosensory, visual, or vestibular systems;
4. Development of sensory strategies for organizing these multiple inputs;
5. Development of internal representations important in the mapping of perception to action;
6. Development of adaptive and anticipatory mechanisms that allow children to modify the way they sense and move for postural control (31).

Apparently, an important part of interpreting senses and coordinating actions for postural control is the presence of an internal representation or *body schema* providing a postural frame of reference. It has been hypothesized that this postural frame of reference is used as a comparison for incoming sensory inputs, as an essential part of interpreting self-motion, and to calibrate motor actions (32).

Development of sensory and motor aspects of postural control has been hypothesized to involve the capacity to build up appropriate internal representations related to posture, which reflect the rules for organizing sensory inputs and coordinating them with motor actions. For example, as the child gains experience moving in a gravity environment, sensory-motor maps would develop. These maps would relate actions to incoming sen-

Table 7.1 Reflex Model of Postural Development

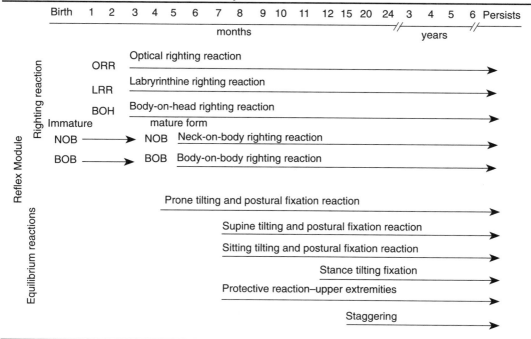

sory inputs from vision, somatosensory, and vestibular systems. In this way, rules for moving would develop and be reflected in altered synaptic relationships. Thus, researchers argue, the path from sensation to motor actions proceeds via an internal representational structure or body schema (32, 33).

ASSESSMENT BASED ON NEWER MODELS

According to these newer theories, assessment of early motor development includes the evaluation of both emerging behavioral motor milestones and the supporting systems for postural control. In addition, evaluation must occur within the context of different tasks and environments. The child's capacity to anticipate and adapt to a changing environment, as evidenced by variability of performance, is also included in an analysis of development. The ability to adapt how we sense and how we move is a critical part of normal development. As a result, it is as crucial to assess as the acquisition of stereotypical motor milestones.

Since different systems affecting postural control develop at different rates, it is important to understand which components are rate-limiting at each developmental stage, or conversely, which ones push the system to a new level of function when they have matured. According to newer models of development, finding the connection between critical postural components and development ultimately guides the clinician in determining which systems should be assessed, and how the contribution of these systems changes at various developmental stages. It also allows the clinician to determine appropriate interventions specific to the system that is dysfunctional.

DEVELOPMENT OF POSTURAL CONTROL: A SYSTEMS PERSPECTIVE

Since Gesell's original studies in 1946 describing the cephalo-caudal nature of development, many researchers have found exceptions to some of his general developmental rules. For example, recent studies have found that infants show control of the legs in kicking and supported walking behaviors well before they can control their head and trunk in space

(34, 35). However, in the area of balance and postural control, it does appear as if development follows a cephalo-caudal sequence.

Emerging Head Control

MOTOR COORDINATION

Heinz Prechtl, a researcher and physician from the Netherlands (36), used ultrasound techniques to study the *spontaneous* postural behavior of infants during prenatal development. He observed spontaneous postural changes and described several different motor patterns responsible for these changes. Positional changes occurred as often as 20 times per hour in the first half of pregnancy, but decreased in later pregnancy, perhaps due to space restriction.

Prechtl (36) also attempted to test responses to *perturbations*, and noted that he was unable to activate vestibular reflexes in utero. He reported that the vestibulo-ocular reflex and the Moro response were absent prenatally but were present at birth, and suggested that these reflexes were inhibited until the umbilical cord was broken, thus preventing the fetus from moving every time the mother turned.

Prechtl also examined *spontaneous* head control in neonates and noted that infants had very poor postural or antigravity control at birth. He hypothesized that this could be due either to lack of muscle strength (a musculoskeletal constraint) or alternatively to lack of maturity of the motor processes controlling posture of the head and neck at this age (motor coordination constraint). To test this, he examined spontaneous head movements using both electromyographic (EMG) recordings and video recordings to determine if coordinated muscle activity was present. He found no organized patterns of muscle activity, which appeared to counteract the force of gravity on any consistent basis. This finding suggests that the lack of head control in newborns is not solely the result of a lack of strength, but also results from a lack of organized muscle activity.

To examine infants' responses to *perturbations* of balance, he placed infants on a rocking table that could be tipped up or down, noting any antigravity responses. Newborns and infants up to 8 to 10 weeks did not respond either to head downwards or upwards tilts. However, by 8 to 10 weeks, with the onset of spontaneous head control, infants showed clear EMG patterns in response to the tilting surface, and this response became consistent at about the third month of age.

This research suggests that the emergence of coordinated postural responses in neck muscles, underlying both spontaneous head control and responses to perturbations, occurs at about 2 months of age. However, it does not give us specific information about the ability of individual sensory systems to drive postural responses in the neck.

SENSORY CONTRIBUTIONS

Babies as young as 60 hours old are able to orient themselves toward a source of visual stimulation, and can follow a moving object by correctly orienting the head (37, 38). These orientation movements appear to be part of a global form of postural control involving the head and entire body.

When do visually controlled postural responses become available to the infant? To examine visual contributions to *spontaneous* control of head movements, Jouen and colleagues (39) performed a study with preterm infants (32 to 34 weeks of gestation), examining head alignment both with and without visual feedback (goggles were worn). They kept the infant's head initially in a midline position, then released it and measured the resulting movements of the head. They found that without vision, there was a significant tendency to turn the head to the right, but with vision, the neonate oriented to midline. Thus, from at least 32 to 34 weeks of gestation, infants show a simple type of head postural control that uses vision to keep the head at midline.

A second study examined the capability of neonates to make responses to visual stimuli giving the illusion of a *postural perturbation* (39, 40). Infants were placed in a room in which a pattern of stripes moved either forward or backward. Postural responses were measured with a pressure-sensitive pillow behind the infant's head. The neonates made postural adjustments of the head in response to the optical flow; for example, when the visual patterns moved backwards, the infants appeared to perceive forward sway of the head, because they moved the head backwards, as if to compensate.

Research has also examined the early development of sensory contributions to antigravity responses in infants. In these experiments, infants of 2.5 or 5 months were placed in a chair that could be tilted to the right or left 25°. During some trials, a red wool ball was placed in the visual field, to catch the infant's attention (41, 42). The infants showed an antigravity response (keeping the head from falling to the side to which the baby was tilted), which improved with developmental level, with the older infants dropping the head less than the younger infants. Interestingly, when the wool ball was placed in the visual field, both age groups tilted the head less, with the effect being strongest in the younger group. The authors conclude that these results show a significant effect of vision on the vestibular antigravity response in the infant and a clear improvement in this response with age. However, in this paradigm it is difficult to determine if the improvement is due to enhanced neck muscle strength, somatosensory/motor processing in neck muscles, or vestibular/motor processing.

RELATING REFLEX TO SYSTEMS THEORY

How consistent are systems and reflex theories in describing the development of head control? Reflex-hierarchical theory suggests that visual-motor coordination appears at approximately 2 months of age and is the result of maturation of the optical righting reaction. Systems theory suggests that certain basic visual-postural mapping is present at birth and with experience in moving, the child develops more refined rules for mapping visual information to action.

Reflex theory suggests that since body-righting reactions acting on the head and labyrinthine-righting reactions also emerge between birth and 2 months, this type of sensory-motor mapping is occurring in these sensory systems as well.

According to a reflex model, the Landau reflex, which requires the integration of all three righting reactions, does not emerge until 4 to 6 months. This finding is consistent with Jouen's findings, which suggest that mapping between vision and vestibular systems for postural action is present at 2 1/2 to 5 months of age. Thus, both theories are consistent in suggesting that mapping of individual senses to action may precede the mapping of multiple senses to action. This type of sensory-to-sensory and sensory-to-motor mapping may represent the beginning of internal neural representations necessary for coordinated postural abilities.

Emergence of Independent Sitting

As infants begin to sit independently, and thus develop trunk control, they must learn to master the control of both spontaneous background sway of the head and trunk and to respond to perturbations of balance. This requires the coordination of sensory-motor information relating two body segments together in the control of posture. To accomplish this, they need to extend the rules they learned for sensory-motor relationships for head postural control to the new set of muscles controlling the trunk. It is possible that once these rules have been established for the neck muscles, they could be readily extended to the control of the trunk muscles.

MOTOR COORDINATION

With the emergence of independent sitting, infants develop the ability to control *spontaneous sway* sufficiently to remain upright. This occurs at approximately 6 to 7 months of age (43).

The ability to respond to postural perturbations with organized postural adjustments appears to develop simultaneously. How do the muscles that coordinate sway responses develop in the neck and trunk? Both cross-sectional and longitudinal studies have been used to explore the development of muscle coordination underlying neck and trunk control in infants 2 to 8 months of age (33, 44). EMGs were used to record muscles in the neck and trunk in infants either seated in an infant seat or sitting independently on a moveable platform, shown in Figure 7.11A. Motion of the platform forward or backward caused a disturbance of the infant's head and trunk posture, requiring a subsequent compensatory adjustment to regain balance.

Two-month-olds did not show consistent, directionally appropriate, responses to the platform perturbations. By 3 to 4 months, infants showed directionally specific responses in the neck muscles 40 to 60% of the time. By 5 months, as infants were beginning to sit independently, coordinated postural activity in the trunk muscles in response to platform motion was occurring approximately 40% of the time. By 8 months of age, muscles in the neck and trunk were coordinated into effective patterns for controlling forward and backward sway in the seated position.

A recent study using similar support surface perturbations to balance (33) has also indicated that platform movements causing backward sway give much stronger and less variable postural muscle response synergies than those causing forward sway. This may be caused by the larger base of postural support in the forward direction in seated infants.

SENSORY CONTRIBUTIONS

Other research has examined the capability of infants sitting unsupported to make responses to visual stimuli, giving the illusion of a postural perturbation (the moving room paradigm) (43, 45, 46). Infants with varying amounts of sitting experience were studied, including infants with 0 to 3 months' experience, 4 to 6 months' experience, and 7 to 12 months' experience. In the 0 to 3 month group, a complete loss of balance was often recorded in response to the visual stimulation, even though the infant could maintain balance when sitting quietly. After the first 3 months of experience sitting, the response amplitude declined. This implies that newly sitting infants rely heavily on visual inputs to maintain dynamic posture, and decrease this dependence, relying more on somatosensory

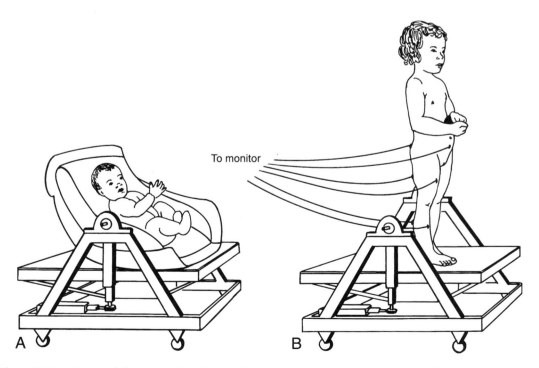

Figure 7.11.   Moving platform posturography used to study postural response patterns in infants in response to a moving surface in **A**, sitting, and **B**, standing.

inputs, with experience in independent sitting.

In addition, Woollacott and coworkers found that taking away visual stimuli did not cause a disruption in muscle activation patterns in response to a moving platform. They concluded that somatosensory and vestibular systems are capable of eliciting postural actions during seated perturbations in isolation from vision in infants first learning to sit (44).

What is the primary sensory system controlling responses to postural perturbations in seated infants? To address this question, experiments were performed in which head orientation was systematically varied, in an effort to change the relationship between inputs related to head motion (vestibular and visual), and proprioceptive inputs from the trunk (33). Coordinated muscle activity stabilizing the trunk did not change regardless of how the head was oriented. This suggests that in the seated position, postural responses to perturbations are largely controlled by somatosensory inputs at the hip joints, not by vestibular or visual stimulation. These results are similar to those found in adults for standing perturbations.

These studies suggest that coordinated postural activity in the neck and trunk develops gradually at about the same time the infant is developing independent head control and the ability to sit independently. First, infants appear to map relationships between sensory inputs and the neck muscles for postural control; this is later extended to include the trunk musculature with the onset of independent sitting. These studies do not tell us whether it is nervous system maturation or experience that allows neck and trunk muscle responses to emerge, since maturation and the refinement of synergies through experience are both gradual, and they seem to occur synchronously.

RELATING REFLEX TO SYSTEMS THEORY

The research we just reviewed suggests that the child's ability to orient the trunk with respect to the head and the support surface occurs at approximately 6 to 8 months of age, coincident to the emergence of independent sitting. These results are quite similar to findings from studies using a reflex-hierarchical approach. In those studies, orientation of the body reportedly emerges at about 6 months of age with the emergence of the mature neck-on-body and body-on-body righting reactions.

While the neck-on-body and body-on-body righting reactions have traditionally been used to describe the emergence of rolling patterns, we have chosen to describe their actions as Magnus did, as they affect body orientation to the head/neck (neck-on-body) and supporting surface (body-on-body). Thus, there appears to be agreement between the two theories concerning the emergence of trunk control, but a difference in the underlying explanation for these emerging behaviors.

Transition to Independent Stance

During the process of learning to stand independently, infants must learn to (*a*) balance within significantly reduced stability limits compared to those used during sitting, and (*b*) control many additional degrees of freedom, as they add the coordination of the leg and thigh segments to those of the trunk and head.

MOTOR COORDINATION

The following sections examine the emergence of this control during both quiet stance and in response to perturbations of balance.

Role of Strength

Several researchers have suggested that a primary rate-limiting factor for the emergence of independent walking is the development of sufficient muscle strength to support the body during static balance and walking (47). Can leg muscle strength be tested in the infant to determine if this is the case?

Researchers have shown that by 6 months of age infants are producing forces well beyond their own body weight (48). These experiments suggest that the ability to support weight against the force of gravity in the standing position occurs well before the emergence of independent stance, and so is probably not the major constraint to emerging stance postural control in infants.

Development of Muscle Synergies

How do postural response synergies compensating for perturbations to balance begin to emerge in the newly standing infant? Longitudinal studies have explored the emergence of postural response synergies in infants from ages 2 to 18 months, during the transition to independent stance (49–52). As

shown in Figure 7.11*B*, infants stood with varying degrees of support on the moving platform while EMGs were used to record muscle activity in the leg and trunk in response to loss of balance.

Figure 7.12 shows EMG responses from one child during the emergence of coordinated muscle activity in the leg and trunk muscles in response to a fall in the backward direction. Infants tested at 2 to 6 months of age, before the onset of pull-to-stand behavior, did not show coordinated muscle response organization in response to threats to balance (Fig.7.12*A*). During early pull-to-stand behavior (7 to 9 months), the infants began to show directionally appropriate responses in their ankle muscles (Fig. 7.12*B*). As pull-to-stand skills improved, muscles in the thigh segment were added and a consistent distal-to-proximal sequence began to

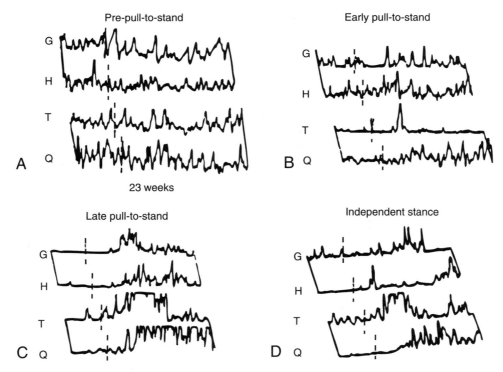

Figure 7.12. EMG responses from one child during the emergence of coordinated muscle activity in the leg and trunk muscles in response to platform perturbations in **A**, pre-pull-to-stand, **B**, early pull-to-stand, **C**, late pull-to-stand, and **D**, independent stance. Abbreviations: *G*, gastrocnemius; *H*, hamstrings; *T*, tibialis anterior; *Q*, quadriceps muscles. (Adapted from Sveistrup H, Woollacott MH. Systems contributing to the emergence and maturation of stability in postnatal development. In: Savelsbergh GJP, ed. The development of coordination in infancy. Amsterdam: Elsevier, 1993:331.)

emerge (Fig. 7.12 C–D) late pull-to-stand and independent stance (9 to 11 months), trunk muscles were consistently activated, resulting in a complete synergy.

To determine if experience is important in the development of postural response characteristics in infants learning to stand, postural responses were compared in two groups of infants in the pull-to-stand stage of balance development (53). One group of infants was given extensive experience with platform perturbations, receiving 300 perturbations over 3 days. The control group of infants did not receive this training.

Infants who had extensive experience on the platform were more likely to activate postural muscle responses, and these responses were better organized. However, onset latencies of postural responses did not change. These results suggest that experience has the capability of influencing the strength of connections between the sensory and motor pathways controlling balance, thus increasing the probability of producing postural responses. However, the lack of a training effect on muscle response latency suggests that neural maturation may be a rate-limiting factor in latency reduction with development. It is probable that the myelination of nervous system pathways responsible for reducing latencies of postural responses during development is not affected by training.

SENSORY CONTRIBUTIONS

Once an infant learns how to organize synergistic muscles for controlling stance in association with one sense, will this automatically transfer to other senses reporting sway? This may not always be the case. It appears that vision maps to muscles controlling stance posture at 5 to 6 months, prior to somatosensory system mapping, and long before the infant has much experience in the standing position (54). This suggests that the infant has to rediscover the synergies when somatosensory inputs are mapped for stance postural control.

EMG responses and sway patterns in response to visual flow created by a moving room were examined in infants and children of varying ages and abilities and compared to those of young adults (54). Figure 7.13 shows an example of an infant positioned in a moving room. The child's sway was recorded through a one-way mirror with a video camera mounted outside the room, and muscle responses were recorded from the legs and hips. Infants who were unable to stand independently were supported by their parents about the hip.

Children as young as 5 months of age swayed in response to room movements; sway amplitudes increased in the pull-to-stand stage, peaking in the independent walkers, and dropped to low levels of sway in experienced walkers (54). Sway responses were associated with clear patterns of muscle responses that pulled the child in the direction of the visual stimulus.

These experiments suggest that the visual system will elicit organized postural responses in standing infants at an earlier time than the somatosensory system, and that the somatosensory system develops postural synergies separately in association with somatosensory inputs signalling sway.

DEVELOPMENT OF ADAPTIVE CAPABILITY

To determine if higher level adaptive processes are available to the infant during pull-to-stand behavior, independent stance, and early walking, the ability of the infants to attenuate postural responses to the visual flow created by the moving room was monitored (54). None of the infants in any of these behavioral categories was able to adapt inappropriate postural responses to low levels, over a period of five trials. The researchers concluded that higher level adaptive processes related to postural control have not yet matured by the emergence of independent walking.

RELATING REFLEX TO SYSTEMS THEORY

Differences in focus between reflex-hierarchical and systems models make it difficult

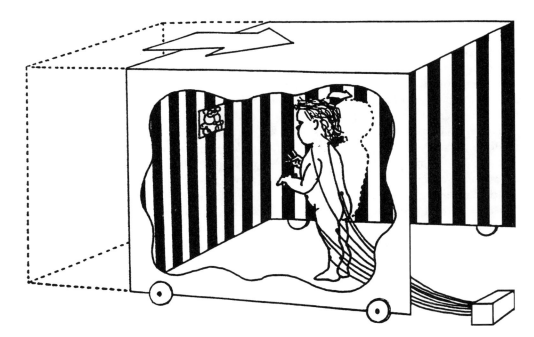

Figure 7.13.   Diagram showing the moving room paradigm used to examine the development of visual contributions to postural control. (From Sveistrup H, Woollacott MH. Systems contributing to the emergence and maturation of stability in postnatal development. In: Savelsbergh GJP, ed. The development of coordination in infancy. Amsterdam: Elsevier, 1993:324.)

to relate findings examining the emergence of independent stance. Reflex-hierarchical theory distinguishes the righting reactions underlying orientation from the tilting and postural fixation reactions essential to the emergence of balance, suggesting different neural mechanisms are involved in these two functions. Studies of tilting and postural fixation reactions have not examined the importance of individual sensory systems to these reactions, nor their capability for adaptation.

Systems-based research suggests that the time-course for emerging stability behaviors is different in each of the sensory systems. Visual inputs relating the body's position in space map to muscular actions controlling the body's position earlier than do inputs from the somatosensory system. It is not known yet how early vestibular inputs map to stance postural actions.

Results from systems-based studies suggest that, for the most part, experience within a specific posture is important for sensory information signalling the body's position in space to be mapped to muscular actions, which control the body's position in space.

Refinement of Stance Control

As children mature, postural adjustments are refined. The emergence of adult levels of control occurs at different times for different aspects of postural control. The following sections review the literature on the refinement of stance postural control.

MOTOR COORDINATION

Quiet Stance

How does the control of spontaneous sway during quiet stance change as children develop? Are children inherently more stable than adults? Children are shorter and therefore closer to the ground. Does their height make balancing an easier task? Anyone who has watched a fearless young child ski down a steep slope with relative ease, falling and bouncing back up might assume that their task is easier. They don't have as far to fall! It turns out that while children are shorter than adults, they are proportioned differently. Children are *top-heavy*. The relative size of the head, in comparison to lower extremities, places the center of mass at about T12 in the child, compared to L5–S1 in the adult. Because of their shorter height, and the difference in the location of their center of mass, children sway at a faster rate than adults. Thus, the task of static balance is slightly more difficult since the body is moving at a faster rate during imbalance (55).

A number of studies have examined changes in spontaneous sway with development (56, 57). One study examining children from 2 to 14 years of age showed that the amplitude of sway decreased with age. There was considerable variability in sway amplitude in the young children. This variance systematically lowered with age and with the children's improved balance. Effects of eye closure were represented by the Romberg quotient (eyes-closed sway expressed as a percentage of eyes-open sway), giving an indication of the contributions of vision to balance during quiet stance. Very low Romberg quotients were recorded for the youngest children who completed the task (4-year-olds) with values less than 100%. This indicates that these children were swaying more with eyes open than with eyes closed (56). Spontaneous sway in children reaches adult levels by 9 to 12 years of age for eyes-open conditions and at 12 to 15 years of age for eyes-closed conditions. Sway velocity also decreased with age, reaching adult levels at 12 to 15 years of age (57).

Compensatory Postural Control

Refinement of compensatory balance adjustments in children 15 months to 10 years of age has been studied by several researchers

using a moveable platform to examine changes in postural control (58–61). Research has shown that compensatory postural responses of young children (15 months of age) are more variable and slower than those of adults (58). These slower muscle responses and the more rapid rates of sway acceleration observed in young children cause sway amplitudes that are bigger and often more oscillatory than those of older children and adults.

Even children of 1 1/2 to three years of age generally produce well-organized muscle responses to postural perturbations while standing (59). However, the amplitudes of these responses are larger, and the latencies and durations of these responses are longer than those of adults. Other studies have also found a longer duration of postural responses in young children and have additionally noted the activation of monosynaptic stretch reflexes in young children in response to platform perturbations. These responses disappear as the children mature (60, 61).

Surprisingly, postural responses in children 4 to 6 years of age are, in general, slower and more variable than those found in the 15-month- to 3-year-olds, 7- to 10-year-olds, or adults, suggesting an apparent *regression* in the postural response organization. Figure 7.14 compares EMG responses in the four age groups.

In these studies, by 7 to 10 years of age, postural responses were basically like those of the adult. There were no significant differences in onset latency, variability, or temporal coordination between muscles within the leg synergy between this age group and adults (59).

Why are postural actions so much more variable in the 4- to 6-year-old child? It may be significant that the variability in response parameters of 4- to 6-year-old children occurs during a period of disproportionate growth with respect to critical changes in body form (59). It has been suggested that discontinuous changes seen in the development of many skills including postural control, may be the result of critical dimension changes in the body of the growing child (62). The system would remain in a state of stability until dimensional changes reached a point where pre-

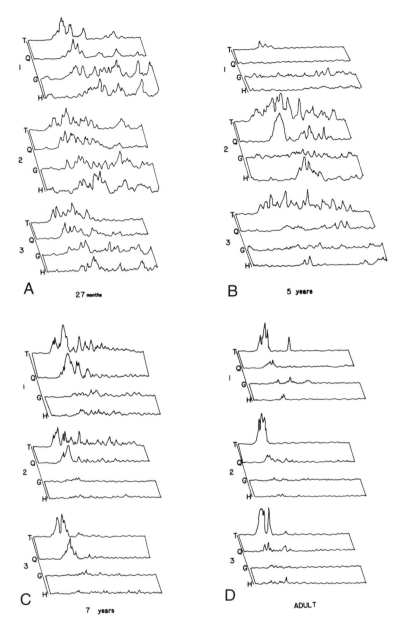

Figure 7.14.   A comparison of muscle activation patterns in leg and trunk muscles in response to forward platform perturbations causing backward sway in four age groups of normal subjects. Three successive responses to platform perturbations are shown for each child. Platform perturbation started at the onset of the electromyogram recording. Abbreviations: *T*, tibialis anterior; *Q*, quadriceps; *G*, gastrocnemius; *H*, hamstring muscles. (From Shumway-Cook A, Woollacott M. The growth of stability: postural control from a developmental perspective. J Motor Behav 1985;17:136.)

vious motor programs were no longer highly effective. At that point, the system would undergo a period of transition marked by instability and variability, and then a new plateau of stability.

Recent work analyzing the movements

of different segments of the body, in response to platform perturbations in both children and adults (63), has shown that the kinematics of passive body movements caused by platform translations are very similar in the 4- to 6-year-old, 7- to 9-year-old, and adult. Thus, it is more probable that changes in response latencies and variability seen in 4- to 6-year-olds represent developmental changes in the nervous system itself.

SENSORY CONTRIBUTIONS

Visual inputs affect balance control in a number of ways. To determine these effects, one can stimulate balance responses with visual inputs. Alternatively, one can remove vision and see if there are any deficits in balance function.

Removing visual inputs with opaque goggles during horizontal platform movements has a surprising effect on the organization of postural responses in children ages 2 to 7 years (44). Previous studies had found that adults wearing opaque goggles showed no significant differences in the organization or timing of muscle responses. In contrast, in 2- to 3-year-olds, postural responses were more likely to be activated with shorter onset latencies. In the 4- to 6-year-olds, muscle response patterns were again more likely to be activated, but the timing of the responses was more variable.

What is the significance of more consistently organized and faster postural responses when vision is removed? It implies that visual cues are not required to activate postural responses in children as young as 2 years of age. In fact, removal of visual cues may actually increase the sensitivity of the postural system to the remaining proprioceptive and vestibular cues. These findings support the concept that vision may be the dominant sense for postural control in the 2- to 3-year-old age group. When vision is removed, a shift occurs from the use of longer latency visual input with eyes open to shorter latency proprioceptive inputs with eyes closed (44).

DEVELOPMENT OF SENSORY ADAPTATION

Postural control is characterized by the ability to adapt how we use sensory information about the position and movement of the body in space to changing task and environmental conditions. The process of organizing and adapting sensory inputs for postural con-

trol involves determining the accuracy of incoming sensory inputs for orientation purposes, and selecting the most appropriate sense for orientation, given the context. This process entails changing the relative weighting of sensory inputs for postural control, depending on their accuracy for orientation (64, 65). How does the CNS learn to interpret information from vision, vestibular, and somatosensory receptors and relate it to postural actions?

We have already described evidence from moving room experiments suggesting that the visual system plays a predominant role in the *development* of postural actions. That is, visual inputs reporting the body's position in space appear to map to muscular actions earlier than other sensory systems. In young children, the invariant use of visual inputs for postural control can sometimes mask the capability of other senses to activate postural actions. Results from the experiments in which children balanced without visual inputs suggest that in certain age groups, postural actions activated by other sensory inputs can be better organized than those associated with vision!

Moving platform posturography in conjunction with a moving visual surround has also been used to examine the development of intersensory integration for postural control. The platform protocols used to study the organization and selection of senses for postural control are described in detail in the previous chapter.

The development of sensory adaptation in children ages 2 to 9 was studied using a modification of this protocol (59). Four- to 6-year-olds swayed more than older children and adults, even when all three sensory inputs were present (condition 1). With eyes closed (condition 2), their stability decreased further, but they did not fall.

Reducing the accuracy of somatosensory information for postural control by rotating the platform surface (condition 3) further reduced the stability of 4- to 6-year-olds, and half of them lost balance. When children 4 to 6 years of age had to maintain balance using primarily vestibular information alone for postural control, all but one fell. In contrast, none of the older children 7 to 9 years of age lost balance. Figure 7.15 compares body sway in children of various ages and adults in these four sensory conditions (59).

These results suggest that children under 7 years are unable to balance efficiently when both somatosensory and visual cues are removed, leaving only vestibular cues to control stability. In addition, children under 7 show a reduced ability to adapt senses for postural control appropriately when one or more of these senses are inaccurately reporting body orientation information.

Development of Anticipatory Postural Actions

Skilled movement has both postural and voluntary components; the postural component establishes a stabilizing framework that supports the second component, that of the primary movement (66). Without this supporting postural framework, skilled action deteriorates, as seen in patients with a variety of motor problems.

The development of reaching in infants shows changes that parallel postural devel-

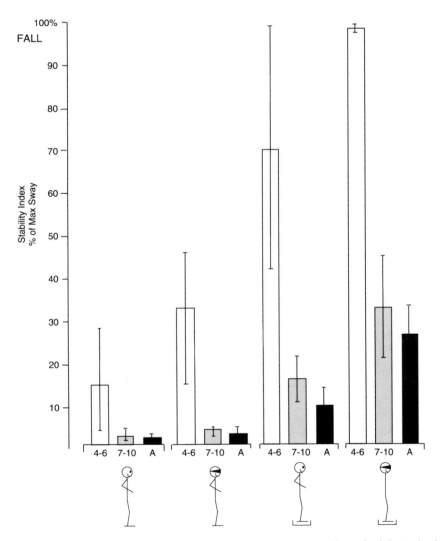

Figure 7.15. A comparison of body sway in 4- to 6-year-olds, 7- to 10-year-olds, and adults in the four sensory conditions. **A**, Eyes open, firm support surface. **B**, Eyes closed, firm support surface. **C**, Eyes open, sway-referenced surface. **D**, Eyes closed, sway-referenced surface. (Adapted from Shumway-Cook A, Woollacott M. The growth of stability: postural control from a developmental perspective. J Motor Behav 1985;17:141.)

Table 7.2   Systems Model of Postural Development

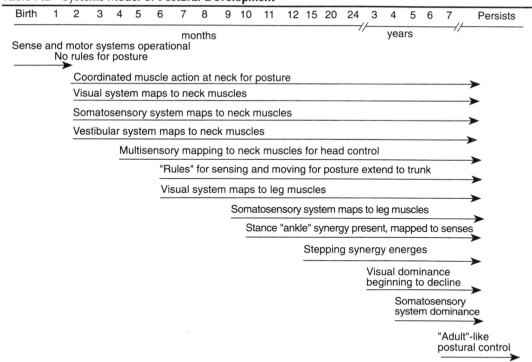

Birth	1	2	3	4	5	6	7	8	9	10	11	12	15	20	24	3	4	5	6	7	Persists
							months								//			years			//

Sense and motor systems operational
No rules for posture

Coordinated muscle action at neck for posture

Visual system maps to neck muscles

Somatosensory system maps to neck muscles

Vestibular system maps to neck muscles

Multisensory mapping to neck muscles for head control

"Rules" for sensing and moving for posture extend to trunk

Visual system maps to leg muscles

Somatosensory system maps to leg muscles

Stance "ankle" synergy present, mapped to senses

Stepping synergy emerges

Visual dominance beginning to decline

Somatosensory system dominance

"Adult"-like postural control

opment. Later sections of this book detail the development of manipulatory function.

Infants as young as 9 months show activation of the postural muscles of the trunk in advance of most but not all reaching movements (67). By the time infants are able to sit independently, and are showing relatively mature reaching movements, they are also showing advance activation of postural muscles to stabilize voluntary movements in the seated position.

Children as young as 12 to 15 months are able to activate postural muscles in advance of arm movements while standing (58). By 4 to 6 years, anticipatory postural adjustments preceding arm movements while standing are essentially mature (68, 69).

Table 7.2 summarizes the emergence of postural control from a systems perspective. By comparing Tables 7.1 and 7.2, you can see the similarities and differences between this model and the reflex-hierarchical model in describing the emergence of posture control in neurologically intact children.

SUMMARY

1. The development of postural control is an essential aspect of the development of skilled actions, like locomotion and manipulation.

2. Consistent with Gesell's developmental principles, postural development appears to be characterized by a cephalo-caudal progression of control.

3. The emergence of postural control can be characterized by the development of rules that relate sensory inputs reporting the body's position with respect to the environment, to motor actions which control the body's position.

   a. Control begins in the head segment. The first sense that is mapped to head control appears to be vision.

   b. As infants begin to sit independently, they learn to coordinate sensory-motor information relating the head and trunk segments, extending the sensorimotor rules for head postural control to trunk muscles.

   c. The mapping of individual senses to action may precede the mapping of multiple senses to action, thus creating internal neural representations necessary for coordinated postural abilities.

4. Anticipatory, or *proactive* postural control, which provides a supportive framework for skilled movements, develops in parallel with *reactive* postural control.

5. Adaptive capabilities that allow the child to modify sensory and motor strategies to changing task and environmental conditions develops later. Experience in using sensory and motor strategies for posture may play a role in the development of adaptive capacities.

6. The development of postural control is best characterized as the continuous development of multiple sensory and motor systems, which manifests behaviorally in a discontinuous step-like progression of motor milestones. New strategies for sensing and moving can be associated with seeming regression in behavior as children incorporate new strategies into their repertoire for postural control.

7. Not all systems contributing to the emergence of postural control develop at the same rate. Rate-limiting components limit the pace at which an independent behavior emerges. Thus, the emergence of postural control must await the development of the slowest critical component.

8. Much debate has occurred in recent years over the relative merits of the reflex-hierarchical vs. systems models in explaining postural development. In many respects, the two models are consistent. Their differences include (*a*) the reflex-hierarchical model views balance control from a reactive perspective, while the systems model stresses the importance or proactive, reactive, and adaptive aspects of the system, and (*b*) the reflex-hierarchical model tends to weight the role of CNS maturation more heavily than experience, while the systems model does not emphasize the role of one over the other.

REFERENCES

1. Amiel-Tison C, Grenier A. Evaluation neurologique du nouveau-ne et du nourrisson. Neurological evaluation of the human infant. New York: Masson, 1980:81.

2. Gesell A. The ontogenesis of infant behavior. In: Carmichael L, ed. Manual of child psychology. NY: John Wiley & Sons, 1946:335–373.

3. McGraw MB. From reflex to muscular control in the assumption of an erect posture and ambulation in the human infant. Child Dev 1932;3:291.

4. Woollacott M, Shumway-Cook A. Changes in postural control across the lifespan—a systems perspective. Phys Ther 1990;70:799–807.

5. Horak F, Shumway-Cook A. In: Duncan P, ed. Balance: Proceedings of the APTA Forum. Alexandria, VA: APTA, 1990:105–111.

6. Magnus R. Some results of studies in the physiology of posture. Lancet 1926;2:531–588.

7. DeKleijn A. Experimental physiology of the labyrinth. J Laryngol Otol 1923;38:646–663.

8. Rademaker GGJ. De Beteekenis der Roode Kernen en van de overige Mesencephalon voor Spiertonus, Lichaamshouding en Labyrinthaire Reflexen. Leiden:Eduarol Ijdo, 1924.

9. Schaltenbrand G. The development of human motility and motor disturbances. Arch Neurol Psychiatr 1928;20:720.

10. Claverie P, Alexandre F, Nichol J, Bonnet F, Cahuzac M. L'activite tonique reflexe du nourisson. Pediatrie 1973;28:661–679.

11. Milani-Comparetti A, Gidoni EA. Pattern analysis of motor development and its disorders. Dev Med Child Neurol 1967;9:625–630.

12. Barnes MR, Crutchfield CA, Heriza CB. The neurophysiological basis of patient treatment. Vol II: Reflexes in motor development. Morgantown, WV: Stokesville Publishing, 1978.

13. Peiper A. Cerebral function in infancy and childhhod. NY: Consultants Bureau, 1963.

14. Ornitz E. Normal and pathological maturation of vestibular function in the human child. In: Romand R, ed. Development of auditory and vestibular systems. NY: Academic Press, 1983:479–536.

15. Cupps C, Plescia MG, Houser C. The Landau reaction: a clinical and electromyographic analysis. Dev Med Child Neurol 1976;18:41–53.

16. Paine RS. The evolution of infantile postural reflexes in the presence of chronic brain syndromes. Dev Med Child Neurol 1964;6:345–361.

17. Martin JP. The basal ganglia and posture. Philadelphia: JB Lippincott, 1967.

18. Bobath B, Bobath K. Motor development in different types of cerebral palsy. London: Heinemann, 1976.

19. Capute AJ, Wachtel RC, Palmer FB, Shapiro BK, Accardo PJ. A prospective study of three postural reactions. Dev Med Child Neurol 1982;24:314–320.

20. Haley S. Sequential analyses of postural reactions in nonhandicapped infants. Phys Ther 1986;66:531–536.

21. Gesell A. Behavior patterns of fetal-infant and child. In: Hooker D, Kare C, eds. Genetics and inheritance of neuropsychiatric patterns. Res Publ Assoc Res Nerv Ment Dis 1954; 33:114–126.

22. Coryell J, Henderson A. Role of the asymmetrical tonic neck reflex in hand visualization in normal infants. Am J Occup Ther 1979; 33:255–260.

23. Larson MA, Lee SL, Vasque DE. Comparison of ATNR presence and developmental activities in 2–4 month old infants. Alexandria, VA: APTA; Conference Proceedings, June, 1990.

24. Fukuda T. Studies on human dynamic postures from the viewpoint of postural reflexes. Acta Otolaryngol (Suppl) 1961;161:1–52.

25. Hellebrandt FA, Schode M, Carns ML. Methods of evoking the tonic neck reflexes in normal human subjects. Am J Phys Med 1962;41:90–139.

26. Hirt S. The tonic neck reflex mechanism in the normal human adult. Am J Phys Med 1967;46:56–65.

27. Tokizane T, Murao M, Ogata T, Kordo T. Electromyographic studies on tonic neck, lumbar and labyrinthine reflexes in normal persons. Jap J Physiol 1951;2:130–146.

28. Campbell SK, Wilhelm IJ. Development from birth to 3 years of age of 15 children at high risk for central nervous system dysfunction. Phys Ther 1985;65:463–469.

29. Molnar GE. Analysis of motor disorder in retarded infants and young children. American Journal of Mental Deficiency 1978; 83:213–222.

30. Van Sant AF. Life-span development in functional tasks. Phys Ther 1990;70:788–798.

31. Woollacott M, Shumway-Cook A, Williams H. The development of posture and balance control. In: Woollacott MH, Shumway-Cook A, eds. Development of posture and gait across the life span. Columbia, SC: University of South Carolina Press, 1989:77–96.

32. Gurfinkel VS, Levik YS. Sensory complexes and sensorimotor integration. Fiziologya Cheloveka 1978;5:399–414.

33. Hirschfeld H. On the integration of posture, locomotion and voluntary movements in hu-

mans: normal and impaired development. Dissertation. Stockholm: Nobel Institute for Neurophysiology, Karolinska Institute, 1992.

34. Thelen E, Ulrich, BD, Jensen JL. The developmental origins of locomotion. In: Woollacott MH, Shumway-Cook A, eds, Development of posture and gait across the life span. Columbia, SC: University of South Carolina Press, 1989:25–47.

35. Forssberg H. Ontogeny of human locomotor control. I: Infant stepping, supported locomotion, and transition to independent locomotion. Exp Brain Res 1985;57:480–493.

36. Prechtl HFR, Prenatal motor develoment. In: Wade MC, Whiting HTA, eds. Motor develoment in children: aspects of coordination and control. Dordrecht: Martinus Nighoff, 1986:53–64.

37. Bullinger A. Cognitive elaboration of sensorimotor behaviour. In: Butterworth G, ed. Infancy and epistemology: an evaluation of Piaget's theory. London: The Harvester Press, 1981:173–199.

38. Bullinger A, Jouen F. Sensibilite du champ de detection peripherique qux variations posturales chez le bebe. Archives de Psychologie 1983;51:41–48.

39. Jouen F, Lepecq JC, Gapenne O. Early visual vestibular relations in newborns. Child Dev, in press.

40. Gapenne O, Jouen F. Effect of visual inputs on head's spontaneous oscillations in newborns. Child Dev, in press.

41. Jouen F. Visual-vestibular interactions in infancy. Infant Behavior and Development 1984;7:135–145.

42. Jouen F. Early visual-vestibular interactions and postural development. In: Bloch H, Bertenthal BI, eds. Sensory-motor organizations and development in infancy and early childhood. Dordrecht: Kluwer, 1990:199–215.

43. Butterworth G, Cicchetti D. Visual calibration of posture in normal and motor retarded Down's syndrome infants. Perception 1978; 7:513–525.

44. Woollacott M, Debu B, Mowatt M. Neuromuscular control of posture in the infant and child: is vision dominant? Journal of Motor Behavior 1987;19:167–186.

45. Butterworth G, Hicks L. Visual proprioception and postural stability in infancy. Perception;6:255–262.

46. Butterworth G, Pope M. Origine et fonction de la proprioception visuelle chez l'enfant. In: de Schonen S, ed. Le developpement dans la

premiere annee. Paris: Presses Universitaires de France, 1983:107–128.

47. Thelen E, Fisher DM. Newborn stepping: an explanation for a "disappearing reflex." Developmental Psychology, 1982;18:760–775.

48. Roncesvalles NC, Jensen J. The expression of weight-bearing ability in infants between four and seven months of age. Sport and Exercise Psychology 1993;15:568.

49. Woollacott M, Sveistrup H. The development of sensori-motor integration underlying posture control in infants during the transition to independent stance. In: Swinnen SP, Heuer H, Massion J, Casaer P, eds. Interlimb coordination: neural, dynamical and cognitive constraints. San Diego, CA: Academic Press, 1993.

50. Sveistrup H, Woollacott MH, Shumway-Cook A, McCollum G. A longitudinal study on the transition to independent stance in children. Neuroscience Abstracts 1990; 16:893.

51. Woollacott MH, Sveistrup H. Changes in the sequencing and timing of muscle response coordination associated with developmental transitions in balance abilities. Human Movement Science 1992;11:23–36.

52. Sveistrup H, Woollacott MH. Systems contributing to the emergence and maturation of stability in postural development. In: Savelsbergh GJP, ed. Advances in psychology: the development of coordination in infancy. Amsterdam: Elsevier, 1993:319–336.

53. Sveistrup H, Woollacott M. Can practice modify the developing automatic postural response? Child Dev, in press.

54. Foster E, Sveistrup H, Woollacott MH. Transitions in visual proprioception: a cross-sectional developmental study of the effect of visual flow on postural control. Journal of Motor Behavior, in press.

55. Zeller W. Konstitution und Entwicklung. Gottingen:Verlag fur Psychologic, 1964.

56. Hayes KC, Riach CL. Preparatory postural adjustments and postural sway in young children. In: Woollacott MH, Shumway-Cook A, eds. Development of posture and gait across the life span. Columbia, SC: University of South Carolina Press, 1989:97–127.

57. Taguchi K, Tada C. Change of body sway with growth of children. In: Amblard B, Berthoz A, Clarac F, eds. Posture and gait: development, adaptation and modulation. Amsterdam: Elsevier, 1988:59–65.

58. Forssberg H, Nashner L. Ontogenetic development of postural control in man: adaptation to altered support and visual conditions during stance. J Neurosci 1982;2:545–552.

59. Shumway-Cook A, Woollacott M. The growth of stability: postural control from a developmental perspective. Journal of Motor Behavior 1985;17:131–147.

60. Berger W, Quintern J, Dietz V. Stance and gait perturbations in children: developmental aspects of compensatory mechanisms. Electroencephalogr Clin Neurophysiol 1985; 61:385–395.

61. Hass G, Diener HC, Bacher M, Dichgans J. Development of postural control in children: short-, medium-, and long latency EMG responses of leg muscles after perturbation of stance. Exp Brain Res 1986;64:127–132.

62. Kugler PN, Kelso JAS, Turvey MT. On the control and coordination of naturally developing systems. In: Kelso JAS, Clark JE, eds. The development of movement control and coordination. NY:John Wiley & Sons, 1982:5–78.

63. Woollacott M, Roseblad B, Hofsten von C. Relation between muscle response onset and body segmental movements during postural perturbations in humans. Exp Brain Res 1988;72:593–604.

64. Horak F, Shupert C. The role of the vestibular system in postural control. In: Herdman S, ed. Vestibular rehabilitation. NY: FA Davis, in press.

65. Berthoz A, Pozzo T. Intermittent head stabilization during postural and locomotory tasks in humans. In: Posture and gait: development, adaptation and modulation. Amblard B, Berthoz A, Clarac F, eds. Amsterdam: Elsevier, 1988;189–198.

66. Gahery Y, Massion J. Coordination between posture and movement. Trends Neurosci 1981;4:199–202.

67. Hofsten von C, Woollacott M. Anticipatory postural adjustments during infant reaching. Neuroscience Abstracts 1989;15:1199.

68. Nashner L, Shumway-Cook A, Marin O. Stance posture control in selected groups of children with cerebral palsy: deficits in sensory organization and muscular coordination. Exp Brain Res 1983;49:393–409.

69. Woollacott M, Shumway-Cook A. The development of the postural and voluntary motor control system in Down's syndrome children. In: Wade M, ed. Motor skill acquisition of the mentally handicapped: issues in research and training. Amsterdam: Elsevier, 1986:45–71.

Chapter 8

AGING AND POSTURAL CONTROL

INTRODUCTION

Why is it that Mr. Jones at the age of 90 is able to run marathons, while Mr. Smith at the age of 68 is in a nursing home, confined to a wheelchair, and unable to walk to the bathroom without assistance? Clearly, the answer to this question is complex. Many factors affect outcomes with respect to health and mobility. These factors contribute to the tremendous differences in abilities found among older adults.

This chapter does not describe all aspects of aging. Rather, the focus is on age-related changes occurring in systems critical to postural control. We review the research examining age-related changes in systems whose dysfunction may contribute to instability among older adults and recent studies that look at the effects of training on improving balance function in these systems. Some introductory comments about research examining changes in older adults are important to keep in mind.

Models of Aging

Though many studies have examined the process of aging and have shown a decline in a number of sensory and motor processes in many older adults, scientists do not agree on how and why we age (1–6). This has led to a number of models of aging (7–9). Two models are shown in Figure 8.1. The first model (Fig. 8.1A) describes the process of aging as a linear decline in neuron function across all levels of the central nervous system (CNS). It predicts that, as the number of neurons declines in a specific part of the CNS, various disease states become evident (8). Alternatively, a second model of aging (Fig. 8.1B) suggests that the CNS continues to function at a relatively high level until death, unless there is a catastrophe or disease that affects a specific part of the CNS. Thus pathology within individual parts of the CNS may result in a rapid decline in a specific neural function (8).

These models lead to very different conclusions regarding the *inevitability* of functional decline with aging. The first model offers a rather pessimistic view of aging, since it suggests that neuronal loss is inevitable, and thus functional loss is an invariant part of growing old. This type of reasoning can lead to self-limiting perceptions on the part of older individuals regarding what they can do (10). These self-limiting perceptions can be inadvertently reinforced by the medical pro-

169

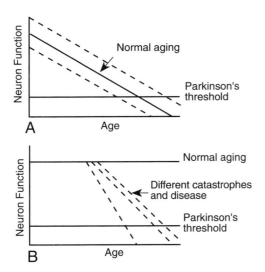

Figure 8.1. Two models of aging. **A,** The first model suggests that aging is associated with an inevitable decline in neuronal function in all systems. **B,** Alternatively, the second model suggests that neuronal function remains optimal with aging unless specific catastrophes or disease affect specific parts of the system. (From Woollacott M. Aging, posture control, and movement preparation. In: Woollacott MH, Shumway-Cook A, eds. Development of posture and gait across the lifespan. Columbia, SC: University of South Carolina Press, 1989:156.)

fessional, who may hold a limited view regarding what older adults can accomplish. For example, when assessing an older adult, a therapist may perceive that the patient's strength is *good, considering the patient's age.* As a result, a strength grade of 3 out of 5, which would never be accepted in a 30-year-old, is often accepted in a 70-year-old as *normal.*

In contrast, the alternative model of aging leads to a more optimistic view (8). In this model, one expects optimal function from the CNS unless unexpected pathology occurs and if optimal experiential factors are present. Experiential factors involve leading a healthy and active life. In this case, when a therapist evaluates an older person, it is anticipated that function will be optimal. If a decline is detected in any area of the nervous system, this perspective will allow the therapist to work on rehabilitation strategies aimed at returning function toward that of a normal young adult.

Primary and Secondary Factors and Aging

Many scientists believe that factors contributing to aging can be considered either primary or secondary (9). **Primary factors,** such as genetics, contribute to the inevitable decline of neuronal function in a system. An example of a genetic predisposition to a condition would be the situation where a person carries the genes for degeneration of auditory neurons and suffers hearing loss in old age. Genetic predisposition can interact with environmental factors. For example, a person who comes from a family with a tendency towards hearing loss and who works in a noisy environment may experience accelerated hearing loss due to a combination of genetic and environmental influences. Primary factors do not necessarily lead to a generalized decline, but rather to a loss of function within specific systems (9).

Research is beginning to suggest that **secondary factors** have a profound effect on aging (10). Secondary, or experiential, factors are more or less under our control. Some of these include nutrition, exercise, insults, and pathologies that affect our mind and body. Environmental factors such as air pollution and carcinogens in our drinking water also fall into this category, though you may not agree that these factors are under your control!

Scientists have shown that proper nutrition results in prolonged and healthier lives (11). Further, animal studies have shown that dietary restriction increases the life span (12, 13). In addition, exercise programs have been shown to improve cardiovascular health, control obesity, and increase physical and mental function. The resultant gains in aerobic power, muscle strength, and flexibility can improve biological age by 10 to 20 years. This can result in delaying the age of dependency and increasing the quality of the remaining years of life (13, 14). This knowledge that how we age is largely determined by how we live leads to an emphasis on preventative health care measures (15). It also has implications for rehabilitation. Therapists work to assist older patients who have experienced pathology to return to optimal life-styles.

Thus, the factors that determine the health and mobility of Mr. Jones vs. Mr. Smith are a combination of *primary aging* factors, primarily genetics, over which they have limited control; and *secondary aging*, primarily experiential factors, over which they have considerable control.

It appears that aging, whether it is primary or secondary, may not necessarily be characterized by an overall decline in all functions. Rather, decline may be limited to specific neural structures and functions. This is consistent with a major theme in this book, that function and dysfunction are not generalized, but emerge through the interaction of the capacities of the individual carrying out tasks within specific environmental contexts.

Heterogeneity of Aging

Certain studies show no change in function of the neural subsystems controlling posture and locomotion with age (16), while others show a severe decline in function in the older adult (17). How can there be such a discrepancy in studies reporting *age-related* changes in systems for posture and gait? This may be due to fundamental differences in the definition that researchers use in classifying an individual as *elderly*.

For example, some researchers have classified the elderly adult as anyone over 60 years of age. When no exclusionary criteria are used in the study of older adults, results can be very different from when researchers use restrictive criteria for including subjects for study. For example, a study on the effects of aging on walking ability selected a group of 71 subjects ranging in age from 60 to 99 years, using no exclusion criteria for possible pathology (17). These researchers noted that the mean walking velocities for their older adults were slower than any other studies had previously reported.

In contrast, another study examined walking in healthy older adults. In this study, 1,187 individuals of 65 years and over were screened to find 32 who were free of pathology, that is, had no disorders of the musculoskeletal, neurological, or cardiovascular systems, or any previous history of falls (16). Interestingly, this study found no significant differences between their younger and older adult groups when comparing four parameters measuring the variability of gait. They thus concluded that an increase in variability in the gait cycle among older adults was not normal, but always due to some pathology.

These types of results suggest that there is much heterogeneity among older adults. This amazing variability reminds us that it is important not to assume that declining physical capabilities occur in all older adults.

BEHAVIORAL INDICATORS OF INSTABILITY

Statistics on injuries and accidents in the older adult indicate that falls are the seventh leading cause of death in people over 75 years of age (18). What are the factors that contribute to these losses of balance? Many early studies on balance loss in the elderly expected to isolate a single cause of falls for a given older adult, such as vertigo, sensory neuropathy, or postural hypotension. In contrast, more current research indicates that falls in the elderly have multiple contributing factors, including intrinsic physiological and musculoskeletal factors and extrinsic environmental factors (19 to 21).

To examine these factors, Lipsitz and his colleagues followed a group of community-dwelling older adults over 70 years of age, for 1 year, and identified all falls that occurred (21). They found that a number of factors were associated with an increased risk of falling, including reduced physical activity, reduced proximal muscle strength, and reduced stability while standing. Other significant factors included arthritis of the knees, stroke, impairment of gait, hypotension, and the use of psychotropic drugs. The conclusions of this study were that most falls in older adults involve multiple risk factors, and that many of these factors may be remediated. Thus, it was suggested that the clinician who is working with an older adult should determine both intrinsic and extrinsic factors associated with a particular fall and reduce or correct as many of these as possible.

The study of intrinsic factors leading to falls has included examining the role of balance control. Several researchers, including Tinetti, from the U.S., Berg, from Canada, and Mathias and colleagues, from England, have measured functional skills related to balance in order to identify people at high risk for falls (19, 22–24). Functional skills include sitting, standing and walking unsupported, standing and reaching forward, performing a 360° turn, and moving from sit to stand position.

A more recent approach to understanding balance function in the elderly examines specific variables relating to normal postural control and determines the extent to which deterioration in their function contributes to loss of stability and mobility in the elderly.

In the remaining sections of this chapter we examine the intrinsic factors related to balance problems in the older adult from a systems perspective. We discuss changes in the motor system, the sensory systems, higher-level adaptive systems, as well as the use of anticipatory postural responses before making a voluntary movement. Studies on the ability of older adults to integrate balance adjustments into the step cycle are covered in the mobility section of this book.

SYSTEMS ANALYSIS OF POSTURAL CONTROL

In previous chapters, we defined postural control as the ability to control the body's position in space for the purpose of stability and orientation, and discussed the many systems that contribute to postural control (refer to Fig. 6.2). What have researchers learned about how changes in these systems contribute to an increased likelihood for falls in the elderly?

Musculoskeletal System

Several researchers have reported changes in the musculoskeletal system in many older adults, including Buchner's and Wolfson's labs from the U.S., and Anniansson's lab from Scandinavia (25–27). Lower extremity muscle strength can be reduced by as much as 40% between the ages of 30 and 80 years (26). This condition is more severe in older nursing home residents with a history of falls (27). In these subjects, the mean knee and ankle muscle strength were reduced two- and fourfold, respectively, compared with non-fallers.

Researchers have shown that the association between strength and physical function is large, with over 20% of the variance in functional status explained by relative strength (25). However, the amount of strength needed for physical function is dependent on the task. For example, it has been suggested that the typical healthy 80-year-old woman is very near, if not at, the

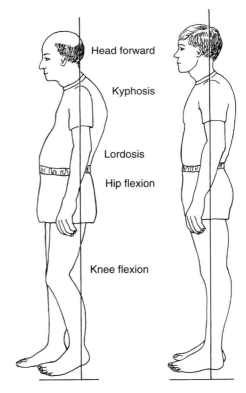

Figure 8.2. Changes in spinal flexibility can lead to a stooped or flexed posture in many elderly people. (Adapted from Lewis C, Bottomley J. Musculoskeletal changes with age. In: Lewis C, ed. Aging: health care's challenge. 2nd ed. Philadelphia: FA Davis, 1990:146.)

threshold value for quadriceps strength necessary to rise from a chair (28). When strength falls below the threshold needed for a task, functional disability occurs.

Decreased range of motion (29) and loss of spinal flexibility in many older adults can lead to a characteristic flexed or stooped posture (Fig. 8.2) (1). This can be associated with other changes in postural alignment, including a shift in the vertical displacement of the center of body mass backwards towards the heels (30). Other conditions, such as arthritis, can lead to decreased range of motion in many joints throughout the body. In addition, pain may limit the functional range of motion of a particular joint (30).

Neuromuscular System

The neuromuscular system contributes to postural control through the coordination of forces effective in controlling the body's position in space.

CHANGES IN QUIET STANCE

Traditional methods for assessing balance function in the older adult have used global indicators of balance control, such as determination of spontaneous sway during quiet stance (31). One of the earliest studies examined the extent to which subjects in age groups from 6 years through 80 years swayed during quiet stance. Subjects at both ends of the age spectrum (ages 6 to 14, and ages 50 to 80) had greater difficulty in minimizing spontaneous sway during quiet stance than the other age groups tested (31). This study tested a great variety of older adults, and did not try to limit subjects in the older groups to those who were free of pathology.

More recent studies have measured spontaneous sway in different age groups using stabilometry, or static force plates. One study examined 500 adults, aged 40 to 80 years, who were free of pathology, and found that postural sway increased with each decade of life. Thus, the greatest amount of spontaneous sway was seen in the 80-year-olds (32).

Similarly, a study examining spontaneous sway in older adults with and without a history of falls found a significant increase in sway in even healthy older adults compared to young adults, with the greatest amount of sway found in older people with a history of recent falls (33). However, not all studies have been consistent in showing increased postural sway among healthy elderly adults (30–37).

Another study by Fernie and colleagues, examined both sway amplitude and velocity in a population of *institutionalized* elderly and determined that sway velocity (but not amplitude) was significantly greater for those who fell one or more times in a year than for those who had not fallen (38).

On the whole, these studies suggest that older adults tend to sway more than young adults during quiet stance. A possible conclusion from these studies is that increased sway is indicative of declining balance control as people age. This is based on the assumption that sway is a good indicator of balance control. It is important to realize that measures of sway are not always good indicators of postural dyscontrol. There are several types of patients with severe neurological disorders, such as Parkinson's disease, vestibular disorders, or peripheral neuropathy, who have normal sway in quiet stance (39). Therefore, caution must be used when interpreting results from studies that use spontaneous sway measures as indicators of balance control.

CHANGES IN MOTOR STRATEGIES DURING PERTURBED STANCE

Is the older adult capable of activating muscle response synergies with appropriate timing, force, and muscle response organization when balance is threatened? Most research addresses this question by using a moving platform to provide an external threat to balance. The organization of muscle responses used to compensate for the induced sway is examined. This approach was described in detail in the chapter on normal postural control.

Remember that when the balance of a

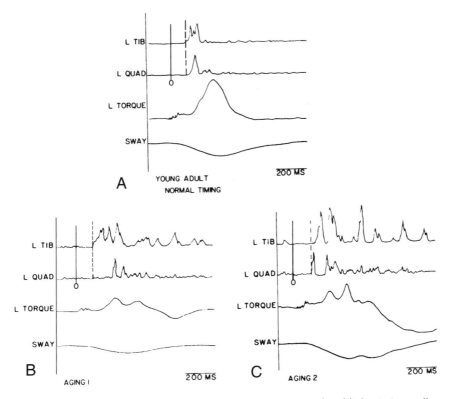

Figure 8.3. Changes in temporal structure of muscle response synergies in the elderly. **A**, Normally coordinated muscle response pattern in a young adult, compared to **B**, a pattern of temporal delay, and **C**, temporal reversal. (Reprinted with permission from Woollacott MH, Shumway-Cook A, Nashner LM. Aging and posture control: changes in sensory organization and muscular coordination. Int J Aging Hum Dev 1986;23:335.)

young adult is disturbed by support surface movements, he or she typically regains stability by using an ankle movement strategy in which sway is focused at the ankle joint, and muscle responses are activated first in the stretched ankle muscle, and then radiate upward to the muscles of the thigh and hip (refer back to Fig. 6.5). How do the postural muscle response characteristics of healthy older adults compare to those of younger adults? Woollacott, Shumway-Cook and Nashner compared the muscle response characteristics of older adults ($n = 12$, aged 61 to 78 years) and younger adults (aged 19 to 38 years), and found that the response organization was generally similar between the older and younger groups, with responses being activated first in the stretched ankle muscle and radiating upward to the muscles of the thigh (35).

However, there were also differences between the two groups in certain response characteristics. The older adults showed significantly slower onset latencies in the ankle dorsiflexors in response to anterior platform movements, causing backward sway (29, 35). In addition, in some older adults, the muscle response organization was disrupted, with proximal muscles being activated before distal muscles. This response organization has also been seen in patients with central nervous system dysfunction (40). Figure 8.3 shows examples of muscle responses to anterior platform movements causing posterior sway in a young adult, temporal delays in an elderly adult, and temporal dyscoordination in another elderly adult.

The older adult group also tended to coactivate the antagonist muscles along with the agonist muscles at a given joint significantly more often than the younger adults. Thus, many of the elderly people studied tended to stiffen the joints more than young adults when compensating for sway perturbations.

ADAPTING MOVEMENTS TO CHANGING TASKS AND ENVIRONMENTS

Several labs, including those of Horak and Woollacott, have found that many older adults generally used a strategy involving hip movements rather than ankle movements significantly more often than young adults (30, 41). Hip movements are typically used by young adults when balancing on a short support surface, which doesn't allow them to use ankle torque in compensating for sway.

It has been hypothesized that this shift towards use of a hip strategy for balance control in older adults may be related to pathological conditions such as ankle muscle weakness or loss of peripheral sensory function (30, 41). With this shift toward a preferential use of the hip strategy, older adults may alter the boundaries for discrete movement strategies within internally mapped stability limits. This concept is shown in Figure 8.4 (30).

Horak has suggested that in older adults some falls, particularly those associated with slipping, may be the result of using a hip strategy in conditions where the surface cannot resist the sheer forces of the feet, which are associated with the use of this strategy, for example, when on ice (30).

In summary, we see that for many older adults, changes in the motor systems affecting postural control can contribute significantly to an inability to maintain balance. Some of these changes include (*a*) impaired range of motion and flexibility, (*b*) weakness, (*c*) impaired organization among synergistic muscles activated in response to instability, and (*d*) limitations in the ability to adapt movements for balance in response to changing task and environmental demands.

Sensory Systems

How do changes in the sensory systems important for posture and balance control contribute to declining stability as people age? The following sections review changes within individual sensory systems and then examine how these changes affect stability in quiet stance, as well as our ability to recover from loss of balance.

CHANGES IN INDIVIDUAL SENSORY SYSTEMS

Somatosensory

Studies have shown that cutaneous vibratory sensation thresholds at the knee are increased in the elderly (70 to 90 years) compared to young adults (42). In this research, the authors reported an inability to record vibratory responses from the ankle because many of the older subjects were not able to perceive sensation there. Sensory neuropa-

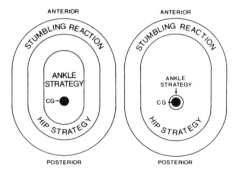

Figure 8.4. A diagrammatic representation of the relationship hypothesized to occur between movements of the center of gravity and the strategies used by a normal subject and older adults with some pathology. (From Horak F, Shupert C, Mirka A. Components of postural dyscontrol in the elderly: a review. Neurobiol Aging 1989;10:745.)

thies and diseases such as cervical spondylosis affect the transmission of sensory information important for balance control.

Vision

Studies on the visual system show similar declines in function. Because of multiple changes within the structure of the eye itself, less light is transmitted to the retina. In addition, there is typically a loss of visual contrast sensitivity, which causes problems in contour and depth perception (43, 44). This information is critical to postural function. Loss of visual acuity can result from cataracts, macular degeneration, and loss of peripheral vision due to ischemic retinal or brain disease.

Vestibular

The vestibular system also shows a reduction in function, with a loss of 40% of the vestibular hair and nerve cells by 70 years of age (45). In young adults, even fairly severe vestibular problems often do not affect balance control significantly because of the availability of other senses providing orientation information to the CNS. Imbalance can become apparent in environments where sensory cues for balance are reduced or inaccurate. For example, when subjects with vestibular loss were asked to balance under conditions with reduced or conflicting somatosensory and visual inputs, they showed excessive sway or loss of balance (30).

Dizziness, an additional consequence of some types of vestibular dysfunction, can also contribute to instability among older adults. Dizziness is a term used to describe the illusion of movement. It can encompass feelings of unsteadiness and imbalance, as well as feelings of faintness or the sense of being lightheaded. Dizziness can be a symptom of a variety of diseases, including those of the inner ear. Partial loss of vestibular function can lead to complaints of dizziness, which can be a significant factor contributing to imbalance in the elderly. Degenerative processes within the otoliths of the vestibular system can produce positional vertigo and imbalance during walking.

Multisensory Deficit

Multisensory deficit is a term used by Brandt (46) to describe the loss of more than one sense important for balance and mobility functions. In many older people with multisensory deficits, the ability to compensate for loss of one sense with alternative senses is not possible because of numerous impairments in all the sensory systems important for postural control (46).

ADAPTING SENSES FOR POSTURAL CONTROL

In addition to showing declines in function within specific sensory systems, research from many labs, including those of Wolfson, Horak, Stelmach, Woollacott, and Brandt, has indicated that some older adults have more difficulty than younger adults in maintaining steadiness under conditions where sensory information for postural control is severely reduced (30, 32, 34–37, 47, 48).

To understand the contribution of vision to the control of sway during quiet stance in older adults, researchers examined sway under altered visual conditions (30, 32, 34–37, 47, 48).When young people close their eyes, they show a slight increase in body sway, and this is also true for healthy older adults (37). However, research is contradictory in this area, since many researchers have found that healthy older adults do not tend to sway more with vision removed than do young adults (36, 37).

In addition, when their eyes are open, healthy older adults are often as steady as young adults when standing on foam, a condition that reduces the effectiveness of somatosensory inputs reporting body sway (37). However, when healthy older adults are asked to stand with their eyes closed on a foam surface, thus using vestibular inputs alone for controlling posture, sway significantly increases compared to young adults (37).

Several studies have examined the ability of healthy older adults to adapt senses to changing conditions during quiet stance using posturography testing (30, 34–36). These studies found that healthy active older adults did not show significant differences from young adults in amount of body sway (Fig. 8.5) except in conditions where *both* ankle joint inputs and visual inputs were distorted or absent (conditions 5 and 6).

When both visual and somatosensory inputs for postural control were reduced (conditions 5 and 6), half of the older adults lost balance on the first trial for these conditions and needed the aid of an assistant. However, most of the older adults were able to maintain balance on the second trial within these two conditions. Thus, they were able to adapt senses for postural control, but only with practice in the condition (35).

These results suggest that healthy older adults do not sway significantly more than

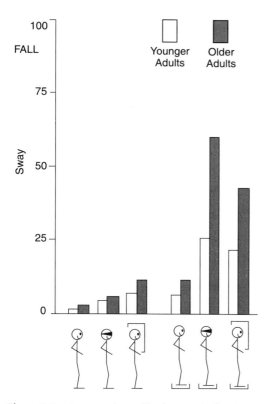

Figure 8.5. A comparison of body sway in the six sensory conditions in young versus a group of active healthy elderly. (Adapted from Woollacott MH, Shumway-Cook A, Nashner LM. Aging and posture control: changes in sensory organization and muscular coordination. Int J Aging Hum Dev 1986;23:340.)

young people when there is a reduction in the availability or accuracy of a single sense for postural control. However, in contrast to young adults, reducing the availability of two senses appears to have a significant effect on postural steadiness in even apparently healthy older adults.

Are the changes summarized above the result of an inevitable decline in nervous system function, or are they the result of borderline pathology in specific subsystems contributing to postural function?

To determine if evidence of borderline pathology existed in subjects who participated in a postural study and who considered themselves fit, active older adults, researchers gave each subject a neurological exam, and then correlated the existence of borderline pathology with performance on the balance tasks (41). Although all the older adults considered themselves to be healthy, a neurologist participating in the study found neural impairment, such as diminished deep tendon reflexes, mild peripheral nerve deficits, distal weakness in tibialis anterior, and gastrocnemius and abnormal nystagmus in many adults in the population. Loss of balance in two subjects accounted for 58% of total losses of balance (41).

These subjects had no history of neurological impairment, but the neurologist diagnosed them as having borderline pathology of central nervous system origin. These results again suggest the importance of pathologies within specific subsystems as contributing to imbalance in the older adult, rather than a generalized decline in performance.

Other researchers have also studied the adaptation of sensory information during quiet stance in older adults (30). One group of older adults was active and healthy and had no previous history of falls (labeled asymptomatic). The second group was symptomatic for falling. Figure 8.6 illustrates some of the results of their study, showing that over 20% of the elderly (both symptomatic and asymptomatic) lost balance when visual information was inaccurate for balance (Condition 3) compared to none of the subjects ages 20 to 39. Forty percent of the asymptomatic elderly

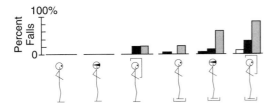

Figure 8.6. A comparison of number of falls in the six sensory conditions in young, elderly non-fallers, and elderly fallers. (*Open box* equals 20–39 years; *black box* equals more than 70 years asymptomatic; *shaded box* equals more than 70 years symptomatic.) (From Horak F, Shupert C, Mirka A. Components of postural dyscontrol in the elderly: a review. Neurobiol Aging 1989; 10:732.)

lost balance in condition 6 when both visual and somatosensory information were inaccurately reporting body sway. By contrast, less than 10% of the normal young adults fell in this condition. The symptomatic elderly had a larger percentage of falls in any condition which was sway-referenced, that is, with misleading somatosensory cues (conditions 4, 5, and 6).

This led researchers to conclude that the ability to select and weight alternative orientation references adaptively is a crucial factor contributing to postural dyscontrol in many older adults. This is especially true for those who are symptomatic for balance problems (30, 48).

Why are there differences among researchers reporting on the capability of older adults to maintain steadiness under altered sensory conditions? These differences may simply be related to the variety of subjects studied. A neurological exam of older adults without obvious signs of pathology, may bring out subtle signs of neural deficits contributing to balance dysfunction.

Another approach to studying adaptation of sensory systems involves the use of rotational movements of a platform. These experiments were described in more detail in earlier chapters. Results from platform rotation studies with older adults found that 50% of the healthy older subjects lost balance on the first trial. However, all but one of the subjects were able to maintain balance on subsequent trials (35). This finding could

suggest a slower ability to adapt postural control in this population.

A propensity for falls in the first trial of a new condition is a recurring finding in many different studies examining postural control in older adults (30, 34–36). Perhaps this means that a slowing occurs, rather than a total lack of adaptability, in many elderly people. A propensity to fall in new or novel situations could also be the result of impaired anticipatory mechanisms. Anticipatory processes related to postural control enable the selection of appropriate sensory and motor strategies needed for a particular task or environment.

ANTICIPATORY POSTURAL ABILITIES

Postural adjustments are often used in a proactive manner, to stabilize the body before making a voluntary movement. Adults in their 70s and 80s may begin to have more difficulty maneuvering in the world because they have lost some of their ability to integrate balance adjustments into ongoing voluntary movements such as lifting or carrying objects. Thus, it is important to study the effects of age on the ability to use postural responses proactively within the context of voluntary movements. It is in these dynamic conditions, including walking, lifting, and carrying objects, that most falls occur.

One of the first researchers to study age-related changes in anticipatory postural adjustments was Man'kovskii, from Russia (49). He compared the characteristics of anticipatory postural responses and prime mover (voluntary) responses for young (ages 19 to 29), medium old (ages 60 to 69), and very old (ages 90 to 99) adults who were asked to do the simple task of flexing one leg at the knee (prime mover response) while using the other leg for support (postural response), both at a comfortable and at a fast speed. Both the medium old adults and very old adults showed a slowing in both the postural (contralateral rectus femoris) and prime mover (ipsilateral biceps femoris) muscle response latencies, for the movements at a comfortable speed, but this slowing did not result in an increased probability of losing balance. However, at the fast speeds, for both medium and very old adults, (*a*) the correlation between the postural and prime mover muscles decreased and (*b*) there was a decrease in the time period between the onset of postural and prime mover muscles. In the very old, postural and prime mover muscles were activated almost simultaneously. This inability to activate postural muscles far enough before the prime mover caused a loss of balance on many trials (49).

In the last chapter, we mentioned that in the normal young adult, the same postural response synergies that are activated during stance balance control are activated in an anticipatory manner before making a voluntary movement while standing. Thus, when a young adult is asked to pull on a handle, first the gastrocnemius is activated, followed by the hamstrings, trunk extensor, and then the prime mover muscle, the biceps of the arm.

A slowing in onset latency or a disruption of the sequence of activation of these postural synergies could affect the ability of an older adult to make such movements as lifting objects. Experiments were performed by the labs of Woollacott, in the U.S., and Frank, in Canada, to explore age-related changes in the ability of older adults to activate postural muscle response synergies in an anticipatory manner (50, 51). In one study, standing young (mean age 26 years) and older (mean age 71 years) adults pushed or pulled on a handle that was adjusted to shoulder level, in response to a visual stimulus. Results of the study showed that the onset latencies of the postural muscles were significantly longer in the older adults than in the younger adults when they were activated in a complex reaction time task. There were large age-related increases in onset times for voluntary muscles. According to a systems perspective, this slowing in voluntary reaction time in the older adult could be caused either by the need for advanced stabilization by the already delayed and weaker postural muscles or to slowing in the voluntary control system itself. Since the absolute differences in onset times between the young and the older adults were

larger for the voluntary muscles than the postural muscles, there may be a slowing in both systems in the older adult (50).

This study also pointed out a number of other interesting differences between this population of elderly and young adults. Muscle response latencies were much more variable in the elderly group than in the young adults. In addition, the organization of muscle synergists was disrupted in the elderly as compared with the young adults.

In a similar study, researchers found that older adults showed more variability in the organization of their postural adjustments than young adults. The majority of older subjects showed a change in the ordering of postural response activation, tonic co-contraction of agonist, and antagonist postural muscles and/or activation of postural muscles following activation of prime mover muscles (51). This was associated with longer reaction times and smaller center of pressure shifts for the older adults in the movement tasks.

These studies suggest that many older adults have problems making anticipatory postural adjustments quickly and efficiently. This inability to stabilize the body in association with voluntary movement tasks such as lifting or carrying may be a major contributor to falls in many elderly people.

COGNITIVE ISSUES AND POSTURE CONTROL

Mrs. Beaulieu, who is 80 years old, normally has no problems with falls. She is walking down a busy sidewalk in the city, talking to a friend, while carrying a fragile piece of crystal she just bought at the department store. Suddenly, a dog runs in front of her, bumping into her. Will she be able to balance in this situation as well as she does when she is walking down a quiet street by herself?

Mrs. Beaulieu's friend, Mr. Champagne, has within the last 6 months recovered from a series of serious falls. These falls have led to a loss of confidence and fear of falling, which has resulted in a reduction in his overall activity level and an unwillingness to leave the safety of his own home. Can fear of falling significantly affect how we perceive and move in relation to balance control? Determining the answer to these and other questions related to the complex role of cognitive issues in postural control may be a key to understanding loss of balance in some older adults.

As we mentioned in the first part of this chapter, the capacity of an individual, the demands of a task, and the strategies the person uses to accomplish a task are important factors that contribute to the ability of a person to function in different environments. As individuals get older, their capacities to perform certain tasks such as balance control may be reduced compared to their abilities at age 20, but they will still be able to function in normal situations where they can focus on the task. However, when they are faced with situations in which they are required to perform multiple tasks at once, such as the one just described, they may not have the capacity to perform both tasks.

Researchers are beginning to explore the question of how our attentional capacities affect our balance abilities in different environments. Theo Mulder, a researcher from the Netherlands, used a rather humorous method for exploring these changes in the elderly (52). He asked both young and older adults to walk at their preferred speed down a walkway, either under normal conditions, while making mental calculations, while wearing scuba diving flippers, or while doing both calculations and wearing the flippers. He noted that the older adults had significantly more problems than the young adults in performing the concurrent tasks, and walked much slower. In fact, he noted that the data of the oldest subjects in this experiment resembled data from amputees who were just starting their rehabilitation. It was as if in both groups the brain had to deal with a breakdown in their normal control strategies and the system became more vulnerable.

Although the single tasks were impaired somewhat in the older adults, the dual tasks were most significantly impaired. He also noticed that the variability in the older adults was great, with some showing performance similar to the young adults and others showing significant impairments. He concluded that dual-task designs were much more sensitive measures of subtle processing deficits across different age groups.

Although many studies have explored the differences in postural performance between *fallers* and *non-fallers*, very few have explored the effect of fear of falling on the control of balance (53). There is now experimental evidence that anxiety and fear of falling affect the performance of older adults on tests of balance control (10, 53). As a result, older adults probably modulate strategies for postural control based on their perception of the level of postural threat. Thus, those older adults who have a great deal of anxiety about falling related to poor perceptions regarding their level of balance skills will move in ways that reflect these perceptions. More work is needed to fully understand the relationship between fear of falling and postural control.

BALANCE RETRAINING

Our review of previous research has shown that there is a significant loss of balance function in many older adults, and that there are specific decreases in function of the different neural and musculoskeletal systems contributing to postural control. Can these losses of balance function be reversed with training? In recent years, many research labs have begun to design and test different training programs with the specific goal of balance improvement. Training programs have included such diverse components as aerobic exercise, strength, and balance training.

One type of balance training program has focused on general aerobic exercise as a way of improving stability. In one study, the exercise program included stretching, walking, reaction time maneuvers, and static and active balance exercises performed for 1 hour, three times a week, for 16 weeks (54). The study did not show significant differences between the exercise and control groups of elderly women when measured on one- and two-legged balance tests with eyes open and eyes closed. It is possible that the study did not find significant improvements in the exercise group because it didn't focus on training a specific subsystem related to balance control, and thus the effects on any single system were too small to be significant.

A second type of training program emphasized muscle strength training to improve balance. One study focused specifically on strengthening the leg muscles, and had considerably greater success than general exercise programs (55). This study used high-resistance weight training of the quadriceps, hamstrings, and adductor muscle groups in frail residents of nursing homes. The authors noted highly significant and clinically meaningful gains in muscle strength in all subjects. In addition, there was a decrease in walking time, and two subjects no longer used canes to walk at the end of the study.

A study from our own laboratory (56, 57) used a balance training protocol that focused on the use of different sensory inputs and the integration of these inputs under conditions in which sensory inputs were reduced or altered. Subjects ranged in age from 65 to 87 years. Differences in the amount of sway of the subject from the beginning to the end of the training period were determined. Significant improvements were found in the training group between the first and the last day of training in five of the eight training conditions.

Although the subjects improved significantly in the training paradigm itself, it was necessary to determine if this training could transfer to other balance tasks. Therefore, the trained and control groups of subjects were also tested up to 4 weeks after the end of training on two other balance tasks. We found the training group lost balance significantly less often than the control group did. In addition, the training group performed significantly better on the two additional tests of balance, including standing on one leg with eyes open and eyes closed. Finally, increased stability in the training group was accompanied by specific changes in muscle response

characteristics to platform perturbations, including significantly less coactivation of antagonist muscles after training than before training when compared with the control group. These experiments suggest that a sensory training program in balance control may result in significant improvements in balance under altered sensory conditions, and this improvement may transfer to other balance tasks.

SUMMARY

1. Two models of aging include (a) the concept that aging involves a linear decline in neuron function across all levels of the central nervous system (CNS); and (b) the concept that during aging, the CNS continues to function well until death, unless there is a catastrophe or disease that affects a specific part of the CNS.

2. Many scientists believe that factors contributing to aging can be considered either primary or secondary. Primary factors, such as genetics, contribute to the inevitable decline of neuronal function in a system. Secondary factors are experiential and include nutrition, exercise, insults, and pathologies.

3. Researchers in all areas find much heterogeneity among older adults, suggesting that assumptions about declining physical capabilities cannot be generalized to all older adults.

4. Falls are the seventh leading cause of death in people over 75 years of age. Falls in the elderly have multiple contributing factors including intrinsic physiological and musculoskeletal factors and extrinsic environmental factors. Understanding the role of declining postural and balance abilities is a critical concern in helping to prevent falls among older adults.

5. Many factors can contribute to declining balance control in older adults who are symptomatic for imbalance and falls. Researchers have documented impairments in all of the systems contributing to balance control; however, there is no one predictable pattern that is characteristic of all elderly fallers.

6. On a positive note, there are many older adults who have balance function that is equivalent to young people, suggesting that balance decline is not necessarily an inevita-

ble result of aging. We suggest that experiential factors such as good nutrition and exercise can aid in the maintenance of good balance and decrease the likelihood for falls as people age.

REFERENCES

1. Lewis C, Bottomley J. Musculoskeletal changes with age. In: Lewis C, ed. Aging: health care's challenge. 2nd ed. Philadelphia: FA Davis, 1990:145–146.
2. Duncan PW, Chandler J, Studenski S, Hughes M, Presott B. How do physiological components of balance affect mobility in elderly men? Arch Phys Med Rehabil 1993; 74:1343–1349.
3. Tinetti ME, Ginter SF. Identifying mobility dysfunctions in elderly patients. JAMA 1988; 259:1190-1193.
4. Kosnik W, Winslow L, Kline D, Rasinski K, Sekuler R. Visual changes in daily life throughout adulthood. J Gerontol Psych Sci 1988;43:63–70.
5. Sloane P, Baloh RW, Honrubia V. The vestibular system in the elderly. Am J Otolaryngol 1989;1:422–429.
6. Aniansson A, Grimby F, Gedberg A. Muscle function in old age. Scan J Rehab Med 1978; 6(Suppl):43–49.
7. Davies P. Aging and Alzheimer's disease: new light on old problems. Paper presented at Neuroscience Society Annual Meeting, New Orleans, LA, 1987.
8. Woollacott, M. Aging, posture control, and movement preparation. In: Woollacott MH, Shumway-Cook A, eds. Development of posture and gait across the lifespan. Columbia, SC: University of South Carolina Press, 1989:155–175.
9. Birren JE, Cunningham W. Research on the psychology of aging: principles, concepts and theory. In: Birren JE, Schaie KW, eds. Handbook of the psychology of aging. 2nd ed. NY: Van Nostrand & Reinholdt, 1985:3–34.
10. Tinetti M, Richman D, Powell L. Falls efficacy as a measure of fear of falling. J Gerontol 1990;45:239–243.
11. Lee I, Manson J, Hennekens C, Paffenbarger R. Body weight and mortality: a 27 year follow up of middle aged men. JAMA 1993; 270:2623–2628.
12. Yu BP, Masossro EJ, McMahan CA. Nutritional influences on aging of Fischer 344 Rats: 1. Physical, metabolic and longevity characteristics. J Gerontol 1985;40:657–670.
13. McCarter RJ, Kelly NG. Cellular basis of aging in skeletal muscle. In: Coe RM, Perry HM, eds. Aging, musculoskeletal disorders and care of the frail elderly. NY: Springer, 1993:45–60.
14. Shephard RJ. Benefits of exercise in the elderly. In: Coe RM, Perry HM, eds. Aging, musculoskeletal disorders and care of the frail elderly. NY: Springer, 1993:228–242.
15. Tinetti M. Performance-oriented assessment of mobility problems in elderly patients. J Am Geriatr Soc 1986;34:119–126.
16. Gabell A, Nayak USL. The effect of age on variability in gait. J Gerontol 1984;39:662–666.
17. Imms FJ, Edholm OG. Studies of gait and mobility in the elderly. Age Ageing 1981; 10:147–156.
18. Ochs AL, Newberry J, Lenhardt ML, Harkins SW. Neural and vestibular aging associated with falls. In: Birren JE, Schaie KW, eds. Handbook of psychology of aging. NY: Van Nostrand & Reinholdt, 1985:378–399.
19. Tinetti ME, Williams TF, Mayewski R. Fall risk index for elderly patients based on numbers of chronic disabilities. Am J Med 1986; 80:429–434.
20. Campbell AJ, Borrie MJ, Spears GF. Risk factors for falls in a community-based prospective study of people 70 years and older. J Gerontol 1989;44:M112–M117.
21. Lipsitz LA, Jonsson PV, Kelley MM, Koestner JS. Causes and correlates of recurrent falls in ambulatory frail elderly. J Gerontol 1991; 46:M114–M122.
22. Mathias S, Nayak USL, Isaacs B. Balance in elderly patients: the "get-up and go" test. Arch Phys Med Rehabil 1986;67:387–389.
23. Berg K, Wood-Dauphinee S, Williams J, Gayton D. Measuring balance in the elderly: preliminary development of an instrument. Physiotherapy Canada 1989;41:304–308.
24. Speechley M, Tinetti M. Assessment of risk and prevention of falls among elderly persons: role of the physiotherapist. Physiotherapy Canada 1990;2:75–79.
25. Buchner DM, deLateur BJ. The importance of skeletal muscle strength to physical function in older adults. Annals of Behavioral Medicine 1991;13:12–21.
26. Anniansson A, Hedberg M, Henning G, et

al. Muscle morphology, enzymatic activity and muscle strength in elderly men: a follow up study. Muscle Nerve 1986;9:585–591.

27. Whipple RH, Wolfson LI, Amerman PM. The relationship of knee and ankle weakness to falls in nursing home residents: an isokinetic study. J Am Geriatr Soc 1987;35:13–20.

28. Young A. Exercise physiology in geriatric practice. Acta Scand 1986;711(Suppl):227–232.

29. Studenski S, Duncan PW, Chandler J. Postural responses and effector factors in persons with unexplained falls: results and methodologic issues. J Am Geriatr Soc 1991;39:229–234.

30. Horak F, Shupert C, Mirka A. Components of postural dyscontrol in the elderly: a review. Neurobiol Aging 1989;10:727–745.

31. Sheldon JH. The effect of age on the control of sway. Gerontology Clinics 1963;5:129–138.

32. Toupet M, Gagey PM, Heuschen S. Vestibular patients and aging subjects lose use of visual input and expend more energy in static postural control. In: Vellas B, Toupet M, Rubenstein L, Albarede JL, Christen Y, eds. Falls, balance and gait disorders in the elderly. Paris:Elsevier, 1992:183–198.

33. Shumway-Cook A, Baldwin M, Kerns K, Woollacott M. The effects of cognitive demands on postural control in elderly fallers and non fallers. Society for Neuroscience Abstracts, 1993;2:257.

34. Wolfson L, Whipple R, Amerman P, Kaplan J, Kleinberg A. Gait and balance in the elderly. Clin Geriatr Med 1985;1:649–659.

35. Woollacott MH, Shumway-Cook A, Nashner LM. Aging and posture control: changes in sensory organization and muscular coordination. Int J Aging Human Dev 1986;23:97–114.

36. Peterka RJ, Black FO. Age-related changes in human posture control: sensory organization tests. Journal of Vestibular Research 1990;1:73–85.

37. Teasdale N, Stelmach GE, Breunig A. Postural sway characteristics of the elderly under normal and altered visual and support surface conditions. J Gerontol 1991;46:B238–B244.

38. Fernie GR, Gryfe CI, Holliday PJ, Llewellyn A. The relationship of postural sway in standing: the incidence of falls in geriatric subjects. Age Ageing 1982;11:11–16.

39. Horak FB. Effects of neurological disorders on disorders on postural movement strategies in the elderly. In: Vellas B, Toupet M, Rubenstein L, Albarede JL, Christen Y, eds. Falls, balance and gait disorders in the elderly. Paris:Elsevier, 1992:137–152.

40. Nashner L, Shumway-Cook A, Marin O. Stance posture control in selected groups of children with cerebral palsy: deficits in sensory organization and muscular coordination. Exp Brain Res 1983;49:393–409.

41. Manchester D, Woollacott M, Zederbauer-Hylton N, Marin O. Visual, vestibular and somatosensory contributions to balance control in the older adult. J Gerontol 1989; 44:M118–M127.

42. Whanger A, Wang HS. Clinical correlates of the vibratory sense in elderly psychiatric patients. J Gerontol 1974;29:39–45.

43. Pitts DG. The effects of aging on selected visual functions: dark adaptation, visual acuity, stereopsis, and brightness contrast. In: Sekular R, Kline D, Dismukes K, eds. Modern aging research: aging and human visual function. NY: Alan R. Liss, 1982: 131–160.

44. Pastalan LA, Mantz RK, Merrill J. The simulation of age-related sensory losses: a new approach to the study of environmental barriers. In: Preiser WFE, ed. Environment design research, vol 1. Stroudsberg, PA: Dowden, Hutchinson & Ross, 1973:383–390.

45. Rosenhall U, Rubin W. Degenerative changes in the human vestibular sensory epithelia. Acta Otolaryngol 1975;79:67–81.

46. Brandt T, Daroff RB. The multisensory physiological and pathological vertigo syndromes. Ann Neurol 1979:7:195–197.

47. Brandt T, Paulus W, Straube A. Vision and posture. In: Blex W, Brandt T, eds. Disorders of posture and gait. Paris:Elsevier, 1986:157–176.

48. Horak FB, Mirka A, Shupert CL. The role of peripheral vestibular disorders in postural dyscontrol in the elderly. In: Woollacott MH, Shumway-Cook A, eds. The development of posture and gait across the lifespan. Columbia, SC: University of South Carolina Press, 1989:253–279.

49. Man'kovskii NB, Mints AY, Lysenyuk VP. Regulation of the preparatory period for complex voluntary movement in old and extreme old age. Human Physiology (Moscow) 1980;6:46–50.

50. Inglin B, Woollacott MH. Anticipatory postural adjustments associated with reaction time arm movements: a comparison between young and old. J Gerontol 1988;43:M105–M113.

51. Frank JS, Patla AE, Brown JE. Characteristics of postural control accompanying voluntary arm movement in the elderly. Society for Neuroscience Abstracts 1987;13:335.

52. Mulder T, Berndt H, Pauwels J, Nienhuis B. Sensorimotor adaptability in the elderly and disabled. In: Stelmach G, Homberg V, eds. Sensorimotor impairment in the elderly. Dordrecht: Kluwer. 1993:413–426.

53. Maki B, Holliday PJ, Topper AK. Fear of falling and postural performance in the elderly. J Gerontol 1991;46:M123–M131.

54. Lichtenstein MJ, Shields SL, Shiavi RG, Burger C. Exercise and balance in aged women: a pilot controlled clinical trial. Arch Phys Med Rehabil 1989;70:138–143.

55. Fiatarone MA, Marks EC, Ryan ND, Meredith CN, Lipsitz LA, Evans WJ. High-intensity strength training in nonagenarians: effects on skeletal muscle. JAMA 1990; 263:3029–3034.

56. Hu M, Woollacott M. Multisensory training of standing balance in older adults. I. postural stability and one-leg stance balance. J Gerontol 1994;49:M52–M61.

57. Hu M, Woollacott M. Multisensory training of standing balance in older adults. II. kinetic and electromyographic postural responses. J Gerontol 1994;49:M62–M71.

Chapter 9

ABNORMAL POSTURAL CONTROL

INTRODUCTION

The recovery of functional independence following a neurological insult is a complex process requiring the reacquisition of many skills. Since controlling the body's position in space is an essential part of regaining functional independence, restoring postural control is a critical part of rehabilitation. Postural control ensures task-specific stability and orientation for functional skills.

In the therapeutic environment, the ability to retrain postural control requires an understanding of the physiological basis for normal postural control, as well as an appreciation for the basis for instability in the neurological patient. Yet, understanding the behaviors related to abnormal postural control seen in our patients is complicated for several reasons.

Hughlings Jackson described upper motor neuron lesions as lesions of cortical and subcortical structures, producing motor dyscontrol because of the presence of abnormal behaviors, so-called positive symptoms, and the loss of normal behaviors, negative symptoms (1). Positive symptoms might include the presence of exaggerated reflexes, hyperkinetic, or associated movements. Negative symptoms may involve inability to generate force, or inappropriate selection of muscles

during performance of a task. In the rehabilitation environment, emphasis is often placed on positive systems, such as abnormalities of muscle tonus, at the expense of negative symptoms, like loss of strength, when attempting to understand performance deficits in the neurological patient (2, 3). In addition, many secondary effects of CNS lesions also contribute to the postural behavior seen in patients. These secondary problems are not the direct result of the CNS lesion, but rather develop as a result of the original problem. For example, the patient with gastrocnemius spasticity due to an upper motor neuron lesion may develop secondary tightness in the achilles tendon, limiting ankle range of motion. Limited range of motion at the ankle joint, which develops secondary to the neurological lesion, may ultimately impair function as much as the original impairment of spasticity (4).

Interpreting patients' behaviors related to posture and movement is further complicated because behaviors (except in the most acute cases) are not solely related to the outcome of the CNS lesion, but most often reflect the CNS's best attempt to compensate for that lesion. Compensatory strategies are alternative approaches to sensing and moving used to accomplish the goal of maintaining the body's position in space (5).

185

An example of a compensatory motor strategy for postural control might be that of the CVA patient who stands with the knee hyperextended because of an inability to generate enough force to keep the knee from collapsing while standing (Fig. 9.1). Standing with the knee in hyperextension ensures that the line of gravity falls in front of the knee joint, keeping the knee passively extended when loaded and preventing knee collapse while standing. Therapeutic interventions designed to keep the patient from hyperextending the knee will not necessarily be effective until the patient either develops sufficient strength to control the knee position, or develops an alternative strategy for preventing knee collapse.

An example of a compensatory sensory strategy might be that of the patient with a loss of vestibular function who learns to rely exclusively on vision for controlling the body's position in space.

Thus, understanding posture and movement behaviors seen in the patient with an upper motor neuron (UMN) lesion is a complicated process. It involves sorting out behaviors (both positive and negative symptoms) that are the direct result of the lesion, those that have developed consequent to the original lesion (secondary factors), and those that are compensatory behaviors.

This chapter reviews the sensory and motor basis for instability in the neurological patient from a systems perspective. Not included in this chapter is a discussion of postural dyscontrol from the perspective of neurological diagnosis, that is, what is the basis for instability in the patient with cerebral vascular accident, or traumatic brain injury, or cerebral palsy. Instead, the chapter uses a problem-based approach to focus on how deficits in the sensory and motor systems important to postural control can contribute to loss of the ability to control the body's position in space.

Postural Dyscontrol: A Systems Perspective

Neurological disorders represent a wide variety of upper motor neuron diseases. Since lesions can occur anywhere in the CNS, there can be many causes of postural dyscontrol in the patient with a neurological insult. In addition, the capacity of the individual to compensate for a neural lesion will also vary. Thus, the patient with a neurological deficit will show a wide range of abilities and disabilities owing to the mixture of type and severity of deficits in the many component systems of posture and movement control.

A systems perspective to postural dyscontrol focuses on identifying the constraints or impairments in each of the systems essential to controlling body posture. **Impairments** are defined as limitations within the individual which restrict sensory and movement strategies for postural control. Impairments can be musculoskeletal, neuromuscular, sensory, perceptual, or cognitive (Fig. 9.2). Our cur-

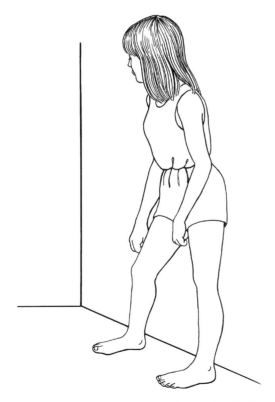

Figure 9.1. Compensatory postural strategies develop to accommodate primary impairments such as weakness. By hyperextending the knee and flexing the trunk, the line of gravity falls in front of the knee joint, preventing collapse of the knee in a hemiparetic patient.

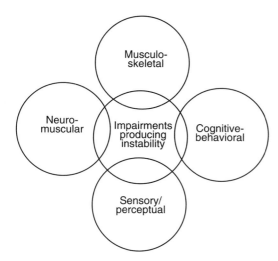

Figure 9.2. Constraints on postural control can be the results of impairments in the musculoskeletal, neuromuscular, sensory, perceptual, and/or cognitive systems.

rent knowledge of the effects of impairments in certain systems on posture control is greater than that of impairments in other systems. For example, we know more about the effects of musculoskeletal impairments on posture control than we do about many cognitive impairments. In addition, impairments arise from interacting deficits; thus, the resulting effect on motor behavior may be complex.

During the recovery of postural control following a neurological lesion, the therapist must help the patient develop a broad range of sensory and motor strategies effective in meeting the postural demands of a task. A key to developing effective strategies for balance is understanding musculoskeletal and neural constraints or impairments that affect the ability to both sense and control the body's position in space. In the following sections we discuss the constraints on motor control resulting from dysfunction in the different systems contributing to posture control.

MUSCULOSKELETAL IMPAIRMENTS

In the patient with upper motor neuron lesions, musculoskeletal disorders develop most often secondary to the neurological lesion. Yet, musculoskeletal problems can be a major limitation to normal postural function in the neurological patient. Atypical postures and movements in sitting (Fig. 9.3*A*) and standing (Fig. 9.3*B*, and *C*) often develop as a result of restrictions in movement associated with shortened muscles.

Musculoskeletal restriction can limit movement strategies used in balance. Since an ankle movement strategy for controlling upright posture requires intact range of motion and strength in the ankle, loss of ankle range or strength will limit the patient's ability to use this movement for postural control. Therapeutic interventions, such as the use of an ankle-foot-orthosis externally constrain motion at the ankle; this may prevent the patient who has adequate ankle range of motion from using it effectively in controlling body sway.

Musculoskeletal impairments constraining the ability to move have been reported in a wide variety of neurologically impaired patients. Loss of spinal flexibility may be a major limitation in capacity to move in patients with Parkinson's disease (6). Changes in spinal flexibility in patients with this disease can also affect the alignment of the center of mass moving it forward with respect to the base of support, which can be seen in Figure 9.4.

Following stroke, paralysis and immobility lead to loss of range of motion and subsequent contracture. Of particular concern is loss of range of motion in the ankle joint due to contractures in the gastrocnemius and soleus muscle groups (7).

Immobilization of a joint decreases the flexibility of the connective tissue, and increases that tissue's resistance to stretch (8). Paralysis and subsequent immobilization also result in disuse atrophy, which affects trophic factors in the muscle itself. This can result in a reduction in sarcomere numbers, a relative increase in connective tissue, and a decreased rate of protein synthesis (9).

Children with cerebral palsy frequently show restricted range of motion in many joints, including the ankle, knee, and hip. Contractures of the hip, knee, and ankle muscles are frequent consequences of disordered

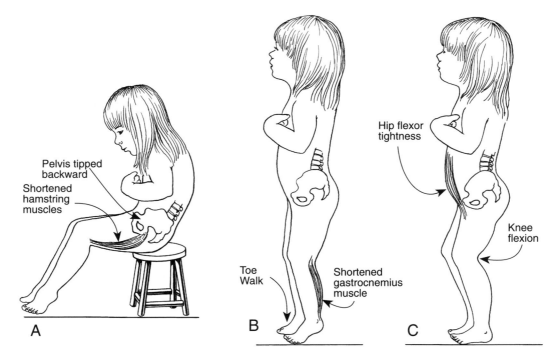

Figure 9.3. Atypical postures due to musculoskeletal impairments. **A,** Excessive posterior tilt of pelvis in sitting accommodates shortened hamstrings. **B,** Shortening of the gastrocnemius muscle results in toe walk. **C,** Hip flexor tightness can result in tilting of the pelvis and flexion of the knee. (Adapted from Reimers J. Clinically based decision making for surgery. In: Sussman M, ed. The diplegic child. Rosemont, IL: American Academy of Orthopedic Surgeons, 1992:155, 156, 158.)

patterns of movement (10). Using a habitual crouched postural pattern during stance and gait results in the subsequent shortening of the hamstring muscles, ensuring the continued use of a habitual crouched posture.

Patients with vestibular abnormalities can show restrictions in cervical range of motion. Often these patients minimize motion of the head in an effort to reduce complaints of dizziness. This strategy leads to secondary cervical dysfunction, which can restrict the patient's ability to move in ways that are necessary to overcome the primary vestibular dysfunction (4).

In summary, musculoskeletal problems, while often not a primary result of a neurological lesion, present a major constraint to normal posture and movement control in many neurologically impaired patients. Loss of range of motion and flexibility can limit the ways in which a patient can move for postural control. In addition, musculoskeletal prob-

lems can contribute to an inability to sustain an ideal alignment of body segments in the upright position, requiring excessive force to counter the effects of gravity and sustain a vertical posture.

NEUROMUSCULAR IMPAIRMENTS

Neuromuscular limitations encompass a diverse group of problems that represent a major constraint on postural control in the patient with neurological dysfunction.

Weakness

Neural lesions affecting the ability to generate forces, both voluntarily and within the context of a postural task, are a major limitation in many neurologically impaired patients. Strength is defined as the ability to generate sufficient tension in a muscle for the

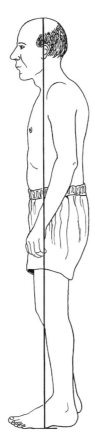

Figure 9.4. In a Parkinson patient, changes in spinal flexibility can also affect the alignment of the center of mass with respect to the base of support. (Adapted from Schenkman M. Interrelationship of neurological and mechanical factors in balance control. In: Duncan P, ed. Balance: proceedings of the APTA forum. Alexandria, VA: APTA, 1990:37.)

purposes of posture and movement (11). Strength results from both properties of the muscle itself (musculoskeletal aspects of strength) and the appropriate recruitment of motor units and the timing of their activation (9, 12–14). Neural aspects of force production reflect (*a*) the number of motor units recruited, (*b*) the type of units recruited, and (*c*) the discharge frequency (12–14).

Weakness, or the inability to generate tension, is a major impairment of function in many patients with upper motor neuron lesions. Several authors have documented the selective atrophy of type I (slow) and II (fast) muscle fibers in patients with a UMN lesion

(15–17). In addition, stroke patients have been shown to have abnormal and reduced firing rates of motor neurons (9). Instability in the weak patient results from an inability to generate sufficient force to counter destabilizing forces, particularly the force of gravity, in the vertical position.

Abnormalities of Muscle Tone

The presence of abnormalities of muscle tone in the patient with upper motor neuron lesions is well known (18–21). However, the exact contribution of abnormalities of muscle tone to functional deficits in posture, locomotion, and movement control is not well understood.

The term spasticity is used clinically to cover a wide range of abnormal behaviors. It is used to describe (*a*) hyperactive stretch reflexes, (*b*) abnormal posturing of the limbs, (*c*) excessive coactivation of antagonist muscles, (*d*) associated movements, (*e*) clonus, and (*f*) stereotyped movement synergies (22). Thus, one word (spasticity) is used to describe many abnormal behaviors often seen in patients with a neurological disorder.

The range of muscle tone abnormalities found within patients who have UMN lesions is broad (Fig. 9.5). At one end of the time spectrum is flaccidity or complete loss of muscle tone. Moving up the tone continuum is hypotonicity, defined as a reduction in the stiffness of a muscle to lengthening. Hypotonicity is described in many different kinds of patients, including those with spinocerebellar lesions (21), and in many developmentally delayed children, such as children with Down syndrome (23).

On the upper end of the tone spectrum is hypertonicity or spasticity. **Spasticity** is defined as "a motor disorder characterized by a velocity-dependent increase in tonic stretch reflexes (muscle tone) with exaggerated tendon jerks, resulting from hyperexcitability of the stretch reflex, as one component of the upper motor neuron syndrome" (24).

Remember, in the chapter on normal postural control, we defined normal muscle tone as the muscle's resistance to being

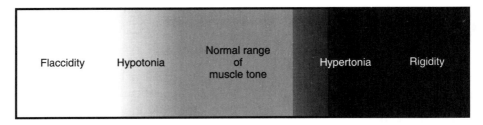

Figure 9.5.   Range of tonus found in a patient with a neurological impairment. On one end of the tonus continuum is flaccidity or low tone. At the other end of the continuum are problems related to hypertonicity including spasticity and rigidity.

lengthened, its *stiffness*. Normal muscle stiffness or tone is the result of both non-neural and neural components. The non-neural components reflect the mechanical-elastic characteristics of the muscle and connective tissue that resist lengthening. The neural basis for stiffness reflects the degree of motor unit activity, most importantly, stretch reflex-generated muscle activity, which resists muscle lengthening. Several mechanisms have been suggested as the basis for spastic hypertonus in the patient with a neurological disorder.

One mechanism for increased muscle stiffness in spastic hypertonia may be changes in the intrinsic properties of the muscle fibers themselves. Researchers analyzing gait in children with cerebral palsy have found that increased tension in the gastrocnemius muscle is not always associated with increased muscle activity in that muscle. Based on these findings, so-called spastic gait (equinus foot position at foot strike) may be partly due to changes in intrinsic properties of the muscle rather than hyperexcitability of the stretch reflex mechanism (25).

The predominant hypothesis regarding the neural mechanism underlying spastic hypertonia is abnormalities within the segmental stretch reflex. Researchers have suggested two possible mechanisms that produce an enhanced reflex response to muscle stretch following a UMN lesion (26).

The first mechanism is an increase in α-motoneuron excitability, which results in an increased response to stretch evoked input. Increased α-motoneuron excitability could occur because the motoneurons are continuously depolarized more than normal and so

are close to their threshold for excitation. Increased depolarization could arise because of (*a*) increased tonic excitatory input from segmental afferents or descending pathways such as the lateral vestibulospinal tracts, and/or (*b*) a tonic reduction in inhibitory synaptic input from the inhibitory interneurons (26).

The second mechanism that could produce an enhanced reflex response to stretch (hypertonicity) is disorder within the stretch reflex mechanism itself. Disorders in the stretch reflex mechanism could be alterations in the threshold and or the gain of the stretch reflex in spastic hypertonicity (26).

Most studies examining alteration in stretch reflex mechanisms with spasticity have been consistent in showing changes in the *setpoint*, or angular threshold of the stretch reflex. It has been shown that the threshold for motoneuron recruitment in response to stretch is reduced in patients with spasticity. As a result, a smaller or slower stretch can reflexly excite the motoneurons. Changes in the threshold of the stretch reflex are purported to result from an enhanced net descending excitatory drive from higher centers, especially vestibulospinal and reticulospinal pathways. It remains unresolved whether this augmented drive is caused solely by increased excitatory descending input from these pathways, or whether it reflects a reduced inflow from descending or regional inhibitory systems (26, 27).

Despite the change in threshold for activating the reflex response to stretch, the gain of the stretch reflex appears to be normal in the spastic muscle. This means the force-length relationship in the *spastic* muscle remains the same as for a normal muscle. It used to be believed that spastic hypertonia was due to hyperactivity of the γ-efferent fibers (so-called γ spasticity), causing an increased sensitivity of the muscle spindle receptor to stretch, and a subsequent change in the gain of the reflex. However, this concept has lost support, since there is no evidence to support the concept of increased dynamic fusimotor activity as the basis for spasticity (26, 27). In summary, spastic hypertonicity in upper motor neuron lesions is probably the result of changes in the threshold of the system to stretch, rather than the gain of the system.

Though we have a greater understanding of the neural mechanisms underlying spastic hypertonicity, there is still no agreement on the role of spastic hypertonicity (a positive sign of UMN disease) in the loss of functional performance (a negative sign) (26, 27).

It has been suggested that spastic hypertonicity limits a patient's ability to move quickly, since activation of the stretch reflex is velocity dependent. Excessive activation of the stretch reflex mechanism would serve to reflexly prevent the lengthening of the antagonist muscle during shortening of the agonist. This has been referred to as *antagonist restraint* (18, 28) or *spastic restraint* (20). It would be expected that evidence for antagonist restraint would appear as coactivation of the agonist and antagonist muscle associated with movement.

A growing number of research studies are finding evidence against this argument. Instead, researchers are arguing that inadequate recruitment of agonist motor neurons, not increased activity in the antagonist, is the primary basis for disorders of motor control following UMN lesions (29–36). Thus, other problems such as inability to recruit motoneurons (weakness), abnormalities of reciprocal inhibition between agonist and antagonist, and dyssynergia may be more disabling to motor control than simply hypertonicity (26).

This research has tremendous implications for clinical practice. It suggests that treatment practices directed primarily at reducing spastic hypertonicity as the major focus in regaining motor control may have limited impact on helping patients regain functional independence. This is because loss of functional independence is often the result of many factors, which may be more limiting to the recovery of motor control than the presence of abnormal muscle tone. Some of those factors include problems within the coordination of synergistic muscles activated in response to instability.

Dyscoordination within Motor Strategies

Neurological lesions also affect the ability to organize multiple muscles into coordinated postural movement synergies.

ALIGNMENT

Alignment of the body refers to the arrangement of body segments to one another, as well as the position of the body with reference to gravity and the base of support (4). Alignment of body segments over the base of support determines to a great extent the effort required to support the body against gravity. In addition, alignment determines the constellation of movement strategies that will be effective in controlling posture (4).

Changes in initial position or alignment are often characteristic of the patient with a UMN lesion. Abnormalities can reflect changes in the alignment of one body part to another. Examples include the patient who sits or stands with the pelvis rotated back posteriorly, with excessive trunk kyphosis and the head in a forward-flexed position (refer back to Fig. 9.3), or the child with cerebral palsy, who uses a habitual crouched postural pattern during stance and gait (10).

Abnormal alignment can also be expressed as a change in the position of the body with reference to gravity and the base of support. For example, asymmetric alignment in sitting and standing is often characteristic of patients with a unilateral neural lesion such as cerebral vascular accident (9). These patients tend to stand with weight displaced towards the noninvolved side. Other patients, most notably, patients with cerebellar lesions, tend to stand with a wide base of support (21).

Finally, many patients stand with the center of mass displaced either forward to backward. For example, it has been reported that elderly patients with a fear of falling tend to stand in a forward lean posture with the center of mass displaced anteriorly (37). (Forward displacement of the center of mass is shown in Fig. 9.4.) However, there are other types of patients who stand with the center of mass displaced posteriorly (4).

Changes in alignment can be viewed as both a musculoskeletal impairment or as a strategy compensating for other impairments. For example, in the elderly person, alignment, which is often characterized by a prominent kyphosis and forward-flexed head position, represents a musculoskeletal impairment that constrains movements necessary for posture and balance (38). In contrast, the asymmetric alignment commonly seen in the hemiplegic patient who sits and stands with weight shifted to the nonhemiplegic side, is often a strategy that develops to compensate for other impairments such as weakness (4). Understanding these differences is important, since achieving a symmetrically aligned position may not be a reasonable goal for the hemiparetic patient until underlying impairments have resolved sufficiently to ensure that the hemiparetic leg will not collapse under the weight of the body.

MOVEMENT STRATEGIES

We divide coordination problems that manifest within postural movement strategies into (a) disorders related to the timing of postural actions, and (b) disorders related to the scaling of postural actions.

Timing Problems

In many patients with neurological disorders, postural dyscontrol is not entirely related to the ability to generate force, but results from an inability to time the application of forces effectively for recovering stability. A number of different timing problems related to postural control have been described, including delays in the onset of a postural response, and problems in the temporal coordination among muscle synergists.

ACTIVE LEARNING MODULE

Let's do another experiment. Get a partner and have him/her stand facing you. Hold your partner by the hips and gently push him/her in the backward direction. Watch the feet, notice how quickly the toes come up as he/she is pushed in the backward direction. Do both feet react at about the same time? For most people, the anterior tibialis in both legs contracts quickly, bringing the toes up symmetrically in both legs. Remember from the chapter on normal postural control, the actual onset time for the tibialis following a perturbation is approximately 100 msec. What would you expect to see if the anterior tibialis in one leg was slow in becoming active? Probably that foot would be slow to come off the ground compared to the other foot when you shift the person in the backwards direction.

Delays in the onset of postural motor activity during recovery of balance result in delayed corrective responses, increased sway, and, in many cases, subsequent loss of balance. To study the timing of muscle activation for postural control, researchers use a moving platform to induce sway in a standing subject and EMGs to record how quickly muscles respond to sway. Using this approach with stroke patients, researchers have found that muscle onset latencies were often very slow, approximately 220 msec compared with 90 to 100 msec found in normal controls (39).

Inability to respond quickly to loss of balance was also found in a number of traumatic brain-injured patients (40). Significantly delayed activation of postural muscles occurred in TBI patients with focal cortical contusions. Interestingly, patients with mild to moderate traumatic cerebral concussions did not show a similar delay in onset latencies of postural muscles.

Significant delays in the onset of postural activity were reported in developmental abnormalities including Down syndrome (41) and some forms of cerebral palsy (42).

Other types of timing problems can affect the coordination of muscles responding synergistically to recover balance. When there is a disruption in the timing among the muscles activated to control the center of body mass, movements become dyscoordinated and can hamper the restoration of equilibrium. Disruption of the timing and sequencing of muscles that work synergistically has been referred to as dyssynergia. **Dyssynergia** is a general term used to describe a variety of problems related to timing or sequencing of muscles for action.

In the rehabilitation literature, the term *synergy* has often been used to describe abnormal or disordered motor control (18, 19). Abnormal synergies are stereotypical patterns of movement that cannot be changed or adapted to changes in task or environmental demands. A variety of abnormal synergies that impair normal movement have been described in hemiplegic patients (9, 19). Figure 9.6 illustrates an example of an abnormal flexor synergy in the arm in supine (*A*), sitting (*B*) and standing (*C*) (19). The process of recovery during stroke rehabilitation has been described as the dissolution of abnormal synergies of movement in favor of independent or selective control (19).

It is important to remember that during the normal control of movement, the CNS makes use of muscular synergies as a way of simplifying the control of movement. As we described in the chapter on normal postural control, a synergy is a group of muscles that are constrained to act together to achieve a functional task. An important feature of normal postural synergies, which distinguishes them from abnormal synergies, is their ability to be modified. Normal synergies are not invariant, that is, immutable, but are assembled to accomplish a task, and are therefore flexible and adaptable to changing demands. In the neurologically impaired patient, dyssynergia, or the absence of normal synergies of movement, constrains the recovery of normal motor control, including postural control.

Timing among postural muscles can be disrupted in a number of different ways. Yet, all types of timing problems are classified as *dyssynergia*. What are some of these problems, and what types of patients typically have these problems?

Dyssynergia has been reported in patients with spastic hemiplegia, either due to cerebral palsy (42), or cerebral vascular accident (39).

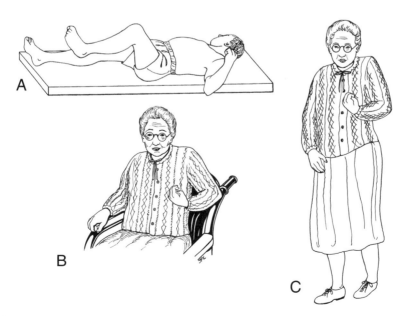

Figure 9.6. Abnormal synergies of movement in a patient with hemiplegia in **A**, supine, **B**, sitting, and **C**, standing. (Adapted from Brunnstrom S. Movement therapy in hemiplegia: a neurophysiological approach. Hagerstown, MD: Harper & Row, 1970:12, 13, 15.)

Using the moving platform technique described in earlier chapters, postural muscle patterns were studied in a group of cerebral palsy children ages 7 to 12 (42). In spastic hemiplegic children, muscle responses in the affected leg were abnormally sequenced primarily due to delayed activation of the distal muscle. When the platform moved backwards, the child swayed forward, and the muscle activation pattern in the nonhemiplegic leg was from distal to proximal, with a 30 to 50 msec delay (Fig. 9.7). In contrast, in the hemiplegic leg, the first set of muscles to become active in response to forward sway was the hamstrings, followed by activation of the gastrocnemius.

This finding was surprising for a number of reasons. On clinical examination, this child showed *spasticity* in the gastrocnemius muscle. Signs included: increased stiffness in response to passive stretch, clonus, equinus gait, and lack of dorsiflexion at the ankle in response to a backwards displacement. One possible explanation for all these clinical findings was a primary impairment of gastrocnemius spasticity.

Given these clinical findings, one might predict a hyperactive response in the gastrocnemius when the child stood on the platform and swayed in the forward direction, since during forward sway the first muscle to be stretched is the gastrocnemius. But during forward sway, imposing a stretch on the *hyperactive gastrocnemius*, the first muscles to respond were the hamstrings! The gastrocnemius muscle was slow to become active, and the amplitude of the muscle activity was low compared to the uninvolved side. These findings are consistent with those of other authors who have noted that one major finding in neurologically impaired patients with spastic hypertonia is an inability to recruit and regulate the firing frequency of motor neurons.

This same disruption was found in response to backward sway, that is, instead of the normal activation of tibialis anterior, quadriceps, and abdominals found in the noninvolved leg, the cerebral palsy hemiplegic children activated the quadriceps muscle first, followed by the tibialis anterior. The biomechanical effect of the disordered sequencing was hyperextension of the knee and forward flexion of the trunk (Fig. 9.8). When seen clinically, this movement pattern is often ascribed to hyperactivity of the gastrocnemius, which prevents appropriate activation of the tibialis anterior (TA) because of antagonist restraint. In the case of the children tested in this study, however, activity in the gastrocnemius muscle was not the cause of this particular movement pattern.

Analysis of postural patterns in adult

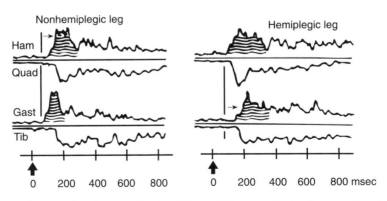

Figure 9.7. Abnormal sequencing of muscles in a hemiplegic child responding to a backward translation of a moving platform. EMG records show an inappropriate activation of muscles responding to forward sway, with proximal muscles firing in advance of the so-called *spastic* distal muscles. (Abbreviations: *Ham,* hamstrings; *Quad,* quadriceps; *Gast,* gastrocnemius; *Tib,* tibialis anterior.) The *arrow* signals platform movement onset. (Adapted from Nashner LM, Shumway-Cook A, Marin D, Stance posture control in select groups of children with cerebral palsy: deficits in sensory organization and muscular coordination. Exp Brain Res 1983;49:401.)

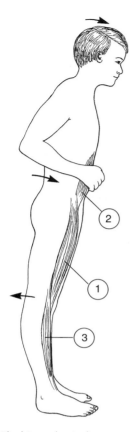

Figure 9.8. The biomechanical consequences of a disruption in the timing of muscles responding to backwards sway includes back-kneeing and forward flexion of the trunk. The numbers represent the order in which the muscles are activated. (Adapted from Shumway-Cook A, McCollum G. Assessment and treatment of balance deficits. In: Montgomery P, Connolly B, eds. Motor control and physical therapy. Hixson, TN: Chattanooga Group, 1991:130.)

stroke patients has also revealed disordered patterns of muscle activity, including abnormal timing and sequencing of muscle activation, excessive cocontraction, and greater variability in the timing of responses among hemiplegic subjects (9). Disorders in initial standing posture also affected the organization of postural strategies in some hemiplegic subjects (43).

Patients with dyssynergia sometimes have abnormally long delays in the onset time of proximal muscle synergists. This type of dyssynergia has been reported in children with Down syndrome (41) and in traumatic brain-injured adults with focal cortical contusions (40). The biomechanical consequences of delayed activation of proximal muscles compared to the distal muscles include excessive motion at the knee and hip. This is because the muscle timing pattern is not efficient in controlling the indirect effects of forces generated at the ankle on more proximal joints.

Dyssynergia can also be characterized by cocontraction of muscles on both anterior and posterior aspects of the body. Researchers have found that Parkinson's patients use a complex movement strategy when responding to threats to balance. (This is shown in Fig. 9.9.) This activation of muscles on both sides of the body results in a stiffening of the body, and is a very inefficient strategy for the recovery of balance, since it is not directionally specific (44).

These results are not consistent with the classic work on Parkinson's patients by Purdue Martin, who reported an absence of equilibrium and righting reactions in Parkinson's patients (45). The rigidity and loss of balance found in patients during tilt tests imply that equilibrium reactions were absent. Placing EMGs on the muscles of Parkinson's patients has allowed researchers to see that Parkinson patients do indeed respond to disequilibrium, but the pattern of muscular activity used is ineffective in recovering balance.

Scaling Problems

Maintaining balance requires that forces generated to control the body's position in space be appropriately scaled to the degree of instability. This means that a small perturbation to stability is met with an appropriately sized muscle response. Thus, force output must be appropriate to the amplitude of instability. Researchers are beginning to examine the physiological mechanisms underlying the scaling of postural responses in neurologically intact subjects. In addition, researchers are looking at the effects of lesions in the cerebellum or basal ganglia on the ability to scale the amplitude of postural responses to different sized perturbations to balance (46, 47). Results from these studies have shown that neurologically intact subjects use a combination of feedforward, or anticipatory, and feedback control mechanisms to scale forces needed for postural stability (46). Grading or scaling force output probably involves anterior portions of the cerebellum, since an inability to anticipate and scale forces appropriate to changes in the size of a postural perturbation was found in patients with anterior cerebellar lesions (47).

Postural responses that are too large are called hypermetric, and are associated with excessive compensatory body sway in the direction opposite the initial direction of instability. For example, patients with unilateral cerebellar pathology affecting the anterior lobe, can show hypermetric responses on the involved side of the body. This will often result in a fall in the direction opposite the affected side due to excessive activity in the hypermetric extremity. By contrast, many hemiparetic patients will fall in the direction of weakness due to an inability to generate sufficient force to counter the destabilizing forces. Patients with hypermetric responses may also show excessive oscillation of the center of mass (4).

MOTOR ADAPTATION PROBLEMS

Normal postural control requires the ability to adapt responses to changing tasks and environmental demands. This flexibility requires the availability of multiple movement strategies and the ability to select the appropriate strategy for the task and environment. The inability to adapt movements to changing task demands is a characteristic of many patients with neurological disorders.

Patients become fixed in stereotypical patterns of movement, showing a loss of movement flexibility and adaptability. The fixed movement synergies seen in the patient with hemiparesis are an example of impairments related to loss of flexibility and adaptability of movements. Infants with cerebral palsy who have trouble dissociating movements of their legs are constrained to kick symmetrically because of these obligatory movement patterns in the legs (48).

Inability to adapt movement strategies

to changes in support has been found in patients with Parkinson's disease (44). In this study, normal controls and a group of Parkinson's patients were asked to maintain stance balance in a variety of situations, including standing on a flat surface, standing across a narrow beam, and sitting on a stool with the feet unsupported. Normal subjects can adapt the muscles used for postural control in response to changing task demands (Fig. 9.9A). In contrast, Parkinson's patients were unable to modify the complex movement strategy used in recovering balance while standing on a flat surface to the beam or seated conditions, showing an inability to modify how they moved in response to changes in environmental and task demands (Fig. 9.9B).

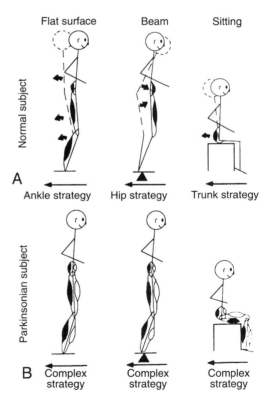

Figure 9.9. Normal and abnormal adaptation. **A,** Normal adaptation of muscle activity in response to three different postural tasks. **B,** By contrast, EMG patterns in Parkinson's patients revealed a complex strategy of muscle activity that did not adapt to changes in task demands. (Adapted from Horak FB, Nashner LM, Nutt JG. Postural instability in Parkinson's disease: motor coordination and sensory organization. Neurology Report 1988;12:55.)

Loss of Anticipatory Postural Control

We have seen that an inability to adapt how we move in response to changing task and environmental conditions can be a source of instability in many neurologically impaired patients. Another source of postural dyscontrol is the loss of anticipatory processes that activate postural adjustments in advance of potentially destabilizing voluntary movements. Anticipatory postural activity is heavily dependent on previous experience and learning.

Inability to activate postural muscles in anticipation of voluntary arm movements has been described in many neurologically impaired patients, including stroke patients (49), children with cerebral palsy (42), children with Down syndrome (41), and Parkinson's patients (50).

Summarizing Motor Problems by Diagnosis

Until now, our discussions of postural dyscontrol in the neurologically impaired patient have focused on presenting a wide variety of motor problems leading to problems in stability and orientation. You can see that the range of problems is great, and this reflects the complexity of problems that affect the central nervous system. In some cases, the same type of problem can be found in patients with very different diagnoses. For example, delayed onset of postural responses can be found in adult hemiplegic patients, in children with Down syndrome, and in elderly people with peripheral neuropathies.

On the other hand, some problems appear to be unique to a diagnosis. For example, a particular type of complex movement strategy used in all task conditions has been found in Parkinson's patients. In most cases, what we don't know about postural dyscontrol in patients far outweighs what we do know! This is because this area of research is only about 20 years old. New information is rapidly becoming available as scientists expand the study of postural control to more groups of patients.

In this next section, we try to summarize some of the research on motor problems related to postural dyscontrol by diagnosis. Several warnings must be stated prior to beginning this section. Remember that even patients with the same diagnosis can be very different. Thus, no two stroke patients look alike because of the difference in type, location, and extent of neural lesion. Other factors such as age, premorbid status, and degree of compensation, also have a profound impact on behavior seen. Nonetheless, we provide a summary here of the kinds of problems one is likely to see in various types of neurologically impaired patients, based on current postural control research. This information is also summarized in Table 9.1.

CEREBRAL VASCULAR ACCIDENT— SPASTIC HEMIPLEGIA

Postural control research has reported the multiple kinds of motor problems in stroke patients with hemiplegia. A number of articles have reviewed the sensory and motor impairments in the patient who has had a stroke (9, 43, 51, 52). Weakness is frequently a primary impairment. Abnormal muscle tone is common, ranging from complete flaccidity to spastic hypertonicity. Postural responses are often delayed. In addition, dyssynergia, or a breakdown in the synergistic organization of muscles, is widely reported. This can include proximal muscles firing in advance of distal muscles, or in some patients, quite late in relationship to distal muscles. Loss of anticipatory activation of postural muscles during voluntary movements is also common, as is an inability to modify and adapt movements to changing task demands. Neuromuscular problems often produce secondary musculoskeletal problems including shortening of the gastrocnemius/soleus muscle groups and loss of ankle range of motion.

PARKINSON'S DISEASE

Motor problems such as bradykinesia and rigidity produce many disabling musculoskeletal problems, including loss of flexibil-

Table 9.1.   Motor Problems by Diagnosis

	Hemiplegic		Cerebellar		
	Adult CVA	Pediatric CP	Adult	Pediatric	Parkinson's
Force Problems					
Weakness	+	+	−	−	−
Abnormal tone	+	+	+/−	+/−	+
Hypermetric response	−	−	+	+	−
Timing Problems					
Delayed onset	+	+	−	+	−
Dysynergia	+	+	−	−	+
Impaired adaptation	+	+	?	?	+
Impaired anticipatory control	+	+	?	?	+
Musculoskeletal problems	+	+	?	?	+

ity and joint range of motion (6, 50, 53, 54). Motor problems do not appear to be the result of muscle weakness (45). Interestingly, despite the fact that bradykinesia or slowed voluntary movement is common in Parkinson's patients, onset latencies of automatic postural responses are reported to be normal (44). EMG studies have found that Parkinson's patients use a complex pattern of muscle activity involving muscles on both sides of the body when responding to instability. This coactivation results in a rigid body and an inability to adequately recover stability. In addition, patients appear to be unable to modify movement patterns in response to changing task demands. Finally, anticipatory postural activity is disrupted in many Parkinson's patients (50, 54).

CEREBELLAR DISORDERS

Signs and symptoms associated with disorders of the cerebellum were first described in the 1920s and 1930s (55). Principal deficits associated with cerebellar disorders include: (*a*) **hypotonia** or decreased resistance of the limb to stretch; (*b*) **ataxia**, which is described as a delay in initiation of movement, or errors in the range, force, or metrics of movement, often referred to as dysmetria or dyssynergia; and (*c*) **action or intention tremor**, particularly at the termination of movement (21). Lesions of the cerebellum tend to produce disorders ipsilateral to the lesion.

In addition, lesions to the various parts of the cerebellum have distinctive signs and symptoms. For example, lesions of the midline vermis and fastigial nuclei affect primarily trunk and upper extremities; they thus can manifest as truncal tremor, wide-based ataxic gait, and dysarthric speech. In contrast, lesions to the anterior lobe (vermis, and leg areas) produce movement disturbances in the legs, which result in poor performance on the heel-shin test, dyssynergia, and abnormal gait (21).

Much of the research on postural control in cerebellar patients has been with patients who have anterior lobe cerebellar degeneration. Thus, findings from these studies may not necessarily be found in patients with lateral hemisphere lesions or vestibulocerebellar lesions. Onset latencies are reported to be normal in adult cerebellar patients, though delayed in cerebral palsy children with cerebellar ataxia. An inability to scale postural activity leading to hypermetric postural responses has also been reported in cerebellar patients (47).

SENSORY DISORDERS

As we mentioned earlier, effective postural control requires more than the ability to generate and apply forces for controlling the body's position in space. In order to know *when* to apply restoring forces, the CNS must have an accurate picture of *where* the body is in space, and whether it is stationary or in motion. As a result, normal postural control requires the organization of sensory information from visual, somatosensory, and vestibular systems about the body's position and movement with respect to the environment, and the coordination of sensory information with motor actions.

Disruptions of sensory information processing may affect postural control in a number of ways (4, 56). First, sensory problems may prevent the development of accurate internal models of the body for postural control. This can affect a patient's ability to accurately determine the orientation of the body with respect to gravity and the environment. Second, disruption of central sensory mechanisms may affect a patient's ability to adapt sensory inputs to changes in task and environmental demands. Third, sensory problems can disrupt motor learning, affecting a patient's ability to adapt to change. Finally, loss of sensory information can impair the ability to anticipate instability, and thus cause a compensatory modification in the strategies a patient uses to sense instability and move.

Misrepresentation of Stability Limits

An important part of interpreting senses and coordinating actions that control the body's position in space appears to be the presence of an internal representation or *body schema*, providing an accurate representation or postural frame of reference. Figure 9.10 provides an example of this concept. Illustrated are the proposed stability limits for the task of independent stance on a firm, flat surface in a neurologically intact adult with normal postural control (Fig. 9.10*A*) (57). Figure 9.10*B*, however, depicts modified stability limits for a hemiplegic patient who requires a cane for support due to unilateral weakness. Stability limits now exclude the left leg, which cannot support the body due to weakness, but include the cane, which serves as an addition to the base of support (5).

It has been suggested that an accurate representation, or model, of stability limits is essential to the recovery of postural control. This allows the development of new sensory and motor strategies while the patient remains within his/her new stability limits, regardless of the impairments resulting from the neurological lesion (5). Thus, the process of recovering postural control after a lesion includes the development of accurate new representations of the body's capability as it relates to postural control. Usually, the indi-

Figure 9.10. Conceptual model of stability limits for stance postural control. **A**, Normal stability limits in a neurologically intact adult, compared to **B**, modified stability limits in a left hemiplegic patient, excludes the weak leg, but includes the cane, which is now part of the patient's base of support. (Adapted from Shumway-Cook A, McCollum G. Assessment and treatment of balance deficits. In: Montgomery P, Connolly B, eds. Motor control and physical therapy. Hixson, TN: Chattanooga Group, 1991:129.)

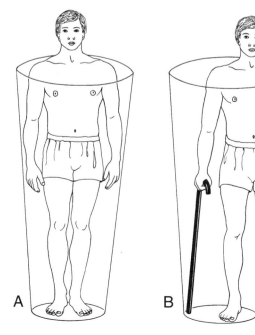

A   B

vidual's model of stability limits are consistent with *actual* stability limits. In many patients, however, perceived stability limits may be inconsistent with actual stability limits, which have changed as a result of sensory and motor limitations following a neurological lesion.

A discrepancy between actual and internal limits of stability can result in instability and potential falls (5). In the drawing in Figure 9.10*B*, the patient's actual stability limits exclude the hemiparetic leg, which is incapable of generating sufficient force to control the body in the upright position. If the patient's internal model of stability limits includes the affected leg as part of the base of support, the patient will have a tendency to fall to that side, when the center of mass shifts to that side.

On the other hand, inaccurate representations of the body with respect to postural control can limit the patient's ability to use new skills for postural control (5). For example, if the hemiplegic patient's internal model of stability limits doesn't change during the course of recovery to reflect new abilities to control the left leg for purposes of support, the patient may continue to stand and walk asymmetrically.

Many patients with neurological disorders fail to develop accurate models of their body related to the dynamics of moving and sensing for postural control (5, 58, 59). Inaccurate internal models result in patterns of moving and sensing that seem inconsistent with the patient's apparent abilities. This aspect of disordered postural control is just beginning to be explored, and much research is needed in this area.

Inability to Adapt Senses

In the neurologically impaired patient, inability to adapt how the senses are used for postural control can result from pathology within individual sensory systems or from damage to central sensory structures important in organizing sensory information for postural control (4, 5).

The loss of somatosensory, kinesthetic, and proprioceptive information is common in many types of cerebral vascular accidents, leaving the hemiplegic patient with hemisensory losses that profoundly affect posture and movement control (60). In addition, many such patients have disorders within the visual system, including impaired ocular motility, visual field defects, and impaired convergence leading to fusional problems (40). Finally, many patients with central neurological disorders have associated problems in peripheral or central vestibular structures (61). Traumatic injury to the head can result in several types of injury to the vestibular system that can complicate the recovery of postural control (61).

In many patients, despite intact peripheral sensation, lesions in a wide variety of central nervous system structures can affect the ability to adapt senses for postural control.

Sensory adaptation problems can manifest as an inflexible weighting of sensory information for orientation, and/or an inability to maintain balance in any environments where sensory information is inaccurately reporting self-motion. The inability to adapt weighting of senses for orientation in different environments is somewhat analogous to the inflexibility in the use of movement strategies seen in many neurologically impaired patients.

Researchers examining the effect of neurological injury on patients' ability to adapt sensory information for postural control have primarily focused on the use of computerized force platforms in conjunction with moving visual surrounds, first developed by Nashner and colleagues (62–66). This approach, described in detail in the chapters on normal postural control, tests the ability of the patient to maintain stance balance under situations where sensory information is lost or made inaccurate for postural control. A classification scheme for identifying different problems related to organizing sensory information for stance postural control has been proposed based on patterns of normal and abnormal sway in six sensory conditions used during dynamic posturography testing (4). Patterns of sway associated with different categories of sensory organization problems are summarized in Figure 9.11.

What is the effect of loss of a sensory input on postural control? It depends! Some important factors include (*a*) the availability of other senses to detect position of the body in space, (*b*) the availability of accurate orientation cues in the environment, and (*c*) the ability to correctly interpret and select sensory information for orientation (4).

As shown in Figure 9.12, patients with loss of vestibular information for postural control may be stable under most conditions as long as alternative sensory information from vision or the somatosensory systems is available for orientation. In situations where vision and somatosensory inputs are reduced, leaving mainly vestibular inputs (the last two conditions in Fig. 9.12) for postural control, the patient may experience a sudden fall (62).

Functionally, patients with this type of postural dyscontrol might perform normally on most tests of balance as long as they are performed in a well-lit environment and on a firm, flat surface. However, performance on balance tasks under ideal sensory conditions will not necessarily predict the patient's likelihood for falls when getting up to go to the

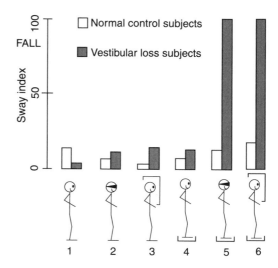

Figure 9.12. A comparison of body sway in the six sensory conditions in neurologically intact adults vs. patients with loss of vestibular function. Results show that instability in patients with loss of vestibular function occurs only in conditions where vision and somatosensory inputs are not available for postural control (conditions 5 and 6). (Adapted from Horak F, Nashner LM, Diener HC. Postural strategies associated with somatosensory and vestibular loss. Exp Brain Res 1990:418.)

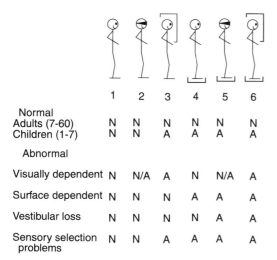

	1	2	3	4	5	6
Normal Adults (7-60)	N	N	N	N	N	N
Children (1-7)	N	N	A	A	A	A
Abnormal						
Visually dependent	N	N/A	A	N	N/A	A
Surface dependent	N	N	N	A	A	A
Vestibular loss	N	N	N	N	A	A
Sensory selection problems	N	N	A	A	A	A

Figure 9.11. A classification scheme for identifying different problems related to organizing sensory information for stance postural control based on patterns of normal and abnormal sway in six sensory conditions used during dynamic posturography testing. (N = normal sway; A = abnormal sway.)

bathroom at night and negotiating a carpeted surface in the dark.

How does disruption of somatosensory information affect postural control? One might expect that a patient with sudden loss of somatosensory information could maintain stability as long as alternative information from vision and vestibular senses were available. A group of researchers examined this question by applying pressure cuffs to the ankles of normal subjects and inflating them until cutaneous sensation in the feet and ankles was lost (63). These neurologically intact subjects were able to maintain balance on all six of the sensory conditions (Fig. 9.13) since they always had an alternative sense available for orientation.

Overreliance on vision for postural control is referred to as a *visual dependence pattern* for sensory organization. In this pattern, sway is abnormally increased in any condition where vision is reduced or inaccurate (conditions 2, 3, 5, and 6 in Fig. 9.11). We saw this type of pattern in very young normal children, as noted earlier in the chapter on normal de-

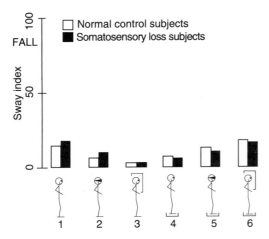

Figure 9.13. Body sway in the six sensory conditions in normal subjects before use of pressure cuffs at the ankle and after subsequent temporary loss of cutaneous sensation with use of pressure cuffs. Loss of somatosensory inputs did not affect the ability of these neurologically intact subjects to maintain balance, due to the availability of alternative senses and the capacity to adapt remaining senses to the changing demands. (Adapted from Horak F, Nashner LM, Diener HC. Postural strategies associated with somatosensory and vestibular loss. Exp Brain Res 1990:418.)

velopment of postural control. A visual dependence pattern has also been reported in other types of neurologically impaired patients, including those with specific types of positional vertigo due to vestibular pathology (66).

Alternatively, some patients may demonstrate an inflexible use of somatosensory inputs for postural control, becoming unstable in conditions where surface inputs do not allow patients to establish and maintain a vertical orientation (56). This type of pattern is referred to as a *surface-dependent pattern*, and is seen in patients who show excessive amounts of body sway in conditions 4, 5, and 6 (Fig. 9.11). Thus, when standing on a compliant surface, like sand or thick carpet, or on a tilted surface, like a ramp, or on a moving surface, like a boat, the position of the ankle joint and other somatosensory and proprioceptive information from the feet and legs does not correlate well with the orientation of the rest of the body (56). An overreliance on somatosensory inputs for postural control in these environments will result in instability.

Inability to appropriately select a sense

for postural control in environments where one or more orientation cues inaccurately report the body's position in space is referred to as a *sensory selection problem* (64, 65). Patients with a sensory selection problem are often able to maintain balance in environments where sensory information for postural control is consistent; however, they are unable to maintain stability when there is incongruity among the senses (64, 65). Patients with a sensory selection problem do not necessarily show a pattern of overreliance on any one sense, but rather appear to be unable to correctly select an accurate orientation reference; therefore, they are unstable in any environment in which a sensory orientation reference is not accurate. This is shown in Figure 9.11, where abnormal sway is seen in conditions 3, 4, 5, and 6.

Sensory selection problems have been reported in stroke patients (60), traumatic brain injury patients (40), and in children with developmental disorders, including cerebral palsy (42), Down syndrome (41), learning disabilities (65) and the deaf (64).

Sensorimotor Adaptation

Sensory problems can affect the ways in which we move for postural control (56). As we mentioned earlier, certain movement strategies for controlling the body's position in space depend on certain senses more than others. When the sense needed for controlling that movement is not available, the ability of the individual to use that movement strategy for postural control is lost. For example, we mentioned earlier that somatosensory inputs are very important when the ankle strategy is used to compensate for support surface movements. Alternatively, visual and vestibular senses appear to be more important when a hip postural movement strategy is used to control balance in this situation.

During the experiments in which pressure cuffs were applied to neurologically intact subjects, thereby reducing the availability of cutaneous inputs for orientation, subjects were able to maintain balance under the six sensory conditions. However, in the absence of somatosensory inputs for orientation, subjects tended to alter how they moved when controlling balance. Instead of using an ankle strategy to control body sway, subjects tended to increase the use of hip movements. This led researchers to suggest that changes in the availability of sensory inputs for orientation result in a change in how people move to control balance (56).

Similarly, patients who have lost visual and/or vestibular inputs for postural control are often unable to use a hip postural movement strategy and are constrained to move only at the ankles (56).

SUMMARY

1. An enormous range of problems can contribute to postural dyscontrol in the neurologically impaired patient. This includes positive and negative signs, which occur as a direct result of the lesion, or problems that occur indirectly or compensatory to the lesion. As a result, understanding posture and movement behaviors seen in such patients is a complicated process.
2. A systems perspective to postural dyscontrol focuses on identifying the constraints or impairments in each of the systems essential to controlling body posture. Impairments are defined as limitations within the individual which restrict sensory and movement strategies for postural control. Impairments can be musculoskeletal, neuromuscular, sensory, perceptual, or cognitive.
3. In the patient with upper motor neuron lesions, musculoskeletal disorders develop most often secondary to the neurological lesion. Yet, musculoskeletal problems can be a major limitation to normal postural function in the neurologically impaired patient.
4. Neuromuscular limitations encompass a diverse group of problems that represent a major constraint on postural control in the patient with neurological dysfunction.
5. Weakness, or the inability to generate tension, is a major impairment of function in many patients with upper motor neuron lesions.
6. Abnormalities of muscle tone are found in many patients with upper motor neuron lesions. The spectrum of muscle tone abnormalities is broad, ranging from flaccidity in the acute stroke patient, to rigidity in the Parkinson patient. Spasticity is defined as a motor disorder characterized by a velocity-dependent increase in tonic stretch reflexes (muscle tone) with exaggerated tendon jerks, resulting from changes in the threshold of the stretch reflex. The exact contribution of abnormalities of muscle tone to functional deficits in posture are not well understood.

7. Other neuromuscular factors contributing to postural dyscontrol include a wide range of abnormalities leading to an inability to organize multiple muscles into coordinated postural movement synergies.
8. Disruptions of sensory information can affect postural control in the following ways: (*a*) sensory problems can prevent the development of accurate internal models of the body for postural control, affecting a patient's ability to accurately determine the orientation of the body with respect to gravity and the environment; (*b*) disruption of central sensory mechanisms can affect a patient's ability to adapt sensory inputs to changes in task and environmental demands; (*c*) sensory problems can disrupt motor learning, affecting a patient's ability to adapt to change; (*d*) loss of sensory information can impair a patient's ability to anticipate instability, modifying the way he or she senses and moves to prevent disruptions to postural control.

REFERENCES

1. Walshe F. Contributions of John Hughlings Jackson to neurology: a brief introduction to his teachings. Arch Neurol 1961;5:119–131.
2. Gordon J. Assumptions underlying physical therapy intervention: theoretical and historical perspectives. In: Carr J, Shepherd R, Gordon J, Gentile AM, Held J, eds. Movement science foundations for physical therapy in rehabilitation. Rockville: Aspen Publications, 1987:1–30.
3. Katz R, Rymer Z. Spastic hypertonia: mechanisms and measurement. Arch Phys Med Rehabil 1989;70:144–155.
4. Shumway-Cook A, Horak F. Balance rehabilitation in the neurologic patient: course syllabus. Seattle: NERA, 1992.
5. Shumway-Cook A, McCollum G. Assessment and treatment of balance deficits. In: Montgomery P, Connolly B, eds. Motor control and physical therapy. Hixson, TN: Chattanooga Group, 1991:123–137.
6. Schenkman M. Interrelationships of neurological and mechanical factors in balance control. In: Duncan P, ed. Balance: proceedings

of the APTA Forum. Alexandria, VA: APTA, 1990:29–41.

7. Shiverick D. Loss of gastrocnemius length in hemiplegic patients. Neurology Report 1990; 3:4–6.

8. Woo SLV, Matthews JV, Akerson WH, et al. Connective tissue response to immobility. Arthritis Rheum 1975;18:257–264.

9. Duncan P, Badke MB. Determinants of abnormal motor control. In: Duncan P, Badke MB, eds. Stroke rehabilitation: the recovery of motor control. Chicago: Year Book Medical Publishers, 1987:135–159.

10. Perry J, Newsam C. Function of the hamstrings in cerebral palsy. In: Sussman M, ed. The diplegic child. Rosemont, IL: American Academy of Orthopedic Surgeons, 1992:299–307.

11. Smidt GL, Rogers MW. Factors contributing to the regulation and clinical assessment of muscular strength. Phys Ther 1982; 62:1283–1290.

12. Buchner DM, DeLateur BJ. The importance of skeletal muscle strength to physical function in older adults. Annals of Behavioral Medicine 1991;13:1–12.

13. Amundsen LR. Isometric muscle strength testing with fixed-load cells. In: Amundsen LR, ed. Muscle strength testing instrumented and non-instrumented systems. New York: Churchill Livingstone, 1990:89–122.

14. Rogers MM. Musculoskeletal considerations in production and control of movement. In: Montgomery P, Connolly BH, eds. Motor control and physical therapy. Hixson, TN: Chattanooga Group, 1991:69–82.

15. Edstrom L. Selective changes in the sizes of red and white muscle fibers in upper motor lesions and parkinsonism. J Neurol Sci 1970; 11:537–550.

16. Edstrom L, Grimby L, Hannerz J. Correlation between recruitment order of motor units and muscle atrophy patterns of upper motor neuron lesions: significance of spasticity. Experientia 1973;29:560–561.

17. Mayer RF, Young JL. The effects of hemiplegia with spasticity. In: Feldman RG, Young RR, Koella WP, eds. Spasticity: disordered motor control. Chicago: Year Book Medical Publishers, 1980:133–146.

18. Bobath B. Adult hemiplegia: evaluation and treatment. London: William Heinemann, 1978.

19. Brunnstron S. Movement therapy in hemiplegia: a neurophysiological approach. Hagerstown, MD: Harper & Row, 1970.

20. Knutson E. Richards C. Different types of disturbed motor control in gait of hemiplegic patients. Brain 1979;102:405–430.

21. Ghez C. The cerebellum. In: Kandel ER, Schwartz JH, Jessell TM, eds. Principles of neural science. NY: Elsevier, 1991:627–646.

22. Horak FB. Assumptions underlying motor control for neurologic rehabilitation. In: Contemporary management of motor control problems. Proceedings of the II Step Conference. Alexandria, VA: APTA, 1991:11–27.

23. Shea A. Motor attainments in Down's syndrome. In: Contemporary management of motor control problems. Proceedings of the II Step Conference. Alexandria, VA: APTA 1991:225–236.

24. Lance JW. Symposium synopsis. In: Feldman RG, Young RR, Koella WP, eds. Spasticity: disordered motor control. Chicago: Year Book Medical Publishers, 1980:485.

25. Berger W, Horstmann GA, Dietz VL. Tension development and muscle activation in the leg during gait in spastic hemiparesis: the independence of muscle hypertonia and exaggerated stretch reflexes. J Neurol Neurosurg Psychiatry 1984;47:1029–1033.

26. Katz RT, Rymer WZ. Spastic hypertonia: mechanisms and measurement. Arch Phys Med Rehabil 1989;70:144–155.

27. Burke D. Critical examination of the case for or against fusimotor involvement in disorders of muscle tone. In: Desmedt JE, ed. Motor control mechanisms in health and disease. NY: Raven Press, 1983:133–150.

28. Davies P. Steps to follow. New York: Springer-Verlag, 1985.

29. Gowland C, deBruin H, Basmajian J, Plews N, Burcea I. Agonist and antagonist activity during voluntary upper-limb movement in patients with stroke. Phys Ther 1992; 72:624–633.

30. Dietz V, Trippel M, Berger W. Reflex activity and muscle tone during elbow movements in patients with spastic paresis. Ann Neurol 1991;6:767–779.

31. Lacquaniti F. Quantitative assessment of somatic muscle tone. Funct Neurol 1990; 5:209–215.

32. Bohannon RW, Andrews AW. Correlation of knee extensor muscle torque and spasticity

with gait seed in patients with stroke. Arch Phys Med Rehabil 1990;71:330–333.

33. Sahrmann SA, Norton BS. The relationship of voluntary movement to spasticity in the upper motoneuron syndrome. Ann Neurol 1977;2:460–465.

34. Tang A, Rymer WZ. Abnormal force-EMG relations in paretic limbs of hemiparetic human subjects. Neurol Neurosurg Psychiatry 1981;44:690–698.

35. McLellan DL. Co-contraction and stretch reflex in spasticity during treatment with baclofen. Neurol Neurosurg Psychiatry 1973; 40:30–38.

36. Whitley DA, Sahrmann SA, Norton BJ. Patterns of muscle activity in the hemiplegic upper extremity. Phys Ther 1982;62:641–651.

37. Maki B, Holliday PJ, Topper AK. Fear of falling and postural performance in the elderly. J Gerontol 1991;46:M123–M131.

38. Lewis C, Phillippi L. Postural changes with age and soft tissue treatment. Phys Ther Forum 1993;9:4–6.

39. Badke M, Duncan P. Patterns of rapid motor responses during postural adjustments when standing in healthy subjects and hemiplegic patients. Phys Ther 1983;63:13–20.

40. Shumway-Cook A, Olmscheid R. A systems analysis of postural dyscontrol in traumatically brain-injured patients. J Head Trauma Rehabil 1990;5:51–62.

41. Shumway-Cook A, Woollacott M. Postural control in the Down's syndrome child. Phys Ther 1985;9:211–235.

42. Nashner LM, Shumway-Cook A, Marin O. Stance posture control in select groups of children with cerebral palsy: deficits in sensory organization and muscular coordination. Exp Brain Res 1983;49:393–409.

43. Badke MB, DiFabio RP, Duncan PW. Laterality of rapid motor responses in hemiplegic subjects during postural adjustments in standing. Phys Ther 1983;63:13–20.

44. Horak FB, Nashner LM, Nutt JG. Postural instability in Parkinson's disease: motor coordination and sensory organization. Neurology Report 1988;12:54–55.

45. Martin JP. The basal ganglia and posture. London: Pitman, 1967.

46. Horak FB, Diener HC, Nashner LM. Influence of central set on human postural responses. J Neurophysiol 1989;62:841–853.

47. Horak FB. Comparison of cerebellar and vestibular loss on scaling of postural responses.

In: Brandt T, Paulus IO, Bles W, et al., eds. Disorders of posture and gait. Stuttgart: George Thieme Verlag, 1990:370–373.

48. Kamm K, Thelen E, Jensen, J. A dynamical systems approach to motor development. In: Rothstein J, ed. Movement science. Alexandria, VA: APTA, 1991:11–23.

49. Horak FB, Anderson M, Esselman P, Lynch K. The effects of movement velocity, mass displaced and task certainty on associated postural adjustments made by normal and hemiplegic individuals. J Neurol Neurosurg Psychiatry 1984;47:1020–1028.

50. Rogers MW. Control of posture and balance during voluntary movements in Parkinson's disease. In: Duncan P, ed. Balance: proceedings of the APTA Forum. Alexandria, VA: APTA, 1990:79–86.

51. Badke MB, DiFabio RP. Balance deficits in patients with hemiplegia: considerations for assessment and treatment. In: Duncan P, ed. Balance: proceedings of the APTA Forum. Alexandria, VA: APTA, 1990:73–78.

52. Duncan PW. Stroke: physical therapy assessment and treatment. In: Contemporary management of motor control problems. Proceedings of the II Step Conference. Alexandria, VA:APTA, 1991:209–217.

53. Cote L, Crutcher MD. The basal ganglia. In: Kandel ER, Schwartz JH, Jessell TM, eds. Principles of neural science. NY: Elsevier, 1991:645–659.

54. Rogers MW. Motor control problems in Parkinson's disease. In: Contemporary management of motor control problems. Proceedings of the II Step Conference. Alexandria, VA: APTA, 1991:195–208.

55. Holmes G. The cerebellum of man. Brain 1939;62:1–30.

56. Horak FB, Shupert CL. Role of the vestibular system in postural control. In: Herdman SJ, ed. Vestibular rehabilitation. Philadelphia:FA Davis, 1994:22–46.

57. McCollum G, Leen T. Form and exploration of mechanical stability limits in erect stance. J Motor Behav 1989;21:225–236.

58. Shumway-Cook A, Horak, F. Vestibular rehabilitation: an exercise approach to managing symptoms of vestibular dysfunction. Seminars in Hearing 1989;10:196–209.

59. Shumway-Cook A, Horak F. Rehabilitation strategies for patients with vestibular deficits. Neurol Clin 1990;8:441–457.

60. DiFabio R, Badke MB. Relationship of sen-

sory organization to balance function in patients with hemiplegia. Phys Ther 1990; 70:543–552.

61. Shumway-Cook A. Vestibular rehabilitation in traumatic brain injury. In: Herdman S, ed. Vestibular rehabilitation. Philadelphia: FA Davis, 1994:347–359.

62. Black FO, Shupert C, Horak FB, Nashner LM. Abnormal postural control associated with peripheral vestibular disorders. In: Pompeiano O, Allum J, eds. Vestibulo-spinal control of posture and movement. Progress in brain research. Amersterdam: Elsevier Science Publishers 1988;76:263–275.

63. Horak FB, Nashner LM, Diener HC. Postural strategies associated with somatosensory and vestibular loss. Exp Brain Res 1990; 82:167–177.

64. Shumway-Cook A, Horak FB, Black FO. Critical examination of vestibular function in motor-impaired learning disabled children. Int J Ped Otorhinolaryngol 1988;14:21–30.

65. Horak FB, Shumway-Cook A, Crowe T, Black FO. Vestibular function and motor proficiency in children with hearing impairments and in learning disabled children with motor impairments. Dev Med Child Neurol 1988;30:64–79.

66. Black FO, Nashner LM. Vestibulo-spinal control differs in patients with reduced versus distorted vestibular function. Acta Otolaryngol (Stockholm) Suppl. 1984;406:110–114.

Chapter 10

ASSESSMENT AND TREATMENT OF PATIENTS WITH POSTURAL DISORDERS

INTRODUCTION

This chapter discusses a task-oriented approach to assessing and treating postural disorders in the patient with neurological dysfunction. In Chapter 5, we introduced a conceptual framework for clinical practice, which incorporated four key elements: the clinical decision-making process, hypothesis-oriented clinical practice, a model of disablement, and a theory of motor control. We referred to this framework as a task-oriented approach. We now combine this approach with our knowledge of normal and abnormal postural control, and show how it is applied to the clinical management of postural disorders. It is important to remember that the development of clinical methods based on a systems theory of motor control is just beginning. As systems-based research provides us with an increased understanding of normal and abnormal postural control, new methods for assessing and treating postural disorders will emerge.

ASSESSMENT

A task-oriented approach assesses postural control on three levels: (*a*) the functional skills requiring posture control, (*b*) the sensory and motor strategies used to maintain posture in various contexts and tasks, and (*c*) the underlying sensory, motor, and cognitive impairments that constrain posture control. The information gained through assessment is used to develop a comprehensive list of problems, establish short- and long-term goals, and formulate a plan of care for retraining posture control. A thorough assessment must include a review of the patient's medical and social history, as well as a review of current symptoms and concerns.

Safety—First Concern

During the course of evaluating postural control, patients will be asked to perform a number of tasks that will likely destabilize them. Safety is of paramount importance. All patients should wear an ambulation belt during testing, and be closely guarded at all times. In determining what tasks and activities cause loss of balance, the patient must be allowed to experience instability. However, the therapist should protect the patient at all times to prevent a fall.

Functional Assessment

A task-oriented approach to evaluating postural control begins with a functional assessment to determine how well a patient can perform a variety of skills that depend on postural control. A functional assessment can provide the clinician with information on the patient's level of performance compared to standards established with normal subjects. Results can indicate the need for therapy, serve as a baseline level of performance, and when repeated at regular intervals, can provide both the therapist and patient with ob-

jective documentation about change in functional status. There are a number of tests available to measure functional skills related to postural control. In addition to the functional assessment, it is good to gather information on number and types of falls and near falls, and to include this in a balance and falls history (see Appendix A).

GET UP AND GO TEST

The Get Up and Go test (1) was developed as a quick screening tool for detecting balance problems in elderly patients. The test requires that subjects stand up from a chair, walk 3 meters, turn around, and return. Performance is scored according to the following scale: 1 normal; 2 very slightly abnormal; 3 mildly abnormal; 4 moderately abnormal; 5 severely abnormal. An increased risk for falls was found among older adults who scored 3 or higher on this test.

The Up and Go test modifies the original test by adding a timing component to performance (2). Neurologically intact adults who are independent in balance and mobility skills are able to perform the test in less than 10 seconds. This test correlates well to functional capacity as measured by the Barthel Index (3). Adults who took greater than 30 seconds to complete the test were dependent in most activities of daily living, and mobility skills.

FUNCTIONAL REACH TEST

The Functional Reach Test (4) is another single item test developed as a quick screen for balance problems in older adults. As shown in Figure 10.1*A*, subjects stand with feet shoulder distance apart, and with the arm raised to 90° flexion. Without moving their feet, subjects reach as far forward as they can while still maintaining their balance (Fig. 10.1*B*). The distance reached is measured and compared to age-related norms, shown in Table 10.1. The Functional Reach Test has established inter-rater reliability, and is shown to be highly predictive of falls among older adults (4).

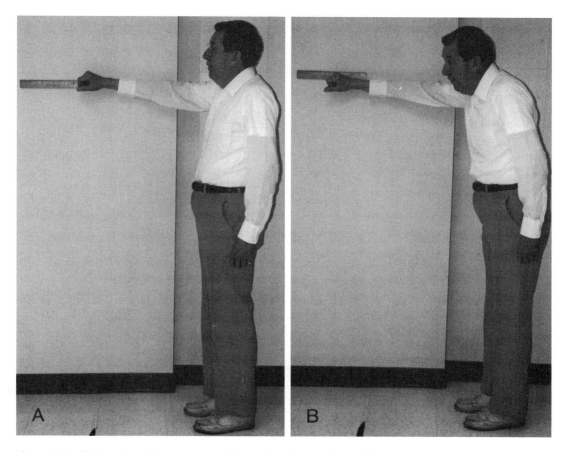

Figure 10.1   The Functional Reach Test. **A,** Subjects begin by standing with feet shoulder distance apart, arm raised to 90° flexion, and reach as far forward as they can while still maintaining their balance.

Table 10.1.   Functional Reach Norms[a]

Norms	Men (in inches)	Women (in inches)
20–40 yrs	16.7 + 1.9	14.6 + 2.2
41–69	14.9 + 2.2	13.8 + 2.2
70–87	13.2 + 1.6	10.5 + 3.5

[a]From Duncan PW, Weiner DK, Chandler J, Studenski S. Functional reach: a new clinical measure of balance. J Gerontol 1990; 45:M195.

PERFORMANCE ORIENTED MOBILITY ASSESSMENT

Mary Tinetti, a physician researcher at Yale University, has published a test to screen for balance and mobility skills in older adults and to determine the likelihood for falls (5, 6). Table 10.2 presents Tinetti's balance and mobility scale, which rates performance on a three-point scale.

FUNCTIONAL BALANCE SCALE

The Functional Balance Scale was developed by Kathy Berg, a Canadian physical therapist (7). This test uses 14 different items, which are rated 0 to 4. The test is shown in Appendix A as part of a comprehensive balance assessment form. The test is reported to have good test-retest and inter-rater reliability; however, to date, there are no norms published for this test.

LIMITATIONS OF FUNCTIONAL ASSESSMENT

As noted in Chapter 5, functional assessments have a number of limitations. These include the inability to (*a*) assess a patient's performance of tasks under changing environ-

Table 10.2.   Balance and Mobility Assessment[a]

I. *Balance Tests*

Initial instructions: Subject is seated in a hard, armless chair. The following maneuvers are tested.

1. *Sitting balance*
   Leans or slides in chair = 0
   Steady, safe = 1

2. *Arises*
   Unable without help = 0
   Able, uses arms to help = 1
   Able without using arms = 2

3. *Attempts to arise*
   Unable without help = 0
   Able, requires >1 attempt = 1
   Able to rise, 1 attempt = 2

4. *Immediate standing balance (first 5 seconds)*
   Unsteady (staggers, moves feet, trunk sway) = 0
   Steady, but uses walker or other support = 1
   Steady without walker or other support = 2

5. *Standing balance*
   Unsteady = 0
   Steady but wide stance (medial heels > 4 inches apart) and uses cane or other support = 1
   Narrow stance without support = 2

6. *Nudged (subject at maximum position with feet as close together as possible,* examiner pushes lightly on subject's sternum with palm of hand 3 times)
   Begins to fall = 0
   Staggers, grabs, catches self = 1
   Steady = 2

7. *Eyes closed (at maximum position no. 6)*
   Unsteady = 0
   Steady = 1

8. *Turning 360 degrees*
   Continuous steps = 0
   Discontinuous steps = 1
   Unsteady steps (grabs, staggers) = 2

9. *Sitting down*
   Unsafe (misjudged distance, falls into chair) = 0
   Uses arms or not a smooth motion = 1
   Safe, smooth motion = 2
   Balance score: /16

II. *Gait Tests*

Initial instructions: Subject stands with the examiner, walks down hallway or across room, first at usual pace, then back at rapid, but safe pace (usual walking aids)

10. *Initiation of gait (immediately after told to "go")*
    Any hesitancy or multiple attempts to start = 0
    No hesitancy = 1

11. *Step length and height*
    a. Right swing foot
       Does not pass left stance foot with step = 0
       Passes left stance foot = 1
       Right foot does not clear floor completely with step = 0
       Right foot completely clears floor = 1
    b. Left swing foot
       Does not pass right stance foot with step = 0
       Passes right stance foot = 1
       Left foot does not clear floor completely with step = 0
       Left foot completely clears floor = 1

12. *Step symmetry*
    Right and left step length not equal (estimate) = 0
    Right and left step appear equal = 1

13. *Step continuity*
    Stopping or discontinuity between steps = 0
    Steps appear continuous = 1

14. *Path (estimated in relation to floor tiles, 12-inch diameter; observe excursion of 1 foot over about 10 ft of the course)*
    Marked deviation = 0
    Mild/moderate deviation or uses walking aid = 1
    Straight without walking aid = 2

15. *Trunk*
    Marked sway or uses walking aid = 0
    No sway, but flexion of knees or back pain or spreads arms out while walking = 1
    No sway, no flexion, no use of arms, and no use if walking aid = 2

16. *Walking time*
    Heel apart = 0
    Heels almost touching while walking = 1

    Gait score: /12
    Balance and gait score: /28

---

[a]From Tinetti, M. Performance-oriented assessment of mobility problems in elderly patients. JAGS 1986;34:119-126.

mental contexts, (b) determine the quality of movement used, and (c) identify specific neuronal or musculoskeletal subsystems within the body responsible for a decline in performance.

Strategy Assessment

The next level of assessment examines the motor and sensory strategies used to control the body's position in space under a variety of conditions.

MOTOR STRATEGIES

Assessment of motor strategies for postural control examines both the alignment of body segments during unperturbed sitting and standing and the patient's ability to generate multi-joint movements, or strategies, which effectively control motion of the center of mass relative to the base of support (8–11).

Alignment in Sitting and Standing

The patient's alignment in sitting and standing is observed. Is the patient vertical? Is weight symmetrically distributed right to left, and forward and backward? A plumb line in conjunction with a grid can be used to quantify changes in alignment at the head, shoulders, trunk, pelvis, hips, knees, and ankles. In addition, the width of the patient's base of support upon standing can be measured and recorded using a tape to measure the distance between the medial malleoli (or alternatively, the metatarsal heads).

Alternative ways to quantify placement of the center of mass in the standing position include the use of static force plates to measure placement of the center of pressure (Fig 10.2), or the use of two standard scales to determine if there is weight discrepancy between the two sides (Fig 10.3).

Movement Strategies

Movement strategies are examined under three different task conditions: self-initiated sway, in response to externally induced

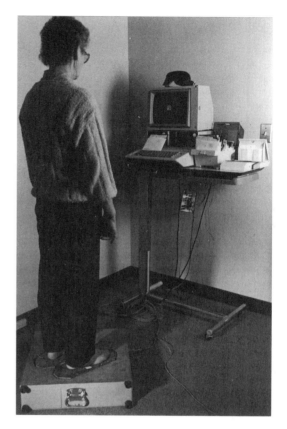

Figure 10.2   The use of a static forceplate can be helpful when quantifying static alignment changes in standing.

sway, and anticipatory to a potentially destabilizing upper extremity movement (10).

Movements used to control self-initiated body sway are observed while the patient voluntarily shifts the weight forward, then backwards, then side to side. The patient is tested both in sitting and in standing. Figure 10.4 illustrates the range of movement patterns seen in a seated neurologically intact individual as he/she shifts the trunk further and further laterally. As weight is transferred to one side of the body, the trunk begins to curve towards the unweighted side, resulting in elongation of the weightbearing side and shortening of the trunk on the unweighted side (Fig. 10.4A). As weight continues to be shifted laterally, maintaining stability requires the patient to abduct the arm and leg in order to keep the trunk mass within the base of support (Fig. 10.4B). Finally, when the center of

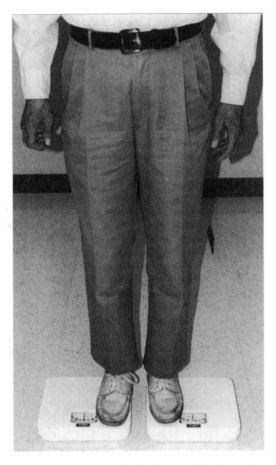

Figure 10.3 Two standard scales can also be used to quantify static asymmetric standing alignment.

mass of the trunk exceeds the base of support, the patient must protectively extend the arm to prevent a fall (Fig. 10.4C).

Figure 10.5 illustrates two types of movement strategies being used to control self-initiated sway in standing. Two patients have been asked to sway forward as far as they can without taking a step. Patient A (Fig. 10.5A) is swaying forward primarily about the ankles, using what has been referred to as an ankle strategy to control center of mass motion. In contrast, Patient B (Fig. 10.5B) is moving primarily the trunk and hips (a hip strategy), which minimizes forward motion of the center of mass.

Movement strategies used to recover from a perturbation are also assessed. Figure 10.6 illustrates one approach to assessing movement patterns used to control sway in response to an external perturbation, or push (10, 12, 13). Holding the patient about the hips, the therapist displaces the patient forward, backward, right, and then left. Figure 10.6A illustrates the use of an ankle strategy used to recover from a small backward displacement.

A larger displacement by the therapist usually results in a greater amount of hip and trunk motion, that is, a hip strategy, as the subject continues to try to keep the center of mass within the base of support and not take a step (Fig. 10.6B). Finally, if the therapist displaces the subject far enough, and the center of body mass moves outside the base of support, the subject will take a step to avoid a fall (Fig. 10.6C) (10).

The most common approach to evaluating multi-joint dyscoordination within task-specific movement strategies is through observation and subjective analysis. For example, the clinician may note that during recovery of stance balance the patient demonstrates excessive flexion of the knees, or asymmetric movements in the lower extremities, or excessive flexion or rotation of the trunk. However, the underlying nature of the dyscoordination, that is, specific timing and or amplitude errors in synergistic muscles responding to instability, cannot be determined without using technical apparatus such as electromyography (8).

Finally, movement strategies used to minimize instability in anticipation of potentially destabilizing movements can be assessed by asking a patient to lift a heavy object as rapidly as possible. If the patient is standing, a small amount of backward sway of the whole body should precede the lift, indicating the presence of anticipatory postural adjustments in the legs. If the patient is sitting independently, one would expect to see backward sway in the trunk, if anticipatory postural adjustments are used. Forward instability is found in patients who do not make anticipatory adjustments (10).

SENSORY STRATEGIES

The Clinical Test for Sensory Interaction in Balance (CTSIB) is one method that

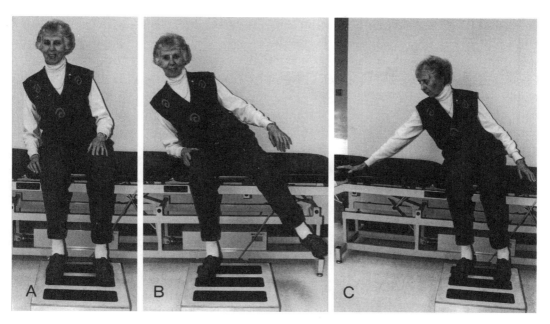

Figure 10.4   Controlling self-initiated trunk movements in sitting. **A,** Small movements produce adjustments at the head and trunk. **B,** Larger movements require counterbalancing with the arms and legs. **C,** When the line of gravity for the head and trunk exceeds the base of support, the arm reaches out to prevent a fall.

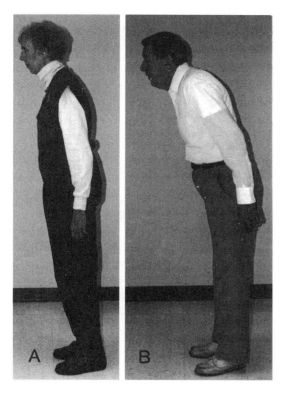

Figure 10.5   Controlling self-initiated sway in stance. Shown are two types of movement strategies being used to control self-initiated sway in standing. **A,** the ankle, and **B,** the hip.

has been proposed for clinically assessing the influence of sensory interaction on postural stability in the standing position (14, 15). The technique uses a 24″ by 24″ piece of medium-density Temper foam in conjunction with a modified Japanese lantern. A large Japanese lantern is cut down the back and attached to a headband. Vertical stripes are placed inside the lantern, and the top and bottom of the lantern are covered with white paper (Fig. 10.7).

The method is based on concepts developed by Nashner (16), and requires the subject to maintain standing balance for 30 seconds under six different sensory conditions that either eliminate input or produce inaccurate visual and surface orientation inputs. These six conditions are shown in Figure 10.8.

Patients are tested in the feet together position, with hands placed on the hips. Using condition 1 as a baseline reference, the therapist observes the patient for changes in the amount and direction of sway over the subsequent five conditions. If the patient is unable to stand for 30 seconds, a second trial is given (15).

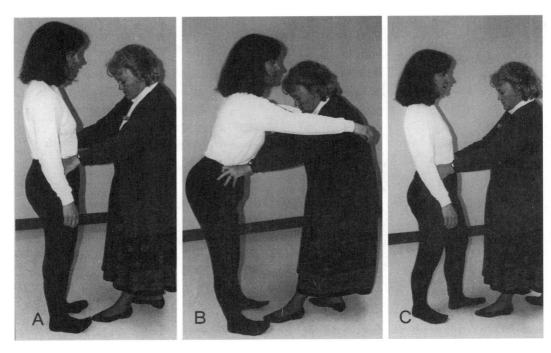

Figure 10.6   Movement strategies used to recover from an external perturbation to balance. **A**, An ankle strategy is used to recover from a small displacement at the hips. **B**, A larger displacement produces a hip strategy. **C**, Movement of the COM outside the base of support requires a step to recovery stability.

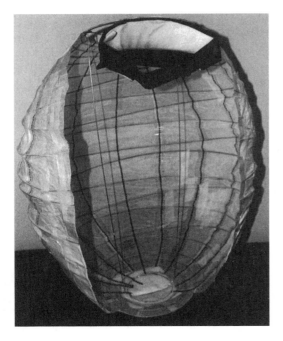

Figure 10.7   A modified Japanese lantern is used to change the accuracy of visual input for postural orientation.

Neurologically intact young adults are able to maintain balance for 30 seconds on all six conditions with minimal amounts of body sway. In conditions 5 and 6, normal adults sway on the average 40% more than in condition 1 (16).

Results from a number of research studies that have used either a moving platform or the CTSIB suggest the following scoring criteria (17–20). A single fall, regardless of the condition, is not considered abnormal. However, two or more falls are indicative of difficulties adapting sensory information for postural control.

A proposed model for interpreting results is summarized in Figure 10.9. This model is in the process of being validated. Patients who show increased amounts of sway or lose balance on conditions 2, 3, and 6 are thought to be *visually dependent*, that is, highly dependent on vision for postural control. Patients who have problems on conditions 4, 5, and 6 are thought to be *surface-*

VISUAL CONDITIONS
NORMAL   BLINDFOLD   DOME

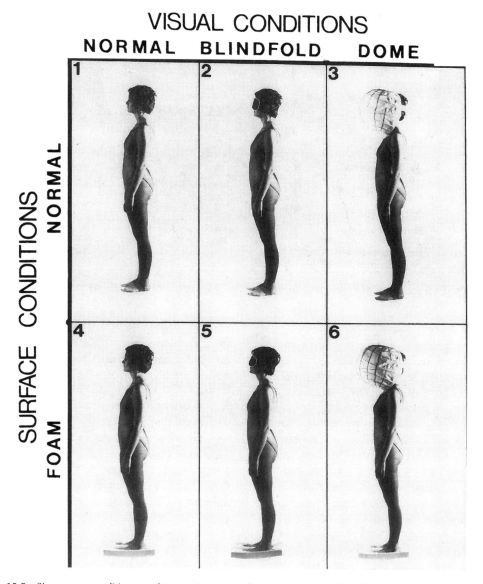

Figure 10.8   Six sensory conditions used to examine postural orientation under altered sensory contexts. The approach tests the ability to adapt how senses are used to maintain orientation. (From Shumway-Cook A, Horak F. Assessing the influence of sensory interaction on balance. Phys Ther 1986;66:1549.)

dependent, that is, dependent primarily on somatosensory information from the feet in contact with the surface, for postural control (9, 10).

However, it is important to remember the following caution when interpreting results showing increased sway on a compliant surface. While we suppose that the primary effect of standing on a foam surface relates to altering the availability of incoming sensory information for postural orientation, additional factors can affect performance in this condition. Standing on foam changes the dynamics of force production with respect to the surface, and this may be a significant factor affecting performance in this condition. There has been no research examining the dynamics of standing on foam, thus clinicians should be

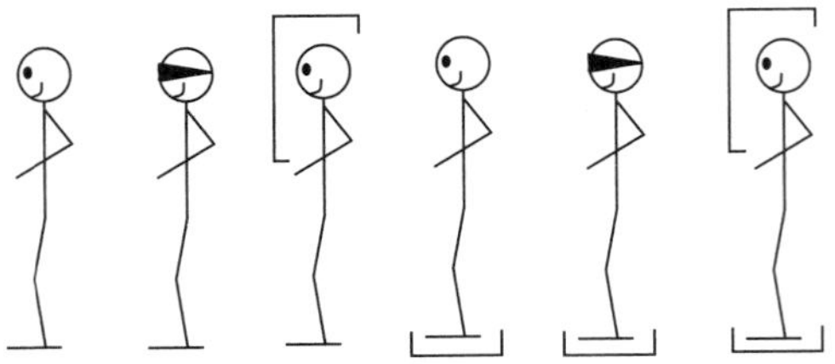

Patterns	1	2	3	4	5	6
Visually Dependent	N	N/A	A	N	N/A	A
Surface Dependent	N	N	N	A	A	A
Vestibular Loss	N	N	N	N	A	A
Sensory Selection	N	N	A	A	A	A

N= Body sway within normal limits
A= Body sway abnormal

Figure 10.9   A proposed model for interpreting the CTSIB test based on information gained through dynamic posturography testing.

careful in interpreting results when using the foam condition.

Patients who sway more, or fall, on conditions 5 and 6 of the CTSIB, demonstrate a *vestibular loss* pattern, suggesting an inability to select vestibular inputs for postural control in the absence of useful visual and somatosensory cues. Finally, patients who lose balance on conditions 3, 4, 5, and 6 are said to have a *sensory selection* problem. This is defined as an inability to effectively adapt sensory information for postural control (10).

Systems Assessment: Identifying Impairments

The next step in a task-oriented assessment involves evaluating the sensory, motor (neural and musculoskeletal), and cognitive subsystems that underlie task-based performance. This allows the clinician to identify the impairments constraining functional abilities.

COGNITIVE SYSTEMS

Understanding cognitive factors is an important part of the assessment process, since these factors can preclude an accurate and valid assessment of a patient's motor abilities. Problems in arousal, attention, memory, and judgment can affect a patient's ability to attend to and perform behaviors being assessed (21). In addition, these factors can affect a patient's ability to comply with a treatment regimen.

During the course of assessment, many aspects of cognitive function are evaluated by the clinician. Some are tested formally; however, more often, cognitive status is judged subjectively, based on observations of the patient's behavior during the course of the assessment process.

Level of Consciousness

The Rancho Los Amigos Scale (22) is probably the most well-known approach to quantifying level of consciousness in the patient with neurological impairments. This scale is shown in Table 10.3. Assessment of level of consciousness, arousal, or *state*, is an essential part of assessing motor control, since motor behavior is very dependent on arousal level (23).

Mental Status

Mental status can be determined informally by determining the patient's orientation

Table 10.3. Rancho Los Amigos Cognitive Scale[a]

I. No response: unresponsive to any stimulus.

II. Generalized response: limited, inconsistent, nonpurposeful responses, often to pain only.

III. Localized response: purposeful responses; may follow simple commands; may focus on presented object.

IV. Confused, agitated: heightened state of activity; confusion, disorientation; aggressive behavior; unable to do self-care; unaware of present events; agitation appears related to internal confusion.

V. Confused, inappropriate; nonagitated; appears alert; responds to commands; distractable; does not concentrate on task; agitated responses to external stimuli; verbally inappropriate; does not learn new information.

VI. Confused, appropriate: goal directed behavior, needs cueing; can relearn old skills as activities of daily living (ADLs); serious memory problems; some awareness of self and others.

VII. Automatic, appropriate: appears appropriate, oriented; frequently robot-like in daily routine; minimal or absent confusion; shallow recall; increased awareness of self, interaction in environment; lacks insight into condition; decreased judgment and problem solving; lacks realistic planning for future.

VIII. Purposeful, appropriate: alert, oriented; recalls and integrates past events; learns new activities and can continue without supervision; independent in home and living skills; capable of driving; defects in stress tolerance, judgment, abstract reasoning persist; many function at reduced levels in society.

[a]Reprinted with permission for Rancho Los Amigos Medical Center, Downy, Calif, USA, Adult Brain Injury Service.

to person, place, and time. A more formal measurement of mental status may be done by using either the Mini-Mental State Exam (24) or the Short Portable Mental Status Questionnaire (25). The Mini-Mental State Exam is shown in the Appendix as part of the comprehensive postural assessment.

Other aspects of cognitive function that are subjectively evaluated include: attention, communication, and motivation. Attention is often evaluated informally through observation of the patient's ability to selectively monitor task-relevant stimuli, while ignoring irrelevant stimuli. Communication abilities, including both receptive and expressive communication skills, are also noted (22).

Determining the patient's motivation and goals are an important part of assessment as well. Remember from the research on motor learning described in Chapter 2, that learning is facilitated by working on tasks that are perceived as important to the learner. What are the patient's goals? How strongly is the patient committed to work towards these goals? Do patients feel that the goals are within their capacity to achieve? The answers to these questions can help a therapist structure a therapeutic program that is both relevant and meaningful to the patient.

MUSCULOSKELETAL SYSTEM

Assessment of the musculoskeletal system includes evaluation of range of motion and flexibility. Alignment, which is often considered an aspect of the musculoskeletal system, was covered earlier under motor strategies for postural control. In addition, strength, which has both non-neural and neural aspects, is discussed as part of the neuromuscular systems in the next section. This chapter does not discuss techniques for assessing the musculoskeletal system in depth; instead, the reader is urged to consult other texts (26–29).

Range of Motion

Range of motion is evaluated using slow passive movements. Passive range of motion (PROM) in a particular joint may vary among normal subjects according to age and sex. PROM can be measured quantitatively using equipment such as a goniometer, or can be described subjectively using a scale similar to the one in Table 10.4 (30).

Evaluation of range of motion can also include active range of motion, that is the joint range achieved by the patient without assistance from the examiner. This is often smaller than PROM. Finally, many clinicians test joint play during an assessment of musculoskeletal parameters of motor control.

Flexibility

Flexibility is sometimes described with reference to loss of mobility in a two-joint

Table 10.4.   Range of Motion Scoring Scale[a]

0 = no movement (ankylosis)
1 = considerable decrease in movement (moderate hypomobility)
2 = slight decrease in movement (mild hypermobility)
3 = normal
4 = slight increase in movement (mild hypermobility)
5 = considerable increase in movement (moderate hypermobility)
6 = severe increase in movement (severe hypermobility)

[a]Adapted from: Jensen GM. Musculoskeletal analysis: introduction. In: Scully RM, Barnes MR, eds. Physical therapy. Philadelphia: JB Lippincott, 1989:331.

muscle (31). Decreased flexibility in a two-joint muscle prevents the simultaneous completion of complete range of motion in related joints. The most common example of decreased flexibility is a gastrocnemius contracture, which limits ankle joint dorsiflexion when the knee is extended. Since the gastrocnemius spans both the ankle and the knee joints, full range of ankle dorsiflexion may be more difficult to achieve with the knee extended than when the knee is flexed and the gastrocnemius is not on stretch. Thus, a joint may be functionally limited in range of motion secondary to loss of muscular flexibility.

Neuromuscular System

Assessment of neuromuscular impairments includes measurement of strength, muscle tone, and nonequilibrium forms of coordination.

Strength

The ability to produce a voluntary contraction depends on both non-neural and neural elements. Strength results from both properties of the muscle itself (musculoskeletal aspects of strength) and the appropriate recruitment of motor units and the timing of their activation (22, 32–34). Although weakness is a predominant feature of upper motor neuron lesions, the measurement of muscle strength in patients with brain lesions is still questioned by many clinicians (35). There is some evidence to support the relationship be-

tween impaired force generation and functional outcomes in patients with CNS lesions, providing justification for including strength testing within a motor control assessment battery (32, 36).

Strength can be measured under three conditions: isometrically, isotonically, or isokinetically (32). However, in the clinic, the most common approach is to examine isometric or isokinetic strength during a shortening contraction (32, 33). Manual muscle testing is the most common clinical approach to testing strength. This test assesses a subject's ability to move a body segment through a range, against gravity, or against externally applied resistance (37). An ordinal scale is used to grade strength from 0, no contraction, to 5, full movement against gravity and maximal resistance (37). A limitation of manual muscle testing is that it does not examine the ability of a muscle to participate in a functional movement pattern (38).

An alternative approach to quantifying strength incorporates the use of hand-held dynamometers, which provide an objective indication of muscle group strength (35, 37). Hand-held dynamometers measure the force required to *break* the patient's position during manual muscle testing (31, 35, 37). Finally, muscle performance can be tested dynamically through the use of instrumented isokinetic systems. Isokinetic testing assesses power, or the ability to generate force throughout the range of motion, at different speeds and over several repetitions (22, 31, 39).

Muscle Tone

Abnormal muscle tone ranging from hypotonicity to hypertonicity may limit a patient's ability to recruit muscles necessary for postural control. The extent to which abnormal muscle tone is a limitation in controlling movements is currently under considerable debate in the rehabilitation literature. Muscle tone is assessed clinically by describing a muscle's resistance to passive stretch. Subjective rating scales, such as the one shown in Table 10.5, are often used to describe alterations in muscle tone (40).

Table 10.5.   Modified Ashworth Scale for Grading Spasticity[a]

0 = No increase in muscle tone
1 = Slight increase in muscle tone, manifested by a slight catch and release or by minimal resistance at the end of the range of motion when the affected part(s) is moved in flexion or extension.
1+ = Slight increase in muscle tone, manifested by a catch, followed by minimal resistance throughout the remainder (less than half) of the range of motion (ROM).
2 = More marked increase in muscle tone through most of the ROM, but affected part(s) easily moved.
3 = Considerable increase in muscle tone, passive movement difficult.
4 = Affected part(s) rigid in flexion or extension.

[a]Adapted from Bohannon RW, Smith MB. Interrater reliability of a modified Ashworth scale of muscle spasticity. Phys Ther 1987; 67:206-207.

Coordination

Tests of coordination have been divided into nonequilibrium and equilibrium tests (41–43). Equilibrium tests of coordination generally reflect the coordination of multijoint movements for posture and gait. Coordination testing related to postural control was discussed in the section on assessing strategies.

Nonequilibrium tests of coordination are important to all aspects of motor control, including posture, mobility, and upper extremity control. These tests are often used to indicate specific pathology within the cerebellum (42). These tests can include: finger to nose, rapid alternating movements, past pointing, heel to shin, finger opposition, tapping (hand or foot), or drawing a circle (hand or foot). Performance is graded subjectively using the following scale: 5 normal, 4 minimal impairment, 3 moderate impairment, 2 severe impairment, 1 cannot perform.

SENSORY SYSTEMS

Postural control requires the organization of vision, somatosensory, and vestibular inputs, which report information about the position of the body relative to external objects, including the support base and gravity.

Assessment of the sensory components begins with an evaluation of the individual senses important to postural control. Particular attention is paid to evaluating somatosensation (muscle, joint, touch, pressure) in the lower extremities. A more in-depth discussion of sensory testing, including commercially available tests to document sensory impairment, is found in the chapter on the clinical assessment of upper extremity control.

Some of the tests used to evaluate somatosensation include:

1. Light touch—using a cotton swab, lightly touch the patient on the face, arm, and legs. The patient should be able to identify when and where the stimulus is being applied.
2. Two-point discrimination—alternately touch one or two points on the patient's skin. Determine whether the patient can feel one or two points, and how much distance between the two points is necessary for the patient to discriminate two points of pressure.
3. Extinction test—touch two corresponding points on different sides of the body simultaneously. Ask the patient to indicate where the touch has occurred. The patient should perceive both touches.
4. Temperature—touch the patient's skin with small containers of hot vs. cold water.
5. Pain—test patient's ability to distinguish sharp from dull, using a pin.
6. Position sense—can be tested in several ways. Most often, the patient's big toe is grasped on the sides and moved up or down. Without looking, the patient is asked to report whether the toe is up or down.
7. Movement sense—move one limb passively, and ask the patient to imitate the motion with the opposite limb.
8. Stereognosis—place a series of common objects in the patient's hand and ask the patient to identify them.
9. Vibration—using a tuning fork on bony prominences such as the malleoli, knee,

or wrist, the patient should be able to identify where the vibration has occurred and when it starts and stops.

In addition, problems in the visual system are noted, such as glaucoma, cataracts, retinal degeneration, decreased visual acuity, diplopia, and peripheral visual field cuts.

ASSESSING PERCEPTIONS RELEVANT TO POSTURAL CONTROL

Two aspects of perception particularly important to postural control are evaluated (9, 10).

Stability Limits

The patient's internal representation of stability limits in sitting and standing is evaluated. In particular, the consistency between the patient's perceived vs. actual limits of stability is subjectively determined. The patient is asked to sway voluntarily as far as possible in all directions without falling. This determines the individual's limits of perceived stability. Alternatively, the patient is asked to reach for an object held at the outer edge of his/her stability limits. The therapist observes the extent to which the patient is willing to move the center of mass, and makes a subjective judgment regarding whether the patient is moving to maximum stability limits in all directions (8—10).

Motion Perception

Motion perception is the conscious sense of whether the body is still or in motion. Dizziness is a misperception of motion (either self or environment) that results when sensory inputs are inconsistent in reporting body motion (9, 44, 45). The term *dizziness* is used by patients to describe a variety of sensations, including spinning (referred to as vertigo), rocking, tilting, unsteadiness, and lightheadedness.

Assessment begins with a careful history to determine the patient's perceptions of whether dizziness is constant or provoked, and the situations or conditions that stimulate dizziness. The Vertigo Positions and Movement Test (9) examines the intensity and duration of dizziness in response to movement and or positional changes of the head while sitting, standing, and walking. The patient is asked to rate the intensity of dizziness on a scale of 0 to 10. In addition, duration of symptoms is timed and recorded, as are the presence of nystagmus and autonomic nervous system symptoms including nausea, sweating, and pallor. For a detailed description of assessment and treatment of dizziness,

Table 10.6.   Task-Oriented Assessment of Postural Control

Levels:	Function	Strategies	Impairment
Tests/measurements: (examples)	Get up/go Functional reach Tinetti Berg	Alignment Sitting Standing Movement Ankle Hip Step Sensory CTSIB Equitest	R.O.M. Strength MMT Dynamometry Tone Passive movement Pendulum test Reflex testing Coordination Individual senses Cognition Mini Mental Test Rancho Scale Perception Stability limits Dizziness

the reader is referred to other sources (9, 44, 45).

In summary, a task-oriented approach to assessing postural control uses a variety of tests, measurements, and observations to: (*a*) document functional abilities related to posture and balance control, (*b*) assess underlying sensory and motor strategies, and (*c*) determine the level of function of underlying sensory, motor, and cognitive systems contributing to postural control. This concept is shown in Table 10.6. In addition, an example of a task-oriented assessment form for assessing an adult patient with an UMN deficit is shown in the Appendix. This particular assessment form is geared to the assessment of an adult patient in a rehabilitation, outpatient, or home health program, rather than an acute care patient.

INTERPRETATION OF ASSESSMENT

Following completion of the assessment, the clinician must interpret the assessment, identify the problems, both at the level of function and impairments, and establish the goals and plan of care.

ACTIVE LEARNING MODULE

Before moving on, take a moment and work on the following case study. Your task is to create a problem list for Phoebe Hines, a 53-year-old patient with right-sided hemiplegia, referred for evaluation of balance 5 weeks following her stroke. (Refer to the evaluation form in Appendix A.) Based on your knowledge of normal and abnormal postural control and the type of problems likely to be found following a stroke, complete the evaluation. Once completed, make a list of problems drawn from all three levels of your assessment. Use this problem list to develop both short- and long-term goals for treatment.

What did you predict? We found that problems drawn from the first level of assessment indicate the patient appears to be having moderate functional balance problems, as indicated by a score of 42/56 on the Functional Balance Scale. Specific functional problems include difficulty with transfers (sit to stand, chair to chair), standing with a reduced base of support, and maintaining balance during dynamic activities such as stepping or turning.

An assessment of the patient's motor strategies indicates an asymmetric alignment, with weight displaced to the left side in both sitting and standing. In addition, movement strategies indicate primary use of a hip strategy to control body sway, inability to use an ankle strategy in the hemiplegic leg, and difficulty taking a step with the noninvolved leg when the center of mass exceeds the base of support.

An assessment of sensory strategies indicates the patient is unable to maintain balance when any sensory information is reduced (falls on conditions 2, 3, 4, 5, and 6 of the CTSIB).

The third level of assessment indicates the following impairments: (*a*) decreased cognitive status; specific problems with orientation to time and place, attention, memory, and emotional lability. In addition, there are moderate problems with receptive and expressive aphasia; (*b*) musculoskeletal impairments, including: 5° of ankle dorsiflexion in the right leg; (*c*) neuromuscular impairments, including: reduced ability to generate force voluntarily (2 ± 5 manual muscle testing in right lower extremity muscles), decreased ability to recruit ankle muscles in the right leg for postural control, and moderate increase in muscle tone in the right elbow flexor and ankle extensors; and (*d*) sensory/perceptual problems, including: decreased sensory discrimination (somatosensation) in the right arm and leg, and right hemianopsia.

With this initial understanding of the patient's problems, the clinician can move ahead to establishing goals and planning treatment. It is difficult to gain an understanding of all of the patient's problems in the first one or two therapy sessions. Rather, understanding and insight continue to grow with each session over the course of treatment. Before we establish goals and a plan of care for Ms. Hines, let's review a task-oriented approach to treating postural dyscontrol.

TREATMENT

The goals of a task-oriented approach to retraining postural control include: to resolve or prevent impairments; to develop effective task-specific strategies, to retrain functional tasks, and to adapt task-specific strategies so that functional tasks can be performed in changing environmental contexts.

Treating at the Impairment Level

The goal of treatments aimed at the impairment level is to correct those impairments that can be changed, and to prevent the development of secondary impairments. Alleviating underlying impairments enables the patient to resume using previously developed strategies for postural control. When permanent impairments make resumption of previously used strategies impossible, new strategies will have to be developed.

COGNITIVE IMPAIRMENTS

Many patients with UMN lesions demonstrate significant cognitive impairments that affect the patient's ability to participate fully in a retraining program. With this in mind, Table 10.7 provides a few suggestions for modifying treatment strategies when working with a patient who has cognitive problems. However, it is not within the scope of this book to discuss in detail issues related to retraining cognitive impairments affecting motor control in the patient with neurological dysfunction.

MUSCULOSKELETAL IMPAIRMENTS

Musculoskeletal problems can be treated using traditional physical therapy techniques, including modalities such as heat, ultrasound, massage, and biofeedback. Passive range of motion exercises are used to improve joint mobility and muscle flexibility. Manual therapies focus on regaining passive range and joint play. Finally, plaster casts and splints are used to passively increase range and flexibility in the patient with neurological impairments. For an in-depth discussion of treatment of this important area of musculoskeletal impairments, the reader is referred to other sources (26–29).

Table 10.7.   Strategies for Working with the Patient with Cognitive Impairments

1. Reduce confusion—make sure the task goal is clear to the patient
2. Improve motivation—work on tasks that are relevant and important to the patient
3. Encourage consistency of performance—be consistent in your goals and reinforce only those behaviors that are compatible with those goals
4. Reduce confusion—use simple, clear, and concise instructions
5. Improve attention—accentuate perceptual cues that are essential to the task, and minimize the number of irrelevant stimuli in the environment
6. Improve problem-solving ability—begin with relatively simple tasks, and gradually increase the complexity of the task-demands
7. Encourage declarative as well as procedural learning—have a patient verbally/and or mentally rehearse sequences when performing a task
8. Seek a moderate level of arousal to optimize learning—moderate the sensory stimulation in the environment; agitated patients require decreased intensity of stimulation (soft voice, low lights, slow touch) to reduce arousal levels; stuporous patients require increased intensity of stimulation (use brisk, loud commands, fast movements, working in a vertical position).
9. Provide increased levels of supervision, especially during the early stages of retraining.
10. Recognize that progress may be slower when working with patients who have cognitive impairments.

NEUROMUSCULAR IMPAIRMENTS

Numerous neuromuscular limitations leading to instability in the patient with a neurological deficit are described in Chapter 9. Since stability requires the ability to generate and coordinate forces necessary for moving the center of mass, upper motor lesions producing limitations in strength, force control, and muscle tone will produce concomitant limitations in stability.

Strength

The ability to produce a voluntary contraction depends on both the characteristics of the muscle itself, and on the appropriate recruitment and timing of motor units. Techniques to improve strength can focus on generating force to move a body segment, or alternatively, the ability to resist a movement.

Progressive resistive exercises are commonly used to increase strength within individual muscles. Isokinetic equipment can also be used to improve a patient's ability to generate force throughout the range of motion, at different speeds of motion, and through repeated efforts within individual and groups of muscles (22). Proprioceptive Neuromuscular Facilitation techniques can be used to improve the timing of force generation, as well as the reciprocal interaction between agonist and antagonist muscles (46).

Biofeedback and functional electrical stimulation can also be used to assist patients in regaining volitional control over isolated muscles and joints. For example, stimulation of the peroneal nerve is commonly performed in hemiplegic patients to improve control over the anterior tibialis muscle during a voluntary contraction.

A number of studies have shown that biofeedback is effective in helping the patient with a neurological impairment learn to initiate, sustain, and/or relax a voluntary muscle contraction (47–49). There is some evidence that improved control over an isolated muscle has some carryover to gait. Thus, patients given therapy related to muscle control increased gait velocity, although this was not trained specifically (47).

Muscle Tone

Considerable effort has been directed at developing therapeutic techniques to alter muscle tone in the patient with neurological impairments. One possible way to alter muscle tone is to change the background level of activity in the motor neuron pool of the muscle. As background level of activity in the motor neuron pool increases so does the likelihood that the muscle will respond to any incoming stimulus, whether from the periphery or as part of a descending command. The opposite is also true; as background levels of activity decrease, the muscle is less likely to fire. What techniques can be used to alter background activity of motor neuron pools?

Sensory stimulation techniques can be used to facilitate or inhibit motor activity, depending on the type of stimulus and how it is applied. For example, ice can facilitate muscle activity when applied quickly, as in a brief sweep over a muscle. Alternatively, prolonged icing is considered inhibitory, decreasing the level of activation.

Vibrators have also been used to either facilitate or inhibit activity in a muscle. High-frequency vibration tends to facilitate muscle activity, while low frequency inhibits muscle activity levels (50, 51).

Techniques such as approximation, which activates joint receptors, have also been used to facilitate muscle activity in the patient with neurological impairments. Joint approximation involves compressing a joint either manually (46), or through the application of weights. Manual techniques that apply traction to a joint are also used to facilitate muscle activity (46).

Quick stretch to a muscle facilitates activation of the muscle through the stretch reflex. In contrast, prolonged stretch (either manually, or through the use of casts, splints, or orthoses) decreases activity levels.

Brisk touch or tapping also facilitates muscle activity. In contrast, slow repetitive touching is considered inhibitory.

Altering a patient's position has also been suggested as a technique that can be used to alter muscle tone and postural tone (54). The underlying assumption, drawn from a reflex hierarchical theory of motor control, is that placing patients in certain positions will alter the distribution of muscle (and postural) tone, primarily through the changes in reflex activity. For example, it has been suggested that placing a patient in the supine position will facilitate extensor tone, while flexor tone is facilitated when the patient is prone, due to the presence of released tonic labyrinthine reflexes in the patient with UMN lesions. The use of a side-lying position is often suggested as an approach to inhibiting the effects of the asymmetric tonic neck reflex on muscle tone, facilitating bilateral symmetric activities (54).

SENSORY IMPAIRMENTS

Often, clinicians tend to view sensory impairments such as loss of limb position sense or somatosensory deficits leading to decreased object recognition, as being permanent, or not modifiable by treatment. However, a number of interesting studies suggest that treatment can affect the patient's ability to process sensory stimuli.

Based on some studies examining the reorganization of somatosensory cortex in primates (55), which were previously discussed in Chapter 4, a number of researchers have developed structured sensory reeducation programs to improve the patient's ability to discriminate and interpret sensory information (56–58). The goal of these interventions is to improve a patient's ability to detect and process information in the environment and thereby improve motor performance. Suggestions for retraining sensory discrimination are presented in more detail in the chapter on retraining upper extremity control.

PERCEPTUAL IMPAIRMENTS

Treatment of dizziness varies, depending on the underlying cause. Vestibular Rehabilitation is an exercise approach to treating symptoms of dizziness and imbalance that result from pathology within the vestibular system. Since there are many potential causes of dizziness, including metabolic disturbances, side-effects of medication, cardiovascular problems, such as orthostatic hypotension, and pathology within peripheral or central vestibular structures, it is essential that the therapist know the underlying diagnosis prior to beginning an exercise-based approach.

Vestibular Rehabilitation uses repeated exercises to habituate symptoms of dizziness. The patient is instructed to repeat the position or movements that provoke dizziness five times in a row, two to three times per day. Exercises are progressive in nature. The patient begins with fairly simple exercises, such as horizontal head movements in the seated position, and progresses to more difficult tasks, such as horizontal head movements integrated into gait. This approach is discussed in more detail elsewhere (9, 44, 45).

Treating at the Strategy Level

The goal of retraining at the strategy level involves helping or guiding patients to recover, or develop, sensory and motor strategies that are effective in meeting the postural demands of functional tasks. To fully retrain strategies, the clinician must understand the inherent requirements of the task being performed.

For example, both seated and stance postural control require that the center of gravity of the body be within the base of support. In the case of standing, the base of support is limited to the feet, unless the patient is using an assistive device. In the case of seated postural control, the trunk mass must stay within the base of support defined by the bottom and feet. Thus, in order to regain the ability to stand or sit independently, the patient must develop movement strategies that are successful in controlling the center of mass relative to the base of support. These include (a) strategies that move the center of mass relative to a stationary base of support, in standing, for example, an ankle or hip strategy, and (b) strategies for changing the base of support when the center of mass moves beyond it, for example, a stepping strategy in standing, or a protective reach in sitting.

ALIGNMENT

The goal when retraining alignment is to help the patient develop an initial position that (a) is appropriate for the task, (b) is efficient with respect to gravity, that is, with minimal muscle activity requirements for maintaining the position, and (c) maximizes stability, that is, places the vertical line of gravity well within the patient's stability limits; this allows the greatest range of movements for postural control. Many tasks utilize a symmetrical vertical position, but this may not always be a realistic goal for all patients (10).

A number of approaches can be used to help patients develop a symmetrically vertical posture. Commonly, verbal and manual cues are used by the clinician to assist a patient in finding and maintaining an appropriate vertical posture. Patients practice with eyes open and closed, learning to maintain a vertical position in the absence of visual cues.

Mirrors can also be used to provide patients with visual feedback about their position in space. The effect of a mirror can be enhanced by having the patient wear a white T-shirt with a vertical stripe down the center, and asking him/her to try to match the stripe on the T-shirt to a vertical stripe on the mirror (Fig. 10.10). The patient can use the mirror and T-shirt approach while performing a variety of tasks, such as reaching for an object, which require that the body be moved away from the vertical line and then reestablish a vertical position.

Another approach to retraining vertical alignment is shown in Figure 10.11, and uses flashlights attached to the patient's body in conjunction with targets on the wall (10). In this task, the patient is asked to bring the light (or lights) in line with the target(s). Lights

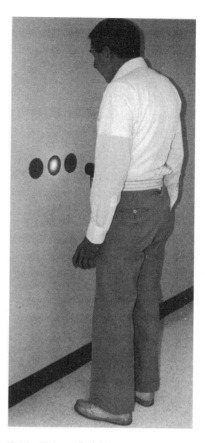

Figure 10.11 Using a flashlight in conjunction with targets on a wall to help a patient learn to control center of mass movements.

can be turned on and off during the task so that visual feedback is intermittent.

Another approach to retraining vertical posture involves having patients stand (or sit) with their back against the wall, which provides enhanced somatosensory feedback about their position in space. This feedback can be further increased by placing a yard stick or small roll vertically on the wall and having the patient lean against it. Somatosensory feedback can be made intermittent by having the patient lean away from the wall, only occasionally leaning back to get knowledge of results (KR).

Kinetic or force feedback devices are often used to provide patients with information about postural alignment and weightbearing status (60–64). Kinetic feedback can be provided with devices as simple as bathroom

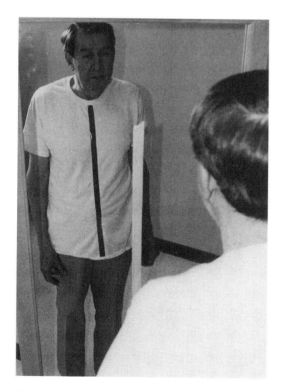

Figure 10.10 Using a mirror when retraining alignment; the patient is asked to line up the vertical stripe on his T-shirt with a vertical stripe on the mirror.

scales (Fig. 10.3). Alternatively, kinetic feedback can be given through either load-limb monitors (60) or forceplate biofeedback systems (Fig. 10.2) (61). Other types of feedback devices include using a feedback cane to improve patients' weightbearing status (63).

Clinicians routinely provide the unsteady patient with assistive devices, such as canes or walkers. What effect does providing an external support such as a cane have on balance? As illustrated in Figure 10.12, an assistive device such as a cane increases the base of support. Since stability requires keeping the center of gravity within the base of support, increasing the base of support makes the task of stability easier. Researchers have studied the effects of a cane on standing balance in patients with hemiparesis, using a forceplate to record changes in center of pressure under various conditions of support. They found that using a cane results in a significant shift in the position of the center of pressure towards the cane side, and a decrease in both anterior-posterior and medial-lateral postural sway. Thus, although using a cane will reduce postural sway, it increases the asymmetric alignment of patients towards the side holding the cane (65).

MOVEMENT STRATEGIES

The goal when retraining movement strategies involves helping the patient develop multijoint coordinated movements that are effective in meeting the demands for posture and balance in sitting and in standing. We retrain strategies within the context of a task, since optimal function is characterized by strategies that are efficient in accomplishing a task goal in a relevant environment (10).

Retraining strategies involves both the recovery of motor strategies and the development of compensatory strategies. As we mentioned in Chapter 2, the term recovery refers to achieving function through original processes, while compensation is defined as behavioral substitution, or the adoption of new strategies to complete a task.

Patients are encouraged and guided to develop strategies for both seated and stance postural control, including the ability to move the body in all directions to accomplish functional tasks. We use as our example of strategy retraining, the development of coordinated ankle, hip, and stepping strategies for stance postural control, and show how these strate-

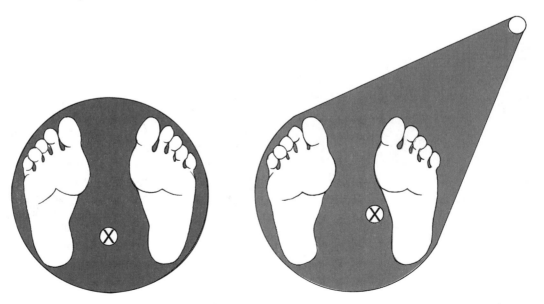

Figure 10.12 The effects of holding a cane while standing include widening the base of support and shifting the mean position of the center of pressure laterally toward the cane side. (Adapted from Milezarek JJ, Kirby LM, Harrison ER, MacLeod DA. Standard and four-footed canes: their effect on the standing balance of patients with hemiparesis. Arch Phys Med Rehabil 1993;74:283.)

gies can be developed within the context of self-initiated voluntary sway, in response to external perturbations, and during tasks requiring anticipatory postural adjustments. Remember, just because we limit our discussion to activities that could be used to retrain strategies for sagittal plane stance postural control, it does not mean that, in actuality, retraining postural control in the patient should be limited to retraining these strategies.

Developing a Coordinated Ankle Strategy

Prior to retraining the use of an ankle strategy for postural control, it is essential to remember that this strategy requires the patient to have adequate range of motion and strength at the ankle (8, 10). In the face of persisting impairments that preclude the use of an ankle strategy, patients would be encouraged to develop the use of alternative strategies, such as the hip or step, when controlling body sway.

When retraining the use of an ankle strategy during *self-initiated sway*, patients are asked to practice swaying back and forth, and side to side, within small ranges, keeping the body straight and not bending at the hips or knees. Knowledge of results regarding how far the center of mass is moving during self-initiated sway can be facilitated using static forceplate retraining systems (10). Flashlights attached to the patient in conjunction with targets on the wall can also be used to encourage patients to move from side to side (refer back to Fig. 10.11).

Patients who are very unsteady or extremely fearful of falling can practice movement while in the parallel bars, or when standing close to a wall, or in a corner with a chair or table in front of them (Fig. 10.13). Modifying the environment (either home or clinic) in this manner allows a patient to continue practicing movement strategies for balance control safely and without the continual supervision of a therapist.

Use of perturbations applied at the hips or shoulders is an effective way to help patients develop strategies for *recovery of bal-*

ance. Small perturbations can facilitate the use of an ankle strategy for balance control, while larger perturbations encourage the use of a hip or step.

Finally, patients are asked to carry out a variety of manipulation tasks, such as reaching, lifting, and throwing, thus helping patients to develop strategies for *anticipatory postural control*. A hierarchy of tasks reflecting increasing anticipatory postural demands can be helpful when retraining patients in this important area. The magnitude of anticipatory postural activity is directly related to the potential for instability inherent in a task. Potential instability relates to speed, effort, degree of external support, and task complexity. Thus, asking a patient who is externally sup-

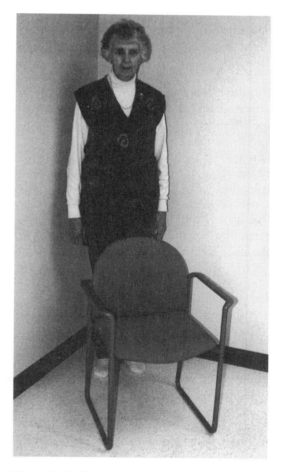

Figure 10.13 Placing a patient near a wall with a chair in front of her increases safety when retraining standing balance in a fearful or unstable patient.

ported by the therapist to lift a light load slowly, requires minimal anticipatory postural activity. Conversely, an unsupported patient who must lift a heavy load quickly, must utilize a substantial amount of anticipatory postural activity to remain stable.

Treatment of Timing Problems

How can a clinician help a patient recover an ankle strategy in the face of coordination problems that affect the timing and scaling of postural movement strategies? When a patient is unable to activate distal muscles quickly enough to recover stability during a postural task, the clinician can use a variety of techniques to facilitate muscle activation. These include icing, tapping, and vibration to the distal muscles while the patient is standing, immediately prior to, and during, perturbations to standing balance, or self-initiated sway (10). This is shown in Figure 10.14.

Biofeedback and electrical stimulation can also be used to improve the automatic recruitment and control of muscles during task-specific movements strategies for posture (67) and gait (62). For example, electrical stimulation in conjunction with a foot switch can be used to decrease onset latencies of postural responses (67). As shown in Figure 10.15, a foot switch can be placed under the heel so that increased weight on the switch triggers a tetanic stimulation of the anterior tibialis muscle. Electrical stimulation to recruit a muscle within a postural movement strategy can be done during self-initiated sway or during perturbed balance.

Several clinicians have combined the use of biofeedback and functional electrical stimulation (FES) during retraining motor control, and found that the combined used of biofeedback and FES was superior to either in isolation (65). One approach we have tried successfully is to use EMG biofeedback on the tibialis anterior muscle, and to link the biofeedback with a functional electrical stimulator whose electrodes were placed on the quadriceps muscle of the same leg (FES). The two units were set up such that a minimal level

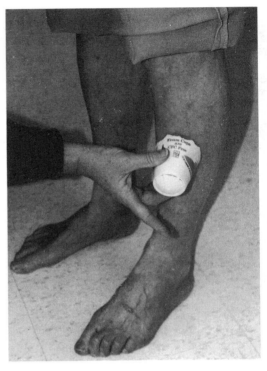

Figure 10.14   The use of ice on the anterior tibialis muscle just prior to a small backward displacement is used to facilitate its activation during recovery of balance.

of tibialis activation was sufficient to trigger stimulation of the quadriceps. This set-up was used in conjunction with external perturbations to balance, and was successful in changing the timing of quadriceps activation within the postural response synergy (66).

There is no established research that provides guidelines to the clinician regarding the optimal frequency and duration of stimulation techniques during postural retraining. We have found through trial and error that 5 minutes of stimulation, twice daily, for 3 to 4 weeks appears to be effective in altering timing parameters. However, further research is needed in this area.

Treatment of Scaling Problems

To produce effective movements of the center of body mass during postural control, the level of muscle activation must be scaled, or graded, appropriate to the amplitude of

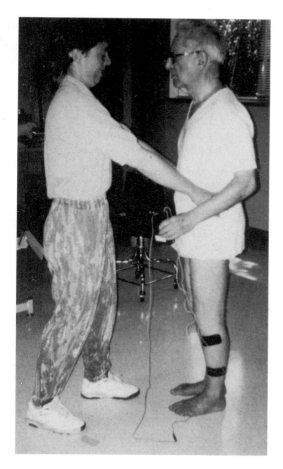

Figure 10.15 Use of electrical stimulation of the distal muscle in conjunction with a foot switch to facilitate activation of the anterior tibialis muscle during stance balance retraining.

body sway. Normal subjects use a combination of feedforward and feedback control mechanisms to scale forces for postural control (68). To improve amplitude scaling of postural synergies, patients may practice responding to perturbations of various amplitudes. Feedback regarding the appropriateness of their response is provided by the clinician. Interestingly, it is easier for many cerebellar patients, who consistently overrespond to small pushes, to appropriately scale postural movements to large perturbations (10).

Static forceplate retraining systems can also be used effectively to retrain scaling problems. Patients are asked to move the center of mass voluntarily to different targets displayed on a screen. Targets are made progressively smaller and are placed closed together, requiring greater precision in force control. Knowledge of results is given with respect to movements that *overshoot* the target, indicating an error in amplitude scaling.

Finally, another approach to treating scaling problems in patients with cerebellar pathology producing ataxia, is to add weights to the trunk or limbs (69, 70). Two rationales are proposed to explain the potential benefits of weighting. The first is that joint compression associated with weights would facilitate coactivation of muscles around a joint, thereby increasing stiffness. The other explanation is mechanical; adding weights increases the mass of the system. In this way, the increased forces generated in the cerebellar patient match the increased mass of the system (69). Researchers have found that adding weights to cerebellar patients has inconsistent effects. Some patients become more stable, while others are destabilized by the weights (69, 70).

Developing a Coordinated Hip Strategy

A hip strategy can be facilitated by asking the patient to maintain balance without taking a step and by using displacements in larger ranges than those used for an ankle strategy. Use of a hip strategy can also be facilitated by restricting motion at the ankle joints either through the use of plaster casts (bivalved so they can be taken on and off) or the use of ankle orthoses (10).

Patients can be asked to maintain various equilibrium positions that require the use of a hip strategy for stability. Possible examples include standing on a narrow beam, standing heel/toe, or adopting a single limb stance (10).

Developing a Coordinated Step Strategy

Stepping to avoid a fall requires the capacity to maintain the body's weight on a single limb momentarily, without collapse of that limb. Stepping is normally used to prevent a fall when the center of mass has (or is rapidly) moving outside the base of support. Traditionally, stepping is taught within the context of step initiation during gait retraining. Unexpected stepping is often viewed by the clinician as a failure on the part of the patient to *maintain* balance. However, learning to step when the center of mass exceeds the base of support is an essential part of postural retraining.

Stepping can be facilitated manually by the clinician by shifting the patient's weight to one side and quickly bringing the center of mass towards the unweighted leg (Fig. 10.16). The clinician can further assist the patient with a step by manually lifting the foot and placing it during the maneuver. To ensure a patient's safety, stepping can be done within the parallel bars, or near a wall. When

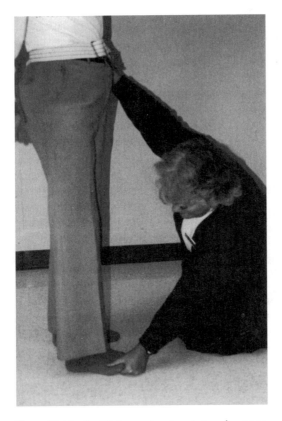

Figure 10.16 Facilitating a stepping strategy by manually shifting the patient's center of mass laterally and manually moving the patient's foot into a step.

helping a patient develop the ability to step for postural control, it is important to tell the patient that the goal of the exercise is to take a step to prevent a fall.

SENSORY STRATEGIES

The goal when retraining sensory strategies is to help the patient learn to effectively coordinate sensory information to meet the demands of postural control. This necessitates correctly interpreting the position and movements of the body in space. Treatment strategies generally require the patient to maintain balance during progressively more difficult static and dynamic movement tasks while the clinician systematically varies the availability and accuracy of one or more senses for orientation (9, 10, 44).

Patients who show increased reliance on vision for orientation are asked to perform a variety of balance tasks when visual cues are absent (eyes closed or blindfolded), or reduced (blinders or diminished lighting). Alternatively, visual cues can be made inaccurate for orientation through the use of glasses smeared with petroleum jelly (shown in Fig. 10.17), or prism glasses. Decreasing a patient's sensitivity to visual motion cues in their environment can be done by asking the patient to maintain balance during exposure to optokinetic stimuli, such as moving curtains with stripes, moving large cardboard posters with vertical lines, or even moving rooms (10, 71).

Patients who show increased reliance on the surface for orientation are asked to perform tasks while sitting or standing on surfaces providing decreased somatosensory cues for orientation, such as carpet or compliant foam surfaces, or on moving surfaces, such as a tilt board.

Finally, to enhance the patient's ability to use remaining vestibular information for postural stability, exercises are given that ask the patient to balance while both visual and somatosensory inputs for orientation are simultaneously reduced, such as standing on compliant foam (Fig. 10.18) or an inclined surface with eyes closed.

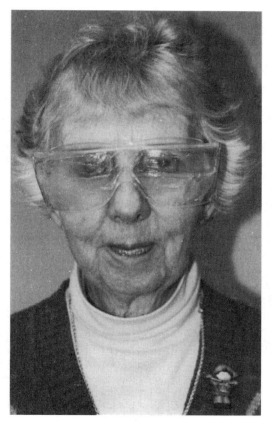

Figure 10.17 Petroleum-covered glasses used to obscure but not completely remove visual cues for postural control.

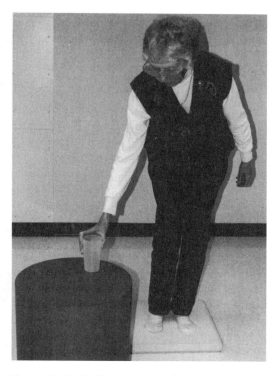

Figure 10.18 Facilitating the use of vestibular inputs for postural control requires that the patient maintain balance when orientation cues from visual and somatosensory systems are reduced or inaccurate by standing on a foam surface and wearing petroleum-covered glasses.

Perceived Limits of Stability

Rehabilitation strategies involving use of postural sway biofeedback have also been used with patients who incorrectly perceive that they have reduced stability limits. Patients are asked to sway using larger and larger areas, in an effort to change perceptions that they cannot move the body safely in space.

In addition, patients may be asked to visualize a space around them with boundaries in which they can move safely when seated or standing. Patients are then asked to practice moving their bodies within and to those boundaries. Boundaries may be gradually expanded with increasing sensory and motor capacities of the patient (8–10, 44).

Treating at the Functional Task Level

Developing adaptive capacities in the patient is also a critical part of retraining postural control. The ability to perform postural tasks in a natural environment requires that the patient modify strategies to changing task and environmental demands. The goal of retraining at the functional level focuses on having patients practice successfully the performance of a wide collection of functional tasks in a variety of contexts.

We began our discussion of task-oriented retraining in the previous section focusing on retraining strategies for postural control during three tasks, self-initiated sway, in response to perturbation, and anticipatory to potentially destablizing movements such as reaching, lifting, or stepping. This concept is now broadened to include having the patient practice a wide variety of functional tasks with varying stability and orientation demands. This could include (*a*) maintaining balance with a reduced base of support, that is, with feet together, in tandem, or on one foot, (*b*) maintaining balance while changing the orientation of the head and trunk, for example, looking over one's shoulder, or leaning over, (*c*) maintaining balance while performing a variety of upper extremity tasks, such as reaching, lifting, pushing, and holding objects with one or both hands.

As we mentioned in Chapter 6, all tasks demand postural control; however, the stability and orientation requirements will vary with the task and the environment. By understanding the postural requirements inherent in various tasks and environments, the clinician can develop a hierarchy of tasks to retrain postural control, beginning with tasks that have relatively few stability demands, and moving to those that place heavy demands on the postural control system. For example, postural demands involved in maintaining an upright seated posture while in a semisupported seated position are relatively few. In contrast, sitting on a moving tilt board while holding a cup of water has fairly rigorous stability requirements, reflecting the changing and unpredictable nature of the task. This task requires constant adaptation of the postural system. Therefore, supported sitting would be a good task to begin with when working with a patient who has severe postural dyscontrol. As the patient improves, more difficult and demanding tasks can be introduced.

SUMMARY

1. A task-oriented approach to assessing postural control uses a variety of tests, measurements and observations to (*a*) document functional abilities related to posture and balance control, (*b*) assess underlying sensory and motor strategies, and (*c*) determine the underlying sensory, motor, and cognitive systems contributing to postural control.
2. Following completion of the assessment, the clinician must interpret the assessment, iden-

tify the problems related to function, strategies, and contributing impairments, and establish the goals and plan of care.
3. The plan of care for retraining posture control in the patient with a neurological deficit will vary widely, depending on the constellation of underlying impairments and the degree to which the patient has developed compensatory strategies that are successful in achieving postural demands in functional tasks.
4. The goals of a task-oriented approach to retraining postural control include (*a*) resolve or prevent impairments, (*b*) develop effective task-specific strategies, (*c*) retrain functional tasks, and (*d*) adapt task-specific strategies so that functional tasks can be performed in changing environmental contexts.
5. The goals of treatments aimed at the impairment level are to correct those impairments that can be changed and prevent the development of secondary impairments.
6. The goal of retraining at the strategy level involves helping patients recover or develop sensory and motor strategies that are effective in meeting the postural demands of functional tasks. This requires that the clinician understand the inherent requirements of the task being performed so that patients can be guided in developing effective strategies for meeting task demands.
7. The goal of retraining at the functional level focuses on having patients practice successfully the performance of a wide collection of functional tasks in a variety of contexts. Since the ability to perform postural tasks in a natural environment requires the ability to modify strategies to changing task and environmental demands, developing adaptive capacities in the patient is a critical part of retraining at the task level.
8. The development of clinical methods based on a systems theory of motor control is just beginning. As systems-based research provides us with an increased understanding of normal and abnormal postural control, new methods for assessing and treating postural disorders will emerge.

REFERENCES

1. Mathias S, Nayak U, Issacs B. Balance in elderly patients: the "Get-up and Go" test. Arch Phys Med Rehabil 1986;67:387–389.
2. Podsiadlo D, Richardson S. The timed "Up

& Go": a test of basic functional mobility for frail elderly persons. J Am Geriatr Soc 1991; 39:142–148.

3. Mahoney RI, Barthel DW. Functional evaluation: the Barthel Index. Md Med J 1965; 14:61–65.

4. Duncan PW, Weiner DK, Chandler J, Studenski S. Functional reach: a new clinical measure of balance. J Gerontol 1990; 45:192–195.

5. Tinetti ME. Performance oriented assessment of mobility problems in elderly patients. J Am Geriat Soc 1986 34;119–126.

6. Tinetti ME, Ginter SF. Identifying mobility dysfunctions in elderly patients: standard neuromuscular examination or direct assessment? JAMA 1988;259:1190–1193.

7. Berg K. Measuring balance in the elderly: validation of an instrment [Dissertation]. Montreal, Canada: McGill University, 1993.

8. Shumway-Cook A, McCollum G. Assessment and treatment of balance disorders in the neurologic patient. In: Montgomery T, Connolly B, eds. Motor control theory and practice. Chattanooga, TN: Chattanooga Corp. 1990:123–138.

9. Shumway-Cook A, Horak F. Rehabilitation strategies for patients with vestibular deficits. Neurology Clinics of North America 1990; 8:441–457.

10. Shumway-Cook A, Horak F. Balance rehabilitation in the neurologic patient: course syllabus. Seattle, NERA, 1992.

11. Woollacott M, Shumway-Cook A. Changes in posture control across the life span—a systems approach. Phys Ther 1990;70:799–807.

12. Carr JH, Shepherd RB. Motor relearning programme for stroke. Rockville, MD: Aspen Publications, 1983.

13. Bobath B. Adult hemiplegia: evaluation and treatment. London: Wm Heinemann Medical Books, 1978.

14. Shumway-Cook A, Horak F. Assessing the influence of sensory interaction on balance. Phys Ther 1986;66:1548–1550.

15. Horak F. Clinical measurement of postural control in adults. Phys Ther 1987; 67:1881–1885.

16. Nashner LM. Adaptation of human movement to altered environments. Trends Neurosci 1982;5:358–361.

17. Peterka RJ, Black FO. Age-related changes in human posture control: sensory organization tests. J Vest Res 1990;1:73–85.

18. DeFabio R, Badke MB. Relationship of sensory organization to balance function in patients with hemiplegia. Phys Ther 1990; 70:542–560.

19. Cohen H, Blatchly C, Gombash L. A study of the clinical test of sensory interaction and balance. Phys Ther 1993;73:346–354.

20. Horak F, Jones-Rycewicz C, Black FO, Shumway-Cook A. Effects of vestibular rehabilitation on dizziness and imbalance. Otolaryngol Head Neck Surg 1992;106:175–180.

21. Duncan PW. Stroke: physical therapy assessment and treatment. In: Contemporary managemment of motor control problems. Proceedings of the II Step Conference. Alexandria, VA: APTA, 1991:209–217.

22. Duncan P, Badke MB. Stroke rehabilitation: the recovery of motor control. Chicago: Year Book Medical Publishers, 1987.

23. Stockmeyer S. Clinical decision making based on homeostatic concepts. In: Wolf S, ed. Clinical decision making in physical therapy. Philadelphia: FA Davis, 1985:79–90.

24. Folstein MF, Folstein SE, McHugh PR. Mini-mental state: a practical method for grading the cognitive states for the clinician. J Psychiatr Res 1975;12:188–198.

25. Pfeiffer E. Short portable mental status questionnaire. J Am Geriatr Soc 1975;23:433–441.

26. Kendall F, McCreary EK. Muscles: testing and function. Baltimore: Williams & Wilkins, 1983.

27. Saunders D. Evaluation, treatment and prevention of musculoskeletal disorders. Minneapolis: Viking Press, 1991.

28. Magee DJ. Orthopedic physical assessment. Philadelphia: WB Saunders, 1987.

29. Kessler RM, Hertling D. Management of common musculoskeletal disorders. Philadelphia: Harper & Row, 1983.

30. Kaltenborn F. Mobilization of the extremity joints. Oslo: Olaf Norlis Bokhandel Universitetsgaten, 1980.

31. Leahy P. Motor control assessment. In: Montgomery P, Connolly BH, eds. Motor control and physical therapy. Hixson, TX: Chattanooga Group, 1991:69–84.

32. Buchner DM, DeLateur BJ. The importance of skeletal muscle strength to physical function in older adults. Annals of Behavioral Medicine 1991;13:1–12.

33. Amundsen LR. Isometric muscle strength testing with fixed-load cells. In: Amundsen

LR, ed. Muscle strength testing instrumented and non-instrumented systems. New York: Churchill Livingstone, 1990:89–122.

34. Rogers MM. Musculoskeletal considerations in production and control of movement. In: Montgomery P, Connolly BH, eds. Motor control and physical therapy. Hixson, TX: Chattanooga Group, 1991:69–82.

35. Bohannon RW. Muscle strength testing with hand-held dynamometers. In: Amundsen LR, ed. Muscle strength testing instrumented and non-instrumented systems. New York: Churchill Livingstone, 1990:69–88.

36. Bohannon RW, Andrews AW. Correlation of knee extensor muscle torque and spasticity with gait speed in patients with stroke. Arch Phys Med Rehabil 1990;71:330–333.

37. Andrews AW. Hand held dynamometry for measuring muscle strength. J Hum Muscle Perform 1991;1:35–50.

38. Lynch L. Manual muscle strength testing of the distal muscles. In: Amundsen LR, ed. Muscle strength testing instrumented and non-instrumented systems. New York: Churchill Livingstone, 1990:25–68.

39. Wilk K. Dynamic muscle strength testing. In: Amundsen LR, ed. Muscle strength testing instrumented and non-instrumented systems. New York: Churchill Livingstone, 1990: 123–150.

40. Bohannon RW, Smith MB. Interrater reliability of a modified Ashworth scale of muscle spasticity. Phys Ther 1987;67:206–207.

41. Schmitz TJ. Coordination assessment. In: O'Sullivan S, Schmitz T, eds. Physical rehabilitation: assessment and treatment. Philadelphia: FA Davis, 1988:121–133.

42. DeJong RN. The neurologic examination. New York: Harper & Row, 1970.

43. Kottke FJ. Krusen's handbook of physical medicine and rehabilitation. Philadelphia: WB Saunders, 1982.

44. Shumway-Cook A, Horak FB. Vestibular rehabilitation: an exercise approach to managing symptoms of vestibular dysfunction. Seminars in Hearing 1989;10:196–205.

45. Herdman S. Vestibular rehabilitation. Philadelphia: FA Davis, 1994.

46. Voss D, Ionta M, Myers B. Proprioceptive neuromuscular facilitation: patterns and techniques. 3rd ed. Philadelphia: Harper & Row; 1985.

47. Binder S, Moll CB, Wolf SL. Evaluation of electromyographic biofeedback as an adjunct to therapeutic exercise in treating the lower extremities of hemiplegic patients. Phys Ther 1981;61:886–893.

48. Baker M, Regenos E, Wolf SL, Basmajian JV. Developing strategies for biofeedback: applications in neurologically handicapped patients. Phys Ther 1977;57:402–408.

49. Krebb DE. Biofeedback. In O'Sullivan S, Schmitz T, eds. Physical rehabilitation: assessment and treatment. Philadelphia: FA Davis, 1988:629–645.

50. Bishop B. Vibration stimulation. I. Neurophysiology of motor responses evoked by vibratory stimulation. Phys Ther 1974; 54:1273.

51. Bishop B. Vibratory stimulation II. Vibratory stimulation as an evaluation tool Phys Ther 1975;55:29.

52. Hagbarth K. Excitatory and inhibitory skin areas for flexor and extensor motoneurons. Acta Physiol Scand 1952;94:1–14.

53. Eldred E, Hagbarth K. Facilitation and inhibition of gamma efferents by stimulation of certain skin areas. J Neurophysiol 1954; 17:59.

54. Bobath K, Bobath B. The neurodevelopmental treatment. In: Scrutton D, ed. Management of the motor disorders of cerebral palsy. Clinics in Developmental Medicine. No 90. London: Heinemann Medical, 1984:6–18.

55. Merzenich MM, Kaas JH, Wall JT, Sur M, Nelson RJ, Felleman DJ. Progression of change following median nerve section in the cortical representation of the hand in areas 3b and 1 in adult owl and squirrel monkeys. Neuroscience 1983;10:639–665.

56. DeJersey MC. Report on a sensory programme for patients with sensory deficits. Aust J Phyiother 1979;25:165–170.

57. Dannenbaum RM, Dyke RW. Sensory loss in the hand after sensory stroke: therapeutic rationale. Arch Phys Med Rehabil 1988; 69:833–839.

58. Carey L, Matyas T, Oke L. Sensory loss in stroke patients: Effective training of tactile and proprioceptive discrimination. Arch Phys Med Rehabil 1993;74:602–611.

59. Lewis C. Phillippi L. Postural changes with age and soft tissue treatment. Physical Therapy Forum 1993;10:4–6.

60. Herman R. Augmented sensory feedback in control of limb movement. In: Fields WS, ed. Neural organization and its relevance to pros-

thetics. New York: Intercontinental Medical Book Corp, 1973.

61. Shumway-Cook A, Anson D, Haller. Postural sway biofeedback, its effect on reestablishing stance stability in hemiplegic patients. Arch Phys Med Rehabil 1988; 69:395–341.

62. Baker MP, Hudson JE, Wolf SL. A "feedback" cane to improve the hemiplegic patient's gait. Phys Ther 1979;59:170–171.

63. DeBacher G. Feedback goniometer for rehabilitation. In: Basmajian JV, ed. Biofeedback: principles and practices for clinicians. Baltimore: Williams & Wilkins, 1983:359–367.

64. Cozean CD, Pease SW, Hubbell SL. Biofeedback and functional electric stimulation in stroke rehabilitation. Arch Phys Med Rehabil 1988;69:401–405.

65. Milezarek JJ, Kirby LM, Harrison ER, MacLeod DA. Standard and four-footed canes: their effect on the standing balance of patients with hemiparesis. Arch Phys Med Rehabil 1993;74:281–284.

66. Shumway-Cook A. Unpublished observation.

67. Shumway-Cook A. Retraining stability and mobility: translating research into clinical practice. Presentation given at the Annual Meeting of the American Physical Therapy Association, Cincinnati, OH, 1993.

68. Horak FB, Diener HC, Nashner LM. Influence of central set on human postural responses. J Neurophysiol 1989;62:841–853.

69. Morgan MH. Ataxia and weights. Physiotherapy 1975;61:332–334.

70. Lucy SD, Hayes KC. Postural sway profiles: normal subjects and subjects with cerebellar ataxia. Physiotherapy Canada 1985;37:140–148.

71. Semont A, Vitte E, Freyss G. Falls in the elderly: a therapeutic approach by optokinetic reflex stimulation. In: Vellas B, Toupet M, Rubenstein L, Albarede JL, Christen Y, eds. Falls, balance and gait disorders in the elderly. Paris: Elsevier, 1992:153–159.

Section III

MOBILITY FUNCTIONS

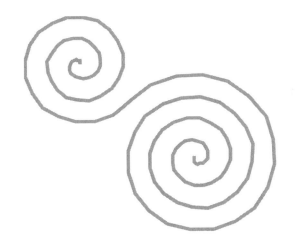

Chapter 11

CONTROL OF NORMAL MOBILITY

INTRODUCTION

A key feature of our independence as human beings is the ability to stand up from a bed or chair, to walk or run, and to navigate through often quite complex environments. During rehabilitation a primary goal of treatment is to help patients regain as much independent mobility as possible. Often, regaining mobility is the primary goal of a patient. This is reflected in the constantly asked question, "Will I walk again?"

In this chapter we discuss many aspects of mobility, including gait, transfers, and stair walking, examining the contributions of the individual, task, and environment to each of these tasks. We begin with a discussion of locomotion, defining the requirements for successful locomotion and discussing the contributions of the different neural and musculoskeletal systems to locomotor control. In addition, we discuss mechanisms essential for the adaptation of gait to a wide variety of task and environmental conditions. Finally, we consider transitions in mobility, including the initiation of gait and transfers.

Gait is an extraordinarily complex behavior. It involves the entire body and therefore requires the coordination of many muscles and joints. In addition, navigating through complex and often cluttered environments requires the use of multiple sensory inputs to assist in the control and adaptation of gait. Because of these complexities, understanding both the control of normal gait and the mobility problems of patients with neurological impairments can seem like an overwhelming task.

To simplify the process of understanding the control of gait, we describe a framework for examining gait which we have found useful. The framework is built around understanding the essential requirements of locomotion and how these requirements are translated into goals accomplished during the different phases of gait. Keeping in mind both the essential requirements of gait, and the conditions that must be met during stance and swing phases of gait to accomplish these requirements, are important when examining both normal and abnormal gait.

ESSENTIAL REQUIREMENTS FOR SUCCESSFUL LOCOMOTION

There are three major requirements for successful locomotion: (*a*) a basic locomotor pattern that can move the body in the desired direction, referred to as the **progression requirement**; (*b*) the ability to maintain stability, including the support of the body against gravity, referred to as the **stability requirement**; and (*c*) the ability to adapt gait to meet the goals of the individual and the demands of the environment, referred to as the **adaptation requirement** (1). These essential characteristics have been called *task invariants*, since they are minimal requirements for locomotion to occur (2).

Human gait can be subdivided into a stance (or support) and swing phase. Certain goals need to be met during each of these phases of gait in order to achieve the three task invariants of successful locomotion (progression, stability, and adaptability). During the support phase of gait, we need to generate both horizontal forces against the support surface, to move the body in the desired direction (progression), and vertical forces, to support the body mass against gravity (stability). In addition, strategies used to accomplish progression and stability must be flexible to accommodate changes in speed, direction, or alterations in the support surface (adaptation).

The goals to be achieved during the swing phase of gait include advancement of the swing leg (progression), and repositioning the limb in preparation for weight acceptance (stability). Both the progression and stability goals require sufficient foot clearance so the toe does not drag on the supporting surface during swing. In addition, strategies used during the swing phase of gait must be sufficiently flexible to allow the swing foot to avoid any obstacles in its path (adaptation).

The movement strategies used by nor-mal subjects to meet the task requirements of locomotion have been well defined. Kinematic studies describing body motions suggest a similarity in movement strategies across subjects. This is consistent with intuitive observations that we all walk somewhat similarly. In contrast, studies that have described the muscles and forces associated with gait, suggest that there is a tremendous variability in the way these gait movements are achieved. Thus, there appears to be a wide range of muscle activation patterns used by normal subjects to accomplish the task requirements of gait.

DESCRIPTION OF THE HUMAN GAIT CYCLE

Let's think about the human body and the control of gait for a moment. We have discussed the essential requirements for normal gait, that is, progression, stability, and adaptability. The normal human perception-action system has developed elegant control strategies for solving these task requirements.

Although other gait patterns are possible (that is, we can skip, hop, or gallop), humans normally use a symmetric alternating gait pattern, probably because it provides the greatest dynamic stability for bipedal gait with minimal control demands (3). Thus, normal locomotion is a bipedal gait in which the limbs move in a symmetrical alternating relationship, which can be described by a phase lag of .5 (4).

A phase lag of .5 means that one limb initiates its step cycle as the opposite limb reaches the midpoint of its own cycle, as you see in Figure 11.1. Thus, if one complete cycle is defined as the time between ipsilateral foot strike (right heel contact to right heel contact (Fig. 11.1), then the contralateral limb begins its cycle midway through the ipsilateral stride cycle.

Traditionally, all descriptions of gait, whether kinematic, EMG, or kinetic are described with reference to different aspects of the gait cycle. Thus, an understanding of the various phases of gait is necessary for understanding descriptions of normal locomotion.

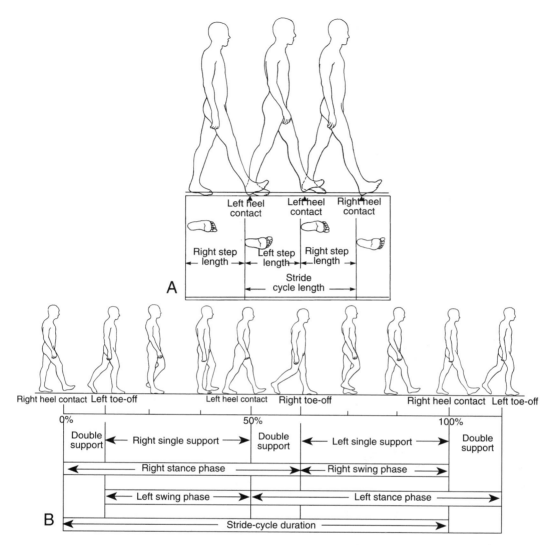

Figure 11.1. Temporal and distance dimensions of the gait cycle. (Adapted from Inman VT, Ralston H, Todd F. Human walking. Baltimore: Williams & Wilkins, 1981.)

Phases of the Step Cycle

As we mentioned earlier, the single limb cycle consists of two main phases: stance, which starts when the foot strikes the ground, and swing, which begins when the foot leaves the ground (Fig. 11.1). At freely chosen walking speeds, adults typically spend approximately 60% of the cycle duration in stance, and 40% in swing. As you see in Figure 11.1, approximately the first and the last 10% of the stance phase are spent in double support, that is, the period of time when both feet are in

contact with the ground. Single-support phase is the period when only one foot is in contact with the ground, and in walking, this consists of the time when the opposite limb is in swing phase (5, 6).

The stance phase is often further divided into five subphases: (*a*) initial contact, (*b*) the loading response (together taking up about 10% of the step cycle, during double-support phase), (*c*) mid-stance, and (*d*) terminal stance (about 40% of stance phase, which is in single support), and (*e*) pre-swing (the last 10% of stance, in double support). The swing phase is often divided into three subphases: initial swing, mid-swing, and terminal swing (all of which are in single support phase and in total make up 40% of the step cycle) (7).

Typically, researchers and clinicians use three techniques to describe different aspects of gait. Kinematic analysis allows an analysis of joint motion; electromyography provides an understanding of muscle activation patterns; and kinetic analysis describes the forces involved in gait. For a review of the technology used to analyze gait from these various perspectives, refer to the learning boxes on pages 124 and 125 of Chapter 6.

Temporal Distance Factors

Gait is often described with respect to temporal distance parameters such as velocity, step length, step frequency (called cadence), and stride length (Fig. 11.1). Velocity of gait is defined as the average horizontal speed of the body measured over one or more strides. In the research literature, it is usually reported in the metric system (for example, cm/sec) (7). In contrast, in the clinic, gait is usually described in nonmetric terms (feet), and in either distance or time parameters. For example, one might report that the patient is able to walk 50 feet, or the patient is able to walk continuously for 5 minutes. Because of this difference in convention between the clinic and the lab, we offer information in both metric and nonmetric terms.

Cadence is the number of steps per unit of time, usually reported as steps per minute. **Step length** is the distance from one foot strike to the foot strike of the other foot. For example, the right step length is the distance from the left heel to the right heel when both feet are in contact with the ground. **Stride length** is the distance covered from, for example, one heel-strike to the following heel-strike, by the same foot. Thus, right stride length is defined by the distance between one right heel-strike and the next right heel-strike (7).

Normal and abnormal gait are often described with reference to these variables. When performing clinical assessment, there is an advantage to measuring step length, rather

than stride length. This is because you won't be able to note any asymmetry in step length if you evaluate only stride length.

How fast do people normally walk? Normal young adults tend to walk about 1.46 m/sec or 3.26 miles per hour, and have a mean cadence (step rate) of 1.9 steps/second (112.5 steps/min) and a mean step length of 76.3 cm (30.05 inches) (8).

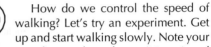

ACTIVE LEARNING MODULE

How do we control the speed of walking? Let's try an experiment. Get up and start walking slowly. Note your cadence (count the number of steps/10 sec) and estimate your step length. Now, walk as fast as you can. What happens to your step length and number of steps/10 sec? As you probably found, walking velocity is a function of step length and step frequency or cadence.

When people increase walking speed, they typically lengthen their step and increase their pace. Thus, there is a linear relationship between step length and step frequency over a wide range of walking speeds (9, 10). However, once an upper limit to step length is reached, continued elevation in speed comes from step rate.

Although normal adults have a wide range of walking speeds, self-selected speeds tend to center around a small range of step rates, with averages of about 110 steps/min for men and about 115 steps/min for women (11, 12). Preferred step rates appear to be related to minimizing energy requirements (13, 14). In fact, it has been found that in locomotion we exploit the pendular properties of the leg and elastic properties of the muscles. Thus, in swing phase there is little energy expenditure. A person's *comfortable* or preferred walking speed is at his/her point of minimal energy expenditure. At slower or higher speeds, pendular models of gait break down, and much more energy expenditure is required (15).

As we increase walking speed, the proportion of time spent in swing and stance changes, with stance phase becoming progressively shorter in relation to swing (16, 17). Finally, the stance/swing proportions shift from the 60/40 distribution of walking to the 40/60 distribution as running velocities are reached. Double support time also disappears during running.

As walking speed slows stance time increases, while swing times remain relatively constant. The double support phase of stance increases most. For example, double support takes up 25% of the cycle time, with step durations of about 1.1 sec, and 50% of the cycle time when cycle duration increases to about 2.5 sec (16). In addition, variability increases at lower speeds, probably due to decreased postural stability during the single support period, which also lengthens with slower speeds.

Within an individual, joint angle patterns and EMG patterns of lower extremity muscles are quite stable across a range of speeds, but the amplitude of muscle responses increases with faster speeds (12, 18, 19). In contrast, joint torque patterns appear more variable, though they also show gain increases as walking velocity increases.

Kinematic Description of Gait

Another way of describing normal vs. abnormal gait is through the kinematics of the gait cycle, that is, the movement of the joints and segments of the body through space. Figure 11.2 shows the normal movements of the pelvis, hip, knee, and ankle in the sagittal, frontal, and transverse planes (7).

The elegant coordination of motion at all the joints ensures the first requirement of gait: the smooth forward progression of the center of body mass. While motion at each individual joint is quite large, the coordinated action of motion across all the joints results in the smooth forward progression of the body, with only minimal vertical displacement of the center of mass (COM) (10, 20, 21).

Next we consider how motion at each of the joints contributes to minimizing vertical motions of the COM. If we look at sagittal plane *hip motion* during gait, we see a large amount of flexion and extension (Fig. 11.2). If gait were accomplished solely through these hip movements, the COM would follow

these large motions of the hip, and you would see large vertical displacements of the COM. This has been called a *compass gait*, and is seen in people who walk with a stiff knee (22).

The addition of *pelvic rotation* about the vertical axis to motion at the hip changes the gait pattern. Stride length increases, and the amplitude of the sinusoidal oscillations of the COM decreases. As a result, the path of the COM becomes smoother and the transition from step to step a little less abrupt.

With the addition of *pelvic tilt* (rotation of the pelvis about an anterior-posterior axis), the path of the COM flattens even further. Pelvic tilt occurs during swing, when the swing hip lowers in preparation for toe-off (22).

In normal gait, there is a lateral shift in the pelvis that occurs as stance is alternately changed from one limb to another. The width of the step contributes to the magnitude of the lateral shift of the COM.

The addition of *knee flexion* significantly improves the coordinated efficiency of gait. During the swing phase of gait, knee flexion shortens the vertical length of the swing limb and allows the foot to clear the ground. Knee flexion during stance further flattens the vertical movements of the COM.

Ankle motion also makes an important contribution to smooth gait (Fig. 11.2). In particular, plantar flexion of the stance ankle allows a smooth transition from step to step and contributes to the initial velocity of the swing limb (22).

Motion at the three major articulations within the foot is also important in the control of progression and stability during gait. The subtalar joint, the junction between the talus and calcaneus, allows the foot to tilt medially (inversion) and laterally (eversion). Eversion of the foot begins as part of the loading response, immediately after heel-strike, and reaches its peak by early mid-stance. Following this, the motion slowly reverses, reaching the peak of inversion at the onset of preswing. During swing, the foot drifts back to neutral and then into inversion just before heel-strike. Subtalar motion is an essential component of shock absorption during limb loading. In addition, rigidity in this area con-

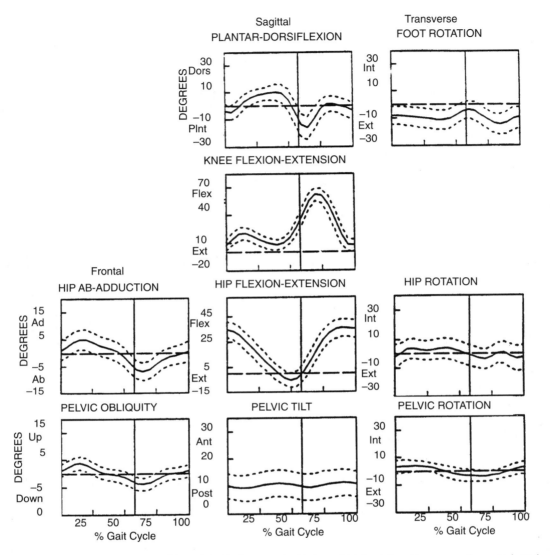

Figure 11.2. Normal movements of the pelvis, hip, knee, and ankle in sagittal, frontal, and transverse planes. (Adapted from DeLuca PA, Perry JP, Ounpuu S. The fundamentals of normal walking and pathological gait. AACP & DM Inst. Course #2. 1992.

tributes to foot stability, as weight is transferred to the forefoot in terminal stance (22).

The mid-tarsal joint is the junction of the hind and forefoot. During loading, the arch flattens quickly, allowing forefoot contact, and thus contributes to shock absorption. Finally, motion at the metatarsophalangeal joints allows the foot to roll over the metatarsal heads rather than the tips of the toes during terminal stance (22).

Thus, you can see that the step cycle is made up of a complex series of joint rotations

which, when coordinated into a whole, provide for a smooth forward progression of the COM, with only minimal vertical displacement. This control strategy reduces the energy cost of walking (20, 23).

Muscle Activation Patterns

Next, we examine the muscle responses during locomotion in terms of their function at each point in the step cycle (7, 24). Despite the variability between subjects and condi-

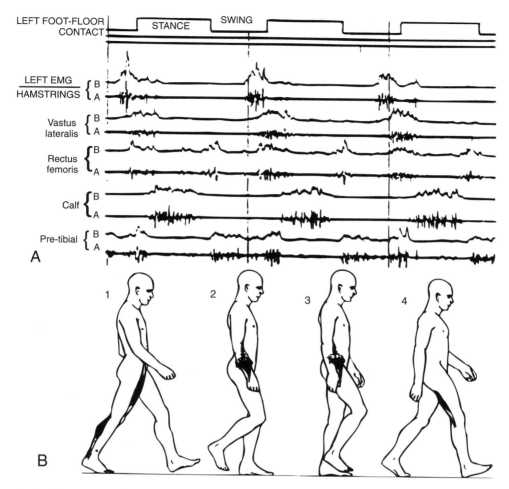

Figure 11.3. Electromyographic patterns associated with the adult step cycle. (*A* Adapted from Murray MP, Mollinger LA, Gardner GM, Sepic SB. Kinematic and EMG patterns during slow, free, and fast walking. J Orthop Res 1984;2:272–280. *B* Adapted from Lovejoy Co. Evolution of human walking. Scientific American 1988; 5.121.)

tions in the electromyographic (EMG) patterns that underlie a typical step cycle, certain basic characteristics have been identified.

In general, muscles in the stance limb act to support the body (stability) and propel it forward (progression). Muscle activity in the swing limb is largely confined to the beginning and end of the swing phase, since the leg swings much like a jointed pendulum under the influence of gravity (21). Typical EMG patterns during the different phases of the step cycle are shown in Figure 11.3.

Remember, there are two goals to be accomplished during the stance phase: (*a*) securing the stance limb against the impact force of foot-strike and supporting the body

against the force of gravity (stability), and (*b*) subsequent force generation, to propel the body forward into the next step (progression).

To accomplish the first goal, that is, force absorption for stability, knee flexion occurs at the initiation of stance, and there is a distribution of the foot-strike impact from heel contact to the foot-flat stance. At the initiation of stance, activity in the knee extensors (quadriceps) controls the small knee flexion wave that is used to absorb the impact of foot-strike. Activity in the ankle dorsiflexors (anterior tibialis) decelerates the foot upon touchdown, opposing and slowing the plantar flexion that results from heel-strike. Both muscle groups initially act to oppose the direction of motion. In addition, stability during the stance phase involves activating extensor muscles at the hip, knee, and ankle, which keeps the body from collapsing into gravity. Activation of the hip extensor muscles controls forward motion of the head, arm, and trunk segments as well. By mid-stance, the quadriceps is predominantly inactive, as are the pre-tibial muscles.

The second goal in the stance phase is generating a propulsive force to keep the body in motion. The most common strategy used to generate propulsive forces for progression involves the concentric contraction of the plantarflexors (gastrocnemius and soleus) at the end of stance phase of gait. The ability of the body to move freely over the foot, in conjunction with the concentric contraction of the gastrocnemius, means the COM of the body will be anterior to the supporting foot by the end of stance, creating a forward fall critical to progression. The hip and knee extensors (hamstrings and quadriceps, respectively) may exhibit a burst of activity late in stance as a contribution to propulsion. This activity, however, typically is less important than the activity observed during the force absorption phase.

The primary goal to be accomplished in the swing phase of gait is to reposition the limb for continued forward progression. This requires both accelerating the limb forward and making sure the toe clears the ground.

Forward acceleration of the thigh in the early swing phase is associated with a concentric contraction of the quadriceps. (Fig. 11.3B, part 1). By mid-swing, however, the quadriceps is virtually inactive as the leg swings through, much like a pendulum driven by an impulse force at the beginning of swing phase. However, the iliopsoas contracts to aid in this forward motion, as shown in Fig. 11.3B, parts 2 and 3. The hamstrings become active at the end of swing to slow the forward rotation of the thigh, in preparation for footstrike. (Fig. 11.4B, part 4). Knee extension at the end of swing in preparation for loading the limb for stance phase occurs, not as the result of muscle activity, but as the result of passive nonmuscular forces (25).

Foot clearance is accomplished through flexion at the hip, knee, and ankle, which results in an overall shortening of the swing limb compared to the stance limb. Again, flexion of the hip is accomplished through activation of the quadriceps muscle. Flexion at the knee is accomplished passively, since rapid acceleration of the thigh will also produce flexion at the knee. Activation of the pre-tibial muscles produces ankle dorsiflexion late in swing to ensure toe clearance and in preparation for the next foot-fall.

Joint Kinetics

Thus far, we have examined the kinematics or movements of the body during the step cycle, and looked at the patterns of muscle activity in each of the phases of gait. What are the typical forces that these movements and muscle responses create during locomotion? The dominant forces at a joint don't necessarily mirror the movements of the joint, as you will see in the discussion that follows.

Determination of the forces generated during the step cycle is considered a kinetic analysis. The kinetic or force parameters associated with the normal gait pattern are less stereotyped than the kinematic or movement parameters. The active and passive muscle forces (called joint moments) that generate locomotion are themselves quite variable.

STANCE PHASE

Remember, the goals during stance phase include stabilizing the limb for weight acceptance and generating propulsive forces for continued motion. During the stance phase of the step cycle, the algebraic sum of the joint moments at the hip, knee, and ankle, called the **support moment** (26), is an extensor torque (Fig. 11.4). This net extensor torque keeps the limb from collapsing while bearing weight, allowing stabilization of the body and thus accomplishing the stability requirements of locomotion.

However, researchers have shown that people use a wide variety of force-generating strategies to accomplish this net extensor

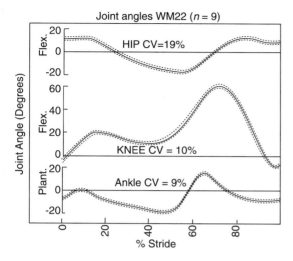

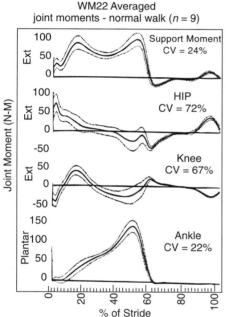

Figure 11.4. Joint torque patterns in the hip, knee, and ankle, and the net support moment associated with the adult step cycle. (Adapted from Winter DA. Kinematic and kinetic patterns of human gait: variability and compensating effects. Human Movement Science 1984; 3:51–76).

torque. For example, one strategy for achieving a net extensor moment involves combining a dominant hip extensor moment, to counter a knee flexor moment. Alternatively, a knee and ankle extensor torque can be combined to counterbalance a hip flexor torque

and still maintain the net extensor support moment (25–27).

Why is it important to have this flexibility in the individual contributions of joint torques to the net extensor moment? Apparently, this flexibility in how torques are generated is important to controlling balance during gait.

David Winter, a well-known Canadian biomechanist, and his colleagues have researched gait extensively and suggest that balance during unperturbed gait is very different from the task of balance during stance (29). In walking, the center of gravity does not stay within the support base of the feet and thus the body is in a continuous state of imbalance. The only way to prevent falling is to place the swinging foot ahead of and lateral to the center of gravity as it moves forward.

In addition, the mass of the head, arms, and trunk, called the HAT segment, must be regulated with respect to the hips, since the HAT segment represents a large inertial load to keep upright. Winter and colleagues propose that the dynamic balance of the HAT is the responsibility of the hip muscles, with almost no involvement of the ankle muscles. They suggest that this is because the hip has a much smaller inertial load to control, that of the HAT segment, as compared to the ankles, which would have to control the entire body. Thus, they propose that balance during ongoing gait is different from stance balance control, which relies primarily on ankle muscles (29).

They note that the hip muscles are also involved in a separate task, that of contributing to the extensor support moment necessary during stance, and view the muscles controlling the HAT segment and those controlling the extensor support moment as two separate synergies. We mentioned earlier that the net extensor moment of the ankle, knee, and hip joints during stance was always the same, but the individual moments were highly variable from stride to stride and individual to individual. One reason for this variability is to allow the balance control system to continuously alter the anterior/posterior motor patterns on a step-to-step basis. However, the hip balance adjustments must be compensated for by appropriate knee torques in order to preserve the net extensor moment essential for stance (28, 29).

SWING PHASE

The major goal during swing is to reposition the limb, making sure the toe clears the ground. Researchers have found that the joint moment patterns during the swing phase are less variable than during stance phase, indicating that adults use fairly similar force-generating patterns to accomplish this task. This is illustrated by the large standard deviations around the mean joint torques during stance (0 to 60% of stride) as compared to the small standard deviations in swing (60 to 100% of stride), shown in Figure 11.4.

For example, at normal walking speeds, early in swing, there is a flexor moment at the hip that contributes to flexion of the thigh. Early hip flexion is assisted by gravity, reducing the need for a large flexor hip joint moment.

Once swing phase has been initiated, it is often sustained by momentum. Then, as swing phase ends, an extensor joint torque may be required to slow the thigh rotation and prepare for heelstrike (30). Thus, even though the thigh is still flexing, there is an extensor torque on the thigh at this point.

What controls knee motions during swing? Interestingly, during swing, joint torque at the knee is basically used to constrain knee motion rather than generate motion. In early swing, an extensor torque slows knee joint flexion and contributes to reversal of the knee joint from flexion to extension. Later in swing, a flexor knee joint torque slows knee extension to prepare for foot placement (19, 26, 30, 31).

At the end of swing phase and during the initial part of stance phase, a small dorsi-flexing ankle torque occurs at the ankle, which helps control plantarflexion at heelstrike. So even though the ankle motion is one of plantarflexion, the ankle joint force is a dorsiflexion torque.

Moving through the stance phase, ankle plantarflexion torque increases to a maximum point just after knee flexion when the ankle begins to plantarflex. The ankle joint torque is the largest of all the torques of the lower limb and is the main contributor to the acceleration of the limb into swing phase.

So, in many of the previous examples, we see that the joint torque is opposite to that of the limb movement itself. In other words, the joint torque shows us that the combined forces may be acting to brake the movement or control foot fall, rather than simply accelerate the limb.

CONTROL MECHANISMS FOR GAIT

How is locomotor coordination achieved? What are the control mechanisms that ensure that the task requirements are met for successful locomotion? Much of the research examining the neural and non-neural control mechanisms essential for locomotion has been done with animals. It is through this research on locomotion in animals that scientists have learned about pattern formation in locomotion, the integration of postural control to the locomotor pattern, the contribution of peripheral and central mechanisms to adaptation and modulation of gait, and the role of the various senses in controlling locomotion.

The following section reviews some of the research on locomotor control in animals, relating it to experiments examining the neural control of locomotion in humans.

Pattern Generators for Gait

Research in the last 25 years has greatly increased our understanding of the nervous system control of the basic rhythmic movements underlying locomotion. Results of these studies have indicated that central pattern generators within the spinal cord play an important role in the production of these movements (32, 33). A rich history of research has enhanced our understanding of the neural basis of locomotion.

In the late 1800s, Sherrington and Mott (34, 35) performed some of the first experiments to determine the neural control of locomotion. They severed the spinal cord of animals to eliminate the influence of higher brain centers and found that the hindlimbs continued to exhibit alternating movements.

In a second set of experiments, in monkeys, they cut the sensory nerve roots on one side of the spinal cord, eliminating sensory inputs to stepping on one side of the body. They found that the monkeys didn't use the deafferented limbs during walking. This led to the conclusion that locomotion required sensory input. A model of locomotor control was created, which attributed the control of locomotion to a set of reflex chains, with the output from one phase of the step cycle acting as a sensory stimulus to reflexly activate the next phase.

Graham Brown performed an experiment only a few years later (36) showing the opposite result. He found that by making bilateral dorsal (sensory) root lesions in spinalized animals, he could see rhythmic walking movements. Why did the two labs get different results? It appears that it is because Sherrington cut only sensory roots on one side of the spinal cord, not both.

In more recent experiments, Taub and Berman (37) found that animals did not use a limb when the dorsal roots were cut on one side of the body, but would begin to use the limb again when dorsal roots on the remaining side were sectioned. Why? Since the animal has appropriate input coming in from one limb, and no sensation from the other, the animal prefers not to use it. Interestingly, researchers have found that they can make animals use a single deafferented limb by restraining the intact limb. These results are the rationale behind a therapy approach called the **forced-use paradigm**. In this approach, hemiplegic patients are forced to use their hemiplegic arm, since the intact side is restrained (38, 39).

Recent studies have confirmed the results of Graham Brown. These studies have found that muscle activity in spinalized cats is similar to that seen in normal cats walking on a treadmill (40), with the extensor muscles of the knee and ankle activated prior to paw contact in stance phase. This demonstrates that extension is not simply a reflex in response to

contact, but is part of a central program. In addition, the spinal cat is capable of fully recruiting motor units within the spinal cord when increasing gait from a walk to a gallop (41).

Can a spinalized cat adapt the step cycle to clear obstacles? Yes. If a glass rod touches the top of the cat's paw during swing phase, it activates a flexion response in the stimulated leg, with simultaneous extension of the contralateral leg. This lifts the swing leg up and over the obstacle and gives postural support in the opposite leg. Interestingly, the exact same stimulation of the dorsal surface of the paw during stance causes increased extension, probably to get the paw quickly out of the way of the obstacle. Thus, the identical stimulus to the skin activates functionally separate sets of muscles during different phases of the step cycle, to appropriately compensate for different obstacles perturbing the movement of the paw (40). Although the spinal pattern generators are able to produce stereotyped locomotor patterns and perform certain adaptive functions, descending pathways from higher centers and sensory feedback from the periphery allow the rich variation in locomotor patterns and adaptability to task and environmental conditions.

Descending Influences

Descending influences from higher brain centers are also important in the control of locomotor activity. Much research has focused on identifying the roles of higher centers in controlling locomotion, through transecting the brain of animals along the neuraxis and observing the subsequent locomotor behavior (1). The three preparations that are most often studied are the spinal, the decerebrate, and the decorticate preparations (Fig. 11.5).

In the **spinal preparation** (which can be made at a level to allow the observation of only the hind limbs or of all 4 limbs as part of the preparation), one needs an external stimulus to produce locomotor behavior. This can be either electrical or pharmacological.

The **decerebrate** preparation leaves the spinal cord, brainstem, and cerebellum intact.

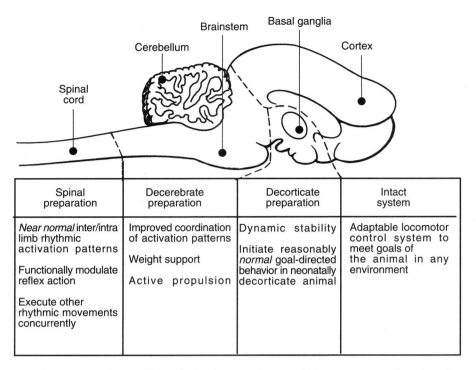

Spinal preparation	Decerebrate preparation	Decorticate preparation	Intact system
Near normal inter/intra limb rhythmic activation patterns Functionally modulate reflex action Execute other rhythmic movements concurrently	Improved coordination of activation patterns Weight support Active propulsion	Dynamic stability Initiate reasonably *normal* goal-directed behavior in neonatally decorticate animal	Adaptable locomotor control system to meet goals of the animal in any environment

Figure 11.5. The different gait capabilities of animal preparations with lesions at various points along the neuraxis. (Adapted from Patla AE. Understanding the control of human locomotion: a prologue. In: Patla AE, ed. Adaptability of human gait. Amsterdam: North-Holland, 1991:7.)

An area in the brainstem called the *mesencephalic locomotor region* appears to be important in the descending control of locomotion. Decerebrate cats will not normally walk on a treadmill, but will begin to walk normally when tonic electrical stimulation is applied to the mesencephalic locomotor region (42). Weight support and active propulsion are locomotor characteristics seen in this preparation.

When spinal pattern generating circuits are stimulated by tonic activation, they produce, at best, a bad caricature of walking due to the lack of important modulating influences from the brainstem and cerebellum. This is because normally, within each step cycle, the cerebellum sends modulating signals to the brainstem that are relayed to the spinal cord via the vestibulospinal, rubrospinal, and reticulospinal pathways, which act directly on motor neurons, to fine-tune the movements according to the needs of the task (43).

The cerebellum also may have a very important role in modulation of the step cycle.

Experiments suggest that two tracts are involved in this modulation. First, the dorsal spinocerebellar tract is hypothesized to send information from muscle afferents to the cerebellum, and is phasically active during locomotion. Second, the ventral spinocerebellar tract is hypothesized to receive information from spinal neurons concerning the central pattern generator output, and to send this information also to the cerebellum (44, 45).

It is also possible that the cerebellum has an additional role in the modulation of the step cycle. It has been hypothesized that the cerebellum may also modulate activity, not to correct error but to alter stepping patterns (46). For example, as an animal crosses uneven terrain, the legs must be lifted higher or lower depending on visual cues about the obstacles encountered. The muscle response patterns may be modulated through the following steps. First, the locomotor rhythm is conveyed to the cerebellum. The cerebellum extrapolates forward in time to specify when the next flexion (or extension) is to occur.

The cerebellum would then facilitate descending commands that originate from visual inputs to alter the flexion (or extension) phase at precisely the correct time (46).

The **decorticate** preparation also leaves the basal ganglia intact, with only the cerebral cortex removed. In this preparation, an external stimulus is not required to produce locomotor behavior, and the behavior is reasonably normal goal directed behavior. However, the cortex is important in skills such as walking over uneven terrain.

Sensory Feedback and Adaptation of Gait

One of the requirements of normal locomotion is the ability to adapt gait to a wide ranging set of environments. Sensory information from all the senses is critical to our ability to modify how we walk. In animals, when all sensory information is taken away, stepping patterns tend to be very slow and stereotyped. The animal can neither maintain balance nor modify its stepping patterns to make gait truly functional. Gait ataxia is a common consequence among patients with sensory loss, particularly loss of proprioceptive information from the lower extremities (47).

There are two ways that equilibrium is controlled during locomotion—reactively and proactively. One uses the reactive mode, when, for example, there is an unexpected disturbance, such as a slip or a trip. One uses the proactive mode to anticipate potential disruptions to gait and modify the way to sense and move in order to minimize the disruption. Like postural control, the somatosensory, visual, and vestibular systems all play a role in reactive and proactive control of locomotion. The next section describes how sensory information is used to modify ongoing gait.

REACTIVE STRATEGIES FOR MODIFYING GAIT

All three sensory systems, somatosensory, visual, and vestibular systems, contribute to reactive or feedback control of gait. Research on animals and humans has contrib-

uted to our understanding of the somatosensory contributions to gait.

Somatosensory Systems

Researchers have shown that animals that have been both spinalized and deafferented can continuously generate rhythmic alternating contractions in muscles of all the joints of the leg, with a pattern similar to that seen in the normal step cycle (43). Does this mean that sensory information plays no role in the control of locomotion? No. Though these experiments have shown that animals can still walk in the absence of sensory feedback from the limbs, the movements show characteristic differences from those in the normal animal. These differences help us understand the role that sensory input plays in the control of locomotion (33).

First, sensory information from the limbs contributes to appropriate stepping frequency. For example, the duration of the step cycle is significantly longer in deafferented cats than in a chronic spinal cat without deafferentation (33).

Second, joint receptors appear to play a critical role in normal locomotion, with the position of the ipsilateral hip joint contributing to the onset of swing phase (33, 48).

Third, cutaneous information from the paw of the chronic spinal cat has a powerful influence on the spinal pattern generator in helping the animal navigate over obstacles, as mentioned earlier (40).

Fourth, the Golgi tendon organ (GTO) afferents (the Ib afferents) from the leg extensor muscles also can strongly influence the timing of the locomotor rhythm, by inhibiting flexor burst activity and promoting extensor activity. A decline in their activity at the end of the stance phase may be involved in regulating the stance to swing transition. Note that this activity of the GTOs is exactly the opposite of their activity when they are activated passively, when the animal is at rest. At rest, the GTOs inhibit their own muscle, and excite the antagonist muscles, while during locomotion they excite their own muscle and inhibit antagonists (49).

Human research, similar to animal research, has shown that reflexes are highly modulated in locomotion during each phase of the step cycle, in order to adapt them functionally to the requirements of each phase (50). Stretch reflexes in the ankle extensor muscles are small in the early part of the stance phase of locomotion, since this is the time that the body is rotating over the foot and stretching the ankle extensors. A large reflex at this phase of the step cycle would slow or even reverse forward momentum (50).

On the other hand, the stretch reflex is large when the center of mass is in front of the foot during the last part of stance phase, since this is the time when the reflex can help in propelling the body forward (50). This phase-appropriate modulation of the stretch reflex is well suited to the requirements of the task of locomotion as compared to stance. Stretch reflex gains are further reduced in running, probably because a high gain reflex response would destabilize the gait in running. Stretch reflex gain changes alter quickly (within 150 msec) as a person moves from stance to walking to running (50).

As was shown in research on cats, cutaneous reflexes actually showed a complete reversal from excitation to inhibition during the different phases of the step cycle. For example, in the first part of swing phase, when the TA is active, the foot is in the air and little cutaneous input would be expected, unless the foot strikes an object. If this happens, a rapid flexion would be needed to lift the foot over the object to prevent tripping. This is when the reflex is excitatory to the TA. However, in the second TA burst, the foot is about to contact the ground, which is a time when a lot of cutaneous input would occur. Limb flexion wouldn't be appropriate at this time, since the limb is needed to support the body. In addition, at this time, the reflex shows inhibition of the TA (50).

These studies have shown that spinal reflexes can be appropriately integrated into different phases of the step cycle to remain functionally adaptive. The same outcome occurs in the integration of compensatory automatic postural adjustments into the step cycle. Studies were performed in which subjects walked across a platform that could be perturbed at different points in the step cycle. Results showed that automatic postural responses were incorporated appropriately into the different step cycle phases (51). For example, postural muscle responses were activated at 100 msec latencies in gastrocnemius when this muscle was stretched faster than normal in response to backward surface displacements pitching the body forward. This helped slow the body's rate of forward progression to realign the center of mass with the backward displaced support foot. Similarly, responses occurred in tibialis anterior when this muscle was shortened more slowly than normal, due to forward surface displacements that displace the body backwards. This helped increase the rate of forward progress to realign the body with the forward displaced foot (51).

VISION

Work with humans suggests that there are a variety of ways in which vision modulates locomotion in a feedback manner. First, visual flow cues help us determine our speed of locomotion (52). Studies have shown that if one doubles the rate of optic flow past persons as they walk, 100% will experience that their stride length has increased. In addition, about half of the subjects will perceive that the force exerted during each step is less than normal. However, other subjects will perceive that they have nearly doubled their stepping frequency (53).

Visual flow cues also influence the alignment of the body with reference to gravity and the environment during walking (54). For example, when researchers tilted the room surrounding a treadmill on which a person was running, it caused the person to incline the trunk in the direction of the tilted room to compensate for the visual illusion of body tilt in the opposite direction (54).

VESTIBULAR SYSTEM

An important part of controlling locomotion is stabilizing the head, since it contains two of the most important sensors for controlling motion: the vestibular and visual systems (55). The otolith organs, the saccule and the utricle, detect the angle of the head with respect to gravity, and the visual system also provides us with the so-called *visual vertical*.

Adults appear to stabilize the head, and thus gaze, by covarying both pitch (forward) rotation and vertical displacement of the head to give stability to the head in the sagittal plane (56, 57). The head is stabilized with a precision (within a few degrees) that is compatible with the efficiency of the vestibulo-ocular reflex, an important mechanism for stabilizing gaze during head movement.

It has been hypothesized that during complex movements, like walking, postural control is not organized from the support surface upward, in what is called a bottom-up mode, but is organized in relation to the control of gaze, in what is called a top-down mode (55). Thus, in this mode, head movements are independent from the movements of the trunk. It has been shown that the process for stabilizing the head is disrupted in patients with bilateral labyrinthine lesions (55).

PROACTIVE STRATEGIES

Proactive strategies for adapting gait focus on the use of sensory inputs to modify gait patterns. Proactive strategies are used to modify and adapt gait in two different ways. First, vision is used proactively to identify potential obstacles in the environment and to navigate around them. Second, prediction is used to estimate the potential destabilizing effects of simultaneously performing tasks like carrying an object while walking, and anticipatory modifications to the step cycle are made accordingly (58).

Proactive visual control of locomotion has been classified into both avoidance and accommodation strategies (58). Avoidance strategies include (*a*) changing the placement of the foot, (*b*) increasing ground clearance to avoid an obstacle, (*c*) changing the direction of gait, when it is perceived that objects can't be cleared, and (*d*) stopping. Accommodation strategies involve longer term modifications, such as reducing step length when walking on an icy surface, or shifting the propulsive power from ankle to hip and knee muscles when climbing stairs (58).

Most avoidance strategies can be successfully carried out within a step cycle. An exception occurs when changing directions, and this requires planning one step cycle in advance. It has been suggested that there are various rules associated with changing the placement of the foot. For example, when possible, step length is increased, rather than shortened, and the foot is placed inside rather than outside of an obstacle, as long as the foot doesn't need to cross the midline of the body (58). Adapting strategies for foot placement does not involve simply changing the amplitude of the normal locomotor patterns, but is complex and task specific.

Non-Neural Contributions to Locomotion

So far, we have looked at neural contributions to the control of locomotion, but there are also important musculoskeletal and environmental contributions. Biomechanical analyses of locomotion in the cat have determined the contributions of both muscular and nonmuscular forces to the generation of gait dynamics (59–63). This involves a type of kinetic analysis called inverse dynamics. To understand more about inverse dynamics, refer to the technology box on the next page.

As we have talked about in earlier chapters, nonmuscular forces, such as gravity, play a role in the construction of all movement. When an inverse dynamics analysis of limb dynamics is used, it is possible to determine the relative importance of the muscular and nonmuscular contributions. For example, during locomotion, each segment of the cat hindlimb is subjected to a complex set of muscular and nonmuscular forces. Changes in speed lead to changes in the interactive patterns among the torque components (59, 63). Very often in cat locomotion, there are high passive extensor torques at a joint, which must be counteracted by active flexor torques generated by the muscles, when the animal is moving at one speed, or in one part of the step cycle. When

---

TECHNOLOGY BOX 1
Kinetic Analysis-Inverse Dynamics

INVERSE DYNAMICS is a process that allows researchers to calculate the joint moments of force (torque) responsible for movement—in this case, locomotion. Researchers begin by developing a reliable model of the body using anthropometric measures such as segment masses, center of mass, joint centers, and moments of inertia. Because these variables are difficult to measure directly, they are usually obtained from statistical tables based on the person's height, weight, and sex (28).

Using extremely accurate kinematic information on the limb trajectory during the step cycle, in combination with a reliable model, researchers can calculate the torque acting on each segment of the body. They can then partition the net torque into components due to gravity, the mechanical interaction among segments (motion-dependent torques), and a generalized muscle torque. This type of analysis allows researchers to assess the roles of muscular and nonmuscular forces in the generation of the movement (27).

---

the speed is increased, or the animal moves to a different part of the cycle, the passive torques that must be counteracted completely change. How does the dialogue between the passive properties of the system and the neural pattern generating circuits occur? This is still unclear, although the discharge from somatosensory receptors plays a role (61–63). What is revealed in the dynamic analysis of limb movements is the intricacies of the interaction among active and passive forces.

The results from these studies suggest that in normal locomotion there is a continuous interaction between the central pattern generators and descending signals. Higher centers contribute to locomotion through feedforward modulation of patterns in response to the goals of the individual and to environmental demands. As noted briefly above, sensory inputs are also critical for feedback and feedforward modulation of locomotor activity in order to adapt it to changing environmental conditions.

INITIATING GAIT AND CHANGING SPEEDS

How do we initiate walking? Before we describe the initiation of gait, let's do an experiment.

ACTIVE LEARNING MODULE

Get up and stand next to a wall, with your shoulder touching the wall. First try to start walking with the foot that is next to the wall. No problem? What muscles did you notice contracting and relaxing? Which way did you notice your body move in the process of preparing to take a step? Now, try to start walking, beginning with the foot that is away from the wall. What happened? Did you notice that you had more problems, because you couldn't easily shift your weight (64)?

Research studies confirm what you no doubt noticed from your own experiment: the initiation of gait from quiet stance begins with the relaxation of specific postural muscles, the gastrocnemius and the soleus (65, 66). In fact, the initiation of gait has the appearance of a simple forward fall and regaining of one's balance by taking a step. This reduction in the activation of the gastrocnemius and soleus is followed by activation of the tibialis anterior, which assists dorsiflexion and moves the COM forward in preparation for toe-off. But, as you noticed, and as recent research on gait confirms, the initiation of gait is more than a simple fall.

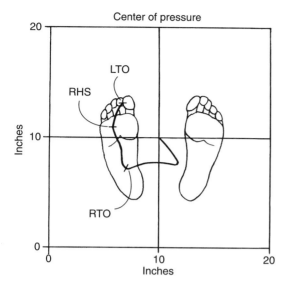

Figure 11.6. Trajectory of the center of pressure during the initiation of gait from a balanced, symmetric stance. Prior to movement, the center of pressure is located midway between the feet. (Adapted from Mann RA, Hagy JL, White V, Liddell D. The initiation of gait. J Bone Joint Surg 1979;61-A:232–239.)

In tracing the center of pressure during the initiation of gait in normal adults, the following sequence of events is evident. Prior to movement onset, the center of pressure is positioned just posterior to the ankle and midway between both feet (Fig. 11.6). As the person begins to move, the center of pressure first moves posteriorly and laterally toward the *swing* limb and then shifts toward the stance limb and forward (67).

Movement of the center of pressure toward the stance limb occurs simultaneously with hip and knee flexion and ankle dorsiflexion as the swing limb prepares for toe-off. Then the center of pressure moves quickly toward the stance limb. Toe-off of the swing limb occurs with the center of pressure shifting from lateral to forward movement over the stance foot. Why do we first shift the center of pressure toward the swing limb when we initiate gait? It has been hypothesized that this is a strategy for setting the center of mass in motion, which would allow the momentum of the center of mass to help create the loss of balance leading to the first step (67).

What neural patterns are correlated with these shifts in center of pressure? As the center of pressure moves posteriorly and toward the swing limb, both limbs are stabilized against backward sway by activation of anterior leg and thigh muscles, the tibialis anterior (TA) and the quadriceps. Subsequent activation of the TA then causes dorsiflexion in the stance ankle, pulling the lower leg over the foot, as the body moves forward in preparation for toe-off. Anterior thigh muscles are activated to keep the knee from flexing so that the leg rotates forward as a unit. Activation of hip abductors counters lateral tilt of the pelvis toward the swing limb side as this limb is unloaded. Also, activation of the peroneals stabilizes the stance ankle. After toe-off, the gastrocnemius and hamstrings muscles in the stance leg are used for propelling the body forward (66, 67). How long after initiation does it take to reach a steady velocity in gait? Steady state is reached within one (68) to three steps (67, 69) depending on the magnitude of the velocity one is trying to achieve.

STAIR-WALKING

Understanding the sensory and motor requirements associated with stair-walking is critical to retraining this skill. Stairs represent a significant hazard even among the nondisabled population. Stair-walking accounts for the largest percentage of falls occurring in public places, with four out of five falls occurring during stair descent (70).

Stair-walking is similar to level-walking in that it involves stereotypical reciprocal alternating movements of the lower limbs (71). Like locomotion, successful negotiation of stairs has three requirements: the generation of primarily concentric forces to propel the body up stairs, or eccentric forces to control the body's descent down stairs (progression), while controlling the center of mass within a constantly changing base of support (stability); and the capacity to adapt strategies used for progression and stability to accommodate changes in stair environment, such as height, width, and the presence or absence of railings (adaptation) (72).

Sensory information is important for controlling the body's position in space (stability), and to identify critical aspects of the stair environment so that appropriate movement strategies can be programmed (adaptation). Researchers have shown that normal subjects change movement strategies used for negotiating stairs when sensory cues about stair characteristics are altered (70, 71).

Similar to gait, stair climbing has been divided into two phases, a stance phase lasting approximately 64% of the full cycle, and a swing phase lasting 36% of the cycle. In addition, each phase of stair-walking has been further subdivided to reflect the objectives that need to be achieved during each phase.

Ascent

During ascent, the stance phase is subdivided into weight acceptance, pull-up, and forward continuance, while swing is divided into foot clearance and foot placement stages.

During stance, weight acceptance is initiated with the middle to front portion of the foot. Pull-up occurs because of extensor activity at the knee and ankle, primarily concentric contractions of the vastus lateralis and soleus muscles. Stair ascent differs from level walking in two ways: (*a*) forces needed to accomplish ascent are two times greater than those needed to control level gait, and (*b*) the knee extensors generate most of the energy to move the body forward during stair ascent (72). Finally, during the forward continuance phase of stance, the ankle generates forward and lift forces; however, ankle force is not the main source of power behind forward progression in stair-walking.

In controlling balance during stair ascent, the greatest instability comes with contralateral toe-off, when the ipsilateral leg takes the total body weight, and the hip, knee, and ankle joints are flexed (72).

The objectives of the swing phase of stair climbing are similar to level gait, and include foot clearance and placing the foot appropriately so weight can be accepted for the next stance phase. Foot clearance is achieved through activation of the tibialis anterior,

dorsiflexing the foot, and activation of the hamstrings, which flex the knee. The rectus femoris contracts eccentrically to reverse this motion by mid-swing. The swing leg is brought up and forward through activation of the hip flexors of the swing leg, and motion of the contralateral stance leg. Final foot placement is controlled by the hip extensors and ankle foot dorsiflexors (72).

Descent

Walking upstairs is accomplished through concentric contractions of the rectus femoris, vastus lateralis, soleus, and medial gastrocnemius. In contrast, walking down stairs is achieved through eccentric contractions of these same muscles, which work to control the body with respect to the force of gravity. The stance phase of stair descent is subdivided into weight acceptance, forward continuance, and controlled lowering, while swing has two phases: leg pull-through and preparation for foot placement (71, 72).

Weight acceptance phase is characterized by absorption of energy at the ankle and knee through the eccentric contraction of the triceps surae, rectus femoris, and vastus lateralis. Energy absorption during this phase is critical, since forces as much as two times body weight have been recorded when the swing limb first contacts the stair. Activation of gastrocnemius *prior* to stair contact is responsible for cushioning the landing (71).

The forward continuance phase reflects the forward motion of the body, and precedes the controlled lowering phase of stance. Lowering of the body is controlled primarily by the eccentric contraction of the quadriceps muscles, and to a lesser degree, the eccentric contraction of the soleus muscle.

During swing, the leg is pulled through, due to activation of the hip flexor muscles. However, by mid-swing, flexion of the hip and knee is reversed, and all three joints extend in preparation for foot placement. Contact is made with the lateral border of the foot, and is associated with tibialis anterior and gastrocnemius activity prior to foot contact.

Adapting Stair-Walking Patterns to Changes in Sensory Cues

Researchers have shown that neurologically intact people adapt the movement strategies they use for going up and down stairs in response to changes in sensory information about the task. Thus, when normal subjects wear large collars obstructing their view of the stairs, anticipatory activation of the gastrocnemius prior to foot contact is reduced. This anticipatory activity is further reduced when the subject is blindfolded (71). In this study, subjects still managed a soft landing by changing the control strategy used to descend stairs. Subjects moved slower, protracting swing time, and using the stance limb to control the landing.

Foot clearance and placement are critical aspects of movement strategies used to safely descend stairs. Good visual information about stair height is critical. When normal subjects wear blurred vision lenses and are unable to clearly define the edge of the step, they slow down and modify movement strategies so that foot clearance is increased and the foot is placed further back on the step to ensure a larger margin of safety (70). Thus, information from the visual system about the step height appears to be necessary for optimal programming of movement strategies used to negotiate stairs.

MOBILITY OTHER THAN GAIT

Although mobility is often thought of solely in relationship to gait or locomotion, there are many other aspects of mobility that are essential to independence in daily life activities. The ability to change positions, whether moving from sit to stand, rolling, rising from a bed, or moving from one chair to another, is a fundamental part of mobility. These various types of mobility activities are often grouped together and referred to as transfer tasks.

Retraining motor function in the patient with a neurological impairment includes the recovery of these diverse mobility skills. This requires an understanding of: (*a*) the essential characteristics of the task, (*b*) the sensory motor strategies that normal individuals typically use to accomplish the task, and (*c*) the adaptations required for changing environmental characteristics.

All mobility tasks share in common three essential task requirements: motion in a desired direction (progression), postural control (stability), and the ability to adapt to changing task and environmental conditions (adaptation). The following sections briefly review some of the research on these other aspects of mobility function. As you will see, compared to the tremendous number of studies on normal gait, there have been relatively few studies examining these other aspects of mobility function.

Transfers

Transfers represent an important aspect of mobility function. One cannot walk if one cannot get out of a chair or rise from a bed. Inability to safely and independently change positions represents a great hindrance to the recovery of normal mobility.

Several researchers have studied transfer skills from a biomechanical perspective. As a result, we know quite a bit about typical movement strategies used by neurologically intact adults when performing these tasks. However, use of a biomechanical approach has provided us with little information about the perceptual strategies associated with these various tasks. In addition, because most often research subjects are constrained to carry out the task in a unified way, we have little insight into ways in which sensory and movement strategies are modified in response to changing task and environmental demands.

Sit-to-Stand

Sit-to-stand (STS) behaviors emerge from an interaction among characteristics of the task, the individual, and constraints imposed by the environment. While the biomechanics of STS have been described, there are many important questions that have not yet been studied by motor control researchers. For example, how do the movements involved in STS vary as a function of the speed of the task, the characteristics of the support, including height of the chair, the compliance of the seat, or the presence or absence of hand rests? In addition, do the requirements of the task vary depending on the nature of the task immediately following? That is, do we stand up differently if we are intending to walk instead of stand still? What perceptual information is essential to establishing efficient movement strategies when performing STS?

The essential characteristics of the STS task include: (*a*) generating sufficient joint torque needed to rise (progression), (2) ensuring stability by moving the center of mass from one base of support (the chair) to a base of support defined solely by the feet (stability), and (*c*) the ability to modify movement strategies used to achieve these goals depending on the environmental constraints, such as chair height, the presence of arm rests, and the softness of the chair (adaptation).

The STS task has been divided into dif-

ferent phases, either two, three or four, depending on the researcher. Each phase has its own unique movement and stability requirements. A four-phase model of STS task is shown in Figure 11.7 (73, 74). This figure also shows the kinematic and EMG data for a normal subject completing this task.

The first phase, called the weight shift, or flexion momentum stage, begins with the generation of forward momentum of the upper body through flexion of the trunk. The body is quite stable during this phase since the center of mass (COM), though moving forward, is still within the base of support of the chair seat and the feet. Muscle activity includes activation of the erector spinae, which contract eccentrically to control forward motion of the trunk (73, 74).

Phase 2 begins as the buttocks leave the seat, and involves the transfer of momentum from the upper body to the total body, allowing lift of the body (74). Phase 2 involves both horizontal and vertical motion of the body, and is considered a critical transition phase. Stability requirements are precise since it is during this phase that the COM of the

Figure 11.7. Diagram of the four phases of the sit-to-stand movement, showing the kinematic and EMG patterns associated with each phase. (Adapted from Millington PJ, Myklebust BM, Shambes GM. Biomechanical analysis of the sit-to-stand motion in elderly persons. Arch Phys Med Rehabil 1992;73:609–617.)

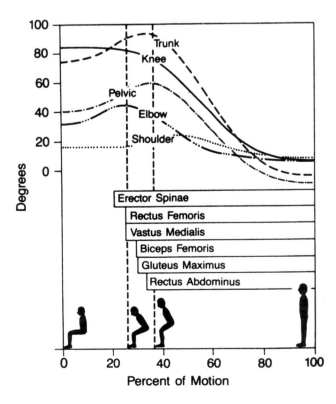

body moves from within the base of support of the chair to that of the feet. The body is inherently unstable during this phase because the COM is located far from the center of force. Because the body has developed momentum prior to lift-off, vertical rise of the body can be achieved with little lower extremity muscle force (74). Muscle activity in this phase is characterized by coactivation of hip and knee extensors, as you see in Figure 11.7.

Phase 3 of the STS task is referred to as the lift or extension phase, and is characterized by extension at the hips and knees. The goal in this phase is primarily to move the body vertically; stability requirements are less than in phase 2 since the COM is well within the base of support of the feet (74).

The final phase of STS is the stabilization phase, and is that period following complete extension, when task-dependent motion is complete and body stability in the vertical position is achieved.

STS requires the generation of propulsive impulse forces in both the horizontal and vertical directions. However, the horizontal propulsive force responsible for moving the COM anterior over the base of support of the foot must change into a braking impulse to bring the body to a stop. Braking the horizontal impulse begins even before lift-off from the seat. Thus, there appears to be a preprogrammed relationship between the generation and braking of forces for the STS task. Without this coordination between propulsive and braking forces, the person could easily fall forward upon achieving the vertical position.

Horizontal displacement of the COM appears to be constant despite changes in the speed of STS (73). Controlling the horizontal trajectory of the COM is probably the invariant feature controlled in STS to ensure that stability is maintained during vertical rise of the body.

This strategy could be referred to as a momentum-transfer strategy, and its use requires (*a*) adequate strength and coordination to generate upper body movement prior to lift-off, (*b*) the ability to eccentrically contract trunk and hip muscles, in order to apply braking forces to slow the horizontal trajec-

tory of the COM, and (*c*) concentric contraction of hip and knee muscles to generate vertical propulsive forces that lift the body (74).

Accomplishing STS using a momentum-transfer strategy requires a trade-off between stability and force requirements. The generation and transfer of momentum between the upper body and total body reduces the requirement for lower extremity force because the body is already in motion as it begins to lift. On the other hand, the body is in a precarious state of balance during the transition stage when momentum is transferred.

An alternative strategy that ensures greater stability but requires greater amount of force to achieve lift-off includes flexing the trunk sufficiently to bring the COM well within the base of support of the feet *prior* to lift-off. However, the body has zero momentum at lift-off. This strategy has been referred to as a zero-momentum strategy, and requires the generation of larger lower extremity forces in order to lift the body to vertical (74).

Another common strategy used by many older adults and people with neurological impairments involves the use of armrests to assist in STS. Use of the arms assists in both the stability and force generation requirements of the STS task.

Understanding the different strategies that can be used to accomplish STS, including the trade-offs between force and stability, will help the therapist when retraining STS in the patient with a neurological deficit. For example, the zero-momentum strategy may be more appropriate to use with a patient with cerebellar pathology who has no difficulty with force generation, but who has a major problem with controlling stability. On the other hand, the patient with hemiparesis, who is very weak, may need to rely more on a momentum strategy to achieve the vertical position. The frail elderly person who is both weak and unstable may need to rely on armrests to accomplish STS.

Supine-to-Stand

The ability to assume a standing position from supine is an important milestone in mobility skills. This skill is taught to a wide range of patients with neurological impairments, from young children with developmental disabilities first learning to stand and walk, to frail older people prone to fall. The movement strategies used by normal individuals moving from supine-to-stand have been studied by a number of researchers. An important theoretical question addressed by these researchers relates to whether rising to stand from supine follows a developmental progression, and whether by the age of 4 or 5 years the mature, or adult-like, form emerges and remains throughout life (75).

Researchers have studied supine-to-stand movement strategies in children, ages 4 to 7 years, and young adults, ages 20 to 35 years (76). These researchers found that while there was a slight tendency towards age-specific strategies for moving supine-to-stance, there was also great variability among subjects of the same age. Their findings do not appear to support the traditional assumption of a single *mature* supine-to-stance pattern, which emerges after the age of 5 years.

The three most common movement strategies for moving from supine-to-stand are shown in Figure 11.8. When analyzing strategies used for moving from supine-to-stand, the body is divided into three components, upper extremities, lower extremities, and axial, which includes trunk and head. Movement strategies are then described in relationship to the various combinations of movement patterns within each of these segments. The research on young adults suggests that the most common pattern used involves symmetrical movement patterns of the trunk and extremities, and the use of a symmetrical squat to achieve the vertical position (Fig. 11.8*A*). However, only one-fourth of the subjects studied used this strategy.

The second most common movement pattern involved asymmetric squat on arising (11.8*B*), while the third most common strategy involved asymmetric use of the upper extremities, a partial rotation of the trunk, and assumption of stance using a half-kneel position (11.8*C*).

Additional studies have characterized movement patterns used to rise from supine in middle-aged adults, ages 30 to 39 years, and found some differences in movement strategies compared to younger adults (77). In addition, this study looked at the effect of physical activity levels on strategies used to stand up. Results from the study found that

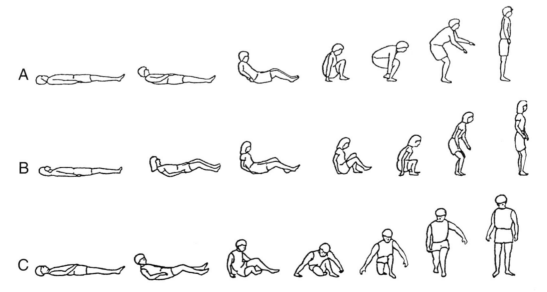

Figure 11.8. Three most common movement strategies identified among young adults for moving from supine to stand. (Adapted from VanSant AF. Rising from a supine position to erect stance: description of adult movement and a developmental hypothesis. Phys Ther 1988;68:185–192.)

strategies used to stand up are influenced by life-style factors, including level of physical activity.

Many factors probably contribute to determining the type of movement strategy used to move from supine-to-stance. Traditionally, nervous system maturation, specifically the maturation of the neck-on-body righting reactions and body-on-body righting reactions, were considered the most significant factors affecting the emergence of a developmentally mature supine-to-stance strategy. However, a switch from an asymmetric rotation to symmetric sit-up strategy may be constrained by the ability to generate sufficient abdominal and hip flexor strength.

Developmental changes in moving from supine-to-stance are considered further in the chapter on age-related aspects of mobility.

RISING-FROM-BED

Clinicians are often called upon to help patients relearn the task of getting out of bed. In therapeutic texts on retraining motor control in the patient with neurological impairments, therapists are instructed to teach patients to move from supine to side-lying, then to push up to a sitting position and from there, to stand up. These instructions are based on the assumption that this pattern represents that typically used to rise from a bed (78, 79).

To test these assumptions, researchers examined movement patterns used by young adults to rise from a bed (80, 81). These studies report that movement patterns used by nondisabled people to rise from a bed are extremely variable. Eighty-nine patterns were found among 60 subjects! In fact, no subject used the same strategy consistently in 10 trials of getting out of bed.

Figure 11.9 shows one of the most common strategies used by young adults to rise from a bed. Essential components of the strategy include pushing with the arms (or grasping the side of the bed and then pushing with the arms), flexing the head and trunk, pushing into a partial sit position, and rolling up into stance. Another common strategy found was

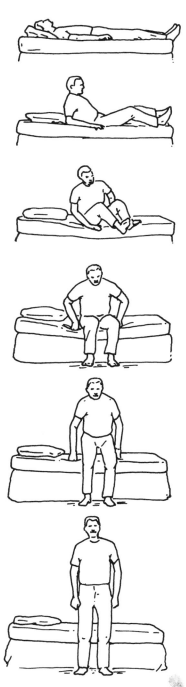

Figure 11.9. Most common movement strategy used by young adults for getting out of bed. (Adapted from Ford-Smith CD, VanSant AF. Age differences in movement patterns used to rise from a bed in subjects in the third through fifth decades of age. Phys Ther 1992;73:305.)

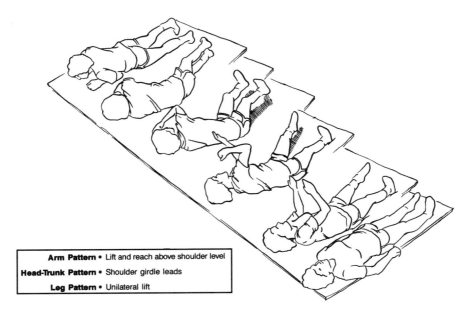

Arm Pattern •	Lift and reach above shoulder level
Head-Trunk Pattern •	Shoulder girdle leads
Leg Pattern •	Unilateral lift

Figure 11.10.   Most common movement strategy used by young adults when rolling from supine to prone. (Adapted from Richter RR, VanSant AF, Newton RA. Description of adult rolling movements and hypothesis of developmental sequences. Phys Ther 1989; 69:63–71.)

a push-off pattern with the arms, rolling to the side and coming to a symmetrical sitting position prior to standing up.

While the authors of this study have not specifically stated the essential features of this task, its similarity to the STS task suggests they share the same invariant characteristics. These include (*a*) the need to generate momentum to move the body to vertical, (*b*) stability requirements for controlling the center of mass as it changes from within the support base defined by the horizontal body to that defined by the buttocks and feet, and finally to a base of support defined solely by the feet; and (*c*) the ability to adapt how one moves to the characteristics of the environment.

In trying to better understand why people move as they do, and in preparation for understanding why patients move as they do, it might be helpful to reexamine descriptions of movement strategies used to rise from a bed in light of these essential tasks characteristics. In doing so, it might be possible to determine common features across diverse strategies that are successful in accomplishing invariant requirements of the task. It would also be possible to examine some trade-offs

between movement and stability requirements in the different strategies. For example, in the roll-off strategy, is motion achieved with greater efficiency at the expense of stability? Alternatively, the come-to-sit pattern may require more force to keep the body in motion, but stability may be inherently greater.

This research demonstrates the tremendous variability of movement strategies used by neurologically intact subjects when getting out of bed. It suggests the importance of helping patients with neurological impairments to learn a variety of approaches to getting out of bed.

Rolling

Rolling is an important part of bed mobility skills and an essential part of many other tasks such as rising from bed (82). Movement strategies used by nonimpaired adults to roll from supine to prone are very variable. Figure 11.10 shows one of the most common movement patterns used by adults to roll from supine to prone (82). Essential features of this strategy include a lift-and-reach arms pattern, with the shoulder girdle initiating motion of the head and trunk, and a unilateral lift of the leg.

A common assumption in the therapeutic literature is that rotation between the shoulders and pelvis is an invariant characteristic in rolling patterns used by normal adults (79); however, in this study on rolling, many of the adults tested did not show this pattern. Similar to the findings from studies on rising from a bed, the great variability used by normal subjects to move from supine to prone suggests that therapists may use greater freedom in retraining movement strategies used by patients with neurological impairments. Clearly, there is no ONE correct way to accomplish this movement.

SUMMARY

1. There are three major requirements for successful locomotion: (*a*) progression, defined as the ability to generate a basic locomotor pattern that can move the body in the desired direction, (*b*) stability, defined as the ability to support and control the body against gravity, and (*c*) adaptability, defined as the ability to adapt gait to meet the individual's goals and the demands of the environment.

2. Normal locomotion is a bipedal gait in which the limbs move in a symmetrical alternating relationship. Gait is divided into a stance and swing phase, each of which has its own intrinsic requirements.

3. During the support phase of gait, horizontal forces are generated against the support surface to move the body in the desired direction (progression), while vertical forces support the body mass against gravity (stability). In addition, strategies used to accomplish both progression and stability must be flexible in order to accommodate changes in speed, direction, or alterations in the support surface (adaptation).

4. The goals to be achieved during the swing phase of gait include advancement of the swing leg (progression), and repositioning the limb in preparation for weight acceptance (stability). Both the progression and stability goals require sufficient foot clearance, so the toe does not drag on the supporting surface during swing. In addition,

strategies used during the swing phase of gait must be sufficiently flexible in order to allow the swing foot to avoid any obstacles in its path (adaptation).

5. Gait is often described with respect to temporal distance parameters such as velocity, step length, step frequency (called cadence), and stride length. In addition, gait is described with reference to changes in joint angles (kinematics), muscle activation patterns (EMG), and the forces used to control gait (kinetics).

6. Many neural and non-neural elements work together in the control of gait. Though spinal pattern generators are able to produce stereotyped locomotor patterns and perform certain adaptive functions, descending pathways from higher centers and sensory feedback from the periphery allow the rich variation in locomotor patterns and adaptability to task and environmental conditions.

7. One of the requirements of normal locomotion is the ability to adapt gait to a wide ranging set of environments, and this involves using sensory information from all the senses both reactively and proactively.

8. An important part of controlling locomotion is stabilizing the head, since it contains two of the most important sensors for controlling motion: the vestibular and visual systems. In neurologically intact adults, the head is stabilized with great precision, allowing gaze to be stabilized through the vestibulo-ocular reflex.

9. Stair-walking is similar to level walking in that it involves stereotypical reciprocal alternating movements of the lower limbs and has three requirements: the generation of primarily concentric forces to propel the body up stairs, or eccentric forces to control the body's descent down stairs (progression), while controlling the center of mass within a constantly changing base of support (stability); and the capacity to adapt strategies used for progression and stability to accommodate changes in stair environment, such as height, width, and the presence or absence of railings (adaptation).

10. Although mobility is often thought of in relationship to gait, many other aspects of mobility are essential to independence. These include the ability to move from sit to stand, rolling, rising from a bed, or moving from one chair to another. These skills are referred to as transfer tasks.

11. Transfer tasks are similar to locomotion in that they share common task requirements: motion in a desired direction (progression), postural control (stability), and the ability to adapt to changing task and environmental conditions (adaptation). Researchers have found great variability in the types of movement strategies used by neurologically intact young adults when performing transfer tasks.

12. Understanding the stability and strength requirements for different types of strategies used to accomplish transfer tasks has important implications for retraining these skills in neurologically impaired patients with different types of motor constraints.

REFERENCES

1. Patla AE. Understanding the control of human locomotion: a prologue. In: Patla AE, ed. Adaptability of human gait. Amsterdam: North-Holland, 1991:3–17.

2. Das P, McCollum G. Invariant structure in locomotion. Neuroscience 1988;25:1023–1034.

3. Raibert M. Symmetry in running. Science 1986;231:1292–1294.

4. Grillner S. Control of locomotion in bipeds, tetrapods, and fish. In: Brooks VB, ed. Handbook of physiology—the nervous system. II. Motor control. Baltimore: Williams & Wilkins, 1981:1179–1236.

5. Murray MP, Mollinger LA, Gardner GM, Sepic SB. Kinematic and EMG patterns during slow, free, and fast walking. J Orthop Res 1984;2:272–280.

6. Rosenrot P, Wall JC, Charteris J. The relationship between velocity, stride time, support time and swing time during normal walking. Journal of Human Movement Studies 1980;6:323–335.

7. DeLuca PA, Perry JP, Ounpuu S. The fundamentals of normal walking and pathological gait. AACP & DM Inst. Course #2. 1992.

8. Craik R. Changes in locomotion in the aging adult. In: Woollacott M, Shumway-Cook A, eds. Development of posture and gait. Charleston, SC: Univ. of South Carolina Press, 1989:176–201.

9. Grieve DW. Gait patterns and the speed of walking. Biomedical engineering 1968; 3:119–122.

10. Inman VT, Ralston H, Todd F. Human walking. Baltimore: Williams & Wilkins. 1981.

11. Finley FR, Cody KA. Locomotive characteristics of urban pedestrians. Arch Phys Med Rehabil 1970;51:423–426.

12. Murray MP, Mollinger LA, Gardner GM, Sepic SB. Kinematic and EMG patterns during slow, free, and fast walking. J Orthop Res 1984;2:272–280.

13. Ralston HJ. Energetics of human walking. In: Herman RM, Grillner S, Stein PSG, Stuart DG, eds. Neural control of locomotion. New York: Plenum, 1976:77–98.

14. Zarrugh MY, Todd FN, Ralston HJ. Optimization of energy expenditure during level walking. Eur J Appl Physiol 1974;33:293–306.

15. Mochon S, McMahon TA. Ballistic walking. J Biomech 1980;13:49–57.

16. Herman R, Wirta R, Bampton S, Finley FR. Human solutions for locomotion I. Single limb analysis. In: Herman R, Grillner S, Stein P, Stuart D, eds. Neural control of locomotion. New York: Plenum, 1976:13–49.

17. Murray MP. Gait as a total pattern of movement. Am J Phys Med 1967;46:290–333.

18. Murray MP, Kory RC, Clarkson BH, Sepic SB. Comparison of free and fast speed walking patterns of normal men. Am J Phys Med 1966;45:8–24.

19. Winter DA. Biomechanical motor patterns in normal walking. Journal of Motor Behavior 1983;15:302–330.

20. Saunders JBdeCM, Inman VT, Eberhart HD. The major determinants in normal and pathological gait. J Bone Joint Surg 1953;35-A:543–558.

21. McMahon TA. Muscles, reflexes and locomotion. Princeton, NJ: Princeton University Press. 1984.

22. Perry J. Gait analysis: normal and pathological function. Thorofare, NJ: Slack, 1992.

23. Eberhart HD. Physical principles of locomotion. In: Herman RM, Grillner S, Stein PSG, Stuart DG, eds. Neural control of locomotion. New York: Plenum, 1976:1–11.

24. Basmajian JV, Deluca CJ. Muscles alive: their functions revealed by electromyography. 5th ed. Baltimore:Williams & Wilkins, 1985.

25. Winter DA. Kinematic and kinetic patterns of human gait: variability and compensating effects. Human Movement Science 1984;3:51–76.

26. Winter DA. Overall principle of lower limb

support during stance phase of gait. J Biomech 1980;13:923–927.

27. Winter DA, Patla AE, Frank, JS, Walt SE. Biomechanical walking pattern changes in the fit and healthy elderly. Phys Ther 1990; 70:340–347.

28. Winter DA. Biomechanics and motor control of human movement. New York: John Wiley & Sons, 1990:80–84.

29. Winter DA, McFadyen BJ, Dickey JP. Adaptability of the CNS in human walking. In: Patla AE, ed. Adaptability of human gait. Amsterdam: Elsevier, 1991:127–144.

30. Woollacott MH, Jensen J. Stance and locomotion. In: S Keele, H Heuer, eds. Handbook of motor skills. In press.

31. Cavanagh PR, Gregor RJ. Knee joint torques during the swing phase of normal treadmill walking. J Biomech 1975;8:337–344.

32. Grillner S. Locomotion in the spinal cat. In: Stein RB, Pearson KG, Smith RS, Redford JB, eds. Control of posture and locomotion. New York: Plenum, 1973:515–535.

33. Smith JL. Programming of stereotyped limb movements by spinal generators. In: Stelmach GE, Requin J, eds. Tutorials in motor behavior. Amsterdam: North-Holland. 1980:95–115.

34. Sherrington CS. Decerebrate rigidity, and reflex coordination of movements. J Physiol (London) 1898;22:319–332.

35. Mott FW, Sherrington CS. Experiments upon the influence of sensory nerves upon movement and nutrition of the limbs. Preliminary communication. Proc R Soc Lond (Biol) 1895;57:481–488.

36. Brown TG. The intrinsic factors in the act of progression in the mammal. Proc R Soc Lond (Biol) 1911;84:308–319.

37. Taub E, Berman AJ. Movement and learning in the absence of sensory feedback. In: Freedman SJ, ed. The neurophysiology of spatially oriented behavior. Homewood, NJ: Dorsey Press, 1968:173–192.

38. Wolf S, LeCraw DE, Barton LA, Jann BB. Forced use of hemiplegic upper extremities to reverse the effect of learned nonuse among chronic stroke and head-injured patients. Exp Neurol 1989;104:125–132.

39. Taub E, Miller NE, Novack TA, et al. Technique to improve chronic motor deficit after stroke. Arch Phys Med Rehabil 1993; 74:347–354.

40. Forssberg H, Grillner S, Rossignol S. Phase dependent reflex reversal during walking in chronic spinal cats. Brain Res 1977;85:121–139.

41. Smith JL, Smith LA, Dahms KL. Motor capacities of the chronic spinal cat: recruitment of slow and fast extensors of the ankle. Neuroscience Abstracts 1979;5:387.

42. Shik ML, Severin FV, Orlovsky GN. Control of walking and running by means of electrical stimulation of the mid-brain. Biophysics 1966;11:756–765.

43. Grillner S, Zangger P. On the central generation of locomotion in the low spinal cat. Exp Brain Res 1979;34:241–261.

44. Arshavsky Yu I, Berkinblit MB, Fukson OI, Gelfand IM, Orlovsky GN. Recordings of neurones of the dorsal spinocerebellar tract during evoked locomotion. Brain Res 1972; 43:272–275.

45. Arshavsky Yu I, Berkinblit MB, Gelfand IM, Orlovsky GN, Fukson OI. Activity of the neurones of the ventral spino-cerebellar tract during locomotion. Biophysics 1972; 17:926–935.

46. Keele S, Ivry R. Does the cerebellum provide a common computation for diverse tasks? A timing hypothesis. In: Diamond A, ed. Developmental and neural bases of higher cognitive function. NY: New York Academy of Sciences. In press.

47. Sudarsky L, Ronthal M. Gait disorders in the elderly: assessing the risk for falls. In: Vellas B, Toupet M, Rubenstein L, Albarede JL, Christen Y, eds. Falls, balance and gait disorders in the elderly. Amsterdam: Elsevier 1992:117–127.

48. Grillner S, Rossignol S. On the initiation of the swing phase of locomotion in chronic spinal cats. Brain Res 1978;146:269–277.

49. Pearson KG, Ramirez JM, Jiang W. Entrainment of the locomotor by group Ib afferents from ankle extensor muscles in spinal cats. Exp Brain Res 1992;90:557–566.

50. Stein RB. Reflex modulation during locomotion: functional significance. In: Patla A, ed. Adaptability of human gait. Amsterdam: North Holland, 1991:21–36.

51. Nashner LM. Balance adjustment of humans perturbed while walking. J Neurophysiol 1980;44:650–664.

52. Lackner JR, DiZio P. Visual stimulation affects the perception of voluntary leg movements during walking. Perception 1988; 17:71–80.

53. Lackner JR, DiZio P. Sensory-motor calibration processes constraining the perception of force and motion during locomotion. In: Woollacott MH, Horak FB, eds. Posture and gait: control mechanisms. Eugene, OR: Univ. of Oregon Books, 1992:92–96.

54. Lee DN, Young DS. Gearing action to the environment. Exp Brain Res Series 15. Berlin: Springer-Verlag, 1986:217–230.

55. Berthoz A, Pozzo T. Head and body coordination during locomotion and complex movements. In: Swinnen SP, Heuer H, Massion J, Casaer P, eds. Interlimb coordination: neural, dynamical and cognitive constraints. San Diego: Academic Press, 1994:147–165.

56. Pozzo T, Berthoz A, Lefort K. Head stabilization during various locomotor tasks in humans. I. Normal subjects. Exp Brain Res 1990;82:97–106.

57. Pozzo T, Levik Y, Berthoz A. Head stabilization in the frontal plane during complex equilibrium tasks in humans. In: Woollacott M, Horak F, eds. Posture and gait: control mechanisms. Eugene, OR: Univ. of Oregon Books, 1992:97–100.

58. Patla AE. The neural control of locomotion. In: Spivack BS, ed. Mobility and gait. NY: Marcel Dekker, in press.

59. Hoy MG, Zernicke RF. Modulation of limb dynamics in the swing phase of locomotion. J Biomech 1985;18:49–60.

60. Hoy MG, Zernicke RF. The role of intersegmental dynamics during rapid limb oscillations. J Biomech 1986;19:867–877.

61. Hoy MG, Zernicke RF, Smith JL. Contrasting roles of inertial and muscle moments at knee and ankle during paw-shake response. J Neurophysiol 1985;54:1282–1294.

62. Smith JL, Zernicke RF. Predictions for neural control based on limb dynamics. Trends Neurosci 1987;10:123–128.

63. Wisleder D, Zernicke RF, Smith JL. Speed-related changes in hindlimb intersegmental dynamics during the swing phase of cat locomotion. Exp Brain Res. In press.

64. Larsson LE. Neural control of gait in man. In: Eccles J, Dimitrijevic MR, eds. Recent achievements in restorative neurology. Basel: Karger, 1985:185–198.

65. Carlsoo, A. The initiation of walking. Acta Anat 1966; 65:1–9.

66. Herman R, Cook T, Cozzens B, Freedman W. In: Stein RB, Pearson KG, Smith RS, Redford JB, eds. Control of posture and locomotion. New York: Plenum, 1973:363–388.

67. Mann RA, Hagy JL, White V, Liddell D. The initiation of gait. J Bone Joint Surg 1979;61-A:232–239.

68. Breniere Y, Do MC. When and how does steady state gait movement induced from upright posture begin? J Biomech 1986; 19:1035–1040.

69. Cook T, Cozzens B. Human solutions for locomotion: III. The initiation of gait. In: Herman RM, Grillner S, Stein PSG, Stuart DG, eds. Neural control of locomotion. New York: Plenum, 1976:65–76.

70. Simoneau GG, Cavanagh PR, Ulbrecht JS, Leibowitz HW, Tyrrell RA. The influence of visual factors on fall-related kinematic variables during stair descent by older women. J Gerontol 1991;46:188–195.

71. Craik RL, Cozzens BA, Freedman W. The role of sensory conflict on stair descent performance in humans. Exp Brain Res 1982; 45:399–409.

72. McFadyen BJ, Winter DA. An integrated biomechanical analysis of normal stair ascent and descent. J Biomech 1988;21:733–744.

73. Millington PJ, Myklebust BM, Shambes GM. Biomechanical analysis of the sit-to-stand motion in elderly persons. Arch Phys Med Rehabil 1992;73:609–617.

74. Schenkman MA, Berger RA, Riley PO, Mann RW, Hodge WA. Whole-body movements during rising to standing from sitting. Phys Ther 1990;10:638–651.

75. VanSant AF. Rising from a supine position to erect stance: description of adult movement and a developmental hypothesis. Phys Ther 1988;68:185–192.

76. VanSant AF. Age differences in movement patterns used by children to rise from a supine positions to erect stance. Phys Ther 1988; 68:1130–1138.

77. Green LN, Williams K. Differences in developmental movement patterns used by active vs sedentary middle-aged adults coming from a supine position to erect stance. Phys Ther 1992; 72:560–568.

78. Carr JH, Shepherd RB. Motor relearning programme for stroke. Rockville: Aspen, 1983.

79. Bobath B. Adult hemiplegia: evaluation and treatment. London: Heinemann, 1978.

80. Sarnacki SJ. Rising from supine on a bed: a description of adult movement and hypoth-

esis of developmental sequences. Richmond, VA: Virginia Commonwealth University, 1985. Master's thesis.

81. McCoy AO, VanSant AF. Movement patterns of adolescents rising from a bed. Phys Ther 1993;73:182–193.

82. Richter RR, VanSant AF, Newton RA. Description of adult rolling movements and hypothesis of developmental sequences. Phys Ther 1989; 69:63–71.

Chapter 12

A LIFE SPAN PERSPECTIVE OF MOBILITY

INTRODUCTION

It is wonderful to see children develop their first mobility skills as they begin to crawl, creep, walk, and run—finally, navigating expertly through complex environments. How do these skills develop? When do they first begin to emerge? What key features of normal locomotor development should we incorporate into our assessment tools so that we can better understand the delayed or disordered development of the child with central nervous system pathology?

Falls, and the injuries that often accompany them, are a serious problem in the older adult. Many of these falls occur during walking. Problems with balance and gait are considered major contributors to falls in the older adult. Nevertheless, not all older adults have difficulties with mobility skills. Much like the study of balance control, it is important to distinguish between *age-related changes* in mobility affecting all older adults and *pathology-*

related changes, which affect only a few. This chapter discusses mobility skills from a life span perspective. We first review the development of mobility skills in neurologically intact children and summarize research from different theoretical perspectives that explore the factors contributing to the emergence of this complex ability. In the latter half of the chapter, we discuss how mobility skills change in the older adult.

DEVELOPMENT OF LOCOMOTION

Independent locomotion may at first seem to be a fairly simple and automatic skill, but it is really a very intricate motor task. A child learning to walk needs to activate a complex pattern of muscle contractions in many body segments to produce a coordinated stepping movement, resulting in *progression*. The child must be strong enough to support body weight, and stable enough to compensate for shifts in balance while walking, to accomplish the goal of *stability*. Finally, the child must develop the ability to *adapt* gait to changing environmental circumstances, allowing navigation around and over obstacles, and across uneven surfaces (1). In the following section, we summarize research evidence suggesting that in the development of locomotion, these three requirements emerge sequentially, during the first years of life. How does this complex behavior develop? What are the origins of this behavior during prenatal development?

Prenatal Development

Researchers have actually traced the origins of locomotor rhythms back to embryonic movements that begin to occur in the first stages of development. Ultrasound techniques have been used to document the movements of human infants prenatally (2). This research has shown that all movements except those observed in the earliest stages of embryonic development (7 to 8 weeks) are also seen in neonates and young infants.

Isolated leg and arm movements develop in the embryo by 9 weeks of age, while alternating leg movements, similar to walking movements seen after birth, develop in the infant by about 16 weeks of embryonic age (2, 3).

Animal research has also explored the prenatal development of locomotor circuitry. Detectable limb movements appear to emerge in a cephalocaudal sequence, with movements in the forelimbs preceding those in the hindlimbs (4). Intralimb coordination develops prior to interlimb coordination, with the first detectable movements occurring at proximal joints, and moving distally with development. Finally, interlimb coordination develops, first with alternating patterns, then with synchronous patterns (5).

Many newborn animals, such as the rat, do not normally show coordinated locomotor movements until about 1 week after birth (6). If, however, rats are placed in water at birth, they swim, demonstrating the maturity of their locomotor system. In addition, adult forms of locomotion can be elicited in 3-day-old kittens by placing them on a treadmill (4). However, gait in kittens is uncoordinated, due to poor postural abilities.

These results suggest that a primary constraint on emerging locomotor behavior is the immaturity of the postural system and thus the inability to achieve upright stability. In addition, these findings remind us to be careful about assuming that because a behavior is not evident, there is no neural circuitry for it.

Early Stepping Behavior

Because locomotor patterns have been developing for some months prenatally, it is not surprising to find that stepping behavior can be elicited in newborns under the right conditions (2, 7, 8). For example, when newborn infants are held under the arms in an upright position, tilted slightly forward, with the soles of the feet touching a surface, they often perform coordinated movements that look much like erect locomotion. Surprisingly, stepping becomes progressively more difficult to elicit during the first month of life, tending to disappear in most infants by about 2 months of age, and reappearing again with the onset of self-generated locomotion, many months later.

This pattern of appearance and disappearance of newborn stepping was found in a study that examined 156 children longitudinally (7). It was found that 94 infants stepped at 1 month, 18 stepped at 3 months, while only two stepped at 4 and 5 months. Then, at 10 months, after a 4- to 8-month period of no stepping, all 156 infants stepped with support and 18 stepped without support. Thus, the stepping pattern appeared to be temporarily lost in 98 to 99% of the infants.

What causes these changes? Different theoretical approaches explain changes in infant behavior in very different ways. From a reflex hierarchy perspective, newborn stepping is thought to result from a stepping reflex. Its disappearance is assumed to be mainly the result of inhibition by maturing higher neural centers. Figure 12.1 illustrates seven

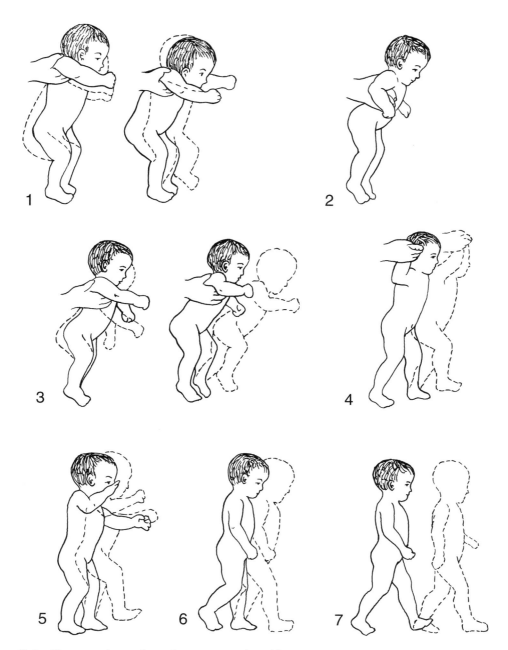

Figure 12.1. The seven phases of erect locomotion. (Adapted from McGraw MB. The neuromuscular maturation of the human infant. NY: Hafner Press, 1945.)

phases in the development of infant locomotion, beginning with the observation of this reflex (phase 1) and its disappearance (phase 2), continuing with its reappearance (phase 3) and the emergence of assisted locomotion (phase 4), and concluding with three phases of erect independent walking in which the hands gradually move from a high guard position (phase 5) down to the side (phase 6), and the trunk and head become more erect (phase 7) (9).

In contrast to a reflex hierarchical model, researchers using a systems approach have examined the emergence of stepping in relationship to the contributions of multiple neural and non-neural systems. In particular, these studies have explored the conditions leading to the emergence of newborn stepping, and the changes that cause its disappearance.

Esther Thelan, a psychologist, and her colleagues have applied a dynamical systems approach to the study of locomotor development (8). This approach views locomotion as an emergent property of many interacting complex processes, including sensory, motor, perceptual, integrative, respiratory, cardiac, and anatomical systems. According to a dynamical systems approach, moving and developing systems have certain **self-organizing** properties, that is, they can spontaneously form patterns that arise simply from the interaction of the different parts of the system.

A dynamical systems model stresses that actions always occur within specific contexts. As a result, a given neural code will produce very different behavioral outcomes, depending on the contributions of the other elements of the system, as in the position of the child with relation to gravity. Thus, dynamical systems researchers suggest that the specific leg trajectory seen in newborn stepping is not coded precisely anywhere in the nervous system. Instead, the pattern emerges through the contributions of many elements. These include the neural substrate, anatomical linkages, body composition, activation or arousal level, and the gravitational conditions in which the infant is kicking (8).

From a dynamical systems perspective, the disappearance of the neonatal stepping pattern at about 2 months of age results from changes in a number of components of the system that reduce the likelihood of seeing this behavior (8). For example, body build changes greatly in the first 18 months of life. Infants add a lot of body fat in the first 2 months of life and then slim down toward the end of the first year. It has been suggested that the stepping pattern goes away at 2 months because infants have insufficient strength to lift the heavier leg during the step cycle (8).

When 4-week-old infants are submerged up to their trunk in water, thus making them more buoyant and counteracting the effects of gravity, stepping increases in frequency (10). This suggests that their weight is a factor that affects the step cycle.

Further support for the weight hypothesis related to the disappearance of newborn stepping comes from research examining newborn kicking patterns. Supine kicking has the same spatial and temporal patterning as newborn stepping. For example, the swing phase of locomotion is similar to the flexion and extension phases of the kick, while the stance phase is similar to the pause between kicks. As stepping speeds up, the stance phase is reduced, and as kicking speeds up, the pause phase is reduced (8).

This suggests that the same pattern generator may be responsible for both supine kicking and newborn stepping. Yet, supine kicking continues during the period when newborn stepping disappears. One explanation for the persistence of supine kicking is that it doesn't require the same strength as stepping, since the infants aren't working against gravity (8, 10).

Hans Forssberg, a Swedish physiologist and pediatrician, examined the nervous system contribution to the emergence of locomotion in more detail. He postulated that human locomotion is characterized by the interaction of many systems with certain hierarchical components (7).

His research suggests that an innate pattern generator creates the basic rhythm of the step cycle, which can be seen in newborn stepping. In the first year, the gradual development of descending systems from higher neural centers gives the child the ability to control this locomotor activity. Adaptive systems for equilibrium control, organized at a higher level than those controlling the pattern generator, develop over a longer period (7).

According to this research, the emergence of walking with support is not the result of critical changes in the stepping pattern per se, but appears to be due to maturation of the equilibrium system. In addition, the gradual emergence of mature gait over the next year is hypothesized to result from a new higher level control system influencing the original lower level network and modifying it (7).

Forssberg's research, using EMG and

motion analysis, has examined how the loco-motor pattern changes over the first 2 years of development (7). Studies using motion analysis techniques have shown a gradual transformation of the locomotor movement from a synchronous pattern of joint move-ments in newborn stepping to a more adult-like dissociated pattern of joint motion by the end of the first year of development. The transformation to adult-like gait patterns hap-pens during the latter part of the second year. At this point, heel-strike begins to occur in front of the body. Figure 12.2 shows the ki-nematics of neonatal vs. adult stepping move-ments.

The EMG analysis supported the find-ings of the motion analysis. For example, in the neonate, the motor pattern was charac-terized by a high degree of synchronized ac-tivity. In other words, the extensor muscles of different joints were active simultaneously, and there was much coactivation of agonist and antagonist muscles at each joint. As with the movement patterns, the EMG patterns also began to look more mature during the latter part of the second year, with asynchro-nous patterns emerging at the different joints (7).

Neonatal locomotion may be similar to that of quadrupeds who walk on the their toes, like cats, dogs, or horses (7). For ex-ample, newborns show high knee/hip flexion and do not have heel-strike. Since extensor muscle activity occurs prior to foot touch-down, it appears to be driven by an innate locomotor pattern generator, as has been found in quadrupeds, rather than being re-flexly activated by the foot in contact with the ground. It has also been suggested that the neural network for stepping must be orga-nized at or below the brainstem level since anencephalic infants (infants born without a cerebral cortex) can perform a similar pattern of infant stepping (11).

Interestingly, some researchers believe that the abnormal gait patterns found in many patients with neurological impairments are actually immature locomotor patterns. Thus, children with cerebral palsy, mentally retarded children, and habitual toe-walkers may persist in using an immature locomotor pattern, while adults with acquired neurological dis-ease may revert to immature locomotion be-cause of the loss of higher center modulation over the locomotor pattern generator (7).

So what are the elements that contrib-ute to the emergence of locomotion in the infant? Remember that in development, some elements of the nervous and musculoskeletal system may be functionally ready before oth-ers, but the system must wait for the matu-ration of the slowest component before the target behavior can appear. A small increase or change in the development of the slowest component can act as the control parameter, becoming the impetus that drives the system to a new behavioral form.

The research we just discussed shows that many of the components that contribute to independent locomotion are functional be-fore the child takes any independent steps. Function of the locomotor pattern generator is present in a limited capacity at birth, and is

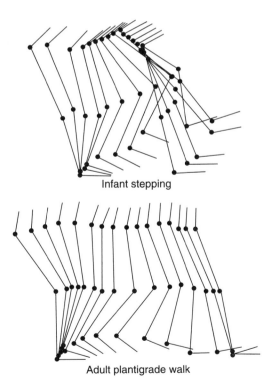

Infant stepping

Adult plantigrade walk

Figure 12.2. Kinematic differences in neonatal vs. adult gait. (Adapted from Forssburg H. Ontogeny of human locomotor control: 1. Infant stepping, supported loco-motion and transition to independent locomotion. Exp Brain Res 1985;67:481.)

improved during the second half of the first year, as the tight intralimb synergies become dissociated and capable of more complex modulation and control. As we noted in the chapter on the development of postural control, infants are able to use optic flow information at birth to modulate head movements, and at least by 5 to 6 months of age for modulation of stance. Motivation to navigate toward a distant object is clearly present by the onset of creeping and crawling, and voluntary control over the limbs is certainly present by this time for many behaviors (8).

So what is the constraint that keeps locomotion from emerging before 9 to 12 months of age? Most researchers believe that it is primarily due to limitations in balance control, and possibly also limitations in strength (7, 8, 12).

For example, when an infant is creeping, one foot can be picked up at a time, so there is always a tripod stance available and, thus, balance is much less demanding. Normal infants who are about to take their first steps have developed motor coordination within the locomotor pattern generator, they have functional visual, vestibular, and somatosensory systems and the motivation to move forward. Infants may also have sufficient muscle strength, at least to balance, if not for use in propelling the body forward. But they won't be able to use these processes in effective locomotion until the postural control system can effectively control the shift of weight from leg to leg, thus avoiding a fall. When these processes hit a particular threshold for effective function, then the dynamic behavior of independent locomotion can emerge.

When looking at the three requirements for successful locomotion: a rhythmic stepping pattern (progression), the control of balance (stability), and the ability to modify gait (adaptation), clearly, a rhythmic stepping pattern develops first. It is present in limited form at birth, and is refined during the first year of life. Stance stability develops second, toward the end of the first year and the beginning of the second year of life. As we discuss in the next section, it appears that adaptability is refined in the first years after the onset of independent walking.

Maturation of Independent Locomotion

Bril and Breniere, two French researchers, studied the emergence of locomotion and hypothesized that learning to walk is a two-stage process (13). In the initial phase, infants learn to control balance, while in the second phase, the locomotor pattern is progressively refined.

They studied children longitudinally during the first 4 years of life to see how gait patterns change as independent locomotion develops. Significant changes in emerging gait patterns are summarized in Figure 12.3 and include a decrease in the double-support phase of gait (Fig. 12.3A), an increase in step length, and a decrease in step width (Fig. 12.3B). The greatest changes occurred in the first 4 months of independent walking (Fig. 12.3A) (13).

In addition, examination of the vertical acceleration of the center of gravity suggested that when infants are first learning to step, they fall into each successive step. By 5 to 6 months this trend has begun to lessen, and continues to improve between the ages of 10 to 40 months as the infant learns to integrate balance into the step cycle (Fig. 12.3C) (13).

Since the changes in step width, step length, and double-support phase appear to relate to the mastery of balance control, their findings support the idea that it is during the first phase of walking that a child learns to integrate posture into locomotor movements.

Studies of changes in EMG characteristics and kinematics from the onset of walking through the mastery of mature forms of gait have been performed by other laboratories as well (14, 15).

In the first days of independent walking, stepping patterns are immature. Push-off motion in the stance phase is absent, the step width is very wide, and the arms are held high. The infant appears to generate force to propel the body forward by leaning forward at the trunk (14). The swing phase is short because the infant is unable to balance on one leg.

By 10 to 15 days of independent walking, the infant begins to reduce cocontrac-

Figure 12.3. Graphs of changes in different walking parameters during the first 4 years of walking. **A,** The relative duration of the double-support phase. **B,** Changes in relative step length and width. **C,** Changes in vertical acceleration of the center of gravity. (Adapted from Bril B, Breniere Y. Posture and independent locomotion in childhood: learning to walk or learning dynamic postural control? In: Savelsbergh GJP, ed. The development of coordination in infancy. Amsterdam: North-Holland, 1993, 337–358.)

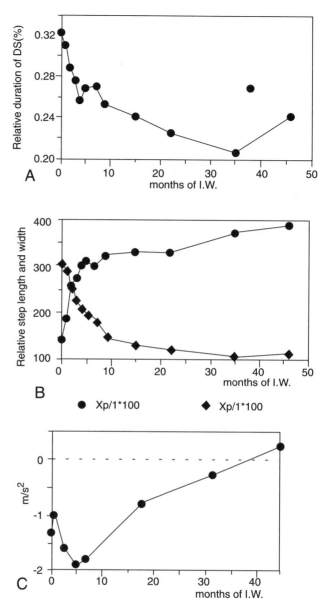

tion, and at 50 to 85 days after walking onset, the muscle patterns begin to show a reciprocal relationship. Interestingly, if infants are supported during walking, the reciprocal relationship between muscles emerges, but, with the additional requirement of stabilizing the body while walking independently, the coactivation returns (14).

Other common gait characteristics in the first year of walking include: a high step frequency, absence of the reciprocal swinging movements between the upper and lower limbs, a flexed knee during stance phase, and an increased hip flexion, pelvic tilt, and hip abduction during swing phase. There is also ankle plantarflexion at foot-strike and decreased ankle flexion during swing, giving a relative foot-drop (15).

By 2 years of age, the pelvic tilt and abduction and external rotation of the hip are diminished. At foot-strike, a knee-flexion wave appears, and reciprocal swing in the upper limb is present in about 75% of the children. The relative foot-drop disappears as the ankle dorsiflexes during swing. By the end of age 2, the infant begins to show a push-off in stance (15).

During the years from 1 until 7, the muscle amplitudes and durations gradually reduce toward adult levels. By the age of 7, most muscle and movement patterns during walking look very similar to that of the adult (15).

Five important characteristics are used to determine mature gait, including (*a*) duration of single limb stance, (*b*) walking velocity, (*c*) cadence, (*d*) step length, and (*e*) the ratio of pelvic span to step width (15).

Duration of single-limb stance increases steadily from 32% in 1-year-olds to 38% in 7-year-olds (39% is a typical adult value). Walking velocity and cadence decrease steadily, while step length increases. Step length is short in the newly walking child due to lack of stability of the supporting limb, and lengthens with increasing balance abilities. Finally, the ratio of pelvic span, which is defined as body width at the level of the pelvis, to step width increases until age 2 1/2, after which it stabilizes. By 3 years of age, the gait pattern is essentially mature, though small improvements continue through age 7 (15).

Table 12.1 summarizes some of the characteristic changes in the step-cycle from the initiation of independent walking through the development of mature patterns at about the age of 3 (16). These changes can be seen more graphically in Figure 12.4.

Run, Skip, Hop, and Gallop

Running is often described as an exaggerated form of walking because it differs from the walk as the result of a brief flight phase in each step. The flight phase that distinguishes a run is seen at about the second year of age. Until this time, the infant's run is more like a fast walk with one foot always in contact with the ground (16). By 4 years of age, most children can hop (33%) and gallop (43%). The development of the gallop precedes the hop slightly. In one study, by 6.5 years, the children were skillful at hopping and galloping. However, only 14% of 4-year-olds could skip (step-hop) (17).

Table 12.1.   Developmental Sequence for Walking[a]

I. Walking:
  A. Initial stage
    1. Difficulty maintaining upright posture
    2. Unpredictable loss of balance
    3. Rigid, halting leg action
    4. Short steps
    5. Flat-footed contact
    6. Toes turn outward
    7. Wide base of support
    8. Flexed knee at contact followed by quick leg extension
  B. Elementary stage
    1. Gradual smoothing out of pattern
    2. Step length increased
    3. Heel-toe contact
    4. Arms down to sides with limited swing
    5. Base of support within the lateral dimensions of trunk
    6. Out-toeing reduced or eliminated
    7. Increased pelvic tilt
    8. Apparent vertical lift
  C. Mature stage
    1. Reflexive arm swing
    2. Narrow base of support
    3. Relaxed, elongated gait
    4. Minimal vertical lift
    5. Definite heel-toe contact
II. Common Problems
  A. Inhibited or exaggerated arm swing
  B. Arms crossing midline of body
  C. Improper foot placement
  D. Exaggerated forward trunk lean
  E. Arms flopping at sides or held out for balance
  F. Twisting of trunk
  G. Poor rhythmical action
  H. Landing flat-footed
  I. Flipping foot or lower leg in or out

[a]From Gallahue DL. Understanding motor development: infants, children, adolescents. Indianapolis: Benchmark Press, 1989:236.

If central pattern generator's (CPGs) control walking, are there separate CPGs for hopping, galloping, and skipping? Probably not. Then why do they emerge in a fixed order of appearance? It is possible to explain their emergence from the dynamical systems perspective (17).

Remember that walking and running are patterns of interlimb coordination in which the limbs are 50% out of phase with one another. This is the easiest stepping pattern to produce, and thus appears earliest. Running appears later than walking, probably due to its increased strength and balance requirements

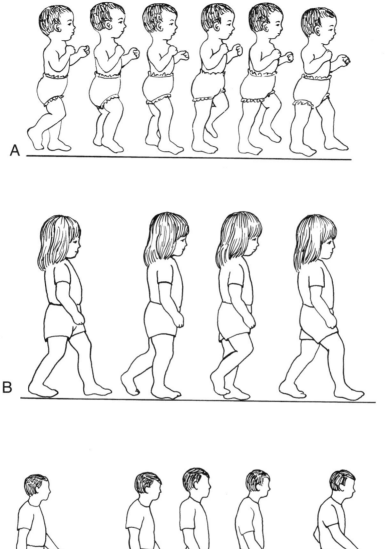

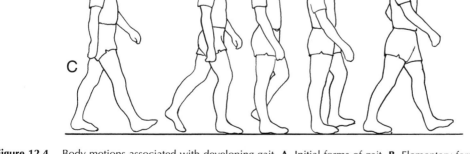

Figure 12.4.   Body motions associated with developing gait. **A**, Initial forms of gait. **B**, Elementary forms of gait. **C**, Mature forms of gait. (Adapted from Gallahue DL. Understanding motor development: infants, children, adolescents. Indianapolis: Benchmark Press, 1989:237.)

compared with walking. Galloping requires that the child produce an asymmetrical gait with unusual timing and a differentiation in force production in each limb, and it may produce additional balance requirements. Hopping emerges next, possibly because it requires the ability to balance the body's weight on one limb and it requires additional force to lift the body off the ground after landing. Skipping (a step-hop) emerges last, possibly because one locomotor coordination pattern is imbedded into another pattern, and thus it requires additional coordination abilities (17).

Development of Adaptation

How do children learn to adapt their walking patterns so they can navigate over and around obstacles? As we mentioned in the previous chapter, both reactive and proactive strategies are used to modify gait to changes in the environment. There has been very little research examining the development of adaptation in normal children. As a result, we know little about how children learn to compensate for disturbances to their gait, nor how they develop proactive strategies to modify gait in advance of obstacles.

REACTIVE STRATEGIES

Reactive strategies for adapting gait relate to the integration of compensatory postural responses into the gait cycle. Researchers have looked at compensatory postural muscle responses to perturbations during locomotion, and compared them to those during perturbed quiet stance (18).

In response to fast velocity stance perturbations, children respond with both an automatic postural response and a monosynaptic reflex response. As children mature, the stretch reflex response gets smaller in amplitude, while the postural response gets faster. In very young children, there is considerable coactivation of antagonist muscles (18).

Perturbations during gait produce a monosynaptic reflex response in children

from 1 to 2.5 years but not in older children. Similar to stance perturbations, automatic postural responses to gait perturbations become faster with age, with mature responses occurring by about 4 years. Coactivation of antagonist muscles also is reduced with age. These changes are shown in Figure 12.5. Changes in the characteristics of compensatory postural activity are associated with increased stability during gait, and increased ability to compensate for perturbations to gait (18). This study suggests that children as young as a year old who are capable of independent locomotion can integrate compensatory postural activity into slow walking when gait is disturbed, though their responses are immature.

PROACTIVE STRATEGIES

Proactive strategies for adapting gait use sensory information to modify gait patterns in advance of obstacles to gait. When do children begin integrating these strategies into the step cycle? It has been suggested that children first learning to walk master feedback control of balance, and then move on to acquire feedforward control (19). The results of experiments by Bril and Breniere (13) support this idea, since children seem to spend the first 4 to 5 months of walking learning to integrate balance into the step cycle. However, there is little research on the development of proactive strategies to help clinicians understand the emergence of this important aspect of mobility.

Head Stabilization During Gait

An important part of controlling locomotion is learning to stabilize the head. Adults stabilize the head with great precision, allowing a steady gaze. Thus, control of the head, arm, and trunk (HAT) segments is a critical part of controlling mobility. How do children control the trunk, arms, and head during locomotion ensuring stabilization of the head and gaze?

Assaiante and Amblard (20) performed experiments in children from early walkers

Figure 12.5. Examples of the gastrocnemius EMG responses of individual children of 1, 2.5, and 4 years of age and of an adult, when their balance is perturbed during walking on a treadmill, by briefly increasing treadmill speed. The left vertical line is the onset of the treadmill acceleration, and the dotted line to its right is the onset of the EMG response. Note that there is a large monosynaptic reflex in the youngest children, before the automatic postural response. This disappears by 4 years of age. (Adapted from Berger W, Quintern J, Dietz V. Stance and gait perturbations in children: developmental aspects of compensatory mechanisms. Electroencephal Clin Neurophysiol 1985;61:385–388.)

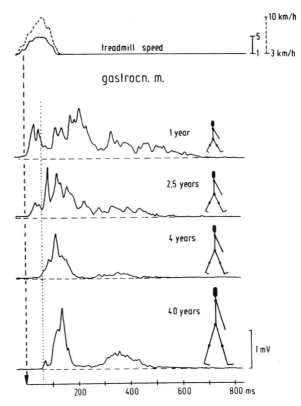

through children 10 years of age, to explore changes in control of these body segments. Based on their findings, balance and locomotion can be organized according to one of two stable reference frames, either the support surface on which the subject stands and moves, or the gravitational reference of vertical.

They noted that when using the support surface as reference, the subject organized balance responses from the feet upward toward the head, using mainly proprioceptive and cutaneous cues. In contrast, when the subject stabilized the head using vestibular information, balance was organized from the head down toward the feet. These researchers explored the changing use of these two strategies in balance control during locomotor development in children (20).

They also noted that the head can be stabilized on the trunk in one of two modes, in an *en bloc* mode, where it moves with the trunk, or in an *articulated* mode, where it moves freely, minimizing movements away from vertical.

This study explored locomotor strategies through kinematic analysis of walking in infants and children up to 8 years of age. The authors found that from the acquisition of stance until about 6 years of age, children organize locomotion in a bottom-up organization, using the support surface as a reference, and controlling head movements in an *en bloc* mode, which serves to reduce the degrees of freedom to be controlled. During this time period, the children gradually learn to stabilize the hip, then the shoulders, and finally the head. At about 7 years of age, with mastery of control of the head, there is a transition, and the head control is changed to an articulated mode, and top-down organization of balance during locomotion becomes dominant. The authors hypothesized that at 7 to 8 years of age, information specifying head position in relation to gravity becomes more available to the equilibrium control centers and thus allows the child to use an articulated mode of head control. They suggest that there may be a transient dominance of vestibular processing in locomotor balance at this age (20).

Development of Other Mobility Skills

The development of postural control underlying the emergence of sitting and standing is covered in detail in Chapter 7. The first part of this chapter describes the emergence of independent locomotion. We now turn briefly to a review of some of the information on the emergence of other mobility behaviors during development, including rolling, prone progression, and movement from lying in a supine position to stance.

There are two approaches to describing motor development in infants and children. One approach relies on normative studies that describe the age at which various motor behaviors emerge. Normative studies have given rise to norm-referenced scales that compare an infant's motor behavior with the performance of a group of infants of the same age. Normative studies can provide clinicians with rough guidelines about the relative ages associated with specific motor milestones. However, they have universally reported that there is incredible variability in the time at which normal children achieve motor milestones (21).

Another approach to describing motor development is with reference to the stages associated with the emergence of a single behavior, such as rolling, or coming to stand. Stages within the emergence of a skill are often used by clinicians as the basis for a treatment progression, with the assumption that a mature and stable adult-like pattern is the last stage in the progression. However, recent research has raised doubts about the concept that there is a consistent stable sequential pattern during the emergence of a particular motor behavior (22, 23).

Given these cautions about timing, variability, and the sequential nature of the emergence of motor skills, we review some of the studies that have examined the stages in the emergence of rolling, prone progression, and the assumption of the vertical position from supine. As we mentioned in the chapter on development of postural control, much of the information we have on the emergence of motor behavior in children is largely the result of efforts in the 1920s and 1930s by two developmental researchers, Arnold Gesell and Myrtle McGraw, who observed and recorded the stages of development in normal children (24).

DEVELOPMENT OF ROLLING

Rolling is an important part of mobility skills because rotation or partial rotation is a part of movement patterns used to achieve supine-to-sit or supine-to-stand behavior. Babies first roll from the side-lying position to the supine position at 1 to 2 months of age and from supine to side-lying at 4 to 5 months. Infants roll from prone to supine at 4 months of age, and then from supine to prone at 6 to 8 months. Infants change their rolling pattern as they mature, from a log-rolling pattern, where the entire body rolls as a unit, to a segmental pattern. By 9 months of age, most infants use a segmental rotation of the body on the pelvis (24, 25).

DEVELOPMENT OF A PRONE PROGRESSION

According to McGraw, the prone progression includes nine phases that take the infant from the prone position to creeping and crawling, and span the months from birth to 10 to 13 months (24). Figure 12.6 illustrates the nine phases reported by McGraw and the relative time in which the behavior was seen. Graphed is the age at which the behavior was seen, and the percent of children in which the behavior was observed. The first phase is characterized by lower extremity flexion and extension in a primarily flexed posture. In phase 2, spinal extension begins, as does the development of head control. In the third phase, spinal extension continues cephalocaudally, reaching the thoracic area. The arms can ex-

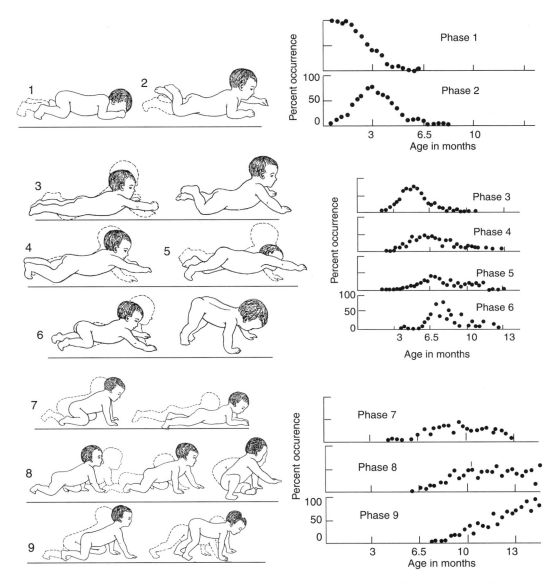

Figure 12.6. The nine phases of prone progression as reported by McGraw. Graphed is the age at which the behavior was seen and the percent of children in which the behavior was observed. See text for details of each stage. (Adapted from McGraw MG. The neuromuscular maturation of the human infant. New York: Hafner Press, 1945.)

tend and support the chest off the surface. Propulsion movements begin in the arms and legs during phases 4 and 5. In phase 6, the creeping position is assumed. Phase 7, is characterized by fairly disorganized attempts at progression; however, by phases 8 and 9, organized propulsion in the creeping position has emerged (24).

Keep in mind that McGraw placed great

emphasis on the neural antecedents of maturing motor behavior. Her emphasis was on describing stages of motor development that could be related to the structural growth and maturation of the central nervous system. Current research has shown that many factors contribute to the emergence of motor skill during development, including but not limited to maturation of the CNS (1, 8).

DEVELOPMENT OF SUPINE-TO-STAND

Just as the pattern used to roll changes as infants age, the movement pattern used to achieve stance from a supine position also undergoes change with development. The pattern initially seen in infants moving from supine to stand includes rolling to prone, then moving into an all-fours pattern, and using a pull-to-stand method to achieve the erect position (24). With development, the child learns to move from the all-fours position to a plantigrade position and from there to erect stance. By the age of 2 to 3 years, the supine-to-prone portion is modified to a partial roll and sit-up pattern, and by ages 4 to 5, a symmetrical sit-up pattern emerges (Fig. 12.7). This is considered a mature or adult-like movement pattern used for this task. But as you remember from the chapter on normal mobility skills, researchers have found tremendous variability in how adults move from supine-to-stand (26). Just as was true for adults, most likely, strength in the abdominals and hip flexors plays a major roll in the type of pattern used by infants when moving from supine-to-stance (26).

LOCOMOTION IN THE OLDER ADULT

Falls and the injuries that often accompany them are a serious problem in the older adult. In fact, falls are the seventh leading cause of death in people over 75 years of age (27). Forty-eight percent of adults over 75 years who have had an injurious fall acquire a fear of falling, and 26% of these people begin avoiding situations that require refined balance skills, thus leading to further decline in walking and balance skills.

Many of the falls experienced by the elderly occur during walking. It is thus important to understand the changes in the systems contributing to normal gait in the elderly to fully understand the cause of increased falls in this population. As we stated in the first section of this chapter, many researchers now believe that balance control is a primary contrib-

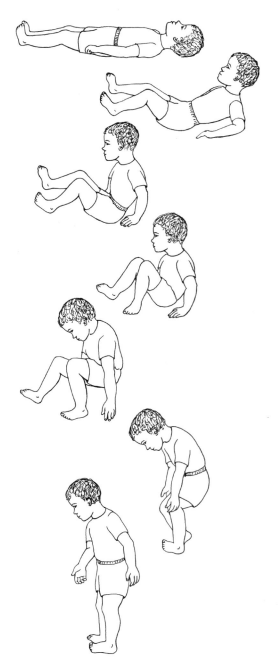

Figure 12.7. Common pattern used to move from supine to stand in children ages 4 to 5. (Adapted from VanSant AF. Age differences in movement patterns used by children to rise from a supine position to erect stance. Phys Ther 1988;68:1130–1138.)

utor to stable walking. In addition, decreased balance control is a major factor affecting loss of independent mobility in many elderly. The following sections describe locomotor changes commonly seen in the older adult and the systems contributing to these changes.

Dysmobility: Aging or Pathology?

Again, age-related changes in locomotion may be due to primary or secondary aging phenomena. Primary factors affecting aging include things like genetics, which result in an inevitable decline of neuronal function within a particular system. Secondary factors are experiential, and include nutrition, exercise, and acquired pathologies, among others.

The extent to which gait disorders in the elderly are due to primary or secondary factors is a very important point to consider as we begin to look at the literature on changes in gait characteristics in the older adult.

The older clinical literature referred to many different walking patterns as age-related gait disorders (28). These diverse gait disorders included: gait apraxia (slow, halting, short-stepped, shuffling, or sliding gait), hypokinetic-hypertonic syndrome (slow, deliberate gait, but without the shuffling or sliding components described above), and marche a petit pas (small, quick shuffling steps, followed by a slow cautious, unsteady gait), vestibular dysfunction gait (difficulties in turning) and proprioceptive dysfunction gait (cautious, with a tendency to watch the feet and make missteps) (28).

As was true in the postural control literature, care must be taken when reviewing studies discussing age-related changes in gait. When interpreting the results of a study, one should examine carefully the population studied, and ask questions such as: What type of criteria were used in selecting older subjects? Did researchers exclude anyone with pathology under the assumption that pathology is not a part of primary aging? Results will vary tremendously depending on the composition of older adults under study.

For example, one study noted that in an unselected group of subjects from 60 to 99 years, walking velocities were much slower than those for young adults, and also slower than other published studies on older adults (29). It is quite possible that the subjects in the study were less fit, and many complained of symptoms likely to impair gait. In contrast, a study that screened 1184 older adults and chose 32 who had no pathology, found no changes in gait parameters tested (30).

Thus, more recent research has begun to indicate that many gait disorders considered to be *age-related*, such as gait apraxia, hypokinetic-hypertonic syndrome, and marche á petit pas, are really manifestations of pathology rather than manifestations of a generalized aging process. However, as we note in the following sections, there appear to be characteristic changes in gait that occur in many, even healthy, older adults.

Temporal-Distance Factors

Studies examining changes in walking patterns with age have used a number of different experimental approaches. In one approach, which we might call a naturalistic approach, adults were observed walking spontaneously in a natural setting. This paradigm was used to try to minimize the constraints on walking style that are often necessary when quantifying gait parameters in a laboratory setting.

In these studies, researchers observed people of different ages walking along the streets of New York City (31) or Amsterdam (32). In the first study, of 752 pedestrians in New York City, as age increased from 20 to 70 years, there was a decrease in walking velocity, step length, and step rate (no statistical analysis was reported). In the second study on 533 pedestrians in Amsterdam, similar results were found. Gender differences were also found; both younger and older women walked with slower velocity, shorter step length, and higher cadence than men (32).

While there are advantages in allowing subjects to walk in a natural environment, the disadvantages include being unable to control for such variables as different walking goals, such as taking a stroll vs. hurrying to work, and relative health of the subjects (28).

Laboratory studies have also repeatedly demonstrated that walking speed decreases with age. One of the earlier studies outlines three stages of age-related changes in walking (33). Stage 1 changes were found in adults between 60 and 72 years of age, and included decreases in walking speed, shorter step length, lower cadence, and less vertical movement of the center of gravity. Subjects between 72 and 86 years old showed stage 2 gait changes, including the disappearance of normal arm-leg synergies, along with an overproduction of unnecessary movements. In stage 3, in subjects ages 86 to 104 years, there was a disintegration of the gait pattern, arrhythmia in the stepping rate, and an absence of arm swing movement (33). It was later pointed out (34) that these changes are not typical of changes seen in healthy older adults, and the study probably included adults with symptoms of Parkinson's disease and other motor pathology.

Kinematic Analysis

Later studies of age-related changes in gait focused on a kinematic analysis of stepping patterns in older adults (34). In one study, subjects were healthy men, with normal strength and range of motion, ranging in age from 20 to 87 years of age. Those over 65 years old were given a neurological exam to exclude the possibility of neurological deficits contributing to the observed changes. Participants were photographed in the laboratory using interrupted-light photography at 20 Hz while walking at their preferred and fast speeds.

Men over 67 years of age showed significantly ($p < .01$) slower walking speeds (118 to 123 cm/sec) than the young adults (150 cm/sec). Stride length was also significantly shorter, especially during fast walking. Vertical movement of the head during the gait cycle was smaller, while lateral movement was larger. Stride width tended to be wider for men over 74. Toeing out was also greater for men over 80. Beyond 65, stance phase was

longer, with a commensurate shortening of time in swing phase (34).

Finally hip, knee, and ankle flexion were less than in young adults, and the whole shoulder rotation pattern was shifted to a more extended position, with less elbow rotation as well. Figure 12.8 is from their study, showing the differences in the limb positions of a younger vs. an older man at heel-strike (34).

Interestingly, the researchers concluded that the men studied did not have a pathological gait pattern. Instead, they said, walking was guarded, possibly with the aim to increase stability. Gait patterns were similar to those used by someone walking on a slippery surface or someone walking in darkness. Doesn't this sound like a postural problem? From reading this description, one might hypothesize that gait changes in the elderly person relate more to the loss of balance control than to changes in the step cycle itself (34).

In a second study (35), age-related changes in gait patterns were investigated in

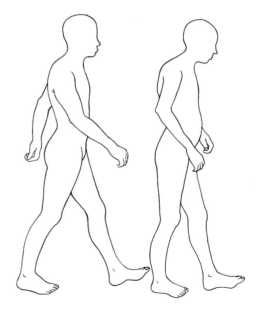

Figure 12.8. Example of the walking pattern of a young adult vs. a healthy older man. (Adapted from Murray MP, Kory RC, Clarkson BH. Walking patterns in healthy old men. J Gerontol 1969;24:169–178.)

women, and similar changes were noted, including reduced walking speeds and shorter steps. These changes occurred in the 60- to 70-year-old age group.

How do these slower walking speeds affect function in daily life? Many of the previous studies report that older adults are unable to walk faster than 1.4 m/min. This is the minimal speed recommended by the Swedish authority to safely pass an intersection. Thus, many of the older adults studied would not be considered functional walkers on city streets with lots of traffic.

Muscle Activation Patterns

The previous studies show clear changes in certain kinematic characteristics of the gait cycle in the average older adult. How do these changes relate to changes in muscle response patterns? In a study comparing patterns of muscle activity in younger (ages 19 to 38 years) and older (ages 64 to 86 years) women, average EMG activity levels in gastrocnemius, tibialis anterior, biceps femoris, rectus femoris, and peroneus longus were higher in the older age group than in the younger group (36).

In addition, there were changes in the activity of individual muscles at specific points in the step cycle. For example, at heel-strike, peroneus longus and gastrocnemius were moderately to highly active in the older women, but showed little or no activity in the younger group. The authors suggested that this increased activity resulted from an effort to improve stability during the stance phase of gait (36). For example, increased coactivation of agonist and antagonist muscles at a joint may be used to improve balance control, by increasing joint stiffness. This is a strategy often seen in subjects who are unskilled in a task, or who are performing in a situation that requires increased control (37).

Kinetic Analysis

We just noted several studies indicating that older adults show higher levels of muscle responses and different activation sequences among leg muscles than young adults during walking. But how do these changes in muscle activation patterns change the dynamics of gait?

Using the method of inverse dynamics, moments of force, as well as the mechanical power generated and absorbed at each joint, can be calculated. This process allows the amount of power generated by muscles to be estimated. Remember from the previous chapter on locomotion that an increase in muscle energy is needed to initiate swing, while a decrease in energy is needed to prepare for heel-strike.

Using inverse dynamics techniques, Winter and colleagues compared the gait patterns of 15 healthy older adults (age range: 62 to 78 years) to 12 young adults (age range: 21 to 28 years) (38). They found that older adults had significantly shorter stride length and longer double-support time than young adults. In addition, in elderly subjects, plantar flexors generated significantly less power at push-off, while the quadriceps muscle absorbed significantly less energy during late stance and early swing.

These researchers concluded that the reduction of plantar flexor power during push-off could explain the shorter step length, flat-footed heel-strike, and increased double-support stance duration. Two alternative explanations were proposed for a weaker push-off in the older adult. One explanation suggested a reduction in muscle strength in the ankle plantar flexors in the older adults could be responsible for the weaker push-off. An alternative explanation argued that reduced push-off could be an adaptive change used to ensure a safer gait, since high push-off power acts upward and forward and is thus destabilizing (38).

In this study, an *index of dynamic balance* was computed to determine the ability to coordinate the anterior/posterior balance of the HAT segment while simultaneously maintaining an appropriate extensor moment in the ankle, knee, and hip during stance phase. It was found that the older adults showed a reduced ability to covary movements at the hip and knee. This means that

Table 12.2.   Summary Gait Changes in the Older Adult

Temporal/distance factors
  Decreased velocity
  Decreased step length
  Decreased step rate
  Decreased stride length
  Increased stride width
  Increased stance phase
  Increased time in double support
  Decreased swing phase
Kinematic changes
  Decreased vertical movement of the center of gravity
  Decreased arm swing
  Decreased hip, knee, ankle flexion
  Flatter foot on heel-strike
  Decreased ability to covary hip/knee movements
  Decreased dynamic stability during stance
Muscle activation patterns
  Increased coactivation (increased stiffness)
Kinetic changes
  Decreased power generation at push-off
  Decreased power absorption at heel-strike

older adults had trouble controlling the HAT segment while simultaneously maintaining an extensor moment in the lower stance limb. In evaluating the older group individually, it was noted that two-thirds were within the normal young adult range, while one-third had very low covariances of moments at the hip and knee. It was concluded that some older adults may have had problems with dynamic balance during locomotion, indicative of balance impairments not detected in their medical history or simple clinical tests (38).

Numerous research studies have described changes in gait patterns found among many older adults. These changes are summarized in Table 12.2.

Changes in Adaptive Control

Many falls by older adults occur while walking and may be due to slipping and tripping. Several research groups have examined proactive adaptive strategies during gait in the elderly. However, there are virtually no studies to date that have examined compensatory postural control in response to perturbed gait in the elderly.

PROACTIVE ADAPTATION

Proactive adaptation depends in large part on the ability to use visual information to alter gait patterns in anticipation of upcoming obstacles (39). One group of researchers asked whether a possible cause of poor locomotor abilities in older adults might be a reduced ability to sample the visual environment during walking (40). They wanted to know whether visual sampling of the environment changed with age.

In their experiment, subjects wore opaque liquid crystal eyeglasses, and pressed a switch to make them transparent whenever they wanted to sample the environment. Subjects walked across a floor that was either unmarked, or that had footprints marked at regular intervals, on which the subjects were supposed to walk. When subjects were constrained to land on the footprints, the young subjects sampled frequently, though for shorter intervals than older subjects, who tended to sample less often, but for longer time periods. Thus, older adults seem to monitor the terrain much more than the young adults (39, 40).

What is the minimum time required to implement an avoidance strategy in the younger vs. older adult? In a second study, healthy young and older adults were asked to walk along a walkway, and when cued by a light at specific points along the walkway, to either lengthen or shorten their stride to match the position of the light (40).

Compared with young adults, older adults had more difficulty in modulating their step length when the cue was given only one step duration ahead. Young adults succeeded 80% of the time, while older adults succeeded 60% of the time when lengthening the step and only 38% of the time when shortening the step. Both groups were equally successful when the cue was given two step durations in advance (40).

The authors suggest that older adults

have more difficulty in shortening a step because of balance constraints. Shortening the step requires regulating the forward pitch of the HAT segment, which if not controlled, could result in a fall. Remember in the review of Winter's study presented earlier, older adults had more trouble than young adults controlling dynamic balance during gait.

These results suggest that the older adult may need to begin making modifications to gait patterns in the step prior to a step requiring obstacle avoidance. This may be one cause of increased visual monitoring.

What strategies do older adults use to avoid obstacles during walking? To answer this question, researchers analyzed the gait of 24 young and 24 older (mean age 71 years) healthy adults while they stepped over obstacles of varying heights (41). Obstacles were made the height of a 1″ or 2″ door threshold or a 6″ curb, and performance was compared to a 0-mm condition (tape marked on the walkway). No age-related changes in foot clearance over the obstacles were found, but older adults used a significantly more conservative strategy when crossing obstacles. Older adults used a somewhat slower approach speed, a significantly slower crossing speed, and a shorter step length. Also, four of the 24 older adults inadvertently stepped on an obstacle, while none of the young adults did (41).

Gait Changes in Fallers vs. Nonfallers

How do the walking characteristics of older adults who fall compare to those with no history of falls? While the previous studies have shown that the gait characteristics of healthy older adults show few differences when compared to younger adults, older individuals with a history of falls show significant differences in walking patterns (42).

Older female subjects with poor balance performance have increased step-width during gait. Other studies reported that step-width measured at the heel was significantly larger in older persons with a history of falls

when they walked at a fast speed of 6 km/hr when compared with subjects without a history of falls (43). It was also noted that older fallers had balance problems unrelated to gait (42) because they were unable to stand as long as non-fallers with feet in tandem position with eyes open. Of course, it is likely that older adults with a history of falls have an undiagnosed pathological condition. Therefore, it is important to carefully examine these subjects, to determine underlying pathology that may contribute to gait disturbances, when performing studies on older adults who fall.

Role of Pathology in Gait Changes in the Elderly

What is the role of secondary aging factors, particularly the role of pathology, in gait abnormalities observed in older adults? In many studies examining apparently healthy older adults, participants are considered pathology-free if they don't have a *known* neurological, cardiovascular, or musculoskeletal disorder. Yet, when this population is examined carefully, many show subtle pathologies. For example, a study on idiopathic gait disorders among older adults found that, on closer medical evaluation, this type of gait pattern could actually be attributed to a number of specific disease processes (44). This suggests that in many instances pathological conditions may be an underlying contributing factor in gait pattern changes seen in older adults. Pathology within a number of systems can potentially affect locomotor skills in the older adult.

COGNITIVE FACTORS

Studies have shown that after repeated falls, older persons develop a fear of falling, and this fear may contribute to changes in gait characteristics as well. For example, it has been shown that preferred walking pace, anxiety level, and depression are good predictors of the extent of fear of falling in community-dwelling older adults (45). Older adults who avoid activities because of a fear of falling tend to walk with a slower pace, and have higher levels of anxiety and depression compared to adults with little fear of falling. This has led several investigators to propose that slowed gait velocity among older adults reflects a conscious strategy used to ensure safe gait, rather than the consequence of specific constraints on walking speed (28, 34, 38).

In other studies examining balance control in older adults with a fear of falling, researchers were not sure whether these adults had real problems with balance control, or whether the fear of falling itself was affecting stability in an artifactual way (46). Thus, it is possible that cognitive factors, such as fear of falling, may contribute to changes in gait patterns in older adults.

SENSORY IMPAIRMENTS

As noted in the chapter on changes in balance control in the older adult, pathologies within visual, proprioceptive, and vestibular systems are common among many older adults, reducing the availability of information from these senses for posture and gait.

Research comparing the perception of vertical and horizontal between six older fallers and six control subjects (ages 67 to 76 years) found that the visual perception of vertical and horizontal showed no differences between the fallers and the controls (47). The research showed, however, that half of the fallers showed problems with recognition of postural tilt when standing on a tilting platform. The older fallers also showed a tendency to lean more heavily on a supporting frame when standing on one leg when compared to control subjects.

These experiments imply that older adults who fall may depend on visual cues to identify postural variations; this suggests that they may have proprioceptive dysfunction. Thus, normal visual cues may be critical for these older adults, as part of altered perceptual strategies to escape additional falls. However, it has also been reported (48) that threshold levels for detection of optical flow associated with normal sway rise in the older adult. If

reduction in sensory function is part of normal aging, it will be important to determine ways to optimize environmental factors and use training to improve stability during walking in older adults.

MUSCLE WEAKNESS

Decreased muscle strength has been indicated as a contributor to locomotor changes in the older adult. In the section on kinetics of the gait cycle, we noted that Winter and colleagues (38) reported a significant decrease in push-off power during gait in healthy older adults, which was possibly related to decreased muscle strength.

Other researchers have studied the strength of the ankle muscles of 111 healthy adults between the ages of 20 and 100 years (49). They found that maximum voluntary muscle strength of the ankle muscles began to drop in adults in their sixties. The older subjects also showed smaller muscle cross-sectional areas and lengthened twitch contraction and half-relaxation times. During maximum voluntary effort, motor nerve stimulation caused no increase in torque in the majority of the older adults. This suggests that healthy older adults are still able to use descending motor pathways in an optimal manner for muscle contraction (49).

Studies have also measured the strength of upper and lower extremities using a simple dynamometer (a modified sphygmomanometer) (50). Results showed that after the age of 75, age is the most significant factor predicting a drop in muscle strength (other factors included were height, weight, and sum of skinfolds). The strength recorded for elbow flexion, grip, knee extension, and dorsiflexion was the best indicator of overall limb strength. Reductions in strength of knee extensor and flexor muscles for both concentric and eccentric contractions have also been reported in a study comparing healthy older women (66 to 89 years old) with younger women (20 to 29 years old) (51). There were fewer age-related differences for eccentric contractions than concentric contractions.

Do these reductions in muscle strength relate to meaningful changes in function? Yes. It has been shown that fallers (mean age 82 years) with no clear pathology showed significantly reduced ability of the ankle and knee muscles to generate peak torque and power when compared to a group of age-matched nonfallers (52). These results suggest that muscle weakness (primarily in the ankle muscles), is a significant contributing factor to balance dysfunction in older adults. High-intensity resistance training has been shown to increase knee extensor muscle strength, muscle size, and to enhance functional mobility in frail older adults in their nineties (53). Mean tandem gait speed was increased in this group by 48% after an 8-week training program. In addition, two of the frail older subjects no longer used canes as an aid in walk at the end of the training period.

In summary, age-related reduction in muscle strength has been found in selected upper and lower extremity muscles. Concentric contraction is more affected in older female subjects than eccentric contraction for knee muscles. Strength training can improve functional mobility in older frail adults. However, since decreased mobility and increased likelihood for falls is the result of many factors, not just weakness, strength training alone may not be sufficient to improve balance and mobility function in many older adults with impaired balance.

Stair-Walking

Research has documented that walking on stairs is associated with the highest proportion of falls in public places, and that most of these falls occur as subjects walk down the stairs. To understand the physical requirements of stair-walking in older adults, characteristics of stair descent were studied in a group of 36 healthy women between the ages of 55 and 70 (55). Participants were asked to walk down a set of stairs under conditions of poor or distorted visual inputs. For example, (*a*) stairs were painted black, (*b*) vision of the stair was blurred (stairs were painted black

and the subject wore a headband with a light-scattering plastic shield), or (*c*) stairs were painted black with a white stripe at the edge of each tread. The stairs were surrounded by a striped corridor.

The results of high-speed film analysis showed significantly slower cadence, larger foot clearance, and more posterior foot placement while subjects walked under the blurred condition as compared to the other two stair color conditions. The authors further observed that foot clearance was larger than that obtained during previous pilot work from their laboratory on young adults. They concluded that older subjects walked with larger foot clearance during stair descent compared to young adults and that gait patterns during stair descent were affected by visual conditions.

Age-Related Changes in Other Mobility Skills

SIT-TO-STAND

Research indicates that 8% of community dwelling older adults over 65 years of age show some problems in rising from a chair or bed. As a result, several studies have examined the sit-to-stand (STS) task in older adults (55, 56).

One study compared movement strategies, forces used, and the time taken to rise from sitting among young adults, older adults able to rise without armrests (old able), and older adults unable to rise from a chair (old unable). Average rise times from a chair were similar in the young and old able groups (1.56 vs 1.83 sec), but significantly longer in the old unable group (3.16 sec). In addition, the hand forces used by the old able group were significantly less than those used by the old unable group.

The old able were mainly different from the young in the amount of time they spent in the initial phase of rising from the chair, which included the time from start to lift-off from the seat. They flexed their legs and trunks more during trials in which they used no hands to help themselves rise.

While all the elderly subjects reported no significant musculoskeletal or neurological impairment, a significantly larger proportion of the old unable group had a history of vertebral fractures, decreased vision, dizziness, poor balance, and falls. Every old unable subject also had muscle weakness in the lower extremity, decreased proprioception in the hands and feet, and spinal and lower extremity deformities such as kyphosis and osteoarthritis (55, 56).

RISING FROM A BED

Are there age-related differences in movement patterns used in rising from a bed? To answer this question, adults ranging in age from 30 to 59 years of age were videotaped while rising from a bed (57). As had been reported for young adults, there was considerable variability in patterns for rising from a bed among the older group, aged 50 to 59. As was mentioned in our previous chapter, the most common patterns of bed rising in the 30- to 39-year-old group involved a grasp and

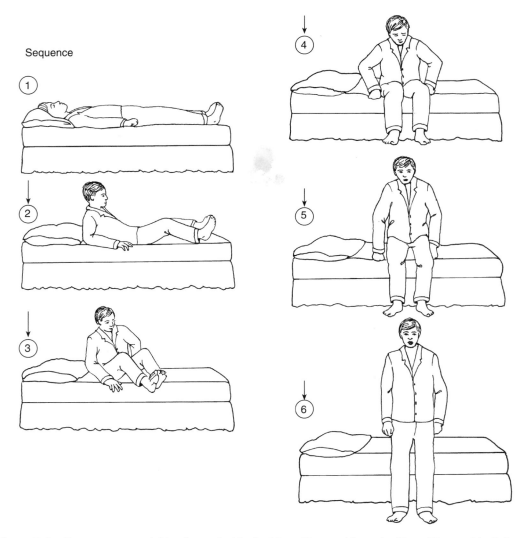

Figure 12.9. Frequent pattern of rising from a bed in the 30- to 39-year-olds vs. the 50- to 59-year-olds. (Adapted from Ford-Smith CD, VanSant AF. Age differences in movement patterns used to rise from a bed in subjects in the third through fifth decades of age. Phys Ther 1993;73:305.)

push pattern with the upper extremities, a roll-off or come-to-sit pattern, and a synchronous lifting of the lower limbs off the bed with one limb extending to the floor in front of the other. The older group, consisting of 50- to 59-year-olds, tended to use a more synchronous lifting pattern, with both legs moved to the floor simultaneously (Fig. 12.9). No studies to date have been published on patterns used by the elderly when rising from the bed. Since many elderly people report falls at night associated with getting out of bed, the need for such a study is essential.

COMPARING GAIT CHARACTERISTICS OF INFANTS AND ELDERLY: TESTING THE REGRESSION HYPOTHESIS

It has been suggested that changes in the gait pattern among the elderly are related to the reemergence of immature walking patterns seen in young infants. Thus, it is hypothesized that, as aging occurs, there is a regression to immature reflex patterns that characterized movement in young infants. This regression is thought to result from loss of higher center control over the primitive reflexes that reemerge in the very old (54). What are the similarities and differences between the gait characteristics of the very young and the very old?

Both groups show a shorter duration of single-limb stance and a greater relative duration of double support. This has been interpreted in both groups as an indication of decreased balance abilities (13, 15, 30, 34).

The gait of young walkers has also been described as having a wide base of support along with toeing-out, a characteristic observed in the elderly as well (13, 34). It has been suggested in both groups that an increased base of support is used to ensure better balance control.

Finally, both young children (7) and older adults (36) show coactivation of agonist and antagonist muscles during gait. This again has been described as a way of increas-

ing joint stiffness, which helps in balance control (37).

Clearly, there are many similarities in the gait characteristics of the young child and the older adult. These similarities appear to relate to difficulties with balance control common to both groups. Thus, it is not necessarily true that similarities between the very old and very young are due to a reappearance of primitive reflexes. In this case, the reason is a functional one: the two groups, for often very different reasons, have difficulties with the balance system, but use similar strategies to compensate for those difficulties.

SUMMARY

1. There are three requirements for successful locomotion: (a) the ability to generate a rhythmic stepping pattern to move the body forward (progression), (b) the control of balance (stability), and (c) the ability to adapt gait to changing task and environmental requirements (adaptation). In the development of locomotion, these three factors emerge sequentially, with the stepping pattern appearing first, equilibrium control next, followed by adaptive capabilities.

2. The emergence of independent gait is characterized by the development of many interacting systems with certain hierarchical components. An innate pattern generator creates the basic rhythm of the step cycle, which can be seen in newborn stepping. In the first year, the gradual development of descending systems from higher neural centers gives the child increasing control over this locomotor behavior. The control of equilibrium, organized at a higher level than that of the pattern generator, develops over a longer period, as do adaptive systems essential to the integration of reactive and proactive strategies into gait.

3. The development of locomotion behavior begins prenatally and continues until the emergence of mature gait at about 7 years of age. Stepping behavior is present at birth and can be elicited in most infants if they are supported and inclined slightly forward. This early behavior resembles quadrupedal stepping, with flexion of the hip and knee, synchronous joint motion, and considerable

coactivation of agonist and antagonist muscles.

4. In many infants, early stepping disappears at about 2 months of age, possibly due to biomechanical changes in the infant's system, such as an increase in relative body weight. Early stepping gradually transforms into a more mature pattern over the first 2 years of life.

5. There seems to be agreement among researchers that the ability to integrate postural control into the locomotor pattern is the most important rate-limiting factor on the emergence of independent walking.

6. The most significant modifications to the gait pattern occur during the first 4 to 5 months of independent walking. Most of these changes reflect the child's growing ability to integrate balance control with locomotion in these first months.

7. Studies characterizing gait patterns in older adults have consistently shown that healthy older adults have reduced walking speed, shorter stride length, and shorter step length than young adults.

8. Proactive locomotor abilities also change with age, with older adults taking more time to monitor the visual environment, more time to alter an upcoming step to avoid an obstacle, and using strategies such as slowing of approach and cross-over time when stepping over obstacles.

9. Changes in the characteristics of gait patterns in older adults are influenced by balance ability, leg muscle strength, and changes in the availability of sensory information. Cognitive factors such as fear of falling and inattention may also be important contributors.

10. When evaluating gait patterns of older people, consideration must be given to the underlying mechanisms contributing to these changes. In this way, one can differentiate between contributions related to pathology vs. aging per se. Only after the systems contributing to walking pattern dysfunction are identified can a clinician design effective and appropriate interventions to improve gait and thus help older adults achieve a safe and independent life-style.

REFERENCES

1. Thelen E, Ulrich BD. Hidden skills: a dynamic systems analysis of treadmill stepping during the first year. Monographs of the Society for Research in Child Development. Serial 223, vol 56, 1991.

2. Prechtl HFR. Continuity and change in early neural development. In: Prechtl HFR, ed. Continuity of neural functions from prenatal to postnatal life. Clinics in Developmental Medicine. No. 94. Oxford: Blackwell Scientific Publications, 1984:1–15.

3. De Vries JIP, Visser GHA, Prechtl HFR. The emergence of fetal behavior. I. Qualitative aspects. Early Human Dev 1982;7:301–322.

4. Bradley NS, Smith JL. Neuromuscular patterns of stereotypic hindlimb behaviors in the first two postnatal months. I. Stepping in normal kittens. Dev Brain Res 1988;38:37–52.

5. Stehouwer DJ, Farel PB. Development of hindlimb locomotor behavior in the frog. Dev Psychobiol 1984;17:217–232.

6. Bradley NS, Bekoff A. Development of locomotion: animal models. In: Woollacott MH, Shumway-Cook A, eds. Development of posture and gait across the lifespan. Columbia, SC: Univ. of South Carolina Press, 1989:48–73.

7. Forssberg H. Ontogeny of human locomotor control: 1. Infant stepping, supported locomotion and transition to independent locomotion. Exp Brain Res 1985;67:480–493.

8. Thelen E, Ulrich B, Jensen J. The developmental origins of locomotion. In: Woollacott MH, Shumway-Cook A, eds. Development of posture and gait across the lifespan. Columbia, SC: Univ. of South Carolina Press, 1989:25–47.

9. McGraw MB. The neuromuscular maturation of the human infant. NY: Columbia University Press, 1945.

10. Thelen E, Fisher DM, Ridley-Johnson R. The relationship between physical growth and a newborn reflex. Infant Behavior and Development 1984;7:479–93.

11. Peiper A. Cerebral functions in infancy and childhood. New York: Consultants Bureau, 1961.

12. Woollacott MH, Shumway-Cook A, Williams H. The development of posture and balance control in children. In: Woollacott MH, Shumway-Cook A, eds. Development of posture and gait across the lifespan. Columbia, SC: Univ. of South Carolina Press, 1989:77–96.

13. Bril B, Breniere Y. Posture and independent locomotion in childhood: learning to walk or

learning dynamic postural control? In: Savelsbergh GJP, ed. The development of coordination in infancy. Amsterdam: North-Holland, 1993, 337–358.

14. Okamoto T, Kumamoto M. Electromyographic study of the learning process of walking in infants. Electromyography 1972; 12:149–158.

15. Sutherland DH, Olshen R, Cooper L, Woo S. The development of mature gait. J Bone Joint Surg 1980;62-A:336–353.

16. Gallahue DL. Understanding motor development: infants, children, adolescents. Indianapolis: Benchmark Press, 1989.

17. Clark JE, Whitall J. Changing patterns of locomotion: from walking to skipping. In: Woollacott MH, Shumway-Cook A, eds. Development of posture and gait across the lifespan. Columbia, SC: Univ. of South Carolina Press, 1989:128–151.

18. Berger W, Quintern J, Dietz V. Stance and gait perturbations in children: developmental aspects of compensatory mechanisms. Electroencephalography and clinical Neurophysiology 1985;61:385–395.

19. Hass G, Diener HC. Development of stance control in children. In: Amblard B, Berthoz A, Clarac F, eds. Development, adaptation and modulation of posture and gait. Amsterdam: Elsevier, 1988:49–58.

20. Assaiante C, Amblard B. An ontogenetic model for the sensorimotor organization of balance control in humans. In press.

21. Palisano RJ. Neuromotor and developmental assessment. In: Wilhelm IJ, ed. Physical therapy assessment in early infancy. New York: Churchill Livingstone, 1993:173–224.

22. Fishkind M, Haley SM. Independent sitting development and the emergence of associated motor components. Phys Ther 1986; 66:1509–1514.

23. Horowitz L, Sharby N. Development of prone extension postures in healthy infants. Phys Ther 1988;68:32–39.

24. McGraw MG. The neuromuscular maturation of the human infant. New York: Hafner Press, 1945.

25. Touwen B. Neurological development in infancy. Clinics in Developmental Medicine, No 58. Philadelphia: JB Lippincott, 1976.

26. VanSant AF. Age differences in movement patterns used by children to rise from a supine position to erect stance. Phys Ther 1988; 68:1130–1138.

27. Ochs AL, Newberry J, Lenhardt ML, Harkins SW. Neural and vestibular aging associated with falls. In: Birren JE, Schaie KW, eds. Handbook of the psychology of aging, NY: Van Nostrand & Reinholdt 1985;378–399.

28. Craik R. Changes in locomotion in the aging adult. In: Woollacott MH, Shumway-Cook A, eds. Development of posture and gait across the lifespan. Columbia, SC: Univ. of South Carolina Press, 1989:176–201.

29. Imms FJ, Edholm OG. Studies of gait and mobility in the elderly. Age Ageing 1981; 10:147–156.

30. Gabell A, Nayak USL. The effect of age on variability in gait. J Gerontol 1984;39:662–666.

31. Drillis R. The influence of aging on the kinematics of gait. The geriatric amputee, publication 919. National Academy of Science, National Research Council, 1961.

32. Molen HH. Problems on the evaluation of gait. [Dissertation]. Amsterdam: Free University, The Institute of Biomechanics and Experimental Rehabilitation, 1973.

33. Spielberg PI. Walking patterns of old people: cyclographic analysis. In: Bernstein NA, ed. Investigations on the biodynamics of walking, running, and jumping. Moscow: Central Scientific Institute of Physical Culture, 1940.

34. Murray MP, Kory RC, Clarkson BH. Walking patterns in healthy old men. J Gerontol 1969;24:169–178.

35. Murray MP, Kory RC, Sepic SB. Walking patterns of normal women. Arch Phys Med Rehabil 1970;51:637–650.

36. Finley FR, Cody KA, Finizie RV. Locomotion patterns in elderly women. Arch Phys Med 1969;50:140–146.

37. Woollacott M. Gait and postural control in the aging adult. In: Bles W, Brandt T, eds. Disorders of posture and gait. Amsterdam: Elsevier, 1986:325–336.

38. Winter DA, Patla AE, Frank JS, Walt SE. Biomechanical walking pattern changes in the fit and healthy elderly. Phys Ther 1990;70:340–347.

39. Patla AE. Age-related changes in visually guided locomotion over different terrains: major issues. In: Stelmach G, Homberg V, eds. Sensorimotor impairment in the elderly. Dordrecht: Kluwer, 1993:231–252.

40. Patla AE, Prentice SD, Martin C, Rietdyk S. The bases of selection of alternate foot placement during locomotion in humans. In: Posture and gait: control mechanisms. Woolla-

cott MH, Horak F, eds. Eugene, OR: Univ. of Oregon Books, 1992: 226–229.

41. Chen H, Ashton-Miller JA, Alexander NB, Schultz AB. Stepping over obstacles: gait patterns of healthy young and old adults. J Gerontol 1991;46:M196–M203.

42. Heitmann DK, Gossman MR, Shaddeau SA, Jackson JR. Balance performance and step width in non-institutionalized elderly female fallers and nonfallers. Phys Ther 1989; 69:923–931.

43. Gehlsen GM, Whaley MH. Falls in the elderly: Part I, gait. Arch Phys Med Rehabil 1990:71:735–738.

44. Sudarsky L, Ronthal M. Gait disorders among elderly patients: a survey study of 50 patients. Arch Neurol 1983;40:740–743.

45. Tinetti ME, Richman D, Powell L. Falls efficacy as a measure of fear of falling. J Gerontol 1990;45:P239–P243.

46. Maki BE, Holliday PJ, Topper AK. Fear of falling and postural performance in the elderly. J Gerontol 1991;46:M123–M131.

47. Brownlee MG, Banks MA, Crosbie WJ, Meldrum F, Nimmo MA. Consideration of spatial orientation mechanisms as related to elderly fallers. Gerontology 1989;35:323–331.

48. Warren WH, Blackwell AW, Morris MW. Age differences in perceiving the direction of self-motion from optical flow. J Gerontol 1989; 44:P147–P153.

49. Vandervoort AA, McComas AJ. Contractile changes in opposing muscles of the human ankle joint with aging. J Appl Physiol 1986; 61:361–367.

50. Rice CL, Cunningham DA, Paterson DH, Rechnitzer PA. Strength in an elderly population. Arch Phys Med Rehabil 1989;70:391–397.

51. Vandervoort AA, Kramer JF, Wharram ER. Eccentric knee strength of elderly females. J Gerontol 1990;45:B125–B128.

52. Whipple RH, Wolfson LI, Amerman PM. The relationship of knee and ankle weakness to falls in nursing home residents: an isokinetic study. J Am Geriatr Soc 1987;35:13–20.

53. Fiatarone MA, Marks EC, Ryan ND, Meredith CN, Lipsitz LA, Evans WJ. High-intensity strength training in nonagenarians. JAMA 1990;263:3029–3034.

54. Shaltenbrand G. The development of human motility and motor disturbances. Arch Neurol Psychiatr 1928;20:720.

55. Simoneau GG, Cavanagh PR, Ulbrecht JS, Leibowitz HW, Tyrrell RA. The influence of visual factors on fall-related kinematic variables during stair descent by older women. J Gerontol 1991;46:M188–M195.

55. Alexander NB, Schultz AB, Warwick DN. Rising from a chair: effect of age and functional ability on performance biomechanics. J Gerontol 1991;46:M91–M98.

56. Millington PJ, Myklebust BM, Shambes GM. Biomechanical analysis of the sit-to-stand motion in elderly persons. Arch Phys Med Rehabil 1992;73:609–617.

57. Ford-Smith CD, VanSant AF. Age differences in movement patterns used to rise from a bed in subjects in the third through fifth decades of age. Phys Ther 1993;73:300–309.

Chapter 13

ABNORMAL MOBILITY

INTRODUCTION

This chapter describes impaired mobility function in the patient with neurological impairments, including abnormalities of gait, stair-walking, and transfers. Using the framework established in our previous chapter on abnormal postural control, we examine problems that affect mobility function in the patient with an upper motor neuron lesion (UMN). We first examine the various types of impairments resulting from a UMN lesion, then look at how impairments affect movement strategies within the stance and swing phases of gait. We also consider how impairments affect the ability to adapt strategies to changes in goals and/or environmental demands. Finally, we list various mobility prob-

lems from a diagnostic perspective, presenting the kinds of mobility problems often found in patients with stroke, Parkinson's disease, and cerebral palsy.

Understanding the effects of sensory, motor, and cognitive impairments on mobility function, as well as the types of patients likely to have these problems, will assist the clinician in assessing and planning treatments that are effective in retraining mobility.

ABNORMAL GAIT

While abnormal gait is a common characteristic of many neurological pathologies, the constellation of underlying problems that produce disordered gait varies from patient to patient, even within the same general area of pathology. A patient's problems with gait will depend on both the type of impairment and the extent to which the patient is able to compensate for that impairment. Understanding the contribution of these two elements to gait dysfunction in the patient with neurological dysfunction can be very difficult. As a result, technology such as EMG, kinematic, and/or kinetic analysis is often necessary to distinguish impairment from compensation. Technology is thus used extensively in studies examining gait dysfunction in the patient with neurological impairments.

There are many people whose research has contributed to our understanding of pathological gait. Among them is Dr. Jacquelin Perry, a noted orthopedic surgeon, who began her work in gait analysis as a practicing physical therapist. Dr. Perry and her colleagues at Rancho Los Amigos Gait laboratory at UCLA have studied gait in many types of patient populations. She has published extensively, including a very comprehensive and detailed book on normal and pathological gait function (1). Much of the knowledge found in this section on abnormal gait is based on research by Dr. Perry and her colleagues (2, 3).

During the recovery of mobility function following a neurological lesion, a primary focus of therapy will be on helping the patient to regain progression, stability, and adaptive functions underlying the control of gait. A key to developing effective mobility function is understanding the musculoskeletal and neural constraints or impairments that affect the patient's ability to walk and perform other mobility skills. In the following sections we discuss the constraints on motor control resulting from dysfunction in the different systems contributing to mobility function.

Musculoskeletal Limitations

Both soft tissue contractures and bony constrictions limit joint range of motion (ROM). This constrains movement and potentially increases the workload on the muscles, thus affecting a patient's ability to meet the requirements of gait. In general, decreased joint mobility during stance restricts forward motion of the body over the supporting foot, thus affecting *progression*. In swing, decreased joint mobility reduces foot clearance, affecting *progression*, and appropriate foot placement for weight acceptance, affecting *stability*. Limited range of motion also limits a patient's ability to modify movement strategies, thus affecting *adaptation*. For example, a patient with limited ankle and knee flexion will be unable to increase limb flexion during the swing phase of gait to step over an obstacle.

As we mentioned in the chapter on abnormal postural control, musculoskeletal limitations found in the patient with neurological dysfunction most often develop secondary to a UMN lesion. Musculoskeletal impairments that particularly affect gait include ankle extensor contractures, knee and hip flexor contractures, and reduced pelvic and spinal mobility.

Neuromuscular Impairments

Many categories of neuromuscular problems affect gait in the patient with neurological impairments. These range from force control problems, including both weakness and abnormalities of muscle tone, to timing problems.

WEAKNESS

Upper motor neuron lesions affect both the non-neural and neural components of force production. Neural lesions can produce a primary neuromuscular impairment affecting the number, type, and discharge frequency of motor neurons recruited during a voluntary contraction, as well as during gait (1, 4). In addition, secondary changes in the muscle fibers themselves affect the patient's ability to generate tension. Muscles act in gait both concentrically to generate motion, and eccentrically to control motion. Thus, weakness can result in both the inability to generate forces to move the body, as well as unrestrained motions such as foot-slap following heel-strike. Foot-slap results from loss of eccentric control by the tibialis anterior and un-controlled plantarflexion (1).

How much does weakness affect the ability to walk independently? This depends on what muscles are weak, and the capacity of other muscles to substitute for weak muscles in achieving the requirements of gait. For example, trunk strength is needed to keep the HAT segment upright. However, no significant trunk deviations occur in gait unless weakness in the trunk muscles is significant, that is, less than a grade 3 on a manual muscle test (1).

Nevertheless, weak hip extensors will have a tremendous impact on the patient's ability to walk when that patient also has a hip flexion contracture, requiring a forward lean posture of the trunk. Strong hip and trunk extensors will be needed to keep the patient's trunk from further flexing under the effects of gravity (1).

The inability to recruit motor units, whether due to weakness or control problems, affects the patient's ability to meet all three requirements of locomotion, that is, progression, stability, and adaptation.

MUSCLE TONE AND CHANGES IN STIFFNESS

As we mentioned in the chapter on abnormal postural control, abnormalities of muscle tone are characteristic of most UMN lesions. The type and severity of muscle tone problems vary, depending on the location and extent of the neural lesion. Spasticity, which is a velocity-dependent increase in the stretch reflex, is the most common manifestation of abnormal muscle tone seen in the patient with a UMN lesion. Spasticity affects gait in a number of ways.

The generation of momentum and the transfer of momentum to adjacent body segments is an important aspect of progression, and results in an energy-efficient gait. Transfer of momentum requires that one joint be able to move freely relative to another joint, changing directions rapidly (5). Therefore, changes in the mechanical properties of the musculoskeletal system, in particular in-creased stiffness of a joint, can affect the free-dom of body segments to move rapidly with regard to one another. This limits the transfer of momentum during gait, affecting the progression requirements of locomotion (5).

Spasticity, or increased stiffness, also manifests as excessive activation of muscles in response to stretch. Stretch-dependent gait abnormalities are primarily apparent in those phases of gait in which the spastic muscle is being lengthened rapidly. For example, rapid knee flexion, just following weight acceptance at the beginning of stance, can result in excessive activation of a spastic quadriceps, due to the rapid lengthening of the muscle.

CONTROL PROBLEMS

We define control problems as muscle activation problems that manifest as task-specific locomotor difficulties, such as the inability to recruit a muscle during gait, even though voluntary force generation may be intact. It is important to note that there is often no clear distinction between problems such as weakness, tone, and control, since they are interrelated in the patient with a neurological disability.

The inability to recruit a muscle during an automatic task such as posture or gait was discussed in the chapter on abnormal posture control. Because a patient has some ability to generate force voluntarily during a manual muscle test does not mean that the muscle will perform normally during movement strategies needed for gait. Therefore, strength is not always a good predictor of performance in locomotion.

Control problems can also be seen as an inappropriate activation of a muscle during gait which is not related to stretch of the muscle and therefore not defined as spasticity. An example is overactivity of the hamstrings in phases of gait when the muscle is not being lengthened (6).

Coactivation of agonist and antagonist muscles around a joint can increase stiffness and decrease motion, thereby affecting progression during gait (1, 6, 7). Some researchers believe that coactivation of muscles during gait does not always represent an impairment, but may be a compensatory strategy to disordered control (7, 8).

Control problems in patients with neurological lesions, particularly in the cerebellum, can produce problems related to scaling the amplitude of muscle activity during gait, producing what is called an ataxic gait pattern. Scaling problems were discussed in more detail in the chapter on abnormal postural control.

Sensory Disorders

Sensation is a critical determinant for maintaining gait in natural environments where we are required to constantly modify how we move in response to changes in our surroundings. Sensory inputs play several important roles in the control of locomotion. They are critical to signaling terminal stance and serve as a trigger for the initiation of swing (9). In addition, sensory inputs are necessary in adapting locomotor patterns to changes in environmental demands. This includes signaling unanticipated disruptions to gait, as well as the ability to predict and anticipate upcoming obstacles.

SOMATOSENSORY DEFICITS

Abnormal somatosensory inputs result in gait ataxia (10). Gait problems in patients with sensory ataxia can be due to interruption of either peripheral or central proprioceptive pathways. When this occurs, the patient is usually no longer aware of the position of the legs in space, or even of the position of the body itself. With mild sensory dysfunction, walking may not appear to be obviously abnormal, if the patient can use vision. However, ataxia is worse when visual cues are reduced or inappropriate. Staggering and unsteadiness increase, and some patients lose the ability to walk (10).

VISUAL DEFICITS

Loss of vision affects primarily stability aspects of gait, reducing the patient's ability to modify gait patterns in response to obstacles in the environment. Visually impaired and blind patients tend to walk more slowly. In addition, they appear able to utilize auditory cues to assist in locating obstacles in space (11).

VESTIBULAR DEFICITS

Patients with vestibular deficits may walk more slowly than normal subjects. Other changes include a prolonged double-support phase, and a 6.5% longer cycle time than normal subjects (12). Interestingly, when vestibular patients were asked to walk at a normal velocity, using a metronome to establish the pace, their double-support phase duration became more normal. It is not clear why vestibular patients seem to prefer a slower gait and whether practicing at faster speeds would improve the kinematics of their gait cycle (12).

It has been reported that these patients may also show impairments in head stabilization during gait, especially when walking in the dark (13–15). Surprisingly, gaze is equally stable for vestibular deficit patients and normal subjects during sitting and standing. However, when walking, the ability to stabilize gaze is impaired and thus patients have complaints of impaired vision and oscillopsia. In addition, eye movements compensate for head movements more effectively during active head rotations than during similar movements made while walking. It has been suggested that this may be due to the predictable nature of active voluntary head movements vs. the passive head movements made during locomotion (14).

When normal subjects walk or run in the dark, the amplitude and velocity of head rotation are decreased compared to head movements during normal walking. However, these parameters increase for subjects with bilateral vestibular deficits when they walk in the dark (15).

MISREPRESENTATION OF STABILITY LIMITS

Many patients with neurological dysfunction have problems with impaired body image. This can result in a number of gait deviations, including ipsilateral trunk lean towards the stance leg, resulting in loss of stability. Impaired body image can also result in inappropriate foot placement, and difficulty in controlling the center of body mass relative to the changing base of support of the feet (1).

ADAPTATION PROBLEMS

Very few studies have focused on the adaptability of the gait cycle in patients with neurological impairments. Adaptability includes the ability to avoid obstacles and to vary the step cycle in unusual terrains to prevent accidents. Clinicians working with patients with neurological impairments are well aware that such problems exist, but there is virtually no research examining exactly how adaptation becomes impaired.

Pain

Pain can also cause the patient to alter movement patterns used for gait. For example, rapid motion of the knee of a patient with intrinsic joint pathology can result in pain. This will limit knee flexion and affect gait in much the same way as when the patient has weakened quadriceps muscles (1).

In addition, pain at the hip is a primary cause of persistent hip flexion and inadequate hip extension during gait. Intra-articular pressure is least at 30° to 40° flexion. As a result, this is the position most often assumed by patients who are experiencing pain (1).

EFFECTS OF IMPAIRMENTS ON PHASES OF GAIT

In the previous section, we reviewed the range of impairments commonly found in patients with neurological dysfunction that can potentially constrain gait. We now look more specifically at how impairments affect progression, stability, and adaptation requirements within each of the phases of gait. Using a problem-based format, we first describe the problem, then discuss the range of impairments that can produce the problem. The dis-

cussion highlights common problems found in the patient with neurological impairments, and is not intended as an exhaustive review of all gait abnormalities. The reader is referred to the extensive review by Perry (1) for further information.

This method of analysis is important preparation for our next chapter, which discusses assessment and treatment of mobility problems. It is the format used for observational gait analysis, the primary clinical tool used to evaluate gait abnormalities. In addition, treatment strategies useful in retraining gait are presented within a problem-based framework.

Stance
FOOT CONTACT/LOADING

The position of the foot when it meets the floor at the beginning of the stance phase of gait has a great impact on both stability and progression. Normally, contact is made with the heel of the foot. This is followed by an eccentric activation of the tibialis anterior (TA), allowing a controlled plantarflexion of the ankle, and a smooth transference of weight to the entire foot. Heel-strike and the subsequent smooth transference of weight to the whole foot are essential to redirecting momentum important to forward progression. In addition, a proper heel-strike foot position secures a stable base of support during weight acceptance, and therefore is important to stability.

Problem 1. Impaired Heel-Strike

Abnormalities at foot-strike and loading are shown in Figure 13.1, and can include: low heel contact, foot-flat contact, forefoot contact, contact made with the medial (or lateral) border of the foot, and foot-slap during loading. A wide range of problems occurring at the ankle, knee, and hip joints can reduce a patient's ability to use a heel-strike strategy during the initiation of stance.

Causes
Ankle joint plantarflexion contractures. During the stance phase of gait, ankle plantarflexor contractions can impair a pa-

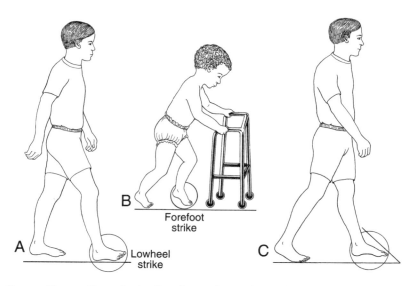

Figure 13.1. Abnormal foot position at heel-strike. Abnormalities at foot-strike include **A**, low-heel contact, **B**, forefoot contact, and **C**, flat-foot contact. (Adapted from Perry J. Gait analysis: normal and pathological function. Thorofare, NJ: Slack, Inc., 1992:315, 324.)

tient's ability to move the limb over the foot. The effect of a plantarflexion contracture on foot-strike will vary, depending on its severity. Fifteen degrees of plantarflexion contracture is common in adults with acquired disability, and usually results in a low heel contact and early flat-foot during loading. A 30° contracture is not uncommon in children with spastic cerebral palsy, and produces a forefoot contact at foot-strike (1).

Gastrocnemius/soleus spasticity. Severe spasticity in the gastrocnemius (G) and soleus muscles results in the continued activation of these muscles during most of gait. Clinically, it can be difficult to distinguish between a spastic G and a contracted G (1). Often, excessive G activity is part of an extensor synergy gait pattern. The strategy for initial contact depends on the knee position. Low heel or flat-foot contact is made with an extended knee, while a flexed knee is associated with a forefoot contact.

If there is no motion available at the ankle, forefoot support continues. Alternatively, if motion at the ankle is possible, the heel drops, but the tibia is driven backwards, resulting in hyperextension or back-kneeing (1, 3).

Inactivity of tibialis anterior. Inability to activate the TA results in a flat-foot at foot-strike, or alternatively, the heel may strike, but the foot drops quickly (foot-slap) due to inadequate eccentric contraction of the anterior tibialis. The presence of a rapid foot-drop following heel-strike suggests that the underlying impairment is an inactive TA rather than a spastic or contracted G or soleus (1, 3).

Inadequate knee extension during terminal swing. Inadequate knee extension, particularly at the end of the swing phase of gait, will keep the knee from fully extending, thus affecting placement of the foot in preparation for stance. Inadequate knee extension can be due to knee flexion contractures, or from overactivity of the hamstrings (1, 3).

Problem 2. Coronal Plane Deviations

Coronal plane deviations at foot-strike include excessive inversion (varus foot) or excessive eversion (valgus foot).

Causes

Excessive varus: spastic invertors. Excessive inversion, referred to clinically as a varus foot, is common in patients with ankle-joint spasticity. Varus is seen clinically as the elevation of the first metatarsal head from the floor with the subsequent foot contact made on the lateral border of the foot only. Excessive varus foot position tends to be seen primarily in spastic patients.

Because of the many muscles that cross the ankle joint, there are potentially many different causes of excessive varus during gait. Inappropriate action of the soleus muscle during terminal swing is one of the most common causes, and results in excessive varus at heel-strike. Excessive inversion in swing is often associated with activation of the anterior tibialis muscle (part of a total flexion synergy) and inactivity of the toe extensors (1, 3).

Causes

Valgus: inactive invertors. Valgus is seen clinically as excessive eversion, with most of the support carried on the medial portions of the foot, in particular, the first metatarsal head. The most common cause of valgus is weakness or inaction by the ankle invertors, for example, a weak or inactive soleus. Thus, a flaccid paralysis tends to lead to a valgus foot posture (1, 3).

MID-STANCE

In mid-stance, the foot is stationary, and tibial advance is controlled by the graded eccentric contraction of the soleus muscle. A smooth progression over the supporting foot requires a minimum of 5° of ankle dorsiflexion. As the stance phase continues, the center of pressure moves forward to the metatarsal heads, and the heel rises. Finally, the center of mass falls beyond the base of support of the stance leg, resulting in an acceleration of the body through free-fall (1).

Problem 1. Excessive Knee Extension

Excessive knee extension can be manifested as either extensor thrust (primitive extensor synergy or spasticity pattern) or hyperextension of the knee. Extensor thrust is defined as a rapid extension of the knee, but not into a hyperextension range, and it usually occurs during loading. Hyperextension, shown in Figure 13.2, occurs when the knee

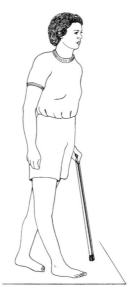

Figure 13.2. Knee hyperextension is a common gait deviation in the patient with neurological dysfunction, and is seen during the stance phase of gait. Knee hyperextension can be the direct result of pathology, such as plantarflexor spasticity, or alternatively used as a compensatory strategy to control the knee in the presence of impaired force control in the quadriceps muscle. (Adapted from Perry J. Gait analysis: normal and pathological function. Thorofare, NJ: Slack, Inc., 1992:324.)

has sufficient mobility to move posteriorly past neutral. This is called **recurvatum**. Knee hyperextension can occur quickly or slowly, and usually begins in mid- or terminal stance and continues into pre-swing. Excessive knee extension means the tibia cannot advance over the stationary foot in the stance phase (1).

Causes

Plantarflexor contractures. Plantarflexor contractures limit tibial advancement over the stationary foot during stance. If the contracture is elastic, that is, able to lengthen in response to body weight, the only result may be an inappropriate foot position at foot contact, since body weight will lengthen the plantarflexors, allowing the tibia to advance (1).

Plantarflexor spasticity. Spasticity can prevent knee flexion during loading, and produce knee hyperextension during the stance phase of gait. Major compensations for loss of progression due to excessive plantar flexion include hyperextension of the knee, and/or forward trunk lean. Patients also compensate by shortening the step length of the other limb. Which compensatory strategy is used will depend on a number of factors. Knee mobility is critical to the hyperextension strategy. In contrast, good hip and trunk extensors are necessary for the trunk flexion strategy (1, 3).

Quadriceps spasticity. In stance, quadriceps spasticity will have its greatest effect during loading. Remember that during weight acceptance, there is a brief flexion of the knee that assists in absorbing the shock of loading. Quadriceps spasticity results in an excessive response to knee flexion and subsequent lengthening of the quadriceps, triggering a stretch reflex response that can limit flexion and result in premature extension of the knee (1, 3).

Compensation for weak quadriceps. A weak quadriceps (grades 3+ to 4) will lead to difficulty controlling knee flexion during loading. A very weak quadriceps (Q) (grades 0 to 3) will lead to trouble stabilizing the knee during mid-stance. The primary compensation for this is hyperextension of the knee during mid-stance, since the forward movement of the body weight will serve as the knee extensor force. When hyperextension is continued into pre-swing, it prevents the knee from freely moving during the swing phase. This can slow progression and result in toe-drag (1, 3).

There are several disadvantages to the use of a knee hyperextension strategy as a compensation for weak Q. First, it limits knee flexion during loading and thus increases the impact of body weight on the structures of the stance limb. In addition, it traumatizes the internal structure of the knee and can damage these structures in the long term. The advantage of the knee hyperextension strategy is that it allows a more stable posture, and therefore may be a reasonable and appropriate strategy for patients with a very weak Q (1).

Pain. Knee flexion during the stance phase of gait may be avoided in patients who have joint pathology to minimize compression of painful joints.

Problem 2. Persisting Knee Flexion

Causes

Inadequate activation of plantarflexors. Inadequate gastrocnemius/soleus activation causes excessive ankle dorsiflexion and can increase knee flexion from 15 to 30°. Persisting knee flexion increases the demands on the Q muscle, which eccentrically contracts to stabilize the knee. In addition, weak or inactive plantarflexors cannot restrain forward motion of the tibia through an eccentric contraction.

Inadequate activation of the soleus also results in loss of heel-rise at terminal stance, and a loss of terminal stance knee extension. As a result, knee flexion persists.

Inadequate activation of the plantarflexors can be caused by: weakness, surgical overlengthening of the achilles tendon, or the use of a fixed ankle-foot orthosis (1, 3).

Knee flexion contracture. Knee flexion contracture can also result in a persisting knee flexion posture during the stance phase of gait.

Hamstrings overactivity. Hamstrings hyperactivity can manifest as either premature or prolonged activation of the hamstrings (1). It was originally thought that hamstrings overactivity was the result of spasticity, that is, velocity-dependent hyperactivity of the stretch reflex. But researchers have subsequently found that performing a dorsal rhizotomy, which involves selectively cutting the sensory nerve roots, does not decrease hamstrings hyperactivity in children with cerebral palsy. This suggests that the basis for hamstrings hyperactivity is abnormal coordination, not a simple hyperactive stretch reflex (1).

Hamstrings activity is often used to substitute for a weak gluteus maximus and adductor magnus. This helps to stabilize the trunk but leads to a mild loss of knee extension in stance.

Problem 3. Excessive Hip Flexion

Causes

Hip flexor spasticity. Spasticity of the hip flexor muscles will result in excessive hip flexion and a forward trunk posture during the stance phase of gait, shown in Figure 13.3.

Hip flexor contracture. Hip flexion contractures result in inadequate hip extension, which can affect both stability and progression. During mid-stance, if the hip can't extend to neutral, the trunk will flex forward, bringing the center of mass anterior to the hip joint. Gravity will pull the trunk forward into more flexion, and this places an additional demand on the hip extensors to prevent collapse of the forward trunk, and loss of stability (1).

Lumbar lordosis is a compensatory posture used to reduce the workload of the hip extensors. Thus, a hip flexion contracture of 15° can be compensated for with increased lordosis, unless there is associated loss of spinal flexibility. A 40° hip flexion contracture in children can be compensated for with increased lumbar lordosis due to the flexibility of the growing spine (1).

An alternative way to compensate for a hip flexion contracture is to flex the knees. This allows the pelvis to be normally aligned despite the hip flexion contracture. Flexion of

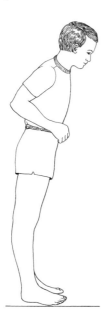

Figure 13.3. Hip flexion and a forward lean trunk posture can result from primary impairments such as hip flexor spasticity or contracture, or from hip extensor weakness. Alternatively, this posture can be an effective strategy to compensate for weak quadriceps, since it brings the line of gravity anterior to the knee joint, thus stabilizing the knee.

the hip and knees is called a crouch gait and is often seen in spastic cerebral palsy as a compensatory gait pattern for inadequate hip extension (1, 3).

However, this compensatory strategy has its own limitations since it increases the demands on the quadriceps muscle to control the knee. Increased knee flexion also requires either excessive ankle dorsiflexion or heel-rise onto the forefoot during stance, and thus constrains progression (1, 3).

Compensation for weak quadriceps. Forward trunk lean brings the body vector anterior to the knee, and is an effective compensatory strategy for stabilizing the knee in response to weak quadriceps. However, it threatens stability.

Hip extensor weakness. Hip extensor weakness can also produce a forward trunk lean that threatens stability.

Pain. Pathologies of the hip joint such as osteoarthritis, producing pain, lead to a forward-flexed posture that minimizes intra-articular pressure (16).

Problem 4. Backward Lean of Trunk

Causes

Compensation for weak hip extensors. Backward lean in stance compensates for hip extensor weakness by bringing the center of mass behind the hips; it is used for stability. However, TA activity is needed to prevent falls in the backward direction (1).

Problem 5. Lateral Lean of Trunk

Lateral lean refers to the lateral lean of the trunk toward the stance leg.

Causes

Causes of lateral lean of the trunk include weak hip abductors and adductor muscle contractures.

Problem 6. Drop in Pelvis

Causes

Contralateral hip abductor weakness. Hip abductor weakness results in a drop of the pelvis on the side contralateral to the weakness. This is shown in Figure 13.4. This can also be seen clinically as excessive adduction of the leg contralateral to the side with the weakness. Medial displacement of the contralateral leg reduces the base of support, impacting stability.

Contralateral hip adductor spasticity. Hip adductor spasticity or contracture can also produce a contralateral drop in the pelvis during stance, as the femur is drawn in medially.

Problem 7. Scissors Gait

Scissors gait is characterized by excessive adduction. During the swing phase of gait, as the hip flexes, excessive adduction produces a severe medial displacement of the entire limb. This results in a reduced base of support affecting stability. In severe cases, the adducted swing leg catches on the stance limb and impedes progression (1, 3).

Causes

Adductor spasticity. Adductor spasticity produces adduction on the ipsilateral side. Excessive adduction can result in medial

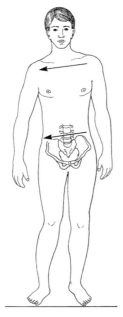

Figure 13.4.   Drop in pelvic position on the contralateral side in response to abductor weakness. (Adapted from Perry J. Gait analysis: normal and pathological function. Thorofare, NJ: Slack, Inc., 1992:270.)

displacement of the thigh past vertical, which will appear as medial displacement of the entire limb.

Abductor weakness. Weak abductor muscles (gluteus medius) result in a contralateral pelvic drop and medial displacement of the entire limb.

TERMINAL STANCE

Problem 1. Lack of Hip Hyperextension

Causes

Hip flexion contractures. Lack of hip extension has a great effect on terminal stance, since it is during this phase that the hip is normally hyperextended. Lack of hip extension produces an anterior pelvic tilt and an inability to move the thigh posterior to the hip. This results in a shortened step length and reduces forward progression of the body.

Problem 2. Inadequate Toe-Off

Causes

Spastic gastrocnemius/soleus. Inadequate toe-off is often the result of an extended knee position into terminal stance. Inability to adequately flex the knee makes toe-off more difficult, and requires the hip and knee flexors to work harder to lift the limb and clear the foot during swing. Toe-drag is the consequence of inadequate knee flexion at pre- and initial swing (1).

Problem 3. Pelvic Retraction

Pelvic retraction is defined as excessive backward rotation of the pelvis (1). Pelvic retraction during terminal stance is shown in Figure 13.5.

Causes

Weak plantarflexors. Dynamic backward rotation occurs in terminal stance and is usually associated with persistent heel contact due to calf muscle weakness. To maintain a reasonable gait velocity, the pelvis is rotated

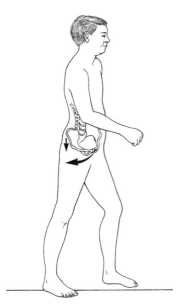

Figure 13.5.   Pelvic rotation in terminal stance is usually associated with persistent heel contact due to calf muscle weakness. To maintain a reasonable gait velocity, the pelvis is rotated backward to lengthen the limb and to avoid a shortened step. (Adapted from Perry J. Gait analysis: normal and pathological function. Thorofare, NJ: Slack, Inc., 1992:271.)

backward to lengthen the limb and avoid a shortened step.

Swing

The goals to be achieved in swing phase include advancement of the swing leg for progression, and repositioning the limb in preparation for weight acceptance for stability. Both goals require adequate foot clearance during swing, which requires that the swing leg be shorter than the stance leg. This is normally accomplished through the action of the hip flexors, which generate enough velocity at initiation of swing to flex the knee, allowing the limb to shorten enough so the foot clears the support surface. An important strategy used to accomplish foot placement involves the transfer of momentum from the forward moving thigh segment to the shank segment. This allows the knee to extend in preparation for the next foot placement with relatively little muscle activity (1, 3).

INITIAL SWING

Problem 1. Inadequate Hip Flexion

Causes

Hip flexor weakness or inability to activate muscles.   Normal gait requires only a grade 2+, (poor plus) muscle strength in the hip flexors (1). Hip flexor weakness, producing inadequate hip flexion, primarily affects the swing phase of gait. Knee flexion is lost in swing when there is inadequate hip flexion; thus, the patient is unable to develop sufficient momentum at the hip to indirectly flex the knee. As a result, toe clearance is reduced or lost. A shortened step is also associated with inadequate hip flexion. A shortened step can affect the position of the foot at heel-strike. When the hip can't be flexed at the initiation of swing, limb advancement and thus progression are hampered. At the same time, placement of the foot in preparation for weight acceptance is affected, challenging stability.

There are several compensatory strategies patients use to achieve foot clearance during swing, despite inadequate hip flexion, and these are shown in Figure 13.6. The first uses a posterior tilt of the pelvis and activation of the abdominal muscles to advance the swing limb (Fig. 13.6A). The second uses circumduction, defined as hip-hike, forward rotation of the pelvis, and abduction of the hip, to advance the limb (Fig. 13.6B). The other strategies used to advance the limb despite hip flexor weakness include contralateral vaulting (Fig. 13.6C), involving coming up onto the forefoot of the stance limb, or leaning the trunk laterally toward the opposite limb (1, 3) (Fig. 13.6D).

Decreased proprioception.   Delayed initiation of swing phase can also result from decreased proprioceptive cues signaling hyperextension in the hip and the termination of stance.

MID-SWING

Problem 1. Inadequate Knee Flexion

Causes

Knee extension contractures.   Contractures of the knee extensors result in an in-

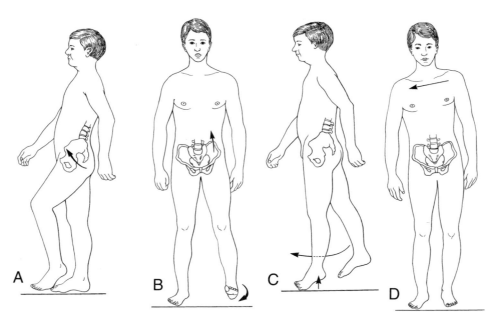

Figure 13.6. Compensatory strategies used to advance the swing leg despite inadequate hip flexion include **A**, activation of the abdominal muscles in conjunction with a posterior tip of the pelvis, **B**, circumduction, **C**, contralateral vaulting, or **D**, leaning the trunk laterally toward the opposite limb. (Adapted from Perry J. Gait analysis: normal and pathological function. Thorofare, NJ: Slack, Inc., 1992:268.)

ability to freely flex the knee in response to the momentum generated, limiting foot clearance and producing toe-drag. This problem is illustrated in Figure 13.7.

Plantarflexor contractures. Plantarflexor contractures also affect foot clearance during swing by preventing sufficient ankle flexion to allow toe clearance.

Plantarflexor spasticity. Spastic plantarflexors, like contractures, affect forward foot clearance during swing. Compensatory strategies include a shortened stride length and reduced gait velocity.

Quadriceps spasticity. During swing, knee flexion can be inhibited by hyperactivity of the stretched quadriceps.

Problem 2. Excessive Adduction

Causes

Compensatory to hip flexor inactivity. Overuse of the adductors to assist with hip flexion can result in excessive adduction of the limb during swing.

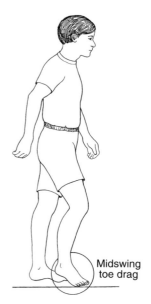

Figure 13.7. Inadequate foot clearance and toe-drag are common gait deviations seen in the patient with neurological dysfunction and can result from many types of impairments. (Adapted from Perry J. Gait analysis: normal and pathological function. Thorofare, NJ: Slack, Inc., 1992:315.)

TERMINAL SWING

Problem 1. Inadequate Knee Extension

Causes

Knee flexion contractures. Knee flexion contractures prevent the knee from fully extending at the end of swing. This affects the patient's ability to place the foot appropriately for weight transfer, reducing stability and increasing the need for muscular action to control the knee (1).

Hamstrings overactivity. Inappropriate activation of the hamstrings muscles during the swing phase of gait is a major cause of inadequate knee extension during terminal swing. While this overactivity occurs during lengthening of the hamstrings, researchers have determined that it is not always due to hyperactivity of the stretch reflex (1).

Flexor synergy. Persistent flexion of the knee throughout the swing cycle is often associated with the use of a flexor synergy, or total flexor pattern at all three joints. Use of the flexor synergy results in an inability to extend the knee while flexing the hip during terminal swing. This is shown in Figure 13.8*B*. Figure 13.8*A* illustrates an extensor synergy.

This concludes our review of some typical problems affecting gait in the neurologically impaired patient, and their potential causes. Later in this chapter we summarize gait problems from a diagnostic perspective, reviewing studies that describe gait patterns in stroke, Parkinson's disease, and cerebral palsy.

STAIR-WALKING

Like level-walking, stair-walking involves reciprocal movements of the legs through alternating stance and swing phases. Climbing up stairs requires the generation of concentric forces at the knee and ankle (mostly the knee) for forward and vertical progression. Stability demands are greatest during the single limb stance phase, when the swing leg is advancing to the next step (17).

In contrast to stair ascent, descent is

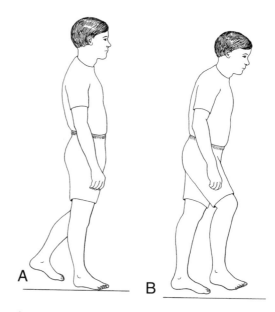

Figure 13.8. Pathological gait patterns resulting from **A**, a total extensor synergy pattern used in stance, and **B**, a flexor synergy pattern used in swing. (Adapted from Gage JR. Gait analysis in cerebral palsy. New York: MacKeith Press, 1991:134.)

achieved largely through eccentric contractions of the hip, knee, and ankle extensors, which control the body position in response to the accelerating force of gravity. Energy absorption and a controlled landing are ensured through anticipatory activation of the gastrocnemius prior to foot contact with the step (17).

This means that in the patient with a neurological deficit, decreased concentric control will primarily affect stair ascent, while decreased eccentric control will primarily affect stair descent.

Patients with an UMN lesion tend to stair-walk slowly, require the use of rails for support and progression, and in severe cases of dyscontrol, are unable to use a reciprocal pattern for stair-walking. Instead, they bring both feet to the same step prior to progressing to the next step.

Impaired visual sensation affects anticipatory aspects of this task. For example, gastrocnemius activity, which precedes foot contact, is less when visual cues are reduced (18).

PATHOLOGY-BASED DESCRIPTIONS OF ABNORMAL GAIT

Stroke

An analysis of temporal distance factors shows that patients who have had a stroke walk 50% more slowly than healthy adults, averaging 37 m/min, compared with 82 m/min for healthy adults. However, the speed of walking depends greatly on the degree of recovery. Researchers have shown a relationship between walking speed and Brunnstrom's stages of recovery following stroke (19). Patients in stage 6, defined by Brunnstrom as the ability to perform isolated joint movements freely in a well-coordinated manner, walk considerably faster (.65 m/sec) than do patients in stage 3, defined as the ability to voluntarily initiate movements only within a full-limb synergy and with marked spasticity (.16 m/sec). Patients who were at stage 1 or 2 were unable to walk (19).

Double-support time in stroke patients is increased, with a decrease in stance time by the involved leg, and a shortened step by the noninvolved leg. This results in a significant step asymmetry.

Many researchers have described gait patterns typically seen in hemiparetic patients. Several problems are quite common among stroke patients; however, EMG studies suggest that the underlying cause may vary from patient to patient (3).

Characteristics of the stance phase of hemiplegic gait include (a) equinovarus foot position, leading to a forefoot or flat-foot strike during loading; (b) knee hyperextension in mid-stance with a forward lean of the trunk; (c) inability to place the hemiparetic leg in a trailing position during terminal stance, allowing the body weight to advance over the forefoot with subsequent heel-rise. Often, the pelvis is retracted on the stance leg and drops on the swing side due to abductor weakness (3).

The most common problems in the swing phase include (a) toe-drag, impeding progression due to inadequate flexion at the hip, knee, and ankle; and (b) inappropriate foot placement, due to incomplete knee extension and ankle dorsiflexion at the end of swing (3).

Researchers have studied muscle patterns in stroke patients to determine the underlying cause of abnormal gait patterns. Despite the similarity in how stroke patients walk, the muscle activation patterns underlying this characteristic gait vary considerably (6). Researchers have classified muscle activation problems into the following categories: (a) a mass synergy pattern, characterized by full limb flexion during swing and extension during stance, (b) premature or prolonged activity that is nonstretch related, (c) stretch-dependent overactivity (spasticity), (d) cocontraction, and (e) increased musculoskeletal restraint, that is, impaired motion in the absence of increased EMG activity (3, 6, 20).

A study examining energy expenditure associated with hemiplegic gait suggests that despite its abnormal appearance, the oxygen cost is quite low. The inefficiency associated with abnormal gait patterns appears to be offset by slow gait speed. This suggests that ambulation is not physiologically stressful for the typical stroke patient unless there are cardiovascular problems as well (2). But this study examined energy costs in stroke patients based on time walked. When distance walked is considered, energy expenditure associated with hemiparetic gait is twice as much as that of normal gait, because it takes stroke patients, who walk at half the velocity of normal adults, twice as long to cover that same distance (3).

Parkinson's Disease

Patients with Parkinson's disease (PD) characteristically show a stooped posture and shuffling gait pattern. They take smaller steps, and usually there is decreased amplitude and speed of movement throughout the body. Studies examining temporal distance factors report that patients with PD walk slower, (33.6 m/min compared with 81.6 m/min in age-matched normals). Step length is asymmetric and decreased, while cycle duration is increased; thus, despite their rapid steps, walking speed is slower than in normals (21–24).

As was true for stroke patients, the degree of gait impairment is related to the severity of the disease progression. Researchers have found a significant relationship between walking velocity in patients with Parkinson's disease and the stages of disability as described by the Schwab Classification of Progression (25) or the Hoehn and Yahr Classification (26, 27).

In addition, joint angular displacement patterns show a smaller range through out the body (21, 28). Specific alterations in the stance phase of gait include: (*a*) lack of heel-strike; instead, patients make contact with the foot flat or with the forefoot; (*b*) incomplete knee extension during mid-stance; (*c*) inability to extend the knee and plantarflex the ankle in terminal stance, resulting in decreased forward thrust of the body; (*d*) forward trunk lean; (*e*) diminished trunk motion; and (*f*) reduced or absent arm swing.

Decreased motion of the joints is apparent in swing phase as well. While dorsiflexion may be exaggerated during the swing phase, decreased hip and knee flexion lead to diminished toe clearance. In addition, reduced speed and amplitude of motion of the swing leg also affect forward thrust of the body (21, 28).

Gait in PD patients is characterized by an inability to control momentum. If a patient is unable to generate sufficient momentum, forward progression is arrested. This is often referred to as a **frozen gait pattern**. In contrast, unrestrained momentum leads to uncontrolled progression, called a **propulsive gait pattern**. Propulsive gait disorders may be due to an exaggerated forward inclination of the body, resulting in an anterior displacement of the center of mass (COM) beyond the supporting foot. In some instances, however, propulsive gait is seen in patients who have normal vertical posture but seem unable to oppose forward momentum (21).

Many researchers consider that the stepping mechanism itself is unimpaired in parkinsonism. It is hypothesized instead that disordered locomotion results from impairments in postural control and/or the ability to control locomotion. These impairments are considered the result of problems in the generation and control of force (29).

EMG studies suggest that gait patterns in PD are associated with three types of muscle activation patterns: (*a*) continuous EMG activity instead of cyclical activity, (*b*) reduced amplitude of muscle activation, and (*c*) abnormal coactivation of muscles.

PD patients often have difficulty in initiating gait. Researchers point out that poor gait initiation is often the result of inadequate weight shift laterally. However, some PD patients are unable to initiate stepping, despite the ability to shift weight (29).

Cerebral Palsy

Cerebral palsy (CP) is a developmental disorder characterized by a wide range of disabilities, all having in common central nervous system pathology occurring pre- or perinatally. CP is classified into several categories of motor abnormalities, including spastic, athetoid, and ataxic, based on the location of the lesion and type of motor abnormality (30). Abnormalities can affect one side of the body (for example, hemiplegia or hemiataxia), all four extremities equally (as in spastic quadriplegia), or primarily the legs (for example, spastic diplegia). The types of sensory, motor, and cognitive impairments found in the patient with cerebral palsy vary widely in each category. In addition, there is much variation among individuals within categories.

Much of the work examining pathological gait in CP has been with children who have spastic hemiplegia or diplegia (7). Temporal distance analysis of CP gait indicates that walking speed is slower, averaging 40 m/min.

Two gait patterns are characteristic of spastic CP: a crouch gait and a genu recurvatum gait pattern (1, 31). A crouch gait pattern is often associated with a bilateral motor control impairment, such as spastic diplegia.

Crouch gait results from excessive hip and knee flexion, excessive ankle plantarflexion, and anterior pelvic tilt during stance and swing phases of gait. Foot-strike is abnormal, with an equinovarus foot posture and most often forefoot contact. This foot position is continued through the stance phase of gait. Excessive plantarflexion and knee and hip flexion are seen during loading and continued through the stance phase of gait. Excessive flexion persists into terminal stance, and the pre-swing phase is minimal or absent due to an inability to extend the hip and knee.

The swing phase of gait also shows excessive ankle, knee, and hip flexion. Often, foot-floor clearance is greater than normal, due to excessive flexion of the swing limb (7, 31).

A genu recurvatum gait pattern presents the opposite clinical picture to the crouch gait pattern. This gait pattern is characterized by knee hyperextension during stance and excessive ankle plantarflexion. Hip flexion and forward lean of the trunk may occur as the patient leans forward to balance over a plantarflexed foot. Loading is onto the forefoot due to inadequate knee extension and excessive plantarflexion during swing. During swing, toe-drag constrains progression, requiring contralateral trunk lean to free the foot and advance the thigh. The genu recurvatum gait pattern is more common in unilateral motor impairments such as in spastic hemiplegia (7, 31).

EMG studies suggest that abnormal gait in spastic CP may be classified into the following problems: (*a*) defective recruitment of motor units, referred to as a paresis or weakness pattern; (*b*) abnormal velocity-dependent recruitment during muscle stretch, the so-called spasticity pattern; (*c*) nonselective activation of antagonist muscles with a loss of a normal reciprocal inhibitory pattern, called the cocontraction pattern, and (*d*) problems associated with musculoskeletal restraint due to changes in mechanical properties of muscles, the non-neural problem pattern (7).

Interestingly, in children with spastic hemiplegic cerebral palsy, a cocontraction pattern of muscle activity was found in both the hemiplegic leg and the noninvolved leg.

Thus, researchers are now considering the possibility that cocontraction represents a compensatory strategy aimed at stiffening a joint to compensate for postural instability or paresis (7, 32, 33).

The particular gait profile seen in an individual will reflect a combination of the factors just listed. Thus, each individual with CP will present a slightly different gait pattern.

Heart rate and oxygen rates are higher in CP children than for age-matched normals. Researchers believe that this is because the flexed posture, which is typical of the crouch gait pattern, requires additional muscle activity for stability. Interestingly, the physiological costs of walking decrease in normal children as they get older. In contrast, the physiological costs of walking increase as children with CP get older. Why does this happen? Increased physiological costs of walking are not due to an increase in motor abnormalities in CP, since it is a nonprogressive disease. Instead, researchers believe that oxygen rates associated with walking increase as CP children get older because changes in body morphology, including increased body weight and size, interact with impaired motor control. This results in an increase in the physiological cost of gait in older children. As a result, the older CP child may walk less and increasingly rely on a wheelchair (2).

DISORDERS OF MOBILITY OTHER THAN GAIT

During the performance of transfer activities such as sit-to-stand (STS), rolling, and rising from a bed, healthy young adults tend to use momentum to move the body smoothly and efficiently from one position to another. A momentum strategy requires the generation of concentric forces to propel the body and eccentric forces to control motion, thus ensuring stability. Momentum generated through movement of the trunk is transferred to the legs, and the body moves smoothly, without stopping, to the new position. The ability to transfer momentum from trunk to lower extremities, which is a characteristic common to most transfer tasks, requires unrestrained motion of the trunk (34, 35).

An alternative strategy that can be used when performing transfer tasks is a force-control strategy. This strategy is characterized by frequent stops. Forces are generated in one body segment to move the body to an interim position of stability. Then force is generated in an adjacent body segment to further propel the body to the new position. For example, when using a force-control strategy to move from STS, the trunk moves forward, bringing the COM over the feet. Then forces are generated to lift the body to the vertical position. The force-control strategy ensures stability, but requires greater forces for progression. In some cases, the arms are used to generate force, assisting with progression and stability (34, 35).

Limitations in the ability to activate muscles concentrically generally affect the progression requirement of mobility skills, that is, the ability to move the body. Inability to activate muscles eccentrically impairs the ability to control motion, affecting stability.

There are many reasons why the neurologically impaired patient tends to use a force-control strategy during transfers. Postural control problems limiting stability, cardiovascular problems such as orthostatic hypotension, and dizziness complaints, all may require a patient to move slowly and make interim stops during the task. For example, when arising from a bed, a patient with orthostatic hypotension would need to sit for a moment on the side of the bed before standing up, or risk a sudden drop in blood pressure and loss of balance. The overreliance on a force-control strategy and upper extremity control during transfer tasks, however, can limit these patients' adaptability in response to changing environmental conditions. For example, they may find it difficult to stand up independently from a chair without arms (34, 35).

There have been many studies examining pathological gait in neurologically dysfunctional patients. In contrast, few studies have systematically explored problems constraining other mobility skills in these patients. Much of the information available comes from anecdotal descriptions of characteristic patterns used by stroke patients to achieve these skills (36–39).

Sit-to-Stand

Many patients with UMN lesions tend to use a force-control strategy to accomplish sit-to-stand (STS) position. Often, this is because of a combination of impairments affecting both stability and progression aspects of the movement. In addition, this is the strategy most commonly taught by clinicians when retraining transfer tasks.

When using a force-control strategy to move from STS, the trunk moves forward, bringing the COM over the feet; then, forces are generated to lift the body to the vertical position. This strategy emphasizes the control of stability, but cannot make use of momentum because of the breaks in the movement. Thus, it is a less efficient approach (34, 35).

Impaired force control affects the STS task in two ways. The inability to activate trunk, hip, and knee muscles concentrically limits the generation of propulsive forces to move and lift the body. Loss of eccentric control limits the patient's ability to control horizontal motions of the center of mass and thus impairs stability (34, 35).

Decreased spinal mobility and diminished motion in the hips, knees, and ankles will restrict a patient's ability to move freely. This affects momentum and force-control strategies, but primarily the momentum control strategy. This is because the ability to transfer momentum from one body segment to another requires freedom of motion in the joints (34, 35).

Decreased postural control impairs the ability to effectively control movements of the COM, and represents a major constraint on the STS task. One of the most frequently seen problems in patients with impaired stability is falling in the backward direction when trying to stand up. This results when the patient prematurely generates propulsive forces to lift the body, before the COM is adequately positioned within the base of support of the feet.

Sensory impairments affect a patient's ability to determine the position of the body in space, particularly placement of the COM with respect to the supporting surface. Force-control problems limit the patient's ability to control horizontal movements of the COM from over the buttocks to the new base of support, the feet.

Perceptual impairments including impaired body image, inappropriate internal representations of stability limits, and abnormal motion perception (dizziness) also affect a patient's ability to safely accomplish STS.

Finally, cognitive impairments can also significantly limit a patient's ability to perform a task safely. For example, a patient may try to sit down before he or she is appropriately positioned with respect to a chair.

Bed Mobility Skills

Bed mobility skills include changing position while in bed (rolling supine to side-lying or prone), and getting out of bed, either to a chair or standing up. Researchers have found that normal young adults use a variety of momentum-related strategies when performing bed mobility skills. There is incredible variety in how people move; in fact, none of the young adults tested used exactly the same strategy twice! In contrast, force-control movement strategies are frequently used by neurologically impaired patients, and are characterized by frequent starts and stops. As mentioned previously, there are many reasons why a force-control strategy may be more appropriate in the neurologically impaired patient than a momentum strategy (36).

The most common approach to rolling shown by normal young adults involves reaching and lifting with the upper extremity, flexing the head and upper trunk, and lifting the leg to roll onto the side, then over to prone. Most healthy young adults did not show rotation between the shoulders and pelvis, assumed by many clinicians to be an invariant feature of rolling (36).

Because bed mobility skills are primarily initiated by movement of the head, upper trunk, and shoulders, impairments that affect these structures (such as weakness and or range of motion limitations) will limit performance of these skills.

SUMMARY

1. While abnormal gait is a common characteristic of many neurological pathologies, the constellation of underlying problems that produce disordered gait will vary from patient to patient depending on (a) primary impairments such as inadequate activation of a muscle, (b) secondary impairments, such as contractures, and (c) compensatory strategies developed to meet the requirements of mobility in the face of persisting impairments.

2. Musculoskeletal impairments constrain movement and increase the workload on the muscles, affecting a patient's ability to meet the requirements of gait. Decreased joint mobility during stance restricts forward motion of the body over the supporting foot, affecting *progression*. In swing, decreased joint mobility reduces foot clearance, affecting *progression*, and appropriate foot placement for weight acceptance, affecting *stability*.

3. Neuromuscular impairments affecting gait include weakness, abnormalities of muscle tone, and task-specific control problems. Task-specific control problems consist of (a) the inability to recruit a muscle during an automatic task such as posture or gait; (b) inappropriate activation of a muscle during gait, which is not related to stretch of the muscle; (c) coactivation of agonist and antagonist muscles around a joint, which increases stiffness and decreases motion; (d) problems related to scaling the amplitude of muscle activity during gait.

4. Sensory disorders can lead to problems in the following areas of locomotor control: (a) signaling terminal stance and thus triggering the initiation of swing, (b) signaling unanticipated disruptions to gait, and (c) detecting upcoming obstacles important for modifying gait to changes in task and environmental conditions.

5. Impairments can manifest as problems affecting the patient's abilities to meet the progression, stability, and adaptation goals inherent in both the stance and the swing phase of gait. A careful analysis of movement patterns can lead the clinician to generate multiple hypotheses about the potential underlying causes of gait problems.

6. During the performance of transfer activities such as sit-to-stand (STS), rolling, and rising

from a bed, healthy young adults tend to use a momentum strategy, which requires the generation of concentric and eccentric contractions to control motion, and ensures stability. In contrast, a force-control strategy, characterized by frequent starts and stops, is frequently used by neurologically dysfunctional patients. This is related to impairments affecting both stability and progression aspects of the movement. This is also the strategy most commonly taught by clinicians when retraining transfer tasks.

REFERENCES

1. Perry J. Gait analysis: normal and pathological function. Thorofare, NJ: Slack Inc., 1992.
2. Waters RL. Energy expenditure. In: Perry J. Gait analysis: normal and pathological function. Thorofare, NJ: Slack Inc., 1992.
3. Montgomery J. Assessment and treatment of locomotor deficits in stroke. In: Duncan PW, Badke MB, eds. Stroke rehabilitation: the recovery of motor control, Chicago: Year Book Medical Publishers, 1987:223–259.
4. Duncan P, Badke MB. Stroke rehabilitation: the recovery of motor control. Chicago: Year Book Medical Publishers, 1987.
5. Oatis CA, Perspectives on the evaluation and treatment of gait disorders. In: Montgomery PC, Connolly, BH, eds. Motor control and physical therapy: theoretical framework and practical applications. Hixson, TN: Chattanooga, 1990:141–155.
6. Knutsson E, Richards C. Different types of disturbed motor control in gait of hemiparetic patients. Brain 1989;102:405–430.
7. Crenna P, Inverno M, Frigo C, Palmieri R, Fedrizzi E. Pathophysiological profile of gait in children with cerebral palsy. In: Forssberg H, Hirshfeld H, eds. Movement disorders in children. Basel: Karger, 1991:186–198.
8. Shumway-Cook A. Equilibrium deficits in children. In: Woollacott MH, Shumway-Cook A. Development of posture and gait across the lifespan. Charleston, SC: University of South Carolina Press, 1989:229–252.
9. Smith JL. Programming of stereotyped limb movements by spinal generators. In: Stelmach GE, Requin J, eds. Tutorials in motor behavior. Amsterdam: North-Holland. 1980: 95–115.
10. Katoka S, Croll GA, Bles W. Somatosensory ataxia. In: Bles W, Brandt T, eds. Disorders of posture and gait. Amsterdam: Elsevier 1986, 177–183.
11. Ashmead DH, Hill EW, Talor CR. Obstacle perception by congenitally blind children. Perception and Psychophysiology 1989; 46:425–433.
12. Kirkpatrick R, Tucker C, Ramirez J, et al. Center of gravity control in normal and vestibulopathic gait. In: Woollacott M, Horak F, eds. Posture and gait: control mechanisms Eugene, OR: University of Oregon Books, 1992:260–263.
13. Takahashi M, Hoshikawa H, Tjujita N, Akiyama I. Effect of labyrinthine dysfunction upon head oscillation and gaze during stepping and running. Acta-Otolaryngol (Stockh) 1988;106:348–353.
14. Grossman GE, Leigh RJ. Instability of gaze during locomotion in patients with deficient vestibular function. Ann Neurol 1990; 27:528–532.
15. Pozzo T, Berthoz A, Lefort L, Vitte E. Head stabilization during various locomotor tasks in humans. II. Patients with bilateral peripheral vestibular deficits. Exp Brain Res 1991; 85:208–217.
16. Eyring EJ, Murray W. The effect of joint position on the pressure of intra-articular effusion. J Bone Joint Surg 1965;47A:313–322.
17. McFadyen BJ, Winter DA. An integrated biomechanical analysis of normal stair ascent and descent. J Biomechanics 1988;21:733–744.
18. Simoneau GG, Cavanagh PR, Ulbrecht JS, Leibowitz HW, Tyrrell RA. The influence of visual factors on fall-related kinematic variables during stair descent by older women, J Gerontol 1991;46:M188–M195.
19. Brandstater M, deBruin H, Gowland C, et al.: Hemiplegic gait: analysis of temporal variables. Arch Phys Med Rehabil 1983;64:583–587.
20. Berger W Altenmueller E, Dietz V. Normal and impaired development of children's gait. Human Neurobiology 1984;3:163–170.
21. Knuttson E. An analysis of Parkinsonian gait. Brain 1972;95:475–486.
22. Murray MP, Sepic SB, Gardner GM, et al. Walking patterns of men with parkinsonism. Am J Phys Med 1978;57:278–294.
23. Blin O, Ferrandez AM, Serratrice G. Quantitative analysis of gait in Parkinson patients: increased variability of stride length. J Neurol Sci 1990;98:91–97.

24. Martin JP, Hurwitz LJ. Locomotion and the basal ganglia. Brain 1962;261–289.

25. Schwab RS. Progression and prognosis in Parkinson's disease. J Nerv Ment Dis 1960; 130:556–572.

26. Hoehn MM, Yahr MD. Parkinsonism: onset, progression and mortality. Neurology 1967; 17:427–435.

27. O'Sullivan S. Parkinson's disease: physical rehabilitation. In: O'Sullivan S, Schmitz T. Physical rehabilitation: assessment and treatment. 2nd ed. Philadelphia: FA Davis, 1988:481–493.

28. Stern GM Franklyn SE, Imms FJ, Prestidge SP. Quantitative assessments of gait and mobility in Parkinson's disease. J Neural Transm Park Dis Dement Sect 1983;19:201–214.

29. Rogers M. Motor control problems in Parkinson's disease. In: Contemporary management of motor control problems: proceedings of the II Step Conference. Alexandria VA: APTA, 1991:195–208.

30. Bobath B. The very early treatment of cerebral palsy. Dev Med Child Neurol 1967; 9:373–390.

31. Gage JR. Gait analysis in cerebral palsy. New York: Mac Keith Press, 1991.

32. Berger W, Quintern J, Dietz V. Pathophysiology of gait in children with cerebral palsy. Electroencephalogr Clin Neurophysiol 1982; 53:538–548.

33. Leonard CT, Hirshfeld H, Forssberg H. The development of independent walking in children with cerebral palsy. Dev Med Child Neurol 1991;33:567–577.

34. Schenkman MA, Berger RA, Riley PO, Mann RW, Hodge WA. Whole-body movements during rising to standing from sitting. Phys Ther 1990;10:638–651.

35. Carr J, Shepard R. Motor relearning programme for stroke. Rockville, MD: Aspen Systems, 1987.

36. Davies P. Steps to follow. London: Heinneman, 1985.

37. Charness A. Stroke/head injury: a guide to functional outcomes in physical therapy management. Rockville, MD: Aspen Systems, 1986.

38. Bobath B. Adult hemiplegia. London: Heinneman, 1978.

35. Millington PJ, Myklebust BM, Shambes GM. Biomechanical analysis of the sit-to-stand motion in elderly persons. Arch Phys Med Rehabil 1992;73:609–617.

36. Richter RR, VanSant AF, Newton RA. Description of adult rolling movements and hypothesis of developmental sequences. Phys Ther 1989; 69:63–71.

Chapter 14

ASSESSMENT AND TREATMENT OF THE PATIENT WITH MOBILITY DISORDERS

INTRODUCTION

This chapter presents a task-oriented approach to assessing and treating the patient with mobility dysfunction. In previous chapters we defined a task-oriented approach with reference to four important concepts: the clinical decision-making process, hypothesis-oriented clinical practice, a model of disablement, and a theory of motor control.

In a task-oriented approach, assessment targets three levels of behavior: (*a*) the functional task level, (*b*) the sensory and motor strategies used to perform functional tasks, and (*c*) the underlying sensory, motor, and cognitive impairments that constrain motor control. The goals of a task-oriented approach to retraining include (*a*) resolve or prevent underlying impairments, (*b*) develop effective task-specific strategies, (*c*) retrain functional tasks, and (*d*) adapt task-specific strategies so that functional tasks can be performed in changing environmental contexts.

An important part of the clinical intervention process is the ability to generate multiple hypotheses about the potential causes of dysfunction in the patient, and to systematically test those hypotheses in order to refine one's understanding of the problems contributing to loss of function.

We now apply this approach to assessment and treatment of mobility problems in patients with upper motor neuron lesions. We begin with a review of some of the tests and measurements that can be used to document functional abilities related to mobility. We then look at the process of observational gait analysis, an approach to assessing gait strategies. (Assessment of sensory, motor, and cognitive systems is described in the chapter on assessment and treatment of the patient with postural disorders.) The last half of the chapter addresses issues related to retraining mobility skills in the patient with neurological impairments.

ASSESSMENT

Assessing at the Functional Level

Performance-based measures quantify the patient's functional walking abilities, but do not address the quality of movement patterns, nor the underlying sensory, motor, and cognitive determinants of function. Performance-based functional assessment can be expressed with reference to the level of assistance a patient requires when performing mobility skills, or in relationship to the temporal and distance characteristics of a patient's gait.

Often, a goal of mobility retraining is to help the patient become a functional community ambulator. But what does this mean?

By what criteria should clinicians determine differences in ambulatory status? What are the minimum distance and velocity requirements for independent community ambulation? As noted in the chapter on normal mobility function, several researchers have examined walking characteristics in neurologically intact adults. These studies have found that normal men between the ages of 20 to 60 years walk about 82 m/min, or 270 ft/min, which is 3.06 miles per hour (mph). Normal women the same age walk slightly slower, between 74 and 78 m/min, or 244 to 257 ft/min, which is 2.76 to 2.91 mph (1–3).

Researchers suggest that in order to be a community ambulator, patients need to be able to walk at greater than 33% of a normal adult's velocity, or about 1.0 mph. In addition, they need to be able to walk a minimum of 300 m, or about 1000 ft. This suggests that the ability to cover 1000 ft in approximately 11½ minutes is a minimum requirement for community ambulation (2, 3).

One study examined the minimum requirements for a range of instrumental activities of daily living (IADL) in the Los Angeles area to determine whether the criteria used by clinicians to judge independence in the community were consistent with actual distances and velocities needed to function independently (4). The results suggest that the following minimum standards may be required to be considered an independent community ambulator:

1. The ability to walk 300 meters, or 1000 feet;
2. The ability to achieve 80 m/min velocity for approximately 13 to 27 m in order to cross a street safely in the normal time allotted by stoplights;
3. The ability to negotiate 7- to 8-inch curbs independently (with assistive devices as needed);
4. The ability to turn the head while walking, without losing balance.

In addition, the study found that clinicians generally underestimated the distance and speed needed to function independently within a residential or commercial community (4). This may be because tests of normal activities of daily living (ADL) skills, for example, the Functional Independence Measure, often define complete independence in locomotor skills as being able to walk 150 ft safely (5). However, this standard may underestimate the requirements for being truly independent within the community.

In carrying out ADL and IADL tasks, the average person walks approximately 300 m (or about 1000 ft) per day, with an average walking speed of 80 m/min, or approximately 3.0 mph (4). Thus, the process of carrying out ADL requires about 4 minutes of walking per day for the average person (6).

Walking must not carry too high a price with respect to cardiovascular output and energy expenditure. The patient who is able to walk 1000 ft but is fatigued to the point of exhaustion afterwards, cannot be considered a functional community ambulator (3).

Finally, safety is an attribute of functional locomotion skills. A patient must be able to meet the stability requirements of locomotion to be functionally independent in gait. This includes (a) the integration of reactive balance strategies into gait to recover stability in response to unexpected perturbations; and (b) the ability to use anticipatory strategies to avoid or accommodate upcoming obstacles. Thus, an essential part of functional locomotion is the ability to adapt gait to both unexpected as well as anticipated disruptions.

The following series of tests are examples of ways in which functional mobility skills can be documented using parameters such as distance, speed, or velocity, cardiovascular efficiency, stability, and adaptability.

THREE-MINUTE WALK TEST

In our clinic, patients who have some locomotor ability are asked to walk at a self-selected speed for a period of 3 minutes. The 3-minute walk test is a variation of the 12-minute walking test, a tool designed to examine exercise tolerance in patients with chronic respiratory disease (7). However, because the 12-minute test is time-consuming and fatiguing to the patient, several researchers examined the validity of a shortened version of the test, determining the performance of patients at 2 and 6 minutes (8). These researchers concluded that, while the 12-minute test has excellent test-retest reliability, the 2-minute test is equally reliable, though slightly less sensitive in discriminating a patient's level of exercise tolerance. They concluded that the use of 12 minutes when assessing exercise tolerance is not critical (8).

In our own clinic, this research has been applied to the development of a 3-minute walk test, assessing walking tolerance in the patient with neurological dysfunction. We use a premeasured established path in corridors that are not subject to heavy amounts of traffic. Standardized instructions are given to patients to walk at a comfortable pace, using whatever assistive device they would use when walking outside their homes, and stopping to rest whenever they need to. Patients are allowed to rest as needed, though the clock is not stopped during the rest period. Thus, an increased number of rest periods is reflected in a shorter distance traveled.

Variables collected during the 3-minute walk test include: distance covered, calculated as self-paced velocity, number of rests required, number of deviations from a 15-inch path, and heart rate before and after the walk.

Self-Paced Velocity

Self-selected velocity represents a cumulative quality score of a patient's ability and confidence in walking (9). Converting the patient's self-selected gait velocity to a percentage of normal (based on a normal score of 82 m/min) can be an effective way to communicate locomotor abilities to patients, their families, and insurers (10). Patients who walk at less than 30% of normal do not usually become community ambulators because it takes too long to cover the required distances involved in IADL (10).

As part of a study examining the effects of exercise on balance mobility and the likelihood for falls in older adults with a history of recurrent falls, scores on the 3-minute walk test were compared between healthy older adults ages 65 to 90 with no neurological impairments and older adults the same age with a history of imbalance and falls. Results from this study found that neurologically intact older adults were able to walk 727±148 ft in 3 minutes with no loss of balance, compared with 323±166 ft in the group of fallers. In addition, the older adults with a history of imbalance lost balance an average of four times during the 3-minute test (11).

Energy Efficiency

Energy cost measurements can quantify the physiological costs of walking (6). Heart rate is a standard indicator for relative exercise intensity and work rate. Heart rate can be monitored through manual palpation or commercially available heart rate monitors. Energy costs associated with walking in the neu-

rologically intact individual are determined by using published tables and charts (3).

Measuring Stability

Stability during nonperturbed gait is documented by reporting the number of deviations from a 15-inch path and/or changes in velocity the patient demonstrates during the 3-minute walk test, and any physical assistance required to prevent a fall. Figure 14.1 gives an example of the scoring for a patient who has completed a 3-minute walk test. The results of his gait assessment suggest that the patient is not a functional community ambulator at this point.

QUANTIFYING TEMPORAL/ DISTANCE FACTORS

A number of authors have advocated the inclusion of other temporal/distance factors such as cadence, step, and stride length, in-

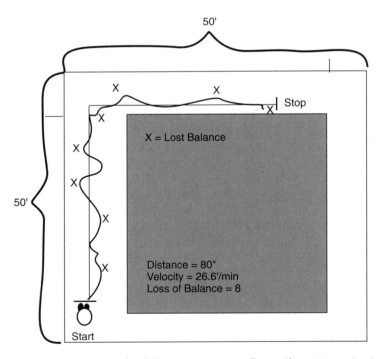

Figure 14.1. Scoring distance, velocity and stability in a 3-minute walk test. Shown is a patient's path along a premeasured course, and the number of times he deviates from a 15-inch path.

cluding right/left asymmetry in step and stride length in the assessment of gait (12, 13). These factors are usually documented during ambulation over a short distance, e.g., 20 to 30 ft. Characteristics of constant velocity gait are determined, and thus the first and last 5 ft are not used in the calculations. Patients are usually given one practice trial, followed by two data collection trials, separated by a rest period.

A number of methods for quantifying temporal/distance factors in the clinic have been suggested, including a footprint analysis using either inked feet and white butcher paper (12) or floor grids (Fig. 14.2) (13). Many clinicians do not have the time to subsequently analyze the results of these tests, and thus unanalyzed rolls of inked butcher block paper are found in closets and storage areas everywhere (14).

Other researchers have suggested that velocity alone can be used as a single measure of functional gait, since it is simple and quick, and appears to be a composite measure of the other temporal/distance variables (9, 15–18). However, as we discussed earlier, functional measures limited to velocity alone do not appear to provide the clinician with sufficient in-

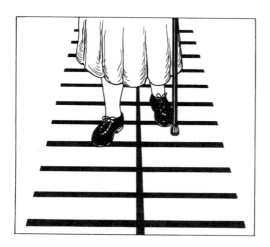

Figure 14.2. An example of a floor grid that can be used to visually guide patients towards better foot placement during gait. (Adapted from Jims C. Foot placement pattern, an aid in gait training. Suggestions from the field. Phys Ther 1977;57:286.)

formation to determine functional mobility capacity.

Scales for Assessing Mobility

Walking in a natural environment is characterized by starts and stops, changes in direction and speed, stepping over and around obstacles, and the integration of multiple tasks such as talking, turning to look at something, or carrying objects during gait. Thus, assessment of functional gait must include not only the evaluation of unimpeded gait, defined as a closed-skill task (18), but also the ability to modify and adapt gait to both expected and unexpected disturbances to locomotion. Several tests are available to examine the patient's ability to adapt gait to changing locomotor demands.

DUKE MOBILITY SKILLS PROFILE

The Duke Mobility Skills Profile (19) quantifies performance on multiple mobility tasks, including unimpeded gait, transfers, and stairs. Skills are scored 0, 1, or 2 based on the criteria shown in Table 14.1. This test is a highly reliable and valid predictor of fall probability in older adults.

FUNCTIONAL INDEPENDENCE MEASURE

The Functional Independence Measure (FIM), is an ADL test that includes measures of mobility function, including locomotion and transfers (5). Patient performance is graded based on the level of assistance required to perform mobility tasks using a 7-point scale. Scores range from 1 for total assistance, to 7, defined as complete independence. Performance is defined relative to distance, effort, and assistance required. For example, complete independence is defined as the ability to walk a minimum of 150 ft without assistive devices. The patient needing total assistance is defined as one who performs with less than 25% effort (meaning that approximately 25% of the work related to this activity is being performed by the patient, and

Table 14.1.   Duke Mobility Skills Profile[a]

1. Can this person walk?
   Yes—go to question three   yes=1
   No—go to question two   no=0 _____
2. Can this person sit upright without human assistance for 60 seconds?   yes=1
                                                                               no=0 _____

3. Does gait meet criteria?   yes=1
   (no device, symmetric, step length twice foot length)   no=0 _____
4. Can this person descend stairs step-over-step without holding railing?   yes=1
                                                                               no=0 _____

                                                                               Total_____

Soc. Sec.#: _____
day : _____

Mobility Skills Protocol
(modified 10/26/89)

Equipment - Straight-back hard-seated chair, tape measure, 12-inch ruler, shoebox, stopwatch, pencil, white tape
1. *Sitting balance*
   Will you sit forward in the chair, arms folded across chest, for 1 minute? (patient sits in
   standardized chair (straight back/kitchen-type chair), without leaning back for 1 minute.
   2 = can sit upright, unsupported for 60 sec.
   1 = can sit upright, independently *with support* for 60 sec. (holding onto arm of chair or leaning
       against back of chair)
   0 = cannot sit upright independently for 60 sec.   _____
2. *Sitting reach*
   Will you reach forward and get this ruler out of my hand? (45° plane-forward—put ruler 12 inches
   beyond dominant hand reach).
   2 = reaches forward and successfully grasps item
   1 = cannot grasp or requires arm support
   0 = does not attempt reach
   C = contraindicated
   R = refused   _____
3. *Transfer*
   Will you show me how to get from your chair to the bed (or to another chair)?
   2 = performs independently (without help from a person), appears steady and safe
   1 = performs independently (without help from a person), but appears unsteady
   0 = cannot do or requires help from a person to complete the task
   C = contraindicated
   R = refused   _____
4. *Rising from a chair*
   a. Will you get up from the chair without using your arms to push up?
      (patient seated in hardback/kitchen chair, arms folded across chest or out in front)
      1 = done on 1st try
      0 = not done on 1st try
      C = contraindicated
      R = refused   _____
   b. Will you get up from the chair using your arms to push up? (subject can put hands on arms of
      chair or on chair seat for assistance; subject can hold onto assistive device if desired as he stands
      up)
           ***** NOTE - (score = 1 if scored 1 on 4a)
      1 = can do independently
      0 = can't do independently
      C = contraindicated
      R = refused   _____

Table 14.1—*continued*

5. *Standing balance*
   a. Will you stand the way you usually stand for 1 minute?
      2 = steady, without holding onto walking aid or other object for support for 60 sec.
      1 = steady, but uses walking aid or other object for support for 60 sec.
      0 = cannot stand upright for 60 sec
      C = contraindicated
      R = refused _____
6. *Picking up object off the floor*
   (drop pencil 1 ft in front of subject (out of base of support), Will you pick this pencil up from the floor?
   2 = performs independently
      (without help from object/person)
   1 = performs with some help (holds on to a table, chair, assistive device, person, etc.) or is
      unsteady (staggers or sways, has to catch self to to keep from falling, etc.)
   0 = unable to pick up object and return to standing
   C = contraindicated
   R = refused _____
7. *Walking*
   (measure 10-ft pathway)
   Will you walk in your usual way (with or without assistive device) from here to here (indicate
   distance to patient—allow 3'–5' for warm-up).
   2 = meets all standards for gait characteristics
   1 = fails any standard or uses assistive device
   0 = unstable, can't do (requires intervention to keep from falling or staggers, trips)
   C = contraindicated
   R = refused _____
   standards for gait (tested only in subject's preferred manner)
   1. symmetrical step length
   2. walks along straight path
   3. distance between stance toe and heel of swing foot at least 1 ft length
8. *Turning*
   Will you walk along the path, then turn and come back?
   2 = no more than three continuous steps, no assistive device
   1 = fails criteria for a score of 2 but completes task without intervention
   0 = unable to turn, requires intervention to prevent falling
   C = contraindicated
   R = refused _____
9. *Abrupt stop*
   Will you walk as fast as you can and stop when I say stop? (walks with subject and announce
   "stop" after 6–8 steps)
   2 = stops within one step without stumbling or grabbing
   1 = cannot stop within one step or stumbles, uses assistive device
   0 = requires intervention to avoid fall
   C = contraindicated
   R = refused _____
10. *Obstacle*
    (place shoebox in walking path)
    Will you walk at your normal pace and step over the shoebox that is in the way?
    2 = steps over without interrupting stride
    1 = catches foot, interrupts stride, uses assistive device
    0 = cannot step over box
    C = contraindicated
    R = refused _____

Table 14.1.—*continued*

11. *Standing Reach*
    (45° plane—forward—put ruler 12 inches beyond dominant hand reach)
    Will you reach forward and get this ruler from me?
    2 = reaches forward and successfully grasps ruler without stepping or holding on
    1 = reaches forward but cannot grasp ruler without stepping or holding on to device
    0 = does not attempt to shift weight
    C = contraindicated
    R = refused   _____

12. *Stairs* (must have at least 2 steps)
    Try to go up and down these stairs without holding on to the railing.
    Ascending
    2 = steps over step, does not hold on to railing or device
    1 = one step at a time, or must hold on to railing or device
    0 = unsteady, can't do
    C = contraindicated
    R = refused   _____
    Descending
    2 = steps over step, does not hold on to railing or device
    1 = one step at a time, or must hold on to railing or device
    0 = unsteady, can't do
    C = contraindicated
    R = refused   _____

13. Preferred assistive device:
    _____ wheelchair (= 1)
    _____ walker (= 2)
    _____ quad cane (= 3)
    _____ straight cane (= 4)
    _____ other_____ (= 5)
    _____ none (= 0)

aReprinted with permission: Duncan P. Duke Mobility Skills Profile. Center for Human Aging, Duke University.

75% is being performed by the therapist), or requires assistance of two people, or does not walk a minimum of 50 ft (5).

DYNAMIC GAIT INDEX

The Dynamic Gait Index (20) evaluates and documents a patient's ability to modify gait in response to changing task demands. This index was developed as part of a profile of tests and measurements effective in predicting likelihood for falls in older adults (21). The test is shown in Table 14.2. Preliminary research has shown that the test has good inter-rater and test-retest reliability and is a valid predictor of falls among the elderly. For example, a population of 15 healthy older adults with no neurological impairments or history of imbalance received a mean score of 21 ± 3 on the Dynamic Gait Index. In contrast, an equal number of older adults with a history of falls and imbalance, but no neurological diagnosis such as stroke or Parkinson's disease, received a mean score of 11 ± 4 (21).

LIMITATIONS OF PERFORMANCE-BASED TEMPORAL/DISTANCE GAIT MEASURES

All performance-based measures, whether of mobility, balance, or general motor control, are indicators of end-product only, and do not provide information about the way performance is achieved. Thus, these measures do not provide insight into underlying impairments that require treatment. However, performance-based measures are good indicators of overall function and, therefore, important indices of change.

Assessing at the Strategy Level

Assessment of gait also includes a systematic description of the strategies used by

Table 14.2. Dynamic Gait Index

1. Gait level surface _____

Instructions: Walk at your normal speed from here to the next mark (20′)

Grading: Mark the lowest category which applies.

  (3) Normal: Walks 20′, no assistive devices, good speed, no evidence for imbalance, normal gait pattern.

  (2) Mild impairment: Walks 20′, uses assistive devices, slower speed, mild gait deviations.

  (1) Moderate impairment: Walks 20′, slow speed, abnormal gait pattern, evidence for imbalance.

  (0) Severe impairment: Cannot walk 20′ without assistance, severe gait deviations, or imbalance.

2. Change in gait speed _____

Instructions: Begin walking at your normal pace (for 5′), when I tell you "go," walk as fast as you can (for 5′). When I tell you "slow," walk as slowly as you can (for 5′).

Grading:

Mark the lowest category that applies.

  (3) Normal: Able to smoothly change walking speed without loss of balance or gait deviation. Shows a significant difference in walking speeds between normal, fast, and slow speeds.

  (2) Mild impairment: Is able to change speed but demonstrates mild gait deviations, or no gait deviations but unable to achieve a significant change in velocity, or uses an assistive device.

  (1) Moderate impairment: Makes only minor adjustments to walking speed, or accomplishes a change in speed with significant gait deviations, or changes speed but loses significant gait deviations, or changes speed but loses balance but is able to recover and continue walking.

  (0) Severe impairment: Cannot change speeds, or loses balance and has to reach for wall or be caught.

3. Gait with horizontal head turns _____

Instructions: Begin walking at your normal pace. When I tell you to "look right," keep walking straight, but turn your head to the right. Keep looking to the right until I tell you, "look left," then keep walking straight and turn your head to the left. Keep your head to the left until I tell you, "look straight," then keep walking straight, but return your head to the center.

Grading: Mark the lowest category which applies.

  (3) Normal: Performs head turns smoothly with no change in gait

  (2) Mild impairment: Performs head turns smoothly with slight change in gait velocity, i.e., minor disruption to smooth gait path or uses walking aid.

  (1) Moderate impairment: Performs head turns with moderate change in gait velocity, slows down, staggers but recovers, can continue to walk.

  (0) Severe impairment: Performs task with severe disruption of gait, i.e., staggers outside 15″ path, loses balance, stops, reaches for wall.

4. Gait with vertical head turns _____

Instructions: Begin walking at your normal pace. When I tell you to "look up," keep walking straight, but tip your head and look up. Keep looking up until I tell you, "look down." Then keep walking straight and turn your head down. Keep looking down until I tell you, "look straight," then keep walking straight, but return your head to the center.

Grading: Mark the lowest category that applies.

  (3) Normal: Performs head turns with no change in gait.

  (2) Mild impairment: Performs task with slight change in gait velocity i.e., minor disruption to smooth gait path or uses walking aid.

  (1) Moderate impairment: Performs task with moderate change in gait velocity, slows down, staggers but recovers, can continue to walk.

  (0) Severe impairment: Performs task with severe disruption of gait, i.e., staggers outside 15″ path, loses balance, stops, reaches for wall.

5. Gait and pivot turn _____

Instructions: Begin walking at your normal pace. When I tell you, "turn and stop," turn as quickly as you can to face the opposite direction and stop.

Grading: Mark the lowest category that applies.

  (3) Normal: Pivot turns safely within 3 seconds and stops quickly with no loss of balance.

  (2) Mild impairment: Pivot turns safely in > 3 seconds and stops with no loss of balance.

  (1) Moderate impairment: Turns slowly, requires verbal cueing, requires several small steps to catch balance following turn and stop.

  (0) Severe impairment: Cannot turn safely, requires assistance to turn and stop.

Table 14.2.—*continued*

6. Step over obstacle _____
Instructions: Begin walking at your normal speed. When you come to the shoe box, step over it, not around it, and keep walking.
Grading: Mark the lowest category that applies.
 (3) Normal: Is able to step over box without changing gait speed; no evidence for imbalance.
 (2) Mild impairment: Is able to step over box, but must slow down and adjust steps to clear box safely.
 (1) Moderate impairment: Is able to step over box but must stop, then step over. May require verbal cuing.
 (0) Severe impairment: Cannot perform without assistance.
7. Step around obstacles _____
Instructions: Begin walking at your normal speed. When you come to the first cone (about 6' away), walk around the right side of it. When you come to the second cone (6' past first cone), walk around it to the left.
Grading: Mark the lowest category that applies.
 (3) Normal: Is able to walk around cones safely without changing gait speed; no evidence of imbalance.
 (2) Mild impairment: Is able to step around both cones, but must slow down and adjust steps to clear cones.
 (1) Moderate impairment: Is able to clear cones but must significantly slow, speed to accomplish task, or requires verbal cueing.
 (0) Severe impairment: Unable to clear cones, walks into one or both cones, or requires physical assistance.
8. Steps _____
Instructions: Walk up these stairs as you would at home (i.e., using the rail if necessary. At the top, turn around and walk down.
Grading: Mark the lowest category that applies.
 (3) Normal: Alternating feet, no rail.
 (2) Mild impairment: Alternating feet, must use rail.
 (1) Moderate impairment: Two feet to a stair; must use rail.
 (0) Severe impairment: Cannot do safely.

patients to meet the requirements inherent in locomotion.

OBSERVATIONAL GAIT ANALYSIS

Observational gait analysis is the tool most frequently used in the clinic to qualitatively evaluate gait patterns (22). Documentation forms have been developed to assist the clinician in observational gait analysis; these forms vary in their degree of complexity and detail.

Prior to discussing some of these forms, we need to understand some key points that are important to note in each of the phases of gait during an observational gait analysis. Table 14.3 summarizes these points. Also summarized are deviations commonly seen in the patient with neurological impairments and a list of the possible impairments that could result in these deviations. This list is not intended to be exhaustive, but rather summarizes some of the major problems commonly found in such patients.

When performing an observational gait analysis using the framework suggested in this table, the clinician observes one phase of gait at a time, noting the action performed at each of the joints, and describing any deviation from a normal gait strategy. The analysis of stance would begin by observing the position of the foot at heel-strike. For example, the clinician might note that the patient with neurological dysfunction makes initial contact at heel-strike with a flat foot.

The possible causes list guides the clinician in forming preliminary hypotheses about the underlying causes of the atypical pattern. In our example, foot-flat position at heel-strike could be the result of plantarflexor contracture, spasticity, or inactivity of the tibialis anterior (TA). These hypotheses guide the next step of assessment, which is to test these hypotheses and thus determine the cause of the patient's gait deviation. In our example, the patient uses a foot-flat heel-strike, due to inactivity of the TA.

With this information, the clinician is

Table 14.3.   Problem-Oriented Observational Gait Analysis

Stance Phase

Ankle

Normal: Dorsiflexed at heel-strike, neutral with respect to eversion/inversion, smooth progression into plantar flexion until the foot is flat, controlled advancement of the tibia over the stable foot (ankle dorsiflexion)

Abnormal	*Possible Causes*
Low heel/foot flat/ or forefoot contact—at heel-strike	Plantarflexor contractures
	Plantarflexor spasticity
	Inactivity of TA
	Poor knee extension-terminal swing
	Use of an extensor synergy
Foot-slap	Inactivity of TA
Lateral border (varus)	Invertor spasticity
Medial border (valgus)	Inactivity of TA
Excessive plantarflexion	As above
Excessive dorsiflexion midstance	Plantarflexor weakness
No heel-rise, no toe-off terminal stance	Plantarflexor spasticity
	Plantarflexor contracture

Knee

Normal: extension followed by brief flexion followed by knee extension until terminal stance when knee begins to flex

Abnormal	*Possible Causes*
Excessive knee extension	Plantar flexor contracture
	Plantar flexor spasticity
	Quadriceps spasticity
	Compensate weak quads
	Use of an extensor synergy
Persistent knee flexion	Plantarflexor inactivity
	Hamstring overactivity

Trunk/Hip

Normal: initial hip flexion with smooth progression to extension by midstance, and hyperextension by terminal stance; trunk remains vertical

Abnormal	*Possible Causes*
Excessive hip flexion/Trunk forward lean	Hip flexor contracture
	Hip flexor spasticity
	Hip extensor weakness
	Compensate weak quads
Hip extension/Trunk backward lean	Compensate weak flexors
	Compensate weak hip extensors
Trunk lateral lean	Weak abductors
Scissors Gait	Abductor weakness—contralateral
	Adductor spasticity—ipsilateral

Pelvis

Normal: neutral with respect to vertical displacement and anterior/posterior tip; forward rotation at heel-strike, smooth progression into posterior rotation through stance phase

Abnormal	*Possible Causes*
Elevated	Abductor weakness—contralateral
Dropped	
Retracted	

Table 14.3.—*continued*

Swing phase

Ankle

Normal: Plantarflexion at toe-off, into dorsiflexion by midswing, continued dorsiflexion into terminal swing

Abnormal	*Possible Causes*
Plantarflexion at ankle	Plantar flexor contracture
	Plantar flexor spasticity
	Inadequate activation of TA
Varus foot position	Spastic invertors
Valgus foot position	Inadequate activation of TA

Knee

Normal: Initial flexion, increased flexion by mid swing, into extension by terminal swing.

Abnormal	*Possible Causes*
Inadequate knee flexion—Initial to mid swing	Knee extensor contracture
	Quadriceps spasticity
	Plantar flexor contracture
	Plantar flexor spasticity
	Use of Extensor synergy
Inadequate knee extension—Terminal swing	Knee flexor contractures
	Hamstring hyperactivity
	Use of flexor synergy

Hip

Normal: General motion is extension into flexion; begins with hyperextension, neutral by midswing, and flexion by terminal swing

Abnormal	*Possible Causes*
Inadequate hip flexion	Inability to activate hip flexors
	Decreased hip proprioception
Circumduction (hip hike/abduction)	Compensate weak hip flexors
Contralateral vaulting	Compensate weak hip flexors

Pelvis

Normal: Pelvis drops slightly during swing, remains neutral with respect to anterior/posterior tilt, rotates from backward to forward position

Abnormal	*Possible Causes*
Posterior tip	Compensate weak hip flexors
Anterior rotation	Compensate weak hip flexors
Elevation	Compensate weak hip flexors

able to develop appropriate treatment strategies to remediate the underlying impairment and improve the gait pattern. In our example, the clinician could use the following treatments: (*a*) a strengthening program targeting eccentric and concentric contractions of the TA; (*b*) facilitation techniques, like icing the TA immediately before and during gait training; (*c*) electrical stimulation during gait to improve activation of the TA, and (*d*) use of an ankle-foot orthosis to control plantarflexion during gait until the patient is able to activate the TA appropriately.

Stance Phase of Gait

Key elements within a normal strategy for controlling the *ankle and foot* during stance include (*a*) smooth unimpeded motion of the body over the foot, (*b*) the foot leading the body at heel-strike but trailing the body at toe-off. This trailing toe-off posture is important for effective generation of propulsive forces.

A clinician might ask several questions when examining ankle-foot control during the stance phase of gait. For example, what is the position of the foot when it contacts the floor at the beginning of the stance phase of gait? During loading and progression to mid-stance, does the tibia advance over the stable foot, reaching vertical by mid-stance? During terminal stance, does the tibia continue its forward advancement, with the ankle dorsi-flexing, even though the hip and knee are ex-tended? Does the heel rise at the end of stance phase as the body rises up onto the forefoot in preparation for toe-off?

Key elements normally observed at the *knee* are (*a*) the position of the knee during weight acceptance, and (*b*) the position and stability of the knee during the course of the stance phase. Normally, the knee is extended at the initiation of stance. Just after contact with the surface, there is a brief flexion, then extension at the knee, which absorbs some of the impact of weight acceptance. The knee re-mains extended, but not hyperextended, dur-ing stance, beginning to flex at toe-off (23).

Is the patient's knee flexed or extended at heel-strike? Is there a brief period of flexion followed by extension as the patient shifts weight to the stance limb? Does the knee move into extension smoothly or abruptly? At mid-stance, is the knee extended to neutral, or does the knee thrust back into hyperexten-sion?

Key elements of normal *hip* control dur-ing stance include (*a*) the smooth progression from flexion into extension by mid-stance and hyperextension by terminal stance, and (*b*) the trunk remains vertical (23).

What is the position of the hip at heel-strike? Is it flexed? Does the hip move smoothly into extension, or remain flexed? Is the hip extended to neutral by mid-stance with the trunk upright and aligned above it? Is the patient able to hyperextend the hip, while at the same time dorsiflexing the ankle, as the stance limb moves posterior?

Normal *pelvic* control includes the fol-lowing key elements: (*a*) a slight elevation of the pelvis during movement to single limb stance; (*b*) smooth rotation of the pelvis from forward to backward position during stance; and (*c*) neutral position of the pelvis with re-spect to anterior and posterior tilt.

What is the position of the pelvis at heel-strike? Is it tipped backward, or alternatively, forward with excessive lordosis? Does the pel-vis move smoothly from a forwardly rotated position to a posterior position as stance pro-gresses? Does the pelvis drop or hike exces-sively?

Swing Phase

Key elements within a normal strategy for controlling the ankle and foot during swing include (*a*) plantarflexion of the foot at toe-off, followed by dorsiflexion of the ankle, which is maintained throughout the rest of swing, and (*b*) foot clearance is normally achieved by less than 1 inch (23).

Is the foot trailing the stance limb at the initiation of swing? Is the heel off the ground during toe-off? Is toe-off accomplished from a forefoot support position? Does the foot clear the ground with no catches during the swing phase? Does the foot move in front of the swing leg toward the end of swing in prep-aration for heel-strike?

Normal control of the knee during swing includes (*a*) flexion of the knee at the beginning of swing, continuing through mid-swing, and (*b*) extension of the knee by ter-minal swing in preparation for heel-strike (23).

Is there a smooth transition from flexion into extension at the knee during the swing phase? Is the patient unable to flex the knee during swing? Is the patient using a flexor syn-ergy pattern to achieve flexion of the swing limb? Is the patient able to extend the knee (in conjunction with hip flexion) at terminal swing?

Key points to observe in normal *hip and trunk* control include (*a*) the general motion at the hip during swing is extension to flexion, (*b*) the hip begins from a hyperextended po-sition at the beginning of gait, moves to neu-tral by mid-swing, and into flexion by the end of swing, and (*c*) the trunk remains vertical (23).

How is the patient advancing the limb? Is foot clearance being achieved? Is the pa-tient using a flexor strategy to bring the limb forward? If flexion is being used, is it within a total flexor synergy pattern? Alternatively, is the patient forced to hike and circumduct the hip to advance the limb? Is vaulting of the contralateral stance limb being used to effect toe clearance? Does the hip start from an extended position? Is the hip flexing with enough force to produce an associated flexion at the knee? Is the trunk vertical, or is it inclined forward, backward, or to one side?

Normal control of the *pelvis* during swing involves (*a*) a slight drop of the pelvis during swing, but the pelvis tends to remain neutral with respect to anterior/posterior tilt. Perry (23) states that if upwards or downwards tilt of the pelvis is apparent, it is always abnormal, since it is not possible to distinguish this motion in normal gait; (*b*) at the beginning of swing, the pelvis is rotated in the backward direction, and rotates smoothly forward during the swing phase (23).

Does the pelvis remain relatively vertical during swing? Is there an obvious tilting motion of the pelvis, either anteriorly or posteriorly? In the beginning of swing, is the pelvis rotated backwards? Is there a smooth progression of the pelvis to an anterior position during swing?

FORMS FOR OBSERVATIONAL GAIT ANALYSIS

There are forms available to help clinicians structure their approach to observational gait analysis. Why would a clinician need to perform both a functional mobility assessment and a gait analysis? Each provides information helpful in establishing a plan of care for the patient. For example, an observational gait analysis can help a clinician determine the extent to which the current strategies a patient is using meet the inherent progression, stability, and adaptation demands of locomotion.

What are the costs and benefits of current strategies; that is, are they effective at meeting demands in one phase of gait, but limit the patient's options in another phase of gait? For example, the use of an extensor synergy pattern during stance to support the

weight of the body during loading may be an effective strategy for stability during stance, but at the same time, an extensor synergy during swing will prevent the forward advancement of the limb, limiting progression (10).

The clinician may use observational gait analysis to document the presence of a hip hike/circumduction movement strategy to advance the limb during the swing phase of gait. But what are the potential effects of using this strategy on this patient's functional performance? First, use of a hip-hike, circumduction strategy to advance the swing leg will slow the patient's gait speed. This will be reflected in decreased distance traveled and velocity, both variables measured on the 3-minute walk test. In addition, it will affect his or her score on the Dynamic Gait Index, since he/she may be unable to adapt this pattern sufficiently to complete the tasks involving walking on uneven surfaces.

The clinician can use information from both functional assessment and gait analysis to determine whether treatment is warranted. Can treatment improve the strategies a patient is using to achieve the demands of locomotion, thereby increasing functional capability?

Some examples of observational gait analysis forms that are helpful in guiding a clinical assessment of gait patterns in the patient with neurological impairments follow.

Rancho Los Amigos Gait Analysis Form

The Gait Analysis Form, shown in Table 14.4, from the physical therapy department, Rancho Los Amigos Hospital, Downey, California, is a comprehensive approach to movement analysis during gait (24).

Mobility Assessment Form

A more simple and less extensive approach to observational gait analysis is represented by the Mobility Assessment Form, part of the Balance and Mobility Assessment Profile proposed by Tinetti (25). This is provided in the chapter on assessment and treatment of postural control.

Table 14.4.   Rancho Los Amigos Gait Analysis Form[a]

GAIT ANALYSIS: FULL BODY

RANCHO LOS AMIGOS MEDICAL CENTER
PHYSICAL THERAPY DEPARTMENT

Reference Limb:
L ☐   R ☐

		Weight Accept		Single Limb Support		Swing Limb Advancement			
☐ Major Deviation		IC	LR	MSt	TSt	PSw	ISw	MSw	TSw
▨ Minor Deviation									
Trunk	Lean: B/F								
	Lateral Lean: R/L								
	Rotates: B/F								
Pelvis	Hikes								
	Tilt: P/A								
	Lacks Forward Rotation								
	Lacks Backward Rotation								
	Excess Forward Rotation								
	Excess Backward Rotation								
	Ipsilateral Drop								
	Contralateral Drop								
Hip	Flexion: Limited								
	Excess								
	Inadequate Extension								
	Past Retract								
	Rotation: IR/ER								
	Ad/Abduction: Ad/Ab								
Knee	Flexion: Limited								
	Excess								
	Inadequate Extension								
	Wobbles								
	Hyperextends								
	Extension Thrust								
	Varus/Valgus: Vr/Vl								
	Excess Contralateral Flex								
Ankle	Forefoot Contact								
	Foot-Flat Contact								
	Foot Slap								
	Excess Plantar Flexion								
	Excess Dorsiflexion								
	Inversion/Eversion: Iv/Ev								
	Heel Off								
	No Heel Off								
	Drag								
	Contralateral Vaulting								
Toes	Up								
	Inadequate Extension								
	Clawed								

MAJOR PROBLEMS:

Weight Acceptance

Single Limb Support

Swing Limb Advancement

Excessive UE Weight Bearing ☐

Name

Diagnosis

© 1991 LAREI, Rancho Los Amigos Medical Center, Downey, CA 90242

[a]Reprinted with permission of Rancho Los Amigos Medical Center's Physical Therapy Department and Pathokinesiology Laboratory, Downey, California.

Gait Assessment Rating Scale (GARS)

The Gait Assessment Rating Scale (GARS), developed by Wolfson and colleagues, is shown in Table 14.5 (26). The scale also allows the quantification and documentation of four categories of gait abnormalities. The scale has been used to document gait problems in healthy elderly, as well as in older adults with a history of falls. The test has been shown to have high inter-rater reliability, and is a sensitive indicator of changes in gait function among older adults.

Finally, clinicians can develop their own form to guide gait analysis. This form can vary in its complexity and depth of analysis, as was shown in the form in Table 14.2. Regardless of the type of form used, the process of gait analysis can be facilitated by videotaping the patient's gait. Though potentially time consuming to perform, in the long run, videotaping provides the clinician more time to observe gait, and therefore increases the reliability and validity of the observational gait analysis. Replaying the tape, particularly with stop-frame and slow-motion features, allows repeated viewing of gait patterns without fatiguing a patient.

LIMITATIONS TO OBSERVATIONAL GAIT ANALYSIS

Studies have shown that a major limitation of most observational gait analysis is poor reliability even among highly trained and experienced clinicians (22). In addition, a detailed qualitative gait analysis is very time-consuming, and often unrealistic in a busy clinical environment. Finally, strong evidence does not exist to indicate that most observational gait analysis forms are sensitive to changes in gait patterns in response to therapy.

An alternative to observational gait analysis is the use of technological systems to quantify movement patterns, muscle activation patterns, and forces used in gait. However, this technology is beyond the reach of the average clinician. In addition to being extremely expensive, this equipment requires considerable time and technical expertise to use.

Gait analysis is an integral part of almost every motor control evaluation in the patient with neurological dysfunction. Gait itself is complex, and understanding the complications of gait is even more difficult. Therefore, it is essential that a clinician have a systematic and consistent approach to observing and analyzing gait. Despite its limitations, an observational gait analysis form provides a framework for systematically observing gait, and is therefore an essential part of the gait assessment process.

Assessing at the Impairment Level

Assessing the impairment level of function was discussed in detail in Chapter 10, and thus is not discussed further in this chapter. The reader is encouraged to refer back to Chapter 10 for a review of principles of assessment at the impairment level of function.

A task-oriented approach to assessing mobility function includes performance-based measures of mobility, assessment of gait strategies, and evaluation and documentation of underlying impairments. There are a range of tests and measurements from which a clinician can draw, in order to assemble a comprehensive mobility assessment tool.

TRANSITION TO TREATMENT

Setting Goals

As is true for goal setting related to other physical skills, clinicians need to establish both long- and short-term goals during mobility retraining which are objective, measurable, and meaningful.

LONG-TERM GOALS

Long-term goals are often stated in terms of functional performance. They usually reflect ambulation outcomes with respect to level of independence. An example of a long-term goal might be: the patient will be able to walk a minimum of 1000 ft independently with the use of a cane and orthosis.

Table 14.5. Components of the Gait Assessment Rating Score (GARS)[a]

A. General Categories
  1. Variability—a measure of inconsistency and arrhythmicity of stepping and of arm movements.
    0 = fluid and predictably paced limb movements;
    1 = occasional interruptions (changes in velocity), approximately <25% of time;
    2 = unpredictability of rhythm approximately 25–75% of time;
    3 = random timing of limb movements.
  2. Guardedness—hesitancy, slowness, diminished propulsion and lack of commitment in stepping and arm swing
    0 = good forward momentum and lack of apprehension in propulsion;
    1 = center of gravity of head, arms and trunk (HAT) projects only slightly in front of push-off, but still good arm-leg coordination;
    2 = HAT held over anterior aspect of foot, and some moderate loss of smooth reciprocation;
    3 = HAT held over rear aspect of stance-phase foot, and great tentativity in stepping.
  3. Weaving—an irregular and wavering line of progression
    0 = straight line of progression on frontal viewing;
    1 = a single deviation from straight (line of best fit) line of progression:
    2 = two to three deviations from line of progression;
    3 = four or more deviations from line of progression.
  4. Waddling—a broad-based gait characterized by excessive truncal crossing of the midline and side-bending
    0 = narrow base of support and body held nearly vertically over feet;
    1 = slight separation of medial aspects of feet and just perceptible lateral movement of head and trunk;
    2 = 3-4" separation feet and obvious bending of trunk to side so that COG of head lies well over ipsilateral stance foot;
    3 = extreme pendular deviations of head and trunk (head passes lateral to ipsilateral stance foot), and further widening of base of support.
  5. Staggering—sudden and unexpected laterally directed partial losses of balance
    0 = no losses of balance to side;
    1 = a single lurch to side;
    2 = two lurches to side;
    3 = three or more lurches to side.
B. Lower Extremity Categories
  1. % Time in Swing—a loss in the percentage of the gait cycle constituted by the swing phase
    0 = approximately 3:2 ratio of duration of stance to swing phase;
    1 = a 1:1 or slightly less ratio of stance to swing;
    2 = markedly prolonged stance phase, but with some obvious swing time remaining;
    3 = barely perceptible portion of cycle spent in swing.
  2. Foot Contact—the degree to which heel strikes the ground before the forefoot
    0 = very obvious angle of impact of heel on ground;
    1 = barely visible contact of heel before forefoot;
    2 = entire foot lands flat on ground;
    3 = anterior aspect of foot strikes ground before heel.
  3. Hip ROM—the degree of loss of hip range of motion seen during a gait cycle
    0 = obvious angulation of thigh backwards during double support (10 deg);
    1 = just barely visible angulation backwards from vertical;
    2 = thigh in line with vertical projection from ground;
    3 = thigh angled forwards from vertical at maximum posterior excursion.
  4. Knee Range of Motion—the degree of loss of knee range of motion seen during a gait cycle
    0 = knee moves from complete extension at heel-strike (and late-stance) to almost 90° (@ 70°) during swing phase;
    1 = slight bend in knee seen at heel-strike and late-stance and maximal flexion at midswing is closer to 45° than 90°;
    2 = knee flexion at late stance more obvious than at heel-strike, very little clearance seen for toe during swing;
    3 = toe appears to touch ground during swing, knee flexion appears constant during stance, and knee angle during swing appears 45° or less.

Table 14.5.—*continued*

C. Trunk, Head, and Upper Extremity Categories
1. Elbow Extension—a measure of the decrease of elbow range of motion
    0 = large peak-to-peak excursion of forearm (approximately 20 deg), with distinct maximal flexion at end of anterior trajectory;
    1 = 25% decrement of extension during maximal posterior excursion of upper extremity;
    2 = almost no change in elbow angle;
    3 = no apparent change in elbow angle (held in flexion);
2. Shoulder Extension—a measure of the decrease of shoulder range of motion
    0 = clearly seen movement of upper arm anterior (15 deg) and posterior (20 deg) to vertical axis of trunk;
    1 = shoulder flexes slightly anterior to vertical axis;
    2 = shoulder comes only to vertical axis, or slightly posterior to it during flexion;
    3 = shoulder stays well behind vertical axis during entire excursion.
3. Shoulder Abduction—a measure of pathological increase in shoulder range of motion laterally
    0 = shoulders held almost parallel to trunk;
    1 = shoulders held 5–10 deg to side;
    2 = shoulders held 10–20 deg to side;
    3 = shoudlers held greater than 20 deg to side.
4. Arm-Heelstrike Synchrony—the extent to which the contralateral movements of an arm and leg are out of phase
    0 = good temporal conjunction of arm and contralateral leg at apex of shoulder and hip excursions all of the time;
    1 = arm and leg slightly out of phase 25% of the time;
    2 = arm and leg moderately out of phase 25-50% of time;
    3 = little or no temporal coherence of arm and leg.
5. Head Held Forward—a measure of the pathological forward projection of the head relative to the trunk
    0 = ear-lobe vertically aligned with shoulder tip;
    1 = ear-lobe vertical projection falls 1″ anterior to shoulder tip;
    2 = ear-lobe vertical projection falls 2″ anterior to shoulder tip;
    3 = ear-lobe vertical projection falls 3″ or more anterior to shoulder tip.
6. Shoulders Held Elevated—the degree to which the scapular girdle is held higher than normal
    0 = tip of shoulder (acromion) markedly below level of chin (1–2″);
    1 = tip of shoulder slightly below level of chin;
    2 = tip of shoulder at level of chin;
    3 = tip of shoulder above level of chin.
7. Upper Trunk Flexed Forward—a measure of kyphotic involvement of the trunk
    0 = very gentle thoracic convexity, cervical spine flat, or almost flat;
    1 = emerging cervical curve, more distant thoracic convexity;
    2 = anterior concavity at mid-chest level apparent;
    3 = anterior concavity at mid-chest level very obvious.

[a]From Wolfsan L, Whipple R, Amerman P, Tobin JN. Gait assessment in the elderly: a gait abnormality rating scale and its relation to falls. J Gerontal 1990; 45:M12–M19.

SHORT-TERM GOALS

Short-term goals for mobility retraining can be expressed in terms of:

1. Changing underlying impairments. One example would be to decrease flexion contractures at the hip by 20°, at the knee by 15°, and at the ankle by 20°.
2. Improving gait patterns. One example would be to decrease forward trunk flexion by 20° and thereby improve upright posture during stance and swing phase of gait.
3. Accomplishing interim steps towards long-term goals. Examples include (*a*) to increase distance walked, with only stand-by assist, from 10 ft to 25 ft; (*b*) to increase speed; patient will be able to walk 200 ft, stand-by assist only, in 45 secs; (*c*) to become independent in the use of a quadruped cane.

Short-term goals usually lead to treatment strategies aimed at resolving underlying impairments, and improving the quality of gait strategies used to achieve the three task requirements of gait, that is, progression, stability, and adaptation. Long-term goals often lead to treatment strategies related to improving the overall performance of ambulation, such as increasing the distance walked or the speed of ambulation. Often, the two are interrelated, as when the goal is to improve a particular aspect of the locomotor pattern to increase the velocity of gait.

In addition, goals related to retraining mobility function can be defined in relationship to the three requirements of gait (20).

DEFINING GOALS BASED ON THE TASK REQUIREMENTS OF GAIT

Progression

Treatment goals related to *progression* concern helping the patient develop the capacity to generate momentum to facilitate forward propulsion of the body. Specific examples include:

1. Improve the range and freedom of motion so that momentum can be transferred freely between body segments. This encompasses improving range of motion, decreasing contractures, reducing spasticity, which limits the velocity of motion, and reducing coactivation of muscles, which increases joint stiffness.

2. Increase the patient's speed of walking because generation of momentum requires, a minimum speed of movement. This includes increasing the speed at which segments are moved. For example, increasing the speed and amplitude of hip flexion during the swing phase of gait will advance the thigh segment quickly. This will facilitate passive knee flexion for toe clearance, and subsequent knee extension for foot placement. This goal requires facilitation of hip flexion in conjunction with knee extension, thus decreasing reliance on a

flexor synergy pattern to accomplish the goals of swing.

3. Work on the goal of helping the patient to achieve a vertical body posture, which allows the center of body mass to move anterior to the stance leg. This will create a forward fall position essential for generating forward momentum. This begins during initial stance with facilitation of graded plantarflexor activity, so that the tibia can advance smoothly over the stationary foot. In addition, during single limb stance, one can encourage the patient to maintain a vertical trunk, with the hip and knee extended. If the trunk is leaning forward and hips are flexed, this position will keep the body vector within the base of support of the foot. One can then progress to helping the patient develop a trailing limb position during terminal stance, facilitating hip and knee extension, knee extension, lifting the heel, and rolling the body weight onto the forefoot.

4. Help the patient develop a strategy that ensures adequate toe clearance during the swing phase of gait. Patients need to learn to advance the swing leg with minimal contact with the surface, since this decreases, or halts, forward momentum.

Stability

Treatment goals related to stability reflect (*a*) the need for a good foot placement, to facilitate weightbearing during initiation of stance, (*b*) the presence of sufficient extensor torque to support the body against gravity during single limb stance, and (*c*) facilitation of hip and trunk extensors to control the hip-arm-trunk (HAT) segment. Thus, working toward stability during gait includes helping the patient:

1. To accomplish a heel first foot-strike, in the absence of coronal plane deviations. This position will allow the body to move smoothly over the foot, and to

take advantage of the full weightbearing surface of the foot, enhancing stability;

2. To develop coordinated extension at the hip and knee, in order to generate an extensor moment to support body weight during single limb stance;

3. To develop a vertical posture of the trunk, with good hip and back extension to control the HAT segment, and adequate activation of the abductors to control the pelvis; and

4. To facilitate extensor moments at the hip and knee while maintaining the capacity to dorsiflex the ankle, thus avoiding use of a total extensor synergy pattern during stance.

Adaptation

Treatment goals related to adaptation require the patient to modify movement and sensory strategies for locomotor control in response to changing task and environmental demands.

Adaptation goals include helping the patient:

1. To develop the ability to integrate compensatory aspects of postural control into the ongoing gait cycle;

2. To develop the ability to utilize visual cues to identify upcoming disturbances to mobility and modify gait strategies in order to minimize their effect. Specific examples include scanning strategies to identify potential obstacles, and stepping over an obstacle safely, without modifying the gait path;

3. To develop the ability to utilize visual cues to identify potential obstacles and alter walking path appropriately so as to avoid obstacles.

With comprehensive and realistic goals established, based on the patient's desires and problems, the clinician can move ahead to planning treatments designed to meet these goals.

TREATMENT OF GAIT

A task-oriented approach to retraining mobility function focuses on helping a patient develop the most effective and efficient strategies for locomotion possible in the face of persisting sensory, motor, and cognitive impairments. Treatment is directed at (*a*) improving or preventing impairments, as possible, (*b*) developing gait strategies that meet the requirements for progression and stability during the stance and swing phases of gait, and (*c*) developing adaptive strategies appropriate to changing task and environmental demands. In addition, treatment may be geared towards preventing the development of secondary impairments.

Treating at the Impairment Level

The goal of treatment aimed at the impairment level is to correct those impairments that can be changed, and prevent the development of secondary impairments. Alleviating underlying impairments enables the patient to resume using previously developed strategies for gait. When permanent impairments make resumption of previously used strategies impossible, new strategies will have to be developed.

In the chapter on assessment and treatment of the patient with postural disorders, we discussed at length various treatment strategies aimed at resolving or preventing underlying musculoskeletal and neuromuscular impairments; thus, this information will not be repeated in this chapter. However, we will briefly discuss the role of training pre-ambulation skills as a part of gait training.

PRE-AMBULATION SKILL TRAINING

Several treatment approaches recommend that during gait training, the patient should begin by practicing skills that are considered *precursors* to ambulation. These skills are thought to lead to successful ambulation, and are thus considered pre-ambulation skills (27–30).

Many of the pre-ambulation gait training sequences are based on having the patient repeat activities that are part of a normal developmental sequence (30, 31). The sequence begins by having patients practice mobility and stability skills in prone and supine positions. This includes such activities as rolling, maintaining prone on elbows or hands, supine bridging, and practicing counter-rotation trunk motions, that is, movements in which the shoulders rotate in the opposite direction from the hips. As motor control in supine and prone positions is recovered, patients begin to practice activities on all fours, then sitting, kneeling, half-kneeling, modified plantigrade position, and finally standing (28–30, 32, 33).

There are a growing number of researchers and clinicians who are questioning the requirement that patients regain mobility skills according to a developmental sequence (34–38). In this book, we present a task-oriented approach to retraining mobility that is not based on a developmental sequence for retraining. Instead, this approach focuses on identifying and remediating underlying impairments, retraining locomotor strategies, and integrating those strategies into the performance of functional mobility tasks. Thus, in this approach to retraining, the patient would not be required to practice maintaining all fours unless this represents a necessary part of their everyday activities.

LIMITATIONS ON IMPAIRMENT LEVEL TRAINING

Though most clinicians develop treatment strategies to remediate underlying impairments, the extent to which these types of improvements carry over to gait is still undetermined. There is mounting evidence to suggest that this type of training does not carry over to gait. For example, researchers have found that, while therapeutic strategies were effective in significantly increasing hip flexion range of motion and improving trunk strength, improvements in these areas did not significantly improve gait speed (39).

Several studies have shown that postural sway biofeedback is an effective way to train patients to control center of mass motions in the standing position (40), but there was no carry-over to improved locomotion (41).

Ostensibly, as the number of gait deviations increases, the patient's level of functional performance should decrease. However, research has not demonstrated a strong relationship between number and types of impairments and functional gait performance. For example, several researchers have shown there is no strong relationship between temporal distance factors such as velocity, used to measure functional performance, and number of gait deviations (9, 17). This has led researchers to suggest that, while there are instances when sensory and motor impairments predict gait performance, they are not valid predictors of functional ambulation outcomes in patients with concomitant cognitive, perceptual, and pain impairments (9, 17).

Considerable time and effort are directed at modifying underlying impairments on the assumption that the result will be improved patterns of gait, and thus increased levels of independence in ambulation. Yet research has raised questions about the effect of retraining components on functional performance of gait, at least as expressed by temporal and distance factors. Thus, resolution of impairments alone may not be enough to ensure recovery of ambulation skills.

Perhaps when retraining mobility skills, more time should be spent on helping patients develop efficient gait strategies that compensate for their impairments, rather than on resolving the impairments themselves. This is especially important when impairments are permanent, making the return to normal gait strategies unreasonable. More research on these issues is critically needed.

Treatment at the Strategy Level

This section discusses therapeutic strategies for retraining gait patterns in the patient with neurological dysfunction according to a problem-based framework. Therapeutic strategies are presented with reference to problems that occur during the stance and swing phase of gait and that limit a patient's ability to achieve the task demands. Techniques suggested are drawn from clinical efforts related to the application of a systems theory of motor control and motor learning, and a wide variety of sources including the neurofacilitation approaches (28, 29, 32, 38, 42). It is important to remember that while these techniques are commonly used by clinicians to retrain gait, they have not been validated through controlled research involving patients with neurological impairments.

Finally, remember the goal of retraining at the strategy level is to assist the patient in developing movement strategies that are effective in meeting the inherent demands of the stance and swing phase of gait and thus the overall demands for progression, stability, and adaptation. While much of gait retraining strives to assist patients in the recovery of previously used normal gait patterns, this may not be a realistic goal in the face of permanent sensory and motor impairments. Thus, a better standard for judging the efficacy of a patient's movement strategies, is to ask, "Are they effective in meeting the demands of the task?"

STANCE PHASE

Impaired Heel-strike

The goals of therapeutic strategies are (*a*) to improve the foot position at heel-strike, (*b*) to improve weight acceptance during loading, (*c*) to improve motion at the ankle and foot, and (*d*) to facilitate smooth motion of the body over the stationary foot. Heel-strike foot contact with a smooth transition to a flat foot position facilitates forward progression and a stable base of support important for stability. The treatment of problems impairing heel-strike depends on the underlying cause.

Plantarflexion contractures. Plantarflexion contractures can be treated with manual stretch to increase range in a tight heel cord. In addition, fixed plaster casts can be used to place the muscle on sustained stretch, thus increasing range (43). Eventually, plaster casts may be bivalved, padded, and used as resting splints during the night and daytime rest periods (10).

Patients are often positioned in the prone position to reduce plantarflexor contractures. Surgery and/or nerve blocks may be needed in response to excessively tight heel cords that cannot be changed in any other way (10, 23).

Plantarflexor spasticity. Impaired heel-strike due to overactivity of the plantarflexors may respond to facilitation techniques to decrease abnormal muscle tone (these were discussed in Chapter 10). An ankle-foot orthosis can be used to prevent plantarflexion at the ankle. However, the loss of plantarflexion results in sustained knee flexion, and thus requires good quadriceps activation to prevent collapse of the stance limb during weight acceptance (10).

Electrical stimulation of the anterior tibialis muscle can be used to reciprocally inhibit activity of the gastrocnemius/soleus. Finally, EMG biofeedback to the gastrocnemius may help the patient to reduce overactivity during the stance and swing phase of gait (44–50).

Inactivity of the tibialis anterior. Inability to activate the tibialis anterior (TA) muscle is a common cause of impaired heel-strike in the patient with neurological impairments. Strengthening exercises to increase force production of the TA are important in making sure the TA is capable of generating force in response to descending commands. Unfortunately, the capacity to generate force does not ensure that the muscle will be recruited during the automatic process of gait. Nonetheless, strengthening is necessary to ensure that force generation capability is at least present.

Biofeedback and/or electrical stimulation of the TA in conjunction with a foot switch placed inside the patient's shoe has been used effectively to increase activation of the TA at heel-strike (44, 49, 50).

Sensory stimulation of the tibialis anterior, such as icing or tapping, during manually assisted step initiation has also been suggested as an approach to facilitate anterior tibialis activation just prior to heel-strike (10). Manually assisted step initiation with heel-strike is shown in Figure 14.3.

Use of an orthotic that has motion at the ankle joint, but a posterior stop is an effective way to control foot-drop in the patient who is unable to recruit the TA. The ankle joint motion of the orthotic allows some dorsiflexion, thus allowing the tibia to advance over the supporting foot (10).

Foot placement can also be assisted by making a grid on the floor, which helps to visually guide patients in establishing a better foot placement pattern on the floor. This was shown in Figure 14.2. The grid is especially helpful for patients who have difficulty with reduced stride length and/or adduction of the leg. Distance between horizontal stripes can be individualized to the patient's desired stride length (51).

Coronal plane foot problems. A varus foot position during gait can be controlled with an ankle-foot orthosis (AFO) with a slight buildup of the lateral border of the foot (10). In addition, electrical stimulation of the toe extensors can reduce varus positioning during stance. A valgus foot position can be controlled with an AFO with a slight buildup of the medial border (10).

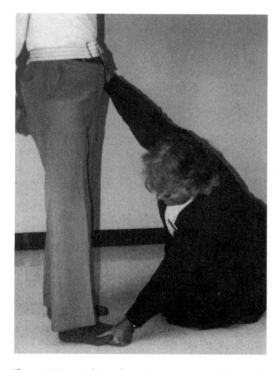

Figure 14.3. Helping the patient to accomplish a heel-first foot strike pattern. This position will allow the body to move smoothly over the foot with a good weightbearing surface, enhancing stability and progression.

Mid-stance Problems

The goals of treatments to improve gait patterns for mid-stance include (*a*) activation of hip and knee extension, to facilitate an extensor support moment for single limb stance, and (*b*) maintenance of a vertical posture and control of the HAT segment.

Knee hyperextension. A common mid-stance problem involves hyperextension of the knee during loading at mid-stance (23). Treatment depends on whether the hyperextension is the primary impairment or compensatory to another problem elsewhere.

If hyperextension is due to hyperactivity of the plantarflexors, then an AFO with plantarflexion stop can be used (10, 43). Alternatively, techniques to decrease muscle tone in the plantarflexors, such as having the patient practice weightbearing with the ankle dorsiflexed, have been recommended (10, 28, 38).

When hyperextension is compensatory to weak quadriceps, preventing knee collapse during loading and mid-stance, strengthening exercises, electrical stimulation, and EMG biofeedback have been recommended to facilitate activation of the quadriceps. Knee hyperextension block orthoses have also been proposed to prevent hyperextension of the knee during gait.

In patients who do not have sufficient knee control to prevent collapse during loading, the knee can be externally supported to prevent collapse, such as with a posterior plaster shell applied to the leg with an ace bandage during stance weightbearing activities or knee brace, as shown in Figure 14.4. While the benefit of bracing the knee into extension is to facilitate weightbearing in the stance phase of gait, the benefit is lost during the swing phase when the patient is required to flex the leg to advance the limb.

Excessive knee flexion. In some patients with neurological dysfunction, problems in mid-stance relate to excessive knee flexion rather than extension. When knee flexion results from weak quadriceps, functional electrical stimulation can be used to activate the quadriceps. Alternatively, (or in combination), a positional feedback device such as

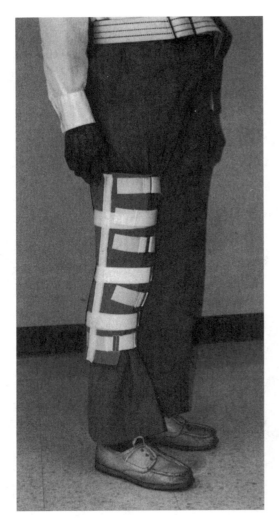

Figure 14.4. In patients who do not have sufficient knee control to prevent collapse during loading, the knee can be externally supported to prevent collapse with a knee brace.

an ELGON can be used to provide kinematic feedback. External devices can also be used to prevent knee flexion (10).

It has also been recommended that patients practice generating an extensor support moment in other tasks such as moving from sit to stand position, or alternatively, standing against a wall and flexing, then extending the knees and hips (27, 28). Again, it is not known whether practicing the generation of an extensor support moment in a task other than gait will carry over to improvements in stability during the stance phase of gait.

Forward-flexed trunk. A forward-flexed trunk posture often accompanies hyperextension of the knee. To facilitate a vertical posture and control of HAT stability over the extended hips, manual cues are given to the patient at the shoulders (shown in Fig. 14.5) or at the hips. Manual assistance can progress from light manual guidance to verbal cuing.

Contralateral pelvic drop. Inadequate activation of the abductors results in a contralateral drop of the pelvis during mid-stance. Treatment suggestions include strengthening exercises for the abductors and having the patients practice maintaining symmetrical pelvic height during single limb stance.

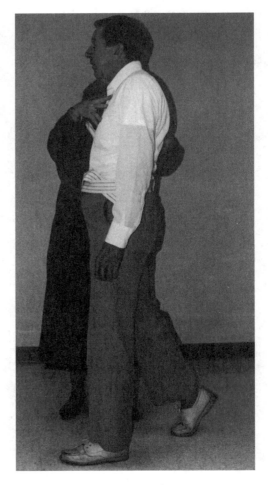

Figure 14.5. Assisting a patient learning to maintain a vertical trunk posture during gait with manual cues.

Terminal Stance

The goals of terminal stance activities are to generate the propulsive forces that are necessary to advance the body, and to provide the momentum to advance the leg.

Inability to advance the weight to the forefoot due to clawing of the toes can be treated with a shoe insert that spreads and extends the toes (10).

The generation of propulsive forces during terminal stance depends on a trailing leg position of the stance limb in which the center of mass is forward of the trailing foot. This requires hip extension in conjunction with knee extension, and plantarflexion of the ankle, with only a small degree of posterior rotation of the pelvis. Patients are often asked to practice assuming and maintaining a trailing leg position initially in a static stance position, as shown in Figure 14.6. This includes practicing lifting the heel and moving the body weight anteriorly over the forefoot, while the hip and knee are extended. Manual cues and assistance are given by the clinician as needed to facilitate this component of gait (27, 28, 38).

SWING

Pre-swing

The goals of pre-swing treatment strategies are (*a*) to improve the ability to generate force in the ankle plantarflexors and hip flexors to power the swing limb and (*b*) to improve activation of hip flexors, and associated knee and ankle flexion for foot clearance. Suggestions for improving the patient's ability to flex the hip during the initiation of swing include manually supporting the swing limb at the foot while the patient generates the force necessary to pull the thigh segment forward.

Mid-swing

The goal is to advance the swing limb, clearing the supporting surface with the foot. This requires facilitation of the hip flexors, to draw the thigh segment forward with sufficient force to passively flex the knee, and con-

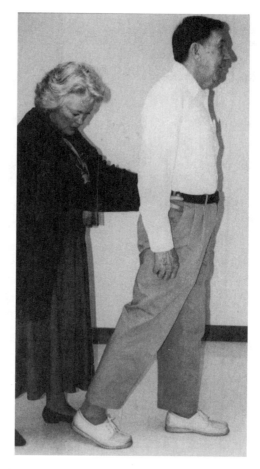

Figure 14.6. Manually assisting a patient to master a trailing limb posture, important in the generation of momentum for progression.

comitant activation of the TA to achieve foot clearance.

Early in gait training, when the patient does not have sufficient control to advance the swing limb using hip and knee flexion, a towel can be placed under the patient's foot to facilitate advancement of the foot (28). This is shown in Figure 14.7. Alternatively, an ace bandage (Fig. 14.8) can be used to prevent ankle plantarflexion and subsequent toe-drag during the swing phase of gait (28).

Terminal Swing

The goals of terminal swing treatment are (*a*) to improve mobility in the knee, (*b*) to improve the ability to extend the knee with

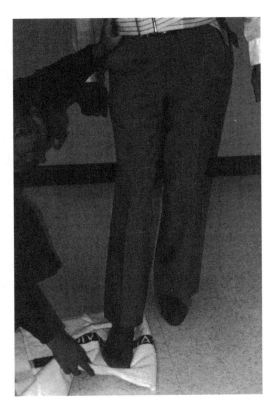

Figure 14.7.   Placing a towel under the hemiparetic leg to facilitate advancement of the swing limb without lateral trunk lean or hip hike.

hip flexed, in preparation for foot-strike, and (*c*) to improve activation of the ankle dorsiflexors, in preparation for heel-strike.

When inadequate knee extension is the result of knee flexion contractures, manual stretching, casting, and splinting can be used to alter mechanical constraints (10). However, contractures will simply recur if the underlying cause is chronic overactivity of the hamstrings muscle during swing. Electrical stimulation of the quadriceps has been used to reciprocally inhibit an overactive hamstrings muscle (10, 48).

Assistive Devices

A variety of assistive devices are available to provide support to patients who are unable to locomote independently. These include standard walkers, rolling walkers, quad canes, straight canes, and various types of crutches.

A number of factors are considered when prescribing an assistive device for a patient with neurological impairments, including extent of physical disability, cognitive impairment, and the patient's personal motivations and desires (30).

Assistive devices contribute to stability by widening the base of support and providing additional support against gravity. Canes are usually held in the hand opposite to the involved extremity, allowing a reciprocal gait pattern, with the opposite arm and involved leg moving together. Base of support can be further widened by choosing a cane with more points of contact with the floor, such as a small- or a large-based quad cane.

Walkers provide the greatest degree of stability during ambulation, further widening the base of support, and improving both lateral and anterior stability. A variety of walkers exist, including straight walkers and rolling walkers with two or four casters. An advan-

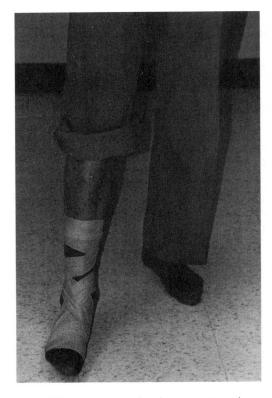

Figure 14.8.   Using an ace bandage to maintain the ankle in dorsiflexion and to facilitate toe clearance.

tage of rolling walkers is that they allow patients to maintain speed, facilitating the generation of momentum, and thereby facilitating progression. However, the disadvantage of rolling walkers is that they have a reduced stability compared with standard pick-up walkers. Further information describing types of assistive devices, procedures for measuring, and techniques for training gait with assistive devices on level surface, curbs, and steps may be found in detail in other sources (30).

It is important to consider the effects of using various assistive devices on factors other than gait skills, such as attentional resources. There appear to be *attentional costs* associated with using an assistive device. Attentional costs refer to the demand for attentional resources for information processing during the performance of a task. The attentional demands can vary depending on the type of assistive device used, and the patient's familiarity with the device. A recent study examined the attentional demands associated with two types of walkers, a standard pick-up walker vs. a rolling walker (52). This study found that, while both a rolling and a standard walker are attention-demanding, a rolling walker is less attentionally demanding than a standard pick-up walker.

Since there is some evidence that competing demands for attentional resources by postural and cognitive systems contribute to instability in the elderly, understanding the attentional requirements of the assistive devices we give patients is an important consideration during gait training (53).

Treatment at the Functional Task Level

The goal of retraining at the functional level focuses on having patients practice walking in a variety of contexts. The ability to walk in a natural environment requires modifying gait strategies to changing task and environmental demands. Thus, developing the ability to adapt is a critical part of retraining mobility skills.

As patients learn to develop strategies

effective in meeting the task requirement of locomotion on a level surface, training is broadened to include locomotor training (*a*) at different speeds of walking, (*b*) on different surfaces, for example, inclines, uneven surfaces, and carpeted surfaces, and (*c*) in a variety of visual conditions such as reduced lighting, or in the presence of visual motion cues in the environment. Adapting gait in anticipation of upcoming obstacles is also practiced, including the ability to step over obstacles of various heights, such as those shown in Figure 14.9, or to step around obstacles, shown in Figure 14.10.

Patients also practice walking under a variety of task conditions such as walking with abrupt stops, walking with quick change in direction, walking with head turns (Fig. 14.11), and walking while carrying a variety of objects (54, 55). In this way, patients learn

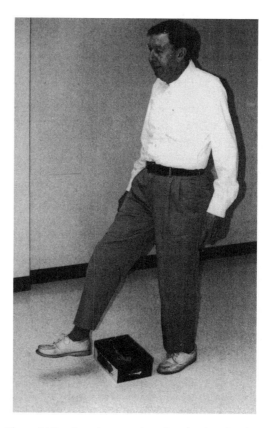

Figure 14.9. Stepping over obstacles of various heights, such as a shoe box, assists patients in learning to modify strategies for gait in anticipation of upcoming obstacles.

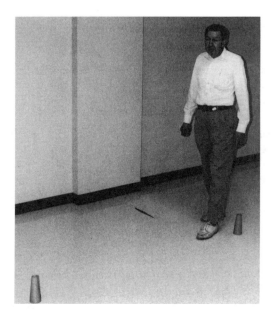

Figure 14.10. The patient is asked to walk around cones placed on the floor to help patients learn to modify gait to avoid obstacles in the gait path.

to modify gait in anticipation of potentially destabilizing threats to balance during gait.

Strategies to retrain compensatory responses to unexpected perturbations to gait have not been identified. One possible approach might be to unexpectedly change the speed of a treadmill while the patient is walking. A harness system would be necessary to safely carry out perturbations to ongoing gait.

TASK-ORIENTED GAIT TRAINING

Recently, there has been a great deal of interest in a strict task-oriented gait retraining program. In this approach, little time is spent on pre-ambulation skills or on retraining gait patterns. The approach is based on the philosophy that, if you want to improve gait, you should practice gait. Thus, patients are exposed early in rehabilitation to a program of ambulation training using reciprocal leg activities on a kinetron and treadmill walking with support provided as needed (56, 57).

Preliminary evidence comparing an intensive task-oriented approach to traditional physical therapy approaches in helping stroke patients learn to walk has found that the task-oriented approach helped patients achieve faster velocities of gait speed. However, the differences between the two groups disappeared after several months (56–58). More research is needed on this approach to therapy. There are increasing numbers of available harness and pulley devices that can be used with and without a treadmill to facilitate early gait training, even in patients who are unable to support the body against gravity (56–58). An example of such a harness and support system is shown in Figure 14.12.

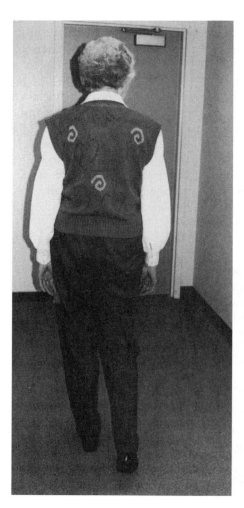

Figure 14.11. The patient practices walking while turning her head to look from side to side in order to retrain gait under altered task conditions.

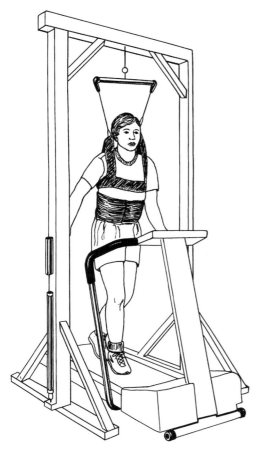

Figure 14.12. An example of a harness and pulley system used in conjunction with a treadmill for assisted task-oriented gait training.

STAIR-WALKING

The patient with neurological impairments with decreased concentric control will have primary problems climbing up stairs, while the patient with difficulty controlling eccentric forces will have primary problems descending stairs. In addition, sensory impairments will affect the patient's ability to clear the step during swing, and place the foot appropriately for the next step. Published strategies for retraining stair-walking have focused primarily on therapeutic strategies with stroke patients.

During stair ascent, the patient is taught to advance the nonhemiplegic leg first. Manual assistance is given as needed to guide and control the involved leg (27, 28, 38). This is shown in Figure 14.13. The clinician helps to control the knee to prevent collapse during the single limb stance phase, and assists with knee and ankle flexion to ensure foot clearance in the swing leg (Fig. 14.14).

During stair descent, shown in Figure 14.15, the stroke patient is taught to advance the hemiplegic leg first. The therapist assists as needed with foot placement and in knee control, to prevent collapse of the leg when the noninvolved leg is advanced during swing (28).

Research has shown that certain stair features are critical in establishing effective movement strategies for stair-walking. Thus, it is possible that accentuating stair features, such as the edge of the step, or the height of the step, and drawing the patient's attention to these features, may enhance the patient's ability to develop effective stair-walking strategies.

RETRAINING OTHER MOBILITY SKILLS

When retraining transfers and other types of mobility skills, it is important to remember that there is no single correct strategy for patients to learn. Research suggests that healthy young people perform such tasks as rising from a bed, standing up from the floor, or rolling, in many different ways. Variability characterizes the movement patterns used by neurologically intact individuals to perform everyday mobility skills. In fact, often the same exact strategy is never repeated. Instead, normal young adults seem to learn the rules for performing a task. This means that they learn what the essential or invariant requirements of a task are, and develop a variety of strategies to accomplish these requirements. This suggests that the goal when retraining transfer skills in the patient with neurological disabilities is to help the patient develop sensory and motor strategies that are effective in meeting the task requirements, despite persisting impairments.

Patients need to learn new rules for moving and sensing, given their impairments,

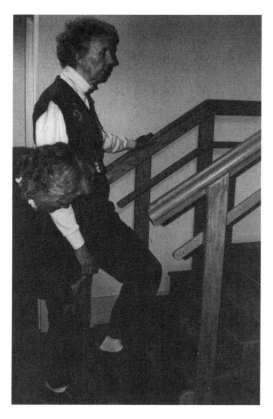

Figure 14.13. Assisting stair-walking, controlling the involved leg for single limb stance in stair ascent.

the extent to which these principles can be applied to the patient with neurological dysfunction.

To assist in the process of exploring movement strategies that are effective in meeting the task demands, conditions of training are varied. For example, during the process of learning to move from sit-to-stand position (STS), the patient may practice standing up from a wheelchair, from the bed, from a chair without arms, and a chair with arms. In addition, patients may learn to embed STS in a variety of other tasks such as stand-up and stop, stand-up and walk, or stand-up and lean-over. This type of variability encourages the patient to adapt the strategy used to stand up in response to changes in the demands of the task and the environment.

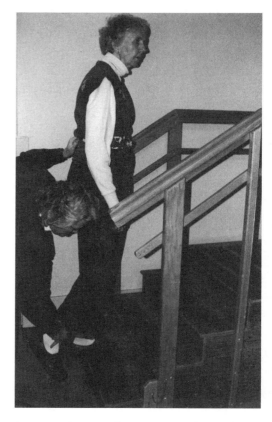

Figure 14.14. Manually assisting with knee and ankle flexion to ensure foot clearance in the swing leg during stair ascent.

rather than learning to use a "normal" pattern of movement. Research with neurologically intact subjects suggests that there is no single template for moving that can be used to train patients. Instead, guided by the clinician, patients learn to explore the possibilities for performing a task. Patients learn the boundaries of what is possible, given the demands of the task and the current constellation of impairments. Again, it is important to remember that the therapeutic strategies suggested in the following sections are attempts to apply a systems theory of motor control and current research in motor learning to retraining mobility skills. These suggestions have not yet been validated through research. In addition, motor learning principles related to the acquisition of a learned skill are largely drawn from research with neurologically intact subjects. Research has not yet determined

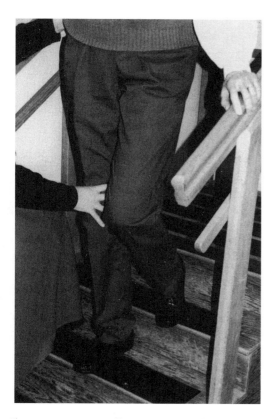

Figure 14.15. Manually assisting control of the knee during stair descent.

This concept of trial and error exploration in the learning of perceptual and motor strategies, which may be quite effective in meeting task goals, has a number of important implications for clinicians. Initial performance may be quite poor as patients learn to explore and to find their own solutions. Patients may not progress as fast as if they were taught a single solution to the task being learned. Short- and long-term therapy goals need to be rewritten to reflect the importance placed on multiple solutions to a task. An example of a new goal would be: the patient will demonstrate the ability to adapt motor responses by performing the sit-to-stand task in three different ways.

With these principles in mind, we will explore some ideas for retraining mobility skills other than gait including STS, rolling, and rising from a bed.

Sit-to-Stand Position

Remember from the chapter on normal mobility skills that there are two basic strategies that can be used separately or in combination to stand up: a momentum strategy and a force-control strategy. The momentum strategy uses concentric forces to propel the body forward and upward, while eccentric forces control the horizontal displacement of the center of mass, necessary for stability. A momentum strategy requires both a minimal speed of movement and that there be no breaks in the motion. This allows the transfer of momentum from the trunk to the whole body.

In contrast, a force-control strategy is characterized by frequent stops. Forces are generated in the trunk to bring the center of mass over the base of support of the feet. Then, forces are generated to lift the body to the vertical position. The force-control strategy ensures stability but requires greater forces for progression. Often, the arms are used to generate force, assisting with progression and stability.

RETRAINING A FORCE-CONTROL STRATEGY

As we mentioned in the chapter on abnormal mobility, patients with neurological dysfunction are most often taught a force-control strategy for STS. In many cases, this is an appropriate response to various types of impairments such as decreased postural control limiting center of mass (COM) control, orthostatic hypotension, and/or vestibular problems that produce dizziness if the patient assumes a vertical position too quickly. When teaching a patient to use a force-control strategy, the patient is taught to bring the buttocks forward towards the edge of the chair. The trunk is brought forward, bringing the "nose over the toes." This is shown in Figure 14.16. This brings the COM over the base of support of the feet. The patient is then cued to stand up. The patient can be encouraged to bring the arms forward, with or without a

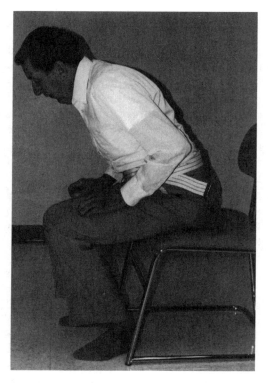

Figure 14.16. Teaching a force-control strategy for accomplishing sit-to-stand position involves asking the patient to move forward to the edge of the chair, incline trunk until the "nose is over the toes," then stand up.

support, to assist in bringing the trunk mass forward; this is shown in Figure 14.17.

Patients whose weakness makes it difficult to achieve a vertical position from a normal-height chair, can begin learning STS from a raised chair, reducing the strength requirement for lifting the body (Fig. 14.18). As the patient improves, seat height can be lowered.

In patients with asymmetrical force production problems, facilitating symmetry is important when possible, since symmetrical weightbearing enhances both progression and stability during the task. A symmetrical weightbearing posture is only possible in patients who can generate sufficient force to control the knee, and prevent collapse of the body when the impaired limb is loaded. When this is not the case, the clinician will have to manually control the knee for the patient, for example as illustrated in Figure 14.19. It is important that when manually assisting knee

control, forward motion of the knee is not blocked as the patient stands up.

ACTIVE LEARNING MODULE

You can try this for yourself. Ask a partner to sit on the edge of a chair. Place your knee so that it is touching the front of your partner's knee, and apply pressure so the knee cannot move forward during the motion. Now ask your partner to stand up. What happens? In most cases, the person will be unable to stand. If your partner succeeds in getting the buttocks off the ground, he or she will often fall backwards. When you're standing, the knee must be allowed to move forward as the patient assumes a vertical position, bringing the center of mass over the feet.

In patients with unilateral motor control problems such as hemiplegia, sensory stimulation techniques have been suggested as an approach to assisting the patient in learning symmetrical weightbearing. Ideas include (*a*) pressure downward applied at the knee to increase the weightbearing sensation of the foot in contact with the support surface (refer back to Fig. 14.19); (*b*) lifting the pa-

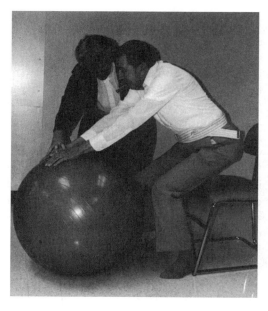

Figure 14.17. Encouraging forward inclination of the trunk during sit-to-stand position (STS) by bringing the arms forward.

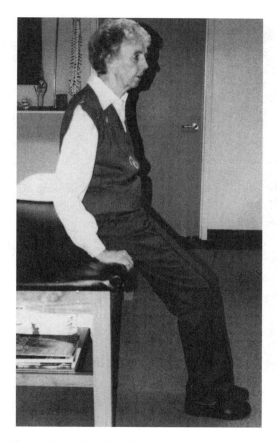

Figure 14.18. Teaching STS from a raised chair reduces the strength requirement for lifting the body and allows the weak patient to accomplish the task.

tient's foot and rubbing the heel on the ground (Fig. 14.20); (*c*) lightly pounding the heel on the ground; or (*d*) using pressure on the dorsum of the foot during the STS movement (27, 28, 32, 38).

It is often easier for a patient to learn to sit down than to stand up because eccentric force control is often gained prior to concentric force control (38, 59). When teaching patients to sit down, the therapist asks the patient to practice flexing the knees in preparation for sitting. This requires eccentric contraction of the quadriceps to control premature collapse of the knee.

RETRAINING A MOMENTUM STRATEGY

A patient should be allowed to explore the possibilities for using momentum when

performing a transfer task, since this strategy is most efficient and requires the least amount of muscular activity. Essential elements of teaching a momentum strategy include encouraging the patient to move quickly, and avoiding breaks in the motion. Figure 14.21 shows a patient using a momentum strategy.

The clinician can verbally instruct the patient to move quickly, with no stops. An appropriate prompt might be, "Now we are going to try standing up again, but this time I want you to move quickly with no stops." Manual cues can be used at the shoulders to set the pace. Patients who have trouble generating force quickly with the trunk can try swinging their arms freely while standing up, to increase momentum generated in upper body segments.

When teaching a momentum strategy, clinicians should be aware of the stringent stability requirements of this strategy, and adequately safeguard a patient with poor postural control to prevent a fall. The risk for a backward fall will be greatest at the beginning of the movement if the patient tries to transfer momentum from the trunk to the legs for a vertical lift before the COM is sufficiently for-

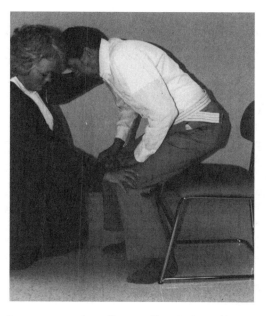

Figure 14.19. Manually controlling the knee when assisting a patient who is moving from sit-to-stand position.

Figure 14.20. Facilitating symmetrical weightbearing in a hemiplegic patient by providing pressure downward applied at the knee and lifting the patient's foot and rubbing the heel on the ground.

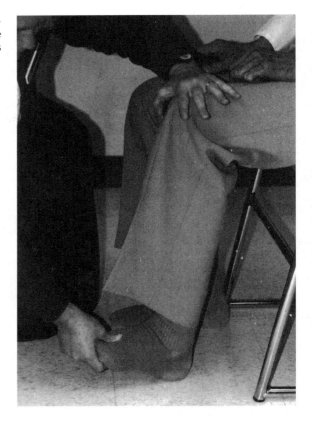

ward over the feet. This is often characteristic of STS in a hemiparetic patient (55). In contrast, the risk for a forward fall will be greatest at the end of the movement in patients who are unable to control horizontal forces affecting the COM. When this occurs, the COM continues to accelerate forward of the base of support of the feet after the patient reaches a vertical position, resulting in a fall forward. This is often characteristic of STS in cerebellar patients who have difficulty scaling forces for movement (55).

The same principles for retraining STS apply to retraining other types of transfers. For example, when learning to transfer from a chair to a chair (or bed, or mat), a patient can learn a standing pivot transfer, which is more consistent with a force-control strategy, or a squat-pivot transfer, which is more consistent with a momentum strategy. In the standing-pivot transfer, the patient moves from the seated position to a vertical stance position, then pivots around, and sits down.

Momentum is lost each time the patient stops to change position.

In contrast, in a squat-pivot transfer, the patient positions the wheelchair at an angle to the bed (or chair), moves to the edge of the chair, and in one swift motion moves the buttocks from one surface to another, keeping the hips, knees, and ankles flexed. This requires good eccentric control of the quadriceps and hip extensors.

It is often surprising to see the number of patients who find it easier to perform a squat-pivot transfer, instead of a standing-pivot transfer, which is often the preferred strategy taught in therapy. For example, a 24-year-old traumatic brain injury patient with cerebellar ataxia was being taught to transfer so that she could go home on leave from the rehabilitation center. She was being taught a standing-pivot transfer, and was unable to perform this independently, due to instability on rising to a vertical position. As a result, she required moderate assistance to transfer

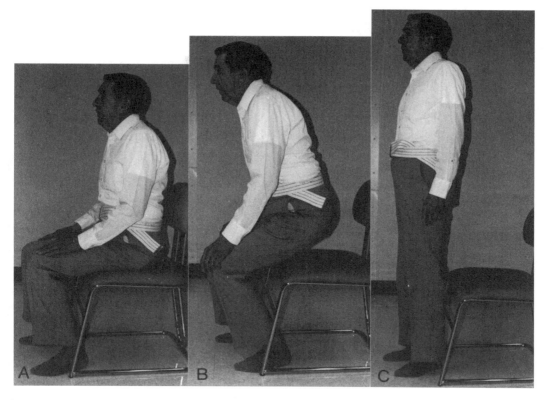

Figure 14.21. Training a momentum strategy involves asking the patient to move quickly and avoid stopping during the move from (**A**) sit to (**C** and **D**) stand positions.

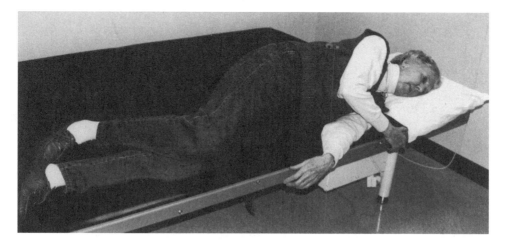

Figure 14.22. Learning to rise from a bed using a force-control strategy breaks the movement into three stages, beginning with rolling to side-lying.

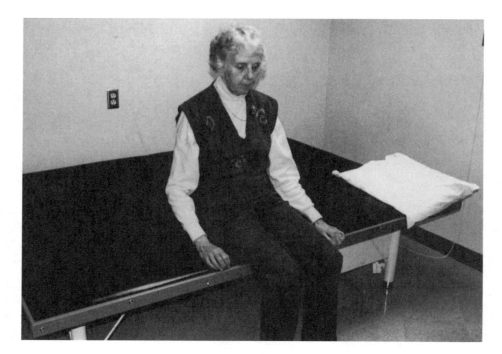

Figure 14.23.   Second stage of a force-control strategy to move from supine-to-stand position is moving into a sitting position.

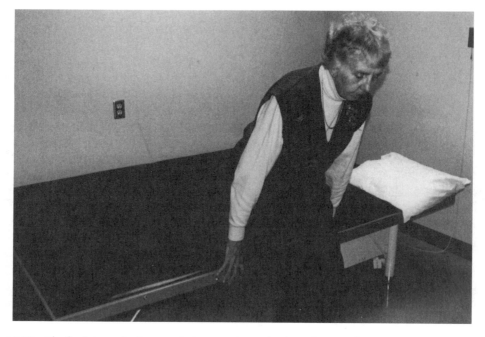

Figure 14.24.   The final stage of a force-control strategy is moving from sit-to-stand position.

safely. Since she had fairly good eccentric control of the knees, but poor balance, it was decided to try letting her experiment with a momentum-driven squat-pivot transfer. To her surprise and ours, she learned to transfer from the bed to her wheelchair independently in one therapy session.

Bed Mobility Skills

Retraining bed mobility skills includes such tasks as changing position while in bed (for example, rolling from the supine position to side-lying or prone), and getting out of bed, either to a chair or standing up. As noted earlier, researchers have found that normal young adults use a variety of momentum-related strategies when performing bed mobility skills. In contrast, force-control movement strategies are frequently used by patients with neurological impairments, and are characterized by frequent starts and stops.

ROLLING

The most common approach to rolling in normal young adults involves reaching and lifting with the upper extremity, flexing the head and upper trunk, and lifting the leg to roll onto the side, then over to prone. However, there were many variations to this pattern. Most healthy young adults did not show rotation between the shoulders and pelvis, assumed by many clinicians to be an invariant feature of rolling.

There are at least two ways to teach a patient to roll over. The first relies more heavily on the generation of momentum to propel the body from supine to prone. Motion is initiated with flexion of the head and trunk. At the same time, the patient reaches over the body with the upper extremity. In addition, the leg is lifted and rotated over the opposite leg, to assist with the generation of momentum, to roll the body to side-lying and on to prone.

An alternative to a momentum-based strategy is a force-control (or combination) strategy. In this approach, the patient is taught to lift one leg and place the foot flat on the bed. Pressure downward by the leg propels the body to side-lying and on to prone. Flexion of the head and trunk and reaching movements of the arms can assist in generating force to roll over (28, 29, 38).

When rolling towards their involved side, stroke patients with hemiparetic arms should be shown how to protect the shoulder by manually protracting and abducting the arm prior to rolling (28).

RISING FROM A BED

Research examining movement patterns used by normal adults to get out of bed again suggests great variability in how this is accomplished. Still, momentum-based strategies are most often used. For example, the movement begins as the person pushes the trunk into flexion with the arms, or alternatively grasps the side of the bed and pulls and pushes into flexion and immediately into a partial sitting position with the weight on one side of the buttocks. Without stopping, the person continues to roll off the bed into a standing position. This strategy has stringent stability requirements, but because there are no breaks in the movement, uses momentum to move the body efficiently. As noted in the chapter on abnormal mobility skills, there are many reasons why this strategy is not appropriate for a patient with neurological dysfunction.

An alternative force-control strategy involves teaching a patient to roll to side-lying (Fig. 14.22), then to push up to a sitting position (Fig. 14.23). After the patient is stable in a symmetrical sitting position with the feet flat on the floor, he/she is taught to stand up (Fig. 14.24) (28, 29, 38).

SUMMARY

1. The key to recovery of mobility skills following neurological injury is learning to meet the task requirements of progression, stability, and adaptability, despite persisting sensory, motor, and cognitive impairments. Research examining mobility strategies in neurologically intact subjects suggests that there is no one right strategy that can, or should, be used to meet these requirements.

2. Retraining the patient with impaired mobility skills begins with an assessment of functional mobility skills, strategies used to accomplish stance and swing requirements of gait, and underlying sensory, motor, and cognitive impairments.

3. Observational gait analysis is the most commonly used clinical tool to aid therapists in systematically analyzing a patient's gait strategies.

4. Treatment focuses on helping patients to resolve impairments, to develop strategies effective in meeting mobility requirements, and to learn how to adapt and modify these strategies so performance can be sustained in a wide variety of settings.

5. There are many approaches to retraining the patient with impaired mobility skills, particularly gait. Some approaches stress the importance of following a strict developmental sequence. This involves learning mobility and stability in developmental postures such as all fours and upright kneel, prior to working on ambulation itself.

6. At the other end of the retraining spectrum are gait retraining approaches that focus solely on retraining locomotion, with no emphasis on training potentially unrelated skills. Often, therapy is started with task-oriented gait training before the patient can sustain weight. Patients are supported by harnesses, and treadmills are used to facilitate walking.

7. Other approaches, such as the one presented in this chapter, stress a balance between therapeutic strategies focused on resolving impairments, retraining movement strategies for gait, and having the patient practice walking under various task and environmental conditions.

8. More research is needed to determine the comparative effectiveness of these approaches in retraining mobility skills in various types of patients with neurological impairments.

REFERENCES

1. Craik R. Changes in locomotion in the aging adult. In: Woollacott MH, Shumway-Cook A, eds. Development of posture and gait across the lifespan. Columbia, SC: University of South Carolina Press, 1989:176–201.

2. Finley FR, Cody KA, Sepic SB. Walking patterns of normal women. Arch Phys Med Rehabil 1970;51:637–650.

3. Waters RL, Lunsford BR, Perry J, Byrd R. Energy-speed relationship of walking: standard tables. J Orthop Res 1988;6:215–222.

4. Lerner-Frankiel MB, Vargas S, Brown MB, Krusell L, Schoneberger W. Functional community ambulation: what are your criteria? Clinical Management 1990;6:12–15.

5. Keith RA, Granger CV, Hamilton BB, Sherwin FS. The functional independence measure: a new tool for rehabilitation. In: Eisentberg MG, Grzesiak RC, eds. Advances in clinical rehabilitation, vol 1. New York: Springer Verlag, 1987:6–18.

6. Waters RL. Energy expenditure. In: Perry J, ed. Gait analysis: normal and pathological function. Thorofare, NJ: Slack Incorporated, 1992:443–490.

7. McGavin CR, Gupta SP, McHardy GJR. Twelve minute walking test for assessing disability in chronic bronchitis. Br Med J 1976;1:822–823.

8. Butland RJA, Pang J, Gross ER, Woodcock AA, Geddes DM. Two-, six-, and 12-minute walking tests in respiratory disease. Br Med J 1982;284:1607–1608.

9. Brandstater M, deBruin H, Gowland C, Clark B. Hemiplegic gait: analysis of temporal variable. Arch Phys Med Rehabil 1983;65:583–587.

10. Montgomery J. Assessment and treatment of locomotor deficits in stroke. In: Duncan PW, Badke MB. Stroke rehabilitation: the recovery of motor control. Chicago: Year Book Publications, 1987:223–259.

11. Shumway-Cook A, Gruber W, Rigby P, Baldwin P. Unpublished observations.

12. Holden MK, Gill KM, Magliozzi MR, Nathan J, Piehl-Baker L. Clinical gait assessment in the neurologically impaired: reliability and meaningfulness. Phys Ther 1984;64:35–40.

13. Robinson JL, Smidt GL. Quantitative gait evaluation in the clinic. Phys Ther 1981;61:351–353.

14. Shumway-Cook, unpublished observations.

15. Murray M, Kory R, Sepic S. Walking patterns of normal women. Arch Phys Med Rehabil 1970;51:637–650.

16. Smidt GL, Mommens MA. System of reporting and comparing influence of ambulatory aids on gait. Phys Ther 1971; 51:9–21.

17. Holden MK, Gill KM, Magliozzi MR. Gait assessment for neurologically impaired pa-

tients: standards for outcome assessment. Phys Ther 1986;66:1530–1539.

18. Gentile A. The nature of skill acquisition: therapeutic implications for children with movement disorders. In: Forssberg H, Hirschfeld H, eds. Movement disorders in children. Med Sport Sci. Basel: Karger, 1992:31–40.

19. Duncan P. Balance dysfunction and motor control theory. Syllabus from a talk. Washington State APTA annual conference, 1993.

20. Shumway-Cook A. Retraining stability and mobility. Cincinnati. Annual conference, APTA, 1993.

21. Shumway-Cook A, Baldwin M, Kerns K, Woollacott M. Reducing the likelihood for falls in the elderly, the effect of exercise. Abstract. Orthop Trans, J Bone Joint Surgery, in press.

22. Krebs DE, Edelstein JE, Fishman S. Reliability of observational kinematic gait analysis. Phys Ther 1985;65:1027–1033.

23. Perry J. Gait analysis: normal and pathological function. Thorofare, NJ: Slack Incorporated, 1992.

24. Rancho Los Amigos Hospital (Gait Analysis Form)

25. Tinetti ME. Performance-oriented assessment of mobility problems in elderly patients. J Am Geriatr Soc 1986;34:119–126.

26. Wolfson L, Whipple R, Amerman P, Tobin JN. Gait assessment in the elderly: a gait abnormality rating scale and its relation to falls. J Gerontol 1990;45:M12–M19.

27. Bobath, B. Adult hemiplegia: evaluation and treatment. London: Heinemann, 1978.

28. Davies, PM. Steps to follow. Berlin: Springer-Verlag, 1985.

29. Voss D, Ionta M, Myers B. Proprioceptive neuromuscular facilitation: patterns and techniques. 3rd ed. Philadelphia: Harper & Row, 1985.

30. Schmitz, TJ. Gait training with assistive devices. In: O'Sullivan S, Schmitz TM, eds. Physical rehabilitation: assessment and treatment. Philadelphia: FA Davis 1988:281–306.

31. Stockmyer S. An interpretation of the approach of rood to the treatment of neuromuscular dysfunction. Am J Phys Med 1967; 46:950–955.

32. Charness, A. Stroke/head injury: a guide to functional outcomes in physical therapy management. Rockville, MD: Aspen Systems, 1986.

33. Brunnstrom S. Movement therapy in hemiplegia: a neurophysiological approach. Hagerstown, MD: Harper & Row, 1970.

34. Forssberg H. Motor learning: A neurophysiological review. In: Berg K, Eriksson B, eds. Children and exercise, vol 9. Baltimore: University Park Press, 1980:13–22.

35. Mayston M. The Bobath concept: evolution and application. In: Forssberg H, Hirschfeld H, eds. Movement disorders in children. Med Sport Sci, Basel: Karger, 1992:1–6.

36. Shumway-Cook A. Equilibrium deficits in children. In: Woollacott M, Shumway-Cook A. Development of posture and gait across the lifespan. Columbia, SC: University of South Carolina Press, 1989:229–252.

37. Woollacott M, Shumway-Cook A, Williams H. The development of posture and balance control. In: Woollacott M, Shumway-Cook A, eds. Development of posture and gait across the lifespan. Columbia SC: University of South Carolina Press, 1989:77–96.

38. Carr JH, Shepard RB. A motor relearning programme for stroke. Rockville, MD: Aspen Systems, 1983.

39. Godges JJ, MacRae PG, Engelke KA. Effects of exercise on hip range of motion, trunk muscle performance and gait economy. Phys Ther 1993;73:468–477.

40. Shumway-Cook A, Anson D, Haller S. Postural sway biofeedback for pretraining postural control following hemiplegia. Arch Phys Med Rehabil 1988;69:395–400.

41. Winstein C, Gardner ER, McNeal DR, Barto PS, Nicholson DE. Standing balance training: effect on balance and locomotion in hemiparetic adults. Arch Phys Med Rehabil 1989;70:755–762.

42. Bobath K, Bobath B. The neurodevelopmental treatment. In: Scrutton D, ed. Management of the motor disorders of cerebral palsy. Clinics in Developmental Medicine, no. 90. London, Heinemann Medical, 1984.

43. Rosenthal RB, Deutsch SD, Miller W, Schumann, Hall JE. A fixed-ankle, below-the-knee orthosis for the management of genu recurvatum in spastic cerebral palsy. J Bone Joint Surg 1975;57A:545–547.

44. Basmajian JV. Kukulka CG, Narayan MD, Takebe K. Biofeedback treatment of footdrop after stroke compared with standard rehabilitation technique: effects on voluntary control and strength. Arch Phys Med Rehabil 1975;56:231–236.

45. Binder S, Moll CB, Wolf SL. Evaluation of electromyographic biofeedback as an adjunct to therapeutic exercise in treating the lower extremities of hemiplegic patients. Phys Ther 1981;61:886–893.

46. Baker M, Regenos E, Wolf SL, Basmajian JV. Developing strategies for biofeedback: applications in neurologically handicapped patients. Phys Ther 1977;57:402–408.

47. Baker MP, Hudson JE, Wolf SL. A "Feedback" cane to improve the hemiplegic patient's gait. Phys Ther 1979;59:170–171.

48. Bogataj U, Gros N, Malezic M, Kelih B, Kljajic M, Acimovic R. Restoration of gait during two to three weeks of therapy with multichannel electrical stimulation. Phys Ther 1989;69:319–327.

49. Takebe D, Kukulka C, Narayan G, Milner M, Basmajian JV. Peroneal nerve stimulator in rehabilitation of hemiplegic patients. Arch Phys Med Rehab 1975;56:237–239.

50. Waters R, McNeal DR. Tasto J. Peroneal nerve conduction velocity after chronic electrical stimulation. Arch Phys Med Rehabil 1975;56:240–243.

51. Jims, C. Foot placement pattern, an aid in gait training. Suggestions from the field. Phys Ther 1977;57:286.

52. Wright DL, Kemp TL. The dual-task methodology and assessing the attentional demands of ambulation with walking devices. Phys Ther 1992;72:306–315.

53. Shumway-Cook A, Baldwin M, Kerns K, Woollacott M. The effects of cognitive demands on postural control in elderly fallers and non-fallers. Abstract. Society for Neuroscience, 1993.

54. Shumway-Cook A, Horak F. Rehabilitation strategies for patients with vestibular deficits. Neurol Clin North Amer 1990;8:441–457.

55. Shumway-Cook A, Horak F. Balance rehabilitation in the neurologic patient: Course Syllabus. Seattle, NERA, 1992.

56. Richards CL, Malouin F, Wood-Dauphinee S, Williams JI, Bouchard JP, Brunet D. Task-specific physical therapy for optimization of gait recovery in acute stroke patients. Arch Phys Med Rehabil 1993;74:612–620.

57. Malouin F, Potvin M, Prevost J, Richards C, Wood-Dauphinee S. Use of an intensive task-oriented gait training program in a series of patients with acute cerebrovascular accidents. Phys Ther 1992;72:781–789.

58. Harburn K, Hill K, Kramer J, Noh S, Vandervoort A, Matheson J. An overhead harness and trolley system for balance and ambulation assessment and training. Arch Phys Med Rehabil 1993; 74:220–223.

59. Duncan PW, Badke MB. Stroke rehabilitation: the recovery of motor control. Chicago: Year Book Publications, 1987.

Section IV

UPPER EXTREMITY CONTROL

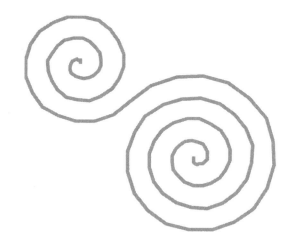

Chapter 15

UPPER EXTREMITY MANIPULATION SKILLS

INTRODUCTION

Mrs. Poirot has just had a stroke and is now in rehabilitation. She has partial paralysis of her right arm with some spasticity. She is having difficulty with many reaching and manipulative activities, including dressing, brushing her teeth, and feeding herself meals. She has difficulty with other tasks that rely on arm function such as controlling her wheelchair, rising from a bed, or pushing herself up from sit-to-stand position. In addition, arm function is affected by movements in other parts of her body. For example, when she walks, her hemiplegic arm draws up into flexion.

Upper extremity, posture, and mobility skills are interwoven. The lack of upper extremity function can affect many aspects of posture and mobility function. Recovery of posture and gait can be facilitated through upper extremity training strategies. In the same way, the recovery of upper extremity function can be enhanced by retraining posture and gait. This interaction broadens the spectrum of treatment strategies available when retraining either function. Clearly, recovery of upper extremity function can be relevant to many aspects of retraining motor control.

Knowing this, what is the best way to determine Mrs. Poirot's main areas of upper extremity dysfunction, and how can we create an optimal rehabilitation program for retraining Mrs. Poirot's problems with upper extremity function?

Before we can answer this question, we need to understand the basic requirements of manipulatory function. This will provide a framework for discussing normal control and the effect of neurological pathology on manipulatory skills. In addition, it will provide the structure for approaching clinical management of upper extremity dysfunction in the patient with neurological impairments.

We suggest that the following components could be considered key elements of upper extremity manipulatory functions: (*a*) locating a target, requiring the coordination of eye-head movements, (*b*) reaching, involving transportation of the arm and hand in space, (c) manipulation, including grip formation, grasp, and release, and (d) postural control.

As we mentioned in earlier chapters, the systems theory of motor control predicts that there are specific neural and non-neural subsystems that contribute to the control of these components of manipulatory function. Musculoskeletal components include such things as joint range of motion, spinal flexibility, muscle properties, and biomechanical relationships among linked body segments. Neural components encompass (a) motor processes, including the coordination of the eye, head, trunk and arm movements; (b) sensory processes, including the coordination of visual, vestibular, and somatosensory systems; (c) internal representations important for the mapping of sensation to action; and (d) higher-level processes essential for adaptive and anticipatory aspects of manipulatory functions.

We begin our discussion of components of normal upper extremity function with a description of the manner in which the eye and head are coupled during target location. We then discuss the components of reach and grasp, including motor aspects, the role of the sensory systems, and higher level adaptive abilities. Finally, we review some of the theories of the control of reaching movements.

LOCATING A TARGET-EYE-HEAD COORDINATION

In a normal reaching movement, the eyes, head, and arm move sequentially. How are reaching movements of the arm coordinated with the movements of the eye and head? Do we move our eyes first to a target, then our head, and finally our hand? Kinematic studies have shown that when an object to be grasped appears in the peripheral visual field, there is normally the following sequence of movements. The eye movement onset has the shortest latency, so it begins first, even before the head. The eyes reach the target first because they move very quickly, so they focus on the target before the head even stops moving (1). However, EMG studies have shown

that activation of neck muscles usually occurs 20 to 40 msec prior to activation of the muscles controlling eye movements. Because the eyes have less inertia than that of the head, the eyes move first, even though the neural signal occurs first in the neck muscles.

When the head is moved to look at an object, is it moved all the way to focus directly on the object? Not necessarily. The amplitude of head movements is usually only about 60 to 75% of the distance to the target (2, 3). However, when arm movements requiring great accuracy are performed, this behavior may be modified. It has been shown that people trained to throw with great accuracy make combined eye-head movements that go most of the distance to the target (4).

Some tasks require eye movements alone, while others require a combination of eye-head movement, and still other tasks require a combination of eye-head-trunk movements. Because of this variability, researchers have argued that eye-head coordination is not controlled by a unitary mechanism, but rather emerges from an interaction of several different neural mechanisms. These could include one neural mechanism that subserves the ability to locate objects in the near periphery, requiring primarily eye movements, with little head motion; a second mechanism to locate objects in the further periphery, controlling combined eye-head movements; and a third mechanism to locate objects in the far peripheral, controlling the movements of eye-head and trunk together (1).

Based on these findings, there are many control mechanisms involved in a normal reach, and thus many possible contributing factors to Mrs. Poirot's problems with reaching. Though the research just noted has focused primarily on understanding normal mechanisms involved in eye-head coordination, we might make the following hypothesis regarding its application to retraining patients with upper extremity problems. For example, when retraining Mrs. Poirot's problems related to the coordination of eye-head movements needed for upper extremity function, the clinician might focus on training the different control systems separately. For example, the clinician might begin by retraining eye movements to targets located within the central visual field, then progress to retraining eye head movements to targets located in the peripheral visual field. Finally, movements involving eye, head, and trunk motions could be practiced as patients learn to locate targets oriented in the far periphery.

From a kinematic perspective, coordination in reaching appears to be characterized by the sequential activation of eye, head, then hand movements. However, an EMG analysis of reaching found that muscles in the eye, head, and arm were activated almost synchronously, not sequentially. In addition, the pattern of muscle activity did not change with regard to target location. What can we learn from these experiments? Apparently, eye, head, and arm movement sequencing are strongly affected by **inertia**.

REACH AND GRASP

Motor Components

When the arm is used to point to an object, all the segments of the arm are controlled as a unit. But when the arm is used to reach for and grasp an object, the hand appears to be controlled independently of the other arm segments, with the arm carrying out movements related to transport, and the hand carrying out movements related to grasping the object. Thus, reaching for an object can be divided into two subcomponents, the reach vs. the grasp component, which appear to be controlled by separate areas of the brain, as you will see in the research described below.

Both reach and grasp involve a complex interaction of musculoskeletal and neural systems. Musculoskeletal components include such things as joint range of motion, spinal flexibility, muscle properties, and biomechanical relationships among linked body segments. In particular, it has been suggested that the following types of joint motion are essential to the ability to move the arm normally: scapular rotation, appropriate movement of the humeral head, the ability to supinate the forearm, shoulder, and elbow

flexion to approximately 100° to 120°, the ability to extend the wrist to slightly beyond neutral, and sufficient mobility in the hand to allow grasp and release (5).

Neuromotor aspects of reaching include appropriate muscle tone, discussed earlier in detail in Chapter 6, muscle strength, and coordination. More specifically, this involves appropriate activation of muscles to stabilize the scapula, rib cage, and humeral head during upper extremity reaching movements, and activation of muscles at the shoulder, elbow, and wrist joint for transport of the arm.

In a patient with neurological deficits it is often not easy to determine the relative contribution of neural vs. musculoskeletal problems to abnormal reaching. Motor control problems that affect the inertial characteristics of the system will give rise to coordination problems, even when the patterns of activation are normal. For example, an increase in stiffness will change the inertial characteristics of the head, arm, and/or trunk, making the initiation of motion more difficult. Thus, we see the important interaction between the biomechanics of movement and the neural control mechanisms.

Two important requirements are necessary for successfully grasping an object. First, the hand must be adapted to the shape, size, and use of the object. Second, the finger movements must be timed appropriately in relation to transport so that they close on the object just at the appropriate moment. If they close too early or too late, the grasp will be inappropriate (1).

During reach and grasp, the shaping of the hand for grasping occurs during the transportation component of the reach (Fig. 15.1A) (6). This pre-grasp hand shaping appears to be under visual control. There are two different categories of properties of objects that affect pre-grasp hand shaping: intrinsic properties, such as the object's size, shape and texture, and extrinsic or contextual properties, such as the object's orientation, distance from the body, and location with respect to the body (1).

Remember that grip formation takes place during the transportation phase (Fig.

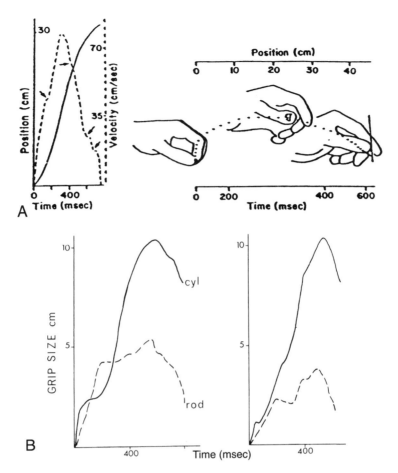

Figure 15.1. Characteristics of the transport phase of reaching. **A**, Changes in hand movement velocity (*solid line*) and grip size (*dotted line*) as a function of time during a reach. (Adapted from Brooks VB. The neural basis of motor control. NY: Oxford University Press. 1986:133.) **B**, Grip size differences for a 2-mm vs. a 10-cm cylinder. (From Jeannerod M. The neural and behavioural organization of goal-directed movements, Oxford: Clarendon Press, 1990:61.)

15.1*A*) and is anticipatory of the characteristics of the object to be grasped. The size of the maximum grip opening is proportional to the size of the object. This relationship is shown in Figure 15.1*B* (1) with a subject reaching for a 2-mm rod vs. a 10-cm cylinder. When subjects change the grip opening, they do it almost entirely with finger movements, while the thumb stays in one place (1). When reaching for an object, as the arm is transported forward, the fingers begin to stretch, and the grip size increases rapidly to a maximum, and then is reduced to match the size of the object.

Subjects show differential hand shaping for different shapes of objects as well. The distance between the thumb and index finger is usually largest during the final slow approach phase. It has been shown that adults with prosthetic hands show this same relationship between grasp and transport phases. Apparently, this relationship isn't due to biomechanical or neural constraints, but may be the most efficient way to reach (1, 7).

If the two components, reach and grasp, are truly controlled independently through different motor programs, then one should be able to modify one component and not affect the other. To test if this were possible, experiments were performed in which a spherical object was transformed into an ellipsoid object, after a reach had begun. Figure 15.2*A* shows the normal differences in hand shape when an ellipse vs. a sphere is the object to be grasped, while Figures 15.2*B* and *C* show an unperturbed reach for a sphere vs. a perturbed reach, where the subject reshapes the grasp to accommodate an ellipsoid. It was noted that the reach component was not affected by the change in shape of the target; however, the grip shape began to change within 540 msec after onset of the perturbation (1).

Studies on both reaching in infants and in patients with specific neural lesions also support the concept that reach and grasp components are controlled separately. Infants of 1 week may intercept moving objects and contact them, but this is done with a hand that is wide open without any grip formation. Grip formation appears to develop at about 10 to 22 weeks (1, 8). In the monkey this is also the case, and it has been shown that the appearance of the grasp component, at 8 months of age, is correlated with the maturation of connections between the corticospinal tract and the motor neurons (9). Children with pyramidal lesions also show similar prob-

lems with the grasp component of reaching, although the transport component may be normal (1).

Though research indicates that these two components of reaching may be controlled independently, they share a common time course, with synchronous changes in the kinematics of the trajectories of the two components. For example, the time of maximal grip size (grasp component) closely corresponds to that of the beginning of arm reacceleration (transport component) (1).

Based on this research, we could hypothesize that in the case of Mrs. Poirot, who has upper extremity paresis complicated by spasticity, both reach and grasp will be affected. We might predict that she will recover the reach phase earlier and more completely than the grasp phase (10). Because the two aspects appear to be controlled separately, they could potentially be trained both separately and together. For example, Mrs. Poirot may begin practicing the reach component by moving her hand towards an object but not actually grasping it. Because even the reach phase is task-dependent, it is important to practice reaching within the context of many

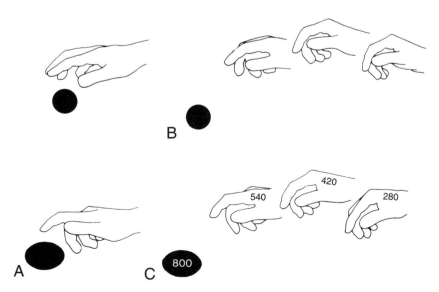

Figure 15.2.   Task-specific changes in hand shaping. **A**, Normal differences in hand shape when an ellipse vs. a sphere is grasped. **B**, An unperturbed reach for a sphere. **C**, A perturbed reach, where the subject reshapes the grasp to accommodate an ellipsoid. The reach begins to change shape at 540 msec after the perturbation onset. (From Jeannerod M. The neural and behavioural organization of goal-directed movements, Oxford: Clarendon Press, 1990:65.)

different types of functional tasks, such as reach and point, reach in preparation for a grasp, reach in preparation for a grasp and lift, or grasp and move.

She may also work on grasp and release of an object close to her hand, alleviating the need for controlling reach. Finally, she may work on combining reach and grasp components.

Role of the Senses

What is the role of sensory information in controlling reach and grasp? You may recall that in Chapter 3, to better understand the function of the different levels of the nervous system, we took a specific upper extremity function task and walked through the pathways of the nervous system that contributed to its planning and execution. We gave the example of being thirsty and wanting to pour some milk from the milk carton in front of you into a glass.

Sensory inputs come in from the periphery to tell you what is happening around you, where you are in space and where your joints are relative to each other: they give you a map of your body in space. Sensory inputs from the visual system go through two parallel pathways involved in goal-directed reaching: one related to "what" is being reached for (object recognition) and the other related to "where" the object is in extrapersonal space (localization). The "what" pathway goes from visual cortex to temporal cortex, while the "where" pathway goes from visual cortex to the parietal lobe.

Higher centers in the cortex take this information (using, possibly, the parietal lobes and pre-motor cortex) and make a plan to act on this information in relation to the goal: reaching for the carton of milk. You make a specific movement plan: you're going to reach over the box of corn flakes in front of you. This plan is sent to the motor cortex, and muscle groups are specified. The plan is also sent to the cerebellum and basal ganglia, and they modify it to refine the movement.

The cerebellum sends an update of the movement output plan to the motor cortex

and brainstem. Descending pathways from the motor cortex and brainstem then activate spinal cord networks, and spinal motor neurons activate the muscles, and you reach for the milk. If the milk carton is full, when you thought it was almost empty, spinal reflex pathways will compensate for the extra weight that you didn't expect and activate more motor neurons. Then the sensory consequences of your reach will be evaluated, and the cerebellum will update the movement—in this case, to accommodate a heavier milk carton.

From this description, you can see that sensory information plays many roles during the control of reaching. Sensory information is used to correct errors during the execution of the movement itself, ensuring accuracy during the final portions of the movement. In addition, sensory information is used proactively in helping to make the movement plan. For a detailed review of the pathways involved in these movements, please see Chapter 3.

VISUAL GUIDANCE IN REACHING

The primary function of visual feedback in reaching appears to be related to the attainment of final accuracy. It has been hypothesized that the constancy of thumb position with relation to the wrist during reaching may be part of a strategy of providing clear visual feedback information regarding the endpoint of the limb (11).

To determine the function of visual feedback in reaching, studies have been performed to compare reaches made with and without vision. Reaches with visual feedback showed a longer duration than those performed without feedback. Absence of visual feedback didn't alter the grasp component of the reach (1).

Can reaching still occur in the absence of visual cortex function? It is usually accepted that destruction of the visual cortex in humans produces total blindness, except for very poor visual perception of illumination changes (1). However, research on monkeys with visual cortex lesions has shown some very interesting results related to visual-motor control (12). Though these monkeys appear to be blind when their visual behavior is tested, they can still reach for objects that appear in or move across their visual field. It has been hypothesized that the superior colliculus in the mid-brain contributes to this residual reaching behavior.

Since the monkey studies were performed, human studies have verified these results (13, 14). In extending the monkey studies to humans, these researchers used a new experimental paradigm that had not been used before in humans. Instead of asking humans with visual cortex lesions if they could see an object, they asked them to try to point to where they "guessed" the target would be. It was shown that subjects did not point randomly; there was a significant correlation between pointing and target position. However, they did show larger constant errors when reaching within their blind visual field. They typically overshot targets when they were within 30° of midline, and undershot them when they were beyond 30° (1).

VISUALLY CONTROLLED REACHES ACROSS THE MIDLINE

Researchers have consistently found that reaching movements across the midline (toward targets in the visual hemifield of the opposite arm) are slower and less accurate than movements to targets on the same side as the arm. Ipsilateral (uncrossed) reaches in these studies were shorter in latency, made with higher maximum velocity and completed more quickly, and made significantly more accurately than contralateral (crossed) reaches (15).

SOMATOSENSORY CONTRIBUTIONS TO REACHING

Is somatosensory input essential for the production of reaching movements? Considerable research (1, 16) has shown that monkeys that were deafferented were still able to perform adequate reaching and grasping movements as soon as 2 weeks after the lesion

was made, as long as vision was available. Researchers noted that the monkeys' movements were awkward at first, with animals only sweeping objects along the floor. Monkeys then developed a primitive grasp with four fingers together and no thumb, and finally redeveloped a crude pincer grasp a few months after the lesion was made (1). Other experiments discussed later in this chapter have shown that deafferented monkeys can still make reasonably accurate single joint pointing movements, even when vision of the arm is occluded, when the pointing task was learned before deafferentation (17). In this case, even displacing the arm before the movement didn't affect terminal accuracy, even though the monkeys couldn't see or feel their arm position! Thus, it was concluded that the monkey is capable of using a central motor program to perform previously learned reaching movements and that kinesthetic feedback isn't required for achieving reasonable accuracy when performing well-learned movements.

Experiments performed with humans with severe peripheral sensory neuropathy in all four limbs have shown similar results (18). One patient was able to perform a wide variety of hand movements, such as tapping movements and drawing figures in the air, even with the eyes closed. However, when he was asked to repeat the movement many times with the eyes closed, the performance deteriorated quickly. Thus, it appears that somatosensory information isn't required for arm movement initiation or execution, as long as the movements are simple or nonrepetitive. However, if subjects have to make complex movements requiring coordination of many joints, or repeat movements, without visual feedback, they are unable to update their central representations of body space and show considerable movement "drift" and problems with coordination (1).

These experiments suggest that certain movements may be carried out without somatosensory feedback. Nevertheless, considerable work has also shown the important contributions of sensory feedback to the fine regulation of movement.

Researchers originally thought that it was mainly joint receptors that controlled position sense during reaching. However, more recent research suggests that joint receptors are mainly active at the extremes of joint motion, but not at mid-position. This would thus make it impossible for these receptors to signal limb position in the mid-working range of joints (1).

More recent work has begun to build evidence for a strong role for muscle spindles in position sense. Experiments have been performed in which tendons were vibrated, specifically activating muscle spindle 1a afferents. Subjects consistently had the illusion that the joint was moving in the direction that it would have been moving if the muscle were being stretched. For example, if the biceps tendon was vibrated, it produced the illusion of elbow extension (19).

Cutaneous afferents are also important contributors to position sense. Mechanoreceptors in the **glabrous** area of the hand are strongly activated by isotonic movements of the fingers (20).

Interestingly, subjects who are recovering from paralysis report that when the muscle is still completely paralyzed, they have no feeling of heaviness in the limb. But as they begin to regain movement ability, they feel as if the limb is being held down by weights. These sensations of heaviness are reduced as movements become easier and strength increases. This could be due to an internal perception of the intensity of motor commands (1).

SENSORY CONTRIBUTION TO ANTICIPATORY ASPECTS OF REACHING

An essential component of all reaching movements is proactive visual and somatosensory control, which is responsible for the correct initial direction of the limb toward the target and the initial coordination between limb segments. In addition, visual information about the characteristics of the object to be grasped is used proactively to preprogram the forces used in precision grip.

It has been hypothesized that visual and somatosensory information is also used to update proprioceptive and visual body maps that allow the accurate programming of reaching movements. To determine the influence of updated maps of the body workspace on the accuracy of a reaching movement, experiments were performed to manipulate visual information regarding hand and target positions *prior to movement*. It was shown that when a subject could not see the hand prior to movement, there were large errors in reaching the target. It was thus concluded that a proprioceptive map of the hand, by itself, was not adequate to appropriately code the hand position in the reaching workspace. This suggests that somatosensory inputs must be calibrated by vision in order for the proprioceptive map and the visual map to be matched (1). No experiments have yet been performed to determine how often the proprioceptive map needs to be updated by visual inputs to ensure accurate movements.

Adaptation of Reach and Grasp

Studies have also been performed (1, 21) to better understand the task-dependent adaptation of reach and grasp. As you will see, this research suggests that the ability to adapt how we reach is a critical part of upper extremity function, since reaching movements vary according to the goals and constraints of the task.

Researchers have shown that the velocity profiles and movement durations of a reach vary, depending on the goal of the task. If the subject was asked to grasp the object, the movement duration of the reach was much longer than if the subject pointed and hit the target. Also, when preparing to grasp an object, the acceleration phase of the reaching movement was much shorter than the deceleration phase, but if the subject was asked to hit the target with the index finger, the acceleration phase was longer than the deceleration phase, with the subject hitting the target at a relatively high velocity (21). This is shown in Figure 15.3.

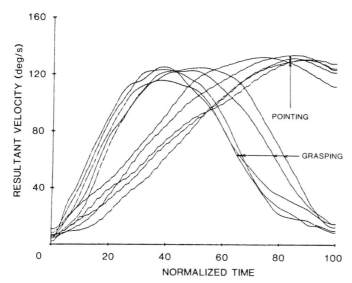

Figure 15.3. The different velocity profiles of the arm for grasping vs. pointing movements. Note that in the grasp, the acceleration phase is shorter than the deceleration phase, while in the point, the reverse is true. (From Jeannerod M. The neural and behavioural organization of goal-directed movements, Oxford: Clarendon Press, 1990:19.)

In addition, if the subject grasped the target, then either fit it in a small box, or alternatively, threw it, movement times and velocity profiles were also different. Movement times were shorter for grasp and throw vs. grasp and fit. In addition, the acceleration phase of the movement was longer for grasp and throw than for grasp and fit. Clearly, the task constraints and goals affect the reaching phase of the movement. This finding has implications for the clinician engaged in retraining the patient with problems related to reach and grasp. Since movements used during reaching for an object vary, depending on the nature of the task, reaching movements need to be practiced within a variety of tasks. For example, these tasks might include practicing reach during reach and point, reach and grasp, reach, grasp, and throw, or reach, grasp and manipulate.

Precision Grip

The types of objects that are picked up during a given day may vary from a light pen to a heavy slick bottle of oil. The nervous system is capable of adapting precision grip so that it accommodates to objects of many different weights and surface characteristics. The control mechanisms underlying these abilities have been carefully investigated (22). It has

been shown that there are discrete phases to any lifting task. These phases are associated with responses in sensory receptors of the hand. The first phase of a lift starts with contact between the fingers and the object to be lifted. When contact has been established, the second phase begins, with the grip force and the load force (load on the fingers) starting to increase. The third phase begins when the load force has overcome the weight of the object and it starts to move. The fourth phase occurs at the end of the lifting task, when there is a decrease in the grip and load force shortly after the object makes contact with the table. (22).

This type of an organizational control scheme has many advantages. For example, it allows great flexibility in lifting objects of different weights. Thus, the duration of the loading phase depends on the object's weight: heavier objects require higher load forces before they move. This also ensures that proper grip forces are used during the load phase. This scheme also requires limited sensory processing, since the end of one phase serves as the trigger for the next.

To ensure a safe grip, the grip-to-load force ratio has to be above a certain level; otherwise, slipping will occur. One cannot assume that two objects of the same weight will require the same grip force, since one may be much more slippery than the other. How does the nervous system choose the correct parameters for grip and load force? It appears to use both previous experience and afferent information during the task. If there is a mismatch between the expected and actual properties of an object, then receptors in the finger pads are activated. Pacinian corpuscles are very sensitive and capable of easily detecting that an object has started to move earlier than expected. In addition, visual and other types of cutaneous cues are important in determining the choice of grip parameters (22).

POSTURAL CONTROL

As was discussed in Chapter 6, postural control, defined as the ability to control the body's position in space for the purpose of stability and orientation, has a strong influence on upper extremity function. The ability to control the body's position in space is essential to being able to move one part of the body, in this case the arms, without destabilizing the rest of the body.

Just as manipulatory control is task-dependent, postural requirements also vary according to the task. For example, postural requirements involved in a seated reaching task will be less stringent than those in a standing task and thus may require only muscles in the trunk. In contrast, postural demands during reaching while standing are greater, requiring more extensive activation of muscles in both the legs and trunk to prevent instability.

Postural demands can affect the speed and accuracy of an upper extremity movement. When postural demands are decreased by providing external support, upper extremity movements are faster, since prior postural stabilization is not necessary (23).

Helping a patient to regain sufficient postural control to meet the postural requirements inherent in a reaching task is essential to retraining that task. The reader is urged to review Chapters 6–10 discussing postural control, its relationship to reaching, and issues related to retraining the patient with postural disorders.

BASIC CHARACTERISTICS OF REACHING TASKS

Until now, we have described the biomechanical and neural contributions to the different components of reach and grasp. However, another approach to studying the control of reaching has come from the field of psychology, where researchers have focused on describing basic characteristics of reaching, and formulated theories about the neural control of reaching based on these characteristics.

Fitts' Law

Some basic characteristics of arm movements that you may find intuitively obvious are that whenever arm movement precision is increased or movement distance is increased, movement time becomes longer. In the 1950s, Fitts (24) quantified these characteristics, in the following experiments. He asked subjects to move a pointer back and forth between an initial position and a target position as quickly as possible. In the set of experiments, he systematically varied the movement distance and the width of the target. He found that he could create a simple equation relating movement time to the distance moved and the target width. This equation, which has become known as Fitts' law, is shown below:

$$MT = a + b \log_2 2D/W$$

a and b are empirically determined constants, MT is movement time, D is distance moved, and W is the width of the target (25). The term $\log_2 2D/W$ has been called the index of difficulty. Movement time increases linearly with the index of difficulty, that is, the more difficult the task, the longer it takes to make the movement.

This equation has come to be known as Fitts' law because its ability to relate movement time to movement accuracy and distance applies to many different kinds of tasks, including discrete aiming movements, moving objects to insert them in a hole, moving a cursor on a screen, small finger movements under a microscope, and even throwing darts. Fitts' law has proven accurate in describing movements made by subjects of all ages, from infants to older adults (25, 26).

What are the constraints of the individual and the task that lead to this particular law regarding movement? It has been suggested that movement time increases with distance and accuracy in part due to the constraints of our visual system. It is difficult to translate our visual perception of the distance to be covered precisely into an actual movement; thus, as the hand approaches the target, time is needed to further update the movement trajectory (25).

Complex Reaching and Bimanual Tasks

In Chapter 1, when we discussed theories of motor control, we mentioned Bernstein's contributions to systems theory (27). Remember that he proposed that a given nervous system program will produce different outcomes in different situations because the response of the body will depend on the initial position of the limbs and on outside forces such as gravity and inertia. When body segments act together, the nervous system must also take into account the forces they generate with respect to each other. Bernstein hypothesized that the nervous system possessed a central representation of the movement that was in the form of a "motor image," representing the form of the movement to be achieved, not the impulses needed to achieve it. He believed that proprioception was important to the final achievement of the movement, not in a reflex-triggering sense, but as it contributed to the central representation of the movement (1). He also suggested that one way of controlling the high number of degrees of freedom involved in any complex movement was to organize the actions in terms of synergies, or groups of muscles or joints that were constrained to act as a unit (27).

In fact, many researchers have now shown that hand movements are organized synergically or through **coordinative struc-**tures. For example, it was shown (28) that when subjects were asked to point at two targets, they moved the hands simultaneously, even if the reaching tasks were very different in difficulty (for example, one was near and large, and the other one was far away and small). Other researchers have noted this same tight bimanual coordination when subjects reached forward to manipulate an object with two hands. Thus, it has been suggested that independent body segments become functionally linked for the execution of a common task (1).

How does the nervous system control complex arm movements to reach targets with speed and elegant precision? This is a complex problem that could be solved in different ways. For example, the nervous system could plan reaching movements with respect to the activation sequences of individual muscles; this has been referred to as a muscle coordinate strategy (29). Alternatively, reaching could be planned in relationship to joint angle coordinates, that is, planning the movements of shoulder, elbow and wrist joints to arrive at the target. This would mean that the nervous system was planning the movement around a set of intrinsic coordinates of the body, expressed in terms of the joint angles. Finally, the nervous system could plan arm movements in terms of the final endpoint coordinates, using extrinsic coordinates in space (29).

Levels of planning could also be considered in terms of a hierarchy, with, for example, both kinematic and kinetic levels of planning. Kinematic levels of planning would be organized around geometry, such as joint angle variables and endpoint variables. Kinetic levels of planning would be organized around forces, such as the forces of muscle activation and joint torques (29).

On the one hand, it seems intuitively obvious that we would need to use some variation on endpoint coordinates planning in order to do something like picking up a glass of water. If we plan a movement using intrinsic coordinates alone, without regard to the actual position of the object in space, the accuracy of the movement with respect to the end position needed is likely to be decreased. But when the nervous system plans according to endpoint coordinates, it needs to make a complex mathematical transformation called an inverse kinematics transformation, which would transform endpoint coordinates into joint angle coordinates. Then it has to create this trajectory by producing the appropriate muscle activation patterns (29).

It has also been proposed that movements are planned in terms of joint angle coordinates, which has the advantage of not requiring an inverse kinematics transformation. This would mean that the organization of movement by the nervous system would be simplified. However, the nervous system would still have to do an inverse dynamics transformation that would transform joint angle coordinates into muscle torques and muscle activation patterns required to make the movement (29).

If trajectories were planned in terms of muscle activation patterns, it would have the advantage of simplifying the inverse kinematics and inverse dynamics problems, but we have also mentioned that muscle activation patterns are only indirectly related to final joint positions. Thus, programming movements in this manner could cause large inaccuracies (29).

How does one go about answering the question of how the nervous system plans movements? Hollerbach, in an excellent review of the research on arm movement planning (29), mentions that Bernstein actually made the following statement (27), which has

guided modern physiologists in their experiments exploring the control of reaching movements.

> If the spatial shape of a trajectory is invariant irrespective of the muscle scheme or the joint scheme, then the motor plan must be closely related to the topology of the trajectory and considerably removed from joints and muscles.

Thus, experimenters have begun to look for invariant characteristics in different variables related to the reach. If invariances are found across different conditions, this could be considered evidence that the nervous system uses this variable to plan movements.

It has been shown (30) that the path of the wrist in an arm movement is unaffected by movement speed, or load (weights held in the hand). In addition, the velocity profiles of a movement are also unaffected by movement speed or load. These findings support the concept that the nervous system uses kinematic variables for planning.

Remember that there are two types of kinematic variables that could be used for movement planning: joint angle coordinates and endpoint coordinates. If the nervous system controls movements in joint angle coordinates, the hand should move in a curved line, because the movements will be about the axis of a joint, as you see in Figure 15.4A. However, if it plans movements with respect to extrapersonal space or endpoint coordinates, the hand would be expected to move in a straight line (Figure 15.4B) (1, 26, 29).

To answer this question, researchers

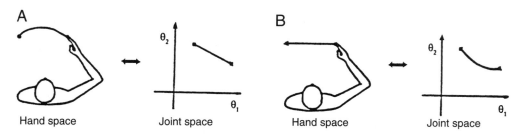

Figure 15.4.   Different variables that can be used for planning arm movements. **A**, If movements are controlled in joint coordinates, hand trajectories are curved. **B**, If movements are controlled in endpoint coordinates, joint space is curved (a complex elbow and shoulder movement is required). (Adapted from Hollerbach JM. Planning of arm movements. In: Osherson DN, Kosslyn SM, Hollerbach JM, eds. Visual cognition and action: an invitation to cognitive science, vol 2. Cambridge, MA: MIT Press, 1990:187.)

(31) asked subjects to point to targets in two-dimensional space (on a surface) and recorded their hand trajectories. They found that subjects tended to move the hand in straight lines, with their joints going through complex angular changes. Even when they were asked to draw curved lines, the subjects tended to draw a series of straight line subunits. These results support the concept that the CNS programs movements according to endpoint coordinates.

Other researchers (29) have explored arm movement control further and have shown that the nervous system can directly control the joints and still produce straight line movements. This is done by varying the onset times for the joint movements, with all joints stopping at the same time. This method of control gives movements with almost straight line paths. This suggests that straight line trajectories can occur even when the CNS is using joint angle coordinates to program movements. Thus, it is not clear whether the CNS programs movements exclusively by one method or the other.

Russian researchers (32) have shown that the elbow and wrist joints are controlled as a synergic unit. When subjects were asked to move the elbow and wrist joint congruently (flexing both together), the subjects could perform this task with ease, with joint motions starting and stopping as a unit. When asked to move the joints incongruently (flexing one and extending the other), they performed the task with considerable difficulty, moving the joints much less smoothly. This is additional evidence for **joint-based planning** (26).

THEORIES ON THE CONTROL OF REACHING

A number of theories on the control of reaching have been formulated to explain some of the reaching characteristics just described. The following section explores these theories. The first group of theories tends to assume that the nervous system is programming *distance* in making movements, while the second group of theories suggests that fi-nal *location* is the parameter being programmed.

Distance vs. Location Programming

What do we mean by programming distance vs. location? According to the distance programming theory, when making an arm movement toward a target, people visually perceive the distance to be covered. Then, they activate a particular set of agonist muscles to propel the arm the proper distance to the target. At a particular point, they turn off the agonist muscles and activate antagonist muscles at the joint in order to provide a braking force to stop the movement (33).

According to the location programming theory, the nervous system programs the relative balance of tensions (or stiffness) of two opposing (agonist and antagonist) muscle sets. According to this theory, every location in space corresponds to a family of stiffness relations between opposing muscles, as we explain later in the chapter. Let's first look at distance programming theories.

DISTANCE THEORIES

Multiple Corrections Theory

It has been shown repeatedly that accuracy of arm movements decreases when vision is absent. For example, when subjects were asked to make arm movements of different durations to a target, movements of 190 msec or less were unaffected by loss of vision, while movements of 260 msec or more were affected by loss of visual feedback (34). Thus, it appears that movement trajectories are corrected based on visual feedback, and that it takes about 200 to 250 msec for vision to be able to update a movement trajectory. Considering that some movement time must occur before the limb is close enough to the target to use visual feedback, one realizes that the visual processing time is slightly shorter. It has been shown (35) that subjects need to see their hand for at least 135 msec during a movement to use vision to improve movement accuracy.

In the 1960s, researchers (36, 37) proposed that aiming movements consisted of a series of submovements, each responding to and reducing visual error. Thus, an initial movement, before any visual correction takes place, covers most of the distance to a target and is independent of final precision. This model predicts a constant b for Fitts' law, which is almost identical to the one that Fitts and Peterson calculated originally (25).

There are, however, some problems with this model. Typically, aiming movements to a target have only one correction, if any, and when corrections are made, they do not have constant durations or proportions of the distance to the target (26).

How might this theory be used to explain problems related to inaccurate reaching movements commonly found in patients with neurological deficits? The multiple corrections theory stresses the importance of visual feedback when making corrections during a movement to increase accuracy. Thus, inaccurate movements could be the result of loss of visual feedback. When retraining a patient using a multiple corrections theory, the clinician could have the patient practice slow movements, requiring a high degree of accuracy, drawing the patient's attention to visual cues relating hand movement to target location.

Schmidt's Impulse Variability Model

Another way of explaining the characteristics of arm movement seen in Fitts' equation is to hypothesize that the initial phase of the movement, involving the generation of a force impulse is more important than later phases of the movement dealing with ongoing control. This would be particularly true in cases where the movement is too fast to utilize visual feedback to aid in accuracy.

Schmidt performed research in which subjects were asked to make fast movements over a fixed distance. These movements required large amounts of force, since high-velocity movements require large forces to generate the movement. He showed that the size of the subject's error increased in proportion to the magnitude of the force used. Thus,

when he asked subjects to make a fast but accurate movement, the large forces required caused increased force variability. This increased variability resulted in a decreased movement accuracy (38). These movement characteristics were described in the following equation:

$$W_e = a + b\, D/MT$$

where We is variation in movement endpoint expressed in standard deviation units, D is distance moved, and MT is movement time. This equation is similar to Fitts' law. It indicates that simply taking into account that faster movement requires more force can explain Fitts' law, without having to factor in a need for visual feedback for movement accuracy (25).

This theory alone cannot be used to explain aiming movements, since as we have seen earlier, many movements, particularly those lasting longer than 250 msec, do use visual feedback for accuracy.

Nonetheless, this theory does have relevance for the clinician involved in retraining upper extremity control. It suggests the importance of practicing fast movements of varying amplitudes during therapy sessions. In this way, the patient learns to program forces appropriately for quick and accurate movements.

Hybrid Model: Optimized Initial Impulse Model

The previous two models deal with two extremes of movement control (*a*) the use of visual feedback to improve accuracy during ongoing portions of slower movements, and (*b*) very fast movements that cannot easily use visual feedback, and thus are controlled only through the amplitude of the initial impulse. In an attempt to create a model to explain the entire range of possible aiming movements, more recent studies (39) have described a hybrid model that combines elements of both of these models. This hybrid model is referred to as the optimized initial impulse model.

Researchers involved in studying this model hypothesized that a subject makes a first movement toward a target, which, if successful, is the sole movement. However, if it is inaccurate, for example, it undershoots or overshoots the target, another movement will be required involving visual feedback during ongoing movement control. Clearly, the subject needs to find a balance between moving quickly, which requires a large initial force, and moving slowly enough to allow corrections to the ongoing movement, thereby ensuring accuracy.

It was found that an equation taking these issues into account was similar to Fitts' law:

$$T = a + b(n(D/W)^{1/n}$$

where T is movement time, D is distance, and W is width of the target, and n is the number of submovements used to reach the target (26).

Since functional activities require a variety of movements, both fast and slow, with varying degrees of accuracy, it is important to retrain a patient's ability to perform a continuum of movements that vary in both speed and accuracy.

LOCATION PROGRAMMING

As we mentioned earlier, there are two ways that the nervous system could program arm movements, through distance programming, or through programming the endpoint location of the movement (25, 40). The example of a cafe-door swinging on springs has sometimes been used to explain the location programming model (33). Figure 15.5A shows the door in a closed position. The movement of the cafe door is described as occurring when there is a reduction in length of one spring and the lengthening of the other spring. When the door is released, the imbalance between the springs causes the door to return to its closed position, where the springs are at their resting length. If you want to keep the door open, you can simply change one spring for another of a different stiffness, and then it will have a new resting position (Fig. 15.5B).

It has been suggested that the agonist/antagonist muscle pairs at the joints are like

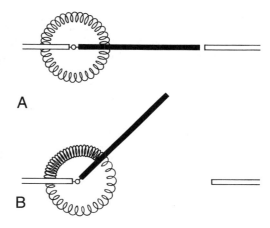

Figure 15.5. The cafe-door model. Simplified explanation of the mass-spring model of motor control. **A,** When a cafe door is at rest, it resembles a joint at midpoint, with both muscles at midlength. **B,** When one spring of a cafe door is shortened and the other is lengthened, the door is open, analogous to one muscle contracting and the other relaxing to allow the joint to flex.

the springs of the cafe door. We can change the position of the joint simply by changing the relative stiffness of the two muscles, through higher or lower relative activation levels. Though this may sound like an unusual way for the nervous system to program reaching movements, experiments have shown that this occurs in many circumstances.

For example, experiments performed on monkeys (17) suggest that many movements may be controlled through location rather than distance programming. In these experiments, the monkeys were trained to make elbow movements to different targets whenever lights above those targets were turned on (Fig. 15.6D). The monkeys wore a large collar that blocked sight of the arm, eliminating visual feedback. In addition, in certain experiments, the dorsal roots of the spinal cord were severed, eliminating kinesthetic feedback from the arm. The accuracy of the monkeys' arm movements was measured with and without visual and kinesthetic feedback. Researchers found that the monkeys' reaching was normal, despite a loss of visual and kinesthetic feedback (Fig. 15.6A) (17).

They then gave a perturbation to the deafferented monkeys' arm, moving it from its original position, just after the target light was turned on, but before the monkey began

Figure 15.6. Experimental set-up to test the mass-spring model of control. The deafferented monkey is pointing to a target, but is unable to see its hand. The hand can be moved to a new position by a torque motor after the target is illuminated, but before the hand starts to move. As you see from the movement traces, the monkey was able to successfully point to the target, even when the hand was perturbed. (From Brooks VB. The neural basis of motor control. NY: Oxford University Press. 1986:138.)

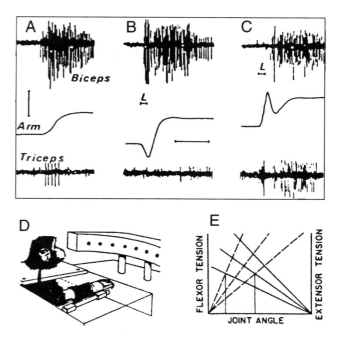

to move. Remember, the monkeys couldn't feel or see their arm position when it was perturbed. Nevertheless, the monkeys reached for the target with reasonable accuracy (Fig. 15.6*B* and *C*). If the monkeys were using distance programming for reaching, this would have been impossible, because they would have applied a fixed force pulse in the elbow muscles to move their arm to the new position. Since the arm had already been perturbed, they should have ended up in the wrong place!

The only way these results can be explained is through the use of endpoint location programming. In this case, what the nervous system would program is the stiffness (or background activity level) settings on the agonist and antagonist muscles of the arm. For example, if the arm was originally in a flexed position, they would have high background activity levels in the elbow flexors and low levels in the extensors. To move the arm precisely to the new location, they would simply change the background activity (stiffness) levels so that the spring constant of the elbow flexors was at a specific lower level, and that of the extensors was at a predetermined higher level (Fig. 15.6*E*). Once this new spring setting was made, it wouldn't matter

where the limb was perturbed, because, just like the cafe door, the limb would swing to its new spring-setting. Thus, the monkey didn't have to know its starting point in order to go to the correct endpoint.

It is interesting that in these experiments (17), the monkeys were not able to continue to make accurate movements when the shoulder position was changed. It appears that without visual or somatosensory feedback from the arm, they could not update a central reference concerning shoulder position changes. These changes then threw off the elbow location programming.

More recent work (41) with humans produced similar results. In this study, subjects were blindfolded, and their fingers were anesthetized by using a pressure cuff. Before testing began, they were trained to move their fingers to a specific position in space. They were then given brief finger perturbations during the course of their finger movement. With complete loss of finger sensation, there was very little difference in terminal error between the perturbed and unperturbed movements.

These results suggest that the nervous system is able to encode the location of body segments in space, in relation to a base body position as varying activation levels of agonist and antagonist muscles. What does this mean? It has been suggested (33) that this could explain why we can perform a skill (such as reaching for a cup or throwing a ball) hundreds of times without repeating exactly the same movement. According to classic programming theory, one would have to make a new program for each movement variation, but according to the mass-spring model, all one would have to do is program the appropriate muscle activity ratios, and the limb would move appropriately to its final position.

Do these results suggest that distance programming is wrong? No. Most likely, both strategies are used for arm movements, depending on the task and the context. For example, it has been shown that when humans make rapid elbow flexion movements (42), they show a triphasic burst of contraction: first the biceps is activated, followed by the triceps (braking the movement), and then the biceps again. This same pattern was found in patients with loss of kinesthetic sensation. However, when subjects were asked to move more slowly and smoothly, they showed continuous biceps activity and no triceps activity. This has led some researchers (25) to argue that the subjects are using mass-spring or location programming for slow movements, and a combination of distance programming and location programming for faster movements.

There are also limitations to the mass-spring model. The model only holds with single-joint, one-plane movements. Most movements involve many joints, are carried out in three-dimensional space, and have to take into account gravity (1).

In summary, research studies appear to indicate that single-joint movements that are shorter than .25 seconds are too short to take advantage of visual feedback, while those longer than about .25 seconds involve visual feedback in the homing-in phase. Slower movements may involve location programming, while faster movements may involve a combination of distance and location programming.

This model would suggest that the capacity to modulate stiffness levels between the agonist and antagonist muscles is an important part of retraining accurate upper extremity movements.

SUMMARY

1. From a kinematic perspective, coordination in reaching is characterized by the sequential activation of eye, head, then hand movements. However, muscle responses in these segments tend to be activated synchronously, not sequentially. Thus, inertial characteristics play an important part in the final movement characteristics.

2. Reach and grasp represent two distinct components that appear to be controlled by different neural mechanisms. Thus, patients with motor control problems can have difficulties in one or both aspects. This has implications for retraining.

3. Certain aspects of the grasp component, such as force of the grasp, are based on the person's perception of the characteristics of the object to be grasped, and thus are programmed in advance.

4. Visual and somatosensory information are also used reactively for error correction during reaching and grasping.

5. Fitts' law expresses the relationship between movement time, distance, and accuracy, stating that when the demands for accuracy increase, movement time will also increase.

6. There are two theories regarding the neural control of reaching: distance programming vs. location theories.

7. According to the distance programming theory, when people make an arm movement toward a target, they visually perceive the distance to be covered, and then they activate a particular set of agonist muscles to propel the arm the proper distance to the target. At a particular point, they turn off the agonist muscles and activate antagonist muscles at the joint to provide a braking force to stop the movement.

8. According to the location programming theory, the nervous system programs the relative balance of tensions (or stiffness) of two opposing (agonist and antagonist) muscle sets. According to this theory, every location in space corresponds to a family of stiffness relations between opposing muscles.

9. It is probably the case that both strategies are used for arm movements, depending on the task and the context.

REFERENCES

1. Jeannerod M. The neural and behavioral organization of goal-directed movements. Clarendon Press: Oxford, 1990.
2. Gresty MA. Coordination of head and eye movements to fixate continuous and intermittent targets. Vision research 1974; 14:395–403.
3. Biguer B, Prablanc C, Jeannerod M. The contribution of coordinated eye and head movements in hand pointing accuracy. Exp Brain Res 1984;55:462–469.
4. Roll JP, Bard C, Paillard, J. Head orienting contributes to directional accuracy of aiming at distant targets. Hum Mov Sci 1986;5:359–371.
5. Charness AL. Management of the upper extremity in the patient with hemiplegia. Course syllabus, Annual Meeting, Washington Physical Therapy Association, 1994.
6. Jeannerod M. The timing of natural prehension movements. J Motor Behav 1984; 16:235–254.
7. Fraser C, Wing A. A case study of reaching by a user of a manually-operated artificial hand. Prosthet Orthot Int 1981;5:151–156.
8. Bruner JS, Koslowski B. Visually pre-adapted constituents of manipulatory action. Perception 1972;1:3–14.
9. Kuypers HGJM. Corticospinal connections: postnatal development in rhesus monkey. Science 1962;138:678–680.
10. De Souza LH, Hewer RL, Miller S. Assessment of recovery of arm control in hemiplegic stroke patients. 1. Arm function tests. Int Rehab Med 1980;2:3–9.
11. Wing AM, Frazer C. The contribution of the thumb to reaching movements. Q J Exp Psychol 1983;35A:297–309.
12. Humphrey NK, Weiskrantz L. Vision in monkeys after removal of the striate cortex. Nature 1969;215:595–597.
13. Weiskrantz L, Warrington ER, Sanders MD, Marshall J. Visual capacity in the hemianopic field following a restricted occipital ablation. Brain 1974;97:709–728.
14. Perenin MT, Jeannerod M. Residual vision in cortically blind hemifields. Neuropsychologia 1975;13:1–7.
15. Fisk JD, Goodale MA. The organization of eye and limb movements during unrestricted reaching to targets in contralateral and ipsilateral visual space. Exp Brain Res 1985; 60:159–178.
16. Taub E, Berman AJ. Movement and learning in the absence of sensory feedback. In: Freedman SJ, ed. The neurophysiology of spatially oriented behavior. Homewood, NJ: Dorsey Press, 1968:173–192.
17. Polit A, Bizzi E. Characteristics of motor programs underlying arm movements in monkeys. J Neurophysiol 1979;42:183–194.
18. Rothwell JC, Traub MM, Day BL, Obeso JA, Thomas PK, Marsden CD. Manual motor performance in a deafferented man. Brain 1982;105:515–542.
19. Goodwin GM, McCloskey DI, Matthews PBC. The contribution of muscle afferents to kinaesthesia shown by vibration induced illusions of movement and by the effects of paralysing joint afferents. Brain 1972;95:705–748.
20. Hulliger M, Nordh E, Thelin AE, Vallbo AB. The responses of afferent fibers from the glabrous skin of the hand during voluntary finger movements in man. J Physiol 1979; 291:233–249.
21. Marteniuk RG, Mackenzie CL, Jeannerod M, Athenes S, Dugas C. Constraints on human arm movements trajectories. Can J Psychol 1987;41:365–368.
22. Johansson RS, Edin BB. Neural control of manipulation and grasp. In: Forssberg H, Hirschfeld H, eds. Movement disorders in children. Basel: Karger, 1992:107–112.
23. Cordo P, Nashner LM. Properties of postural adjustments associated with rapid arm movements. J Neurophysiology 1982;47:287–302.
24. Fitts PM. The information capacity of the human motor system in controlling the amplitude of movement J Exp Psychol 1954; 47:381–391.
25. Keele SW. Behavioral analysis of movement. In: Brooks VB, ed. Handbook of physiology: section I: The nervous system, vol 2. Motor control, part 2. Baltimore: Williams & Wilkins, 1981:1391–1414.
26. Rosenbaum DA. Human motor control. San Diego: Academic Press. 1991.
27. Bernstein N. The coordination and regulation of movements. Oxford: Pergamon Press, 1967.
28. Kelso JAS, Southard DL, Goodman D. On the coordination of two-handed movements. J Exp Psychol [Hum Percept] 1979;5:229–238.
29. Hollerbach JM. Planning of arm movements. In: Osherson DN, Kosslyn SM, Hollerbach

JM, eds. Visual cognition and action: an invitation to cognitive science, vol 2. Cambridge, Mass: MIT Press. 1990:183–211.

30. Atkeson CG, Hollerbach JM. Kinematic features of unrestrained vertical arm movements. J Neuroscience 1985;5:2318–2330.

31. Morasso P. Spatial control of arm movements. Exp Brain Res 1981;42:223–227.

32. Kots YM, Syrovegin AV. Fixed set of variants of interactions of the muscles to two joints in the execution of simple voluntary movements. Biophysics 1966;11:1212–1219.

33. Keele SW. Motor control. In: Kaufman L, Thomas J, Boff K, eds. Handbook of perception and performance. New York: John Wiley & Sons, 1986:30.1–30.60.

34. Keele SW, Posner MI. Processing visual feedback in rapid movement. J Exp Psychol 1968; 77:155–158.

35. Carlton LG. Processing visual feedback information for movement control. J Exp Psychol [Hum Percept] 1981;7:1019–1030.

36. Crossman ERFW, Goodeve PJ. Feedback control of hand-movement and Fitts' law. Q J Exp Psychol 1983;35A:251–278.

37. Keele SW. Movement control in skilled motor performance. Psychol Bull 1968;70:387–403.

38. Schmidt RA, Zelaznik HN, Hawkins B, Frank JS, Quinn JT, Jr. Motor output variability: a theory for the accuracy of rapid motor acts. Psychol Rev 1979;86:415–452.

39. Meyer DE, Abrams RA, Kornblum S, Wright CE, Smith JEK. Optimality in human motor performance: ideal control of rapid aimed movements. Psychol Rev 1988;95:340–370.

40. Feldman AG. Change in the length of the muscle as a consequence of a shift in equilibrium in the muscle-load system. Biofizika 1974;19:534–538.

41. Kelso JAS, Holt KJ. Exploring a vibratory systems analysis of human movement production. J Neurophysiol 1980;43:1183–1196.

42. Hallett M, Shahani BT, Young RR. EMG analysis of stereotyped voluntary movements in man. J Neurol Neurosurg Psychiatry 1975; 38:1154–1162.

Chapter 16

UPPER EXTREMITY MANIPULATION SKILLS: CHANGES ACROSS THE LIFE SPAN

INTRODUCTION

The development of reaching and manipulation skills is complex and actually involves the development of many behaviors, each of which emerges progressively over time in association with maturation of different parts of the nervous and musculoskeletal systems and with experience. For example, the infant's ability to transport the arm towards an object precedes the ability to grasp. The ability to grasp emerges at 4 to 5 months, preceding the infant's ability to explore objects, which does not emerge until about the first year of life. Thus, the development of mature reaching and manipulation occurs gradually over the first few years of life.

This chapter explores the research on the development of reaching abilities in infants and children as well as the changes in reaching abilities that occur in older adults. We first discuss some of the early hypotheses concerning the development of reaching, which propose that reaching either results from the inhibition of primitive reflexes or the integration of those reflexes into voluntary movement (1). We also discuss the relative contributions of genetics vs. experience to the emergence of reaching in the neonate. We then review more recent studies that come from newer theories of motor control such as the ecological, dynamical, and systems approaches.

Role of Reflexes in Development of Reaching Behaviors

Is early reaching reflexly controlled? This is a question that has been debated in the developmental literature for many years. Early theories of the development of reaching argued that reflexes provide the physiological substrate for complex voluntary movements such as reaching (1). According to these theories, the transition from reflexes to voluntary reaching is a continuous process, with newborn reflexes gradually being incorporated into a hierarchy of complex coordinated actions (2). A review of eye-hand coordination development mentions that early developmental theoreticians may have overlooked another possibility regarding the development of reaching: that eye-hand coordination may emerge concurrently with the maturation of reflex function rather than emerging from the modification of reflex function (2). Thus, such reflexes as the grasp reflex may develop separately from the eye-hand coordination system, and may underlie different functions.

Reaching Behaviors: Innate or Learned?

A second question that has intrigued researchers concerns the extent to which the integration of sensory and motor systems underlying eye-hand coordinations is genetically predetermined and/or experientially determined.

If the integration of eye-hand coordination were completely genetically predetermined, it would imply that the nervous system has a ready-made map of visual space and one of manipulative space laid out in a one-to-one correspondence. Thus, just by seeing an object, an infant would know exactly where to reach. If it were completely experientially determined, experience would be required to "map" visual space onto motor space.

The first hypothesis implies that once the nervous system's sensory and motor pathways for visually guided reaching have matured, the infant will be able to reach accurately for an object, with little or no prior experience. The second hypothesis predicts that a learning period is required in development, during which the infant creates, through trial and error, the visual map that overlays the motor map for reaching.

In the 1950s, Piaget's research on child development led him to believe that though nervous system maturation is a requirement for the appearance of a behavior, experience is responsible for its coordination with the senses. He believed that only through repeatedly and simultaneously looking at and touching an object would the visual and manipulative impressions be associated (3).

Other researchers gave further support to this concept when they noted that neonates showed both visual and manual activity in the first few weeks after birth, but these movements were apparently unrelated (4). Thus, in the 1960s, many researchers in development supported the theory that visual and hand control systems are unrelated at birth.

In the 1970s, a group of scientists (5, 6) presented interesting evidence that they believed supported the opposite concept: that there was clear coordination of eye and hand in the newborn. They reported that infants between 7 and 14 days of age showed arm movements that were clearly directed toward the object in the visual field. They said a significant proportion of reaches were within 5° to 10° of the object and that in 30 to 40% of the reaches, the hand closed around the object. They also observed that infants differentiated between graspable (small object) and nongraspable (large object at large distance) objects: they reached for the first but not the second.

Many researchers initially had difficulty replicating these experiments, and thus the results were questioned (7). However, more recent studies indicate that an early form of eye-hand coordination does exist in the neonate, although reaching doesn't seem to be as accurate or coordinated as originally indicated (8, 9).

In 1980, Amiel-Tison and Grenier, two researchers from France, wrote a surprising article on neonatal abilities (10). They showed that when the heads of neonates were stabilized, giving them postural support, amazing coordination of other behaviors was seen. For example, they showed that chaotic movements of the arms became still and the infants appeared to be able to reach forward toward objects (Fig. 16.1). Their article is one example of recent research that supports the hypothesis that infants are born with certain innate abilities or behaviors, which have sometimes been termed pre-reaching behaviors (10).

In the late 1970s and 1980s, Claes von Hofsten, a psychologist from Sweden, began exploring the development of eye-hand coordination in the neonate (11). He placed infants in an infant seat and moved an object in

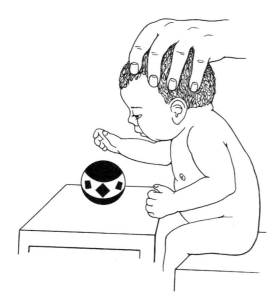

Figure 16.1. The release of reaching movements in a neonate by stabilizing the head. (Adapted from Amiel-Tison C, Grenier A. Evaluation neurologique du nuveau-ne et du nourrisson. Paris: Masson, 1980:95.)

front of them, as you see in Figure 16.2, and carefully documented the number and accuracy of reaches that he observed. He observed the infants' arm movements with and without an object present. He showed that the number of extended movements performed when the infants were visually fixating on the object was twice as high as when the object wasn't fixated. The reaching movements weren't very accurate. However, those that were made while the infants fixated on the target were aimed an average of 32° laterally and 25° vertically toward the target, while those that were made without fixation were only within 52° laterally and 37° vertically. Though these reaching movements weren't as accurate as had previously been postulated, they were clearly aimed at the target, since they were significantly more accurate than the nonvisually fixated movements. These results thus showed a clear effect of vision on forward directed movements (11).

Von Hofsten noted that the system works from hand to eye as well. Several times the infant accidentally touched the object and immediately turned the eyes toward it. Neo-

nates also have proprioceptive control of hand movements: they reach toward their mouth without vision, in a goal-directed way. If they miss at first, they move to the mouth using proprioceptive feedback (11, 12).

Thus, this research suggests that some aspects of reaching, in particular, the ability to locate objects in space and transport the arm, may be present in rudimentary form at birth, while other components, such as grasp, develop later in the first year of life. These findings suggest support for the hypothesis that at least some aspects of reaching are innate.

In the next sections we follow the progression of the development of reaching and manipulation skills through the first few years of life, exploring the emergence of various aspects of reaching and manipulation behaviors. We have already seen that location of an object in space is possible in the neonate, and that the ability to transport the arm toward the object is also available at birth. However, as you will see, the grasp component of reaching does not develop until 4 to 5 months of age, with pincer grasp developing at 9 to 13 months. Higher cognitive aspects of reaching begin to emerge at about 1 year of age. Throughout development, there appears to be a repetitive shift between visually triggered (or proactively guided reaching) and visually guided (or feedback-controlled) reaching.

EARLY DEVELOPMENT OF EYE-HAND COORDINATION

During the first year of life, there are a number of clear transitions in the infant's eye-hand coordination abilities. The first transformation in reaching skills appears to occur at about 2 months of age (11, 12). Until this time, whenever the infant extends the arm, the hand opens in extension at the same time, so that it is difficult to grasp an object. At 2 months, the extension synergy is broken up, so that the fingers flex as the arm extends: the probability of seeing this behavior goes from 10 to 70% of reaches, from shortly after birth to 2 months. At 2 months, head-arm movements become coupled very strongly as the

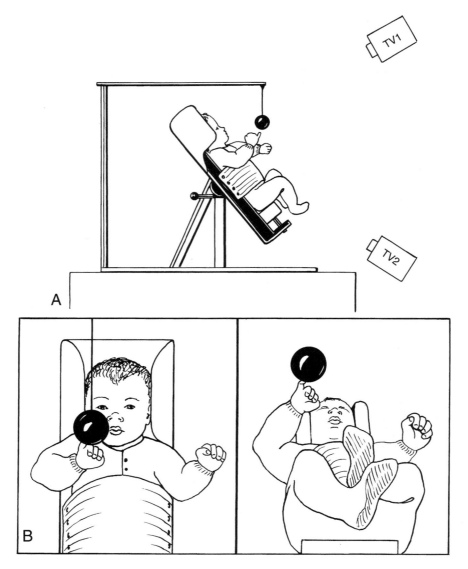

Figure 16.2. **A**, Experimental set-up used to study reaching in neonates. The infant is placed in an infant seat (50° angle) that has head support on the back and sides, but allows the arms freedom to move. **B**, Diagram of the outline of the infant as it touched the object, taken from single frames from the two video cameras seen in A. (Adapted from Hofsten C von. Eye-hand coordination in the newborn. Developmental Psychology 1982;18:452.)

infant gains control over the neck muscles (11, 12).

Over the next 2 months, there is an increased uncoupling of head and arm movements, which allows more flexibility in eye-hand coordination. At about 4 months, infants begin to gain trunk stability, so they have a more stable base for reaching movements.

A number of developmental changes thus converge at about 4 months of age, all of which are essential for the emergence of successful reaching. This supports the concept that the emergence of successful reaching is not due to the maturation of a single system, but to contributions of multiple maturing systems (11, 12).

At about 4 months, infants enter a new developmental phase, involving integration of the newly developed skill of eye-hand coordination. Reaches of 4-month-olds typically consist of several steps, and the final approach toward the object is crooked and awkward. In the next 2 months, the approach path straightens and the number of steps in the reach are reduced in number, with the first part of the reach getting longer and more powerful. By 6 months of age, the trajectory of most reaches appears to be adult-like (11, 12).

Visually Triggered vs. Visually Guided Reaching

Remember from the last chapter that reaching movements in adults have two different phases: the transport phase and the grasp phase. It has been hypothesized that the beginning of the reach is visually triggered. That is, visual location of the target is used to initiate the movement. Thus, the position of the object is defined visually, while the position of the arm is defined proprioceptively. In contrast, the last part of the reach is considered visually guided. In this case, the position of the arm is defined visually with reference to the target, allowing precise adjustments to be made to ensure the accuracy of the reach (13).

Newborns seem able to use the visually triggered mode reasonably well, since they are able to initiate a reach aimed toward the target (8). However, they do not appear to be proficient in the visually guided mode, since they are still very inaccurate in their reaches. Visually guided reaching requires the ability to attend to the hand as it moves toward the object, as well as the ability to attend to the object. It also requires the ability to anticipate possible errors.

Research indicates that the visually guided mode of reaching emerges between the 4th and the 5th month of life just as trunk control and arm coordination are also improving (2, 12).

In order to study the development of visually guided reaching in infants, researchers have fitted infants with special glasses with prism lenses to give an apparent lateral shift in the target position as the infants reached for small toys (2). By 5½ months, when the infant's hand comes into view, he/she is able to perceive the discrepancy between hand position and target position and correct the trajectory. This suggests that by 5½ months, visually guided reaching is evident in most infants. Visually guided reaching, or the ability to make corrections to a trajectory based on visual information, peaks at around 7 months, and then is gradually replaced by a ballistic style of reach, though infants can still use visual guidance when needed. In a ballistic style of reach, corrections are made at the end of the movement instead of during the ongoing movement. Once the movement is completed, the error between hand position and target position is used to correct the position of the hand in space.

Emergence of Hand Orientation

When do infants first begin to orient their hands to the position and shape of the object? To answer this question, researchers placed brightly colored rods either horizontally or vertically in front of the infant and recorded the characteristics of their reaching movements, as you see in Figure 16.3. Preparatory adjustments of hand orientation (vertical vs. horizontal, depending on object orientation) occurred when infants first began to grasp objects, as early as 4½ to 5 months of age (14). However, the adjustments of the hand to the orientation of the object became more precise with age. Adjustments of the hand were often done before or during the early part of the reach, though they could also be seen during the approach phase.

To reach smoothly for an object, the infant must time the grasp appropriately with relationship to encountering the object. If the hand closes too late, the object will bounce off the palm of the infant, and if the hand closes too early, the object will hit the knuckles. This type of planning requires visual control, since tactile control would not allow the hand to close until after touching the object (14). In experiments in which the kinematics of reaching of 5-, 6-, 9-, and 13-month-olds were compared to those of adults, it was shown that infant grasping was visually con-

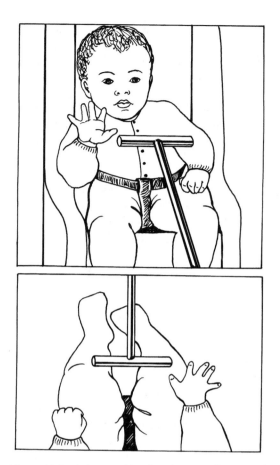

Figure 16.3. Infant reaching for a horizontally oriented bar (Adapted from Hofsten C von, Fazel-Zandy S. Development of visually guided hand orientation in reaching. J Exp Child Psychol 1984;38:210.)

with research performed on the anatomic development of the primate motor system. In primates, it has been shown that neural pathways controlling movements of the arm are different from those that control the fine movements of the fingers and hand. The two systems develop at different times. Arm control, which appears to be mainly coordinated at the brainstem level, develops earlier than hand and finger control, which appears to be coordinated at the cortical level (16, 17).

Researchers found that infant monkeys show arm movements toward objects early in development, but do not show independent finger and hand movements until they are 3 months old (12, 18). It has also been shown that at about 9 to 13 months of age, with the development of the pyramidal tract, infants are able to control fractionated finger movements and thus develop more difficult grasping skills such as the pincer grasp (12). At about 14 to 16 months of age, the infant develops the ability to adapt reaching to the weight of objects, using shape and size as indicators of weight (19).

Learning to Grasp Moving Objects (Catching)

Studies have also been performed to determine the emergence of the ability of infants to reach for and grasp a moving object; this could be considered a rudimentary form of catching behavior (20). Researchers have shown that by the time infants could reach successfully for nonmoving objects, they were also successful at reaching for moving objects. Infants as young as 18 weeks could catch objects moving at 30 cm/sec. Fifteen-week-olds could intercept the object, but were not yet able to grasp it. These results suggest that infants are able to predict where the object will be at a future point in time because they must start reaching early to intercept it in its path. It was noted that the infants didn't automatically reach toward every object that passed by. Rather, they seemed to be able to detect in advance whether they had a reasonable chance to reach it (20).

trolled as early as 5 to 6 months of age, with the hand starting to close in anticipation of reaching the object. Also, the opening of the hand was related to the size of the object for the 9- and 13-month-olds, but not in the younger group. Finally, the 13-month-olds initiated the grasp farther away from the target than the younger groups, with timing of the grasp similar to that seen in adults. The grasp component of the reach is still not mature in the 13-month-old, however, since, unlike adults, they do not yet correlate the onset of closing of the hand with the size of the object to be grasped (15).

These developmental changes related to reaching and grasping skills correlate well

Development of the Pincer Grasp

There are two different ways that objects can be grasped. They can be grasped in a power grip, using the palm and palmar surface of the fingers, with the thumb reinforcing this grip, or they can be grasped in a precision grip, between the terminal pads of the finger and the thumb. The precision grip requires that the fingers be moved independently, and is a prerequisite for accurate and skilled movement of objects (21, 22).

In the first months after birth, infant grasping movements are controlled by tactile and proprioceptive reflexes. Thus, when an object contacts the palm, the fingers close. Also, when the arm flexes, the hand closes, as part of a flexor synergy. At about 4 months of age, with the onset of functional reaching, the palmer grasp is used exclusively by the infant. With subsequent development, first the thumb and then the fingers begin to operate independently, and at about 9 to 10 months of age, pincer grasp develops (22).

Recent experiments have followed the development and refinement of precision grasp in human infants and children ranging in age from 8 months to 15 years. Remember from our last chapter that when an adult is asked to lift an object, as soon as his/her fingers touch the object, cutaneous receptors activate a centrally programmed response that consists of an increase in grip forces and load forces, designed to lift the object without letting it slip through the fingers. In adults, these two forces are always programmed in parallel, to prevent slips and to avoid squeezing the object too hard (22).

This parallel programming of grip and load forces was not found in human infants. In fact, until 5 years of age, the children pushed the object into the table as they increased the grip force, showing a reversed coordination between the two forces. In these children, the grip force had to be very high before the load force increase occurred. In addition, the timing and sequencing of the different phases of lifting were much longer in the infants. For example, the time between first and second finger contact was three times

as long in 10-month-olds, and two times as long in children up to 3 years of age, compared with adults. It was common in the younger children to have several touches by the thumb and index finger before the object was properly gripped. Also, any finger could be the first to contact the object (22).

Emergence of Object Exploration

When do infants first begin to change their manipulative activities in relation to the characteristics of the objects grasped? During the first year, the actions infants perform with objects tend to be mouthing, waving, shaking, or banging. Rigid objects tend to be banged, while spongy objects are squeezed or rubbed (23). In studies on 6-, 9-, and 12-month-olds, it was noted that mouthing activity decreased with age and that object rotation, transferring the object between hands and looking at and fingering the object, increased (19, 24).

At about 1 year of age, infants begin to acquire the understanding of how to use objects, but even before this age, they can discover simple functional relationships if these require little precision. Thus, an infant first uses a spoon for banging or shaking before using it for eating. The infant establishes the relationships between spoon and hand, spoon and mouth, and spoon and plate as subroutines before putting them together for the act of eating, in which the spoon is filled at the plate, and transported to the mouth with an anticipatory mouth opening (25).

At about 16 to 19 months of age, infants begin to understand that certain objects go together culturally, such as a cup in a saucer. Finally, at the end of the second year, they begin to perform symbolic actions like pretending to eat or drink (19).

After 1 year of age, infants begin to develop skills requiring more precision of movement and closer relationships between objects, such as fitting one object into another. At 13 to 15 months, infants begin piling two cubes on top of each other; at 18 months, three cubes; at 21 months, five cubes; and at 23 to 24 months, six cubes. This shows that the infant is gradually developing coordinated reaching and manipulation, so that objects can be placed and released carefully (19, 26).

ROLE OF EXPERIENCE IN THE DEVELOPMENT OF EYE-HAND COORDINATION

Remember that in humans, reaching behavior has two aspects, a visually triggered portion and a visually guided portion. These two aspects of eye-limb coordination are also found in cats. Elegant studies on the development of these two aspects of eye-limb coordination have shown that movement-produced visual feedback experience is essential for the visually guided portion to develop (27).

In these experiments, kittens were raised in the dark until 4 weeks of age and then allowed to move freely for 6 hours each day in a normal environment. But during this time, they wore lightweight opaque collars that kept them from seeing their limbs and torso. This is shown in Figure 16.4A. For the rest of the day, they remained in the dark. After 12 days of this treatment, the animals were tested for the presence of visually triggered vs. visually guided placing reactions. This was accomplished by lowering the kitten toward a continuous surface (requires only visually triggered placing, since accuracy is not required) vs. a discontinuous surface, made up of prongs (requires visually guided placing to hit the prong). All animals showed a visually triggered placing reaction, in which they automatically extended the forelimb toward a continuous surface. But they showed no greater than chance hits for a placing reaction to a pronged surface (Fig. 16.4B). However, after removal of the collar, the animals only required 18 hours in a normal environment before showing visually guided placing. It was thus concluded that visually triggered paw extension develops without sight, but visually guided paw placing requires prolonged viewing of the limbs (27).

The researchers then asked: what kind of contact with the environment is important for visually guided behavior? Is passive contact

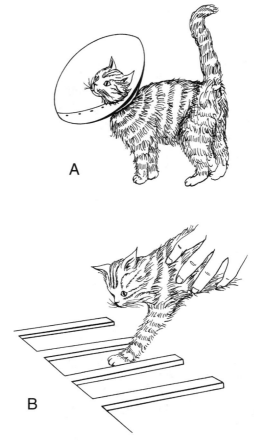

Figure 16.4.   **A**, Experimental collar worn by kittens to block their view of their paws during early development. **B**, Pronged apparatus for testing visually guided reaching. (Adapted from Hein A, Held R. Dissociation of the visual placing response into elicited and guided components. Science 1967;158:391.)

sufficient, or must it be active (28)? To answer this question, they tested 10 pairs of kittens. One kitten of each pair was able to walk freely in a circular room, pulling a gondola, and the other kitten was placed in the gondola and was passively pulled around the room. This is shown in Figure 16.5. Thus, both kittens had similar visual feedback and motion cues, but for the kittens who walked, the cues were active and for the kittens who rode, they were passive.

The kittens had experience with the apparatus for 3 hours a day. At the end of the experiment, the active animals showed normal visually guided placing reactions and re-

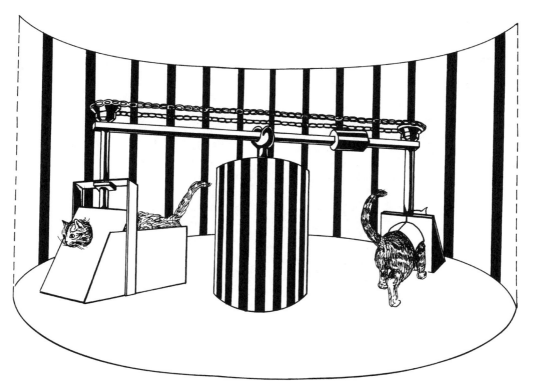

Figure 16.5. Experimental apparatus in which one cat actively pulls the second cat, which is passively pulled in the gondola. (Adapted from Held R, Hein A. Movement-produced stimulation in the development of visually guided behavior. Journal of Comparative and Physiological Psychology 1963;56:873.)

sponses to a visual cliff test, in which a normal animal does not walk out over an illusory cliff, but the passive animals did not. Thus, the researchers concluded that self-produced movement is necessary for the development of visually guided behavior. However, once again, after 48 hours in a normal environment, the passive group of animals showed normal visually guided paw placement (28).

Eye-Head-Hand Coordination Development

In our last chapter, we mentioned that the eye, head, and hand are coordinated when adults reach, such that the eyes move first, followed by the head, and then the arm. How does eye, head, and hand coordination develop in children? Little research has been performed in this area. However, research by Laurette Hay, a developmental psychologist

from Marseille, France, has begun to explore these developmental changes in children from 6 to 11 years of age. Remember from our last chapter that, in adults, when a target is placed to the side, both eye and hand reaction time increase, compared to when it is at midline. This is also true of reaction times for the eye and hand for children 6 to 11 years of age (29). However, in children under 8 years of age, when the head must also turn to look at the target as the child reaches, the head movement seems to interfere with the hand movement, and slows the reaction time, compared to movements with the head held fixed. Head movements also seemed to interfere with the ability to intercept a moving target in children of this age (29).

Reaction-Time Reaching Tasks

A great deal of research has been performed on developmental changes in reaction-time (RT) tasks. In general, it has been shown that for simple RT tasks, reaction times become faster as children mature. The greatest changes occur until about 8 to 9 years of age, with slower changes occurring subsequently, until reaction times reach adult levels at 16 to 17 years. However, when children are asked to perform more complex movements as part of the RT task, these developmental changes vary according to the task. For example, in a study in which 2- to 8-year-old children were asked to make target aiming movements, a decrease in RT was observed from 2 to 5 years of age, followed by a stabilization in RT (29, 30).

Movement time in these reaction time tasks also changes as a function of age. Remember from our last chapter that movement time depends on the accuracy and distance requirements of a task (31). Strategies for programming movements also vary, depending on whether the movement requires an accurate stop or not. If an accurate stop is required, the individual must use a braking action controlled by antagonist muscles. Alternatively, if the movement can be stopped automatically by hitting a target, antagonist muscle activation isn't required. Studies analyzing movement time in children from 6 to 10 years of age, for either type of movement, have shown a reduction in movement time with increased age. As might be expected, movements that require an accurate stop are slower at all ages. However, the difference between the speed of the two types of movements is about three times higher at 6 years of age than at 8 to 10 years of age. It has been hypothesized that this could be due to a difficulty experienced by the 6-year-olds in modulating the braking action of the antagonist muscle system (29, 32).

Fitts' Law

Remember from our last chapter that Fitts' law shows a specific relationship between the time to make a movement and the amplitude and accuracy of that movement. The difficulty of the task is related both to the accuracy and the amplitude requirements, and is represented by the following equation:

$$ID = log_2(2A/W)$$

where A = amplitude of the movement; W = width of the target, and ID = index of difficulty (29, 31).

Studies testing the extent to which Fitts' law applies to children have found that movement time decreases with age. This decrease is in general a linear change, except for a regression, which appears to occur at about 7 years of age (29, 33). Remember that in the development of postural control, there is also a regression, as indicated by an increase in postural response latencies, between 4 and 6 years of age (34). A study examining 5- to 9-year-olds has shown that these developmental decreases and regressions in movement time are not related to any changes in biomechanical factors, such as growth of the bones of the arm (35).

Using Fitts' law, one can plot movement time as a function of index of difficulty for different age groups. This relationship is shown in Figure 16.6. The intercept of the line with the y axis reflects the general efficiency of the motor system, while the slope of the line reflects the amount of information that can be processed per second by the motor system (29). Almost all studies have shown that the y-intercept decreases with age, indicating increased efficiency. However, age-related improvements in slope appear to depend on the task involved, and appear to be more evident in discrete rather than serial movements (36).

Movement Accuracy

To determine developmental changes in children's use of visual feedback in making reaching movements, studies were performed in which they were asked to make movements with or without visual feedback. Laurette Hay has shown that there are interesting changes in the use of visual information by children between 4 and 11 years of age (37). Children between 4 and 6 years of age can make movements without visual feedback with reasonable accuracy, as you see in Figure 16.7. (Note that, although 5-year-olds may appear to be more accurate than adults, there are no

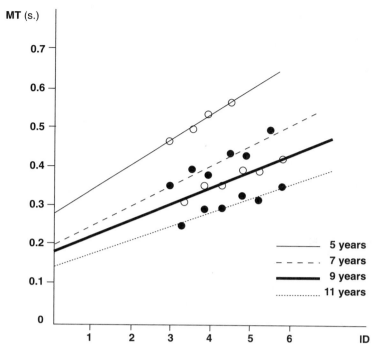

Figure 16.6.   Graph showing the relationship between movement time (*y* axis) and the index of difficulty (*ID*) of a task, for four age groups of children. (Adapted from Hay L. Developmental changes in eye-hand coordination behaviors: preprogramming versus feedback control. In: Bard C, Fleury M, Hay L, eds. Development of eye-hand coordination across the lifespan. Columbia, SC: University of South Carolina Press, 1990:227.)

significant differences between these groups.) However, at age 7, there is an abrupt reduction in this ability, as seen in the increased errors made in reaching without visual feedback. The accuracy then begins to increase again, reaching adult levels by 10 to 11 years of age. As we describe in the next section, this reduction in accuracy is reflected in an increased dependence on visual feedback at the age of 7 years.

Kinematics of Reaching Movements

In our last chapter, we described studies on the kinematics of reaching movements in adults, and showed that reaches consist of an initial ballistic, distance-covering phase, followed by a homing-in phase, which uses visual feedback. In studies of children from 5 to 9 years of age performing *reciprocal tapping* tasks, it was determined that the ballistic

phase remains constant in duration as children develop. However, the accuracy or closeness of approach to the target at the end of this phase increases (29, 38). This increase in accuracy results in a reduction in the number of corrections required in the homing-in phase.

However, on *discrete reaching* tasks, this developmental change starts only at the age of 7 to 8 years, while the opposite developmental trend occurs between 6 and 7 to 8 years (39). This is thus one more piece of research to support the hypothesis that the age of 7 is a transition time in the development of reaching (29).

Other studies analyzing the kinematics of reaching movements without visual feedback in children ages 5 to 11 also support this hypothesis (40). Figure 16.8 shows that 5-year-olds produce mainly ballistic movements, with sharp decelerations at the end of the movement (*black bars*), while this pattern shows a sharp decrease at age 7. At this age,

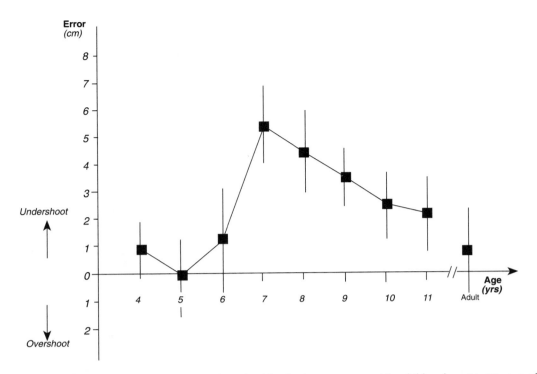

Figure 16.7.   Graph showing pointing errors when visual feedback was not present for children from 4 to 11 years of age, compared to adults. (Adapted from Hay L. Developmental changes in eye-hand coordination behaviors: preprogramming versus feedback control. In: Bard C, Fleury M, Hay L, eds. Development of eye-hand coordination across the lifespan. Columbia, SC: University of South Carolina Press, 1990:228.)

a ramp and step pattern increases (*stippled bars*). At the same time, ballistic patterns with a smooth deceleration at the end of the movement increase and continue to increase through 9 years of age (*striped bars*). It has been hypothesized that this could be due to the increased use of proprioceptive feedback control in 7-year-olds, and the progressive restriction of feedback control to the final homing-in phase in older children, possibly the result of increased efficiency of the movement braking system (29).

For a closer look at developmental changes in the use of visual feedback in reaching movements in children, experiments were performed in which children ages 5 to 11 were asked to make reaches while wearing prismatic lenses, which make an illusory shift in the image of the object (40). These experiments are similar to those described earlier, examining the use of visual feedback in reaching in neonates and infants. As you see in Figure 16.9*A*, as the children make a reach, the kinematics of the hand movement show a curved, rather than a straight line trajectory toward the object. This occurs as the hand shifts from an initially incorrect path, due to the shift in the visual image caused by the prismatic lenses, to a correct path when the hand comes into view, based on visual information of the relative hand and target positions. The length of the visually corrected path indicates the amount of visual feedback used in the movement.

As evident in Figure 16.9*A* and *B*, 5-year-old children corrected the movement late in its trajectory, and in fact, the majority of these children did not make a correction until they reached the virtual target, indicating minimal use of visual feedback. Thus, in this age group, visual control occurs mainly after, rather than during, reaching movements. This is correlated with highly stereotyped movement times seen in this age group (29).

The 7-year-old children corrected the

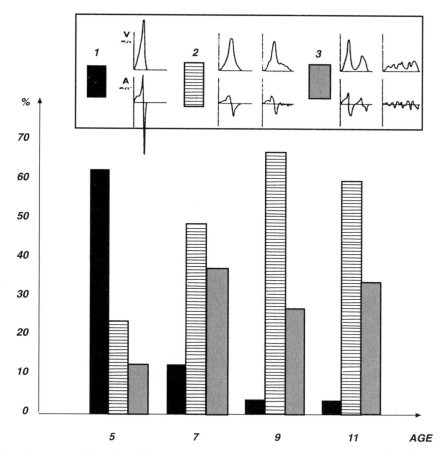

Figure 16.8.   Percentage of time three different reaching movement patterns were seen in children from 5 to 11 years of age. 1 = ballistic pattern with sharp accelerations/decelerations; 2 = ballistic patterns with smooth decelerations; 3 = step and ramp patterns. (Adapted from Hay L. Developmental changes in eye-hand coordination behaviors: preprogramming versus feedback control. In: Bard C, Fleury M, Hay L, eds. Development of eye-hand coordination across the lifespan. Columbia, SC: University of South Carolina Press, 1990:231.)

movements earlier than any other group, indicating a strong use of visual feedback. While this gives rise to an increased flexibility in reaching behavior, it is coupled with increased variability in movement times, and decreased accuracy when visual feedback is not present.

The 9- and 11-year-olds showed an intermediate level of trajectory correction, indicating a shift in the use of visual control toward the final phase of the movement trajectory. Thus, between 5 and 9 years of age there appears to be a reorganization in the programming of reaching movements from mainly feed-forward or anticipatory activation of reaching, to predominant feedback control, and finally to an integration of the feed-forward and feedback control, resulting in

fast, accurate movements by 9 years of age (29).

CHANGES IN OLDER ADULTS

As we have noted in our previous chapters on age-related changes in postural control and mobility skills, there are specific changes in these skills with age. These can be divided into (*a*) time-related changes, such as slowing of onset latencies for postural response or decreased movement speed in locomotion; (*b*) coordination factors, related to changes in movement or muscle activation patterns; and (*c*) changes in the use of feedback and feedforward control of both postural and mobility skills.

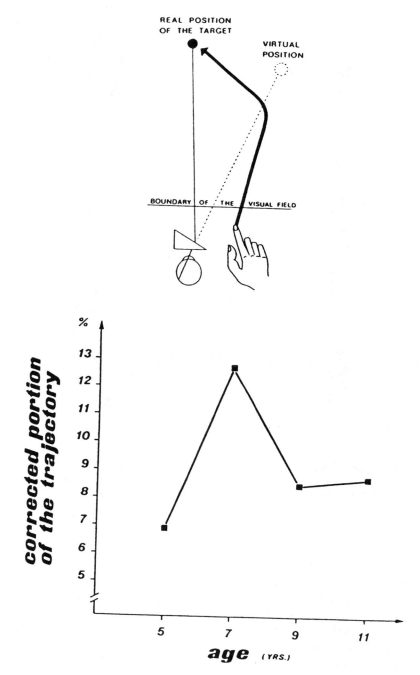

Figure 16.9. **A**, Diagram of reaching movements of children who wore prismatic lenses, displacing the apparent position of the target in the visual field. **B**, Corrected portion of the reaching trajectory for 5-, 7-, 9-, and 11-year-olds. (Adapted from Hay L. Spatial-temporal analysis of movements in children: motor programs versus feedback in the development of reaching. Journal of Motor Behavior 1979;11:196, 198.)

Unfortunately, the literature on changes in eye-hand coordination characteristics in the older adult is very limited compared to the extensive research on the development of eye-hand coordination in children. Research on age-related changes in eye-hand coordination has focused more on changes in reaction time and movement time in reaching tasks of various levels of complexity, rather than on changes in the kinetics of reaching and grasping movements. In the sections that follow, we review the literature in these research areas.

Changes in Reaching Movement Time with Age

A review of studies examining changes in the speed of reaching movements with age has shown that discrete reaching movements show a range of 30 to 90% reduction in velocity with aging, depending on the ages compared and the task performed. For example, one study examining changes in the speed of discrete arm movements showed a 32% reduction between the ages of 50 and 90 years, while another showed a reduction in movement speed of 90% when comparing subjects from 20 to 69 years performing a repetitive tapping task (41, 42).

What are some of the age-related changes in different systems of the body that might contribute to this slowing in reaching movements? Different systems that could contribute to the slowing include (*a*) sensory and perceptual systems, such as the visual system's ability to detect the target, (*b*) central processing systems, (*c*) motor systems, and (*d*) arousal and motivational systems (41).

Welford, an English psychologist, performed an experiment to determine if changes in central mechanisms contribute to the slowing in reaching speed in older adults. In these experiments, subjects were asked to keep a pointer (which they could move with a handle) in line with a target that continuously moved from side to side, in an irregular sinusoidal fashion, with the movement varying in both speed and extent. He found that as the speed of the target movement was in-

creased, the subjects could follow it less easily, until at some point it was impossible to follow.

However, there was a difference between the older and younger subjects. As you see in Figure 16.10, the older adults dropped off in their ability to follow the movements sooner than the young adults. Welford hypothesized that the limitation in the performance of the older adults wasn't due to problems with the motor system because they could move faster if they were not following the target. He hypothesized that the limitation wasn't sensory because the older adults could easily see the target. Therefore, he concluded that the limitation was in central processing abilities, that is, in the older adults' ability to match the target and pointer and react quickly to changes in target direction. This implies that the time spent in actual movement itself slows little compared to the time taken to make decisions about the next part of the movement sequence (43).

It has also been shown that hand steadiness decreases with age during reaching tasks (42). When older adults were asked to insert a small stylus in slots of different diameters (½- to ⅛-inch), steadiness dropped by 77% from the 50s to the 90s. Steadiness deteriorated faster in the nonpreferred hand than in the preferred hand.

Based on the literature, there appears to be little change in performance speed for reaching movements with age, if subjects are asked to repeat the same simple action, like tapping a pencil between two targets, or performing a simple reaction time (SRT) task (41, 43). In this case, the slowing may be as little as 16%. But if the complexity of the task is increased, by making the target smaller, using successive targets, or using a choice reaction time (CRT) task, then slowing can range from 86 to 276%. Table 16.1 gives examples of these differences in slowing of the performance of reaching movements with complexity of the task. The largest slowing in performance was in tasks involving symbolic translations (using a code to relate a stimulus to a response) or spatial transpositions (for example, a light cue on the left requiring a reach

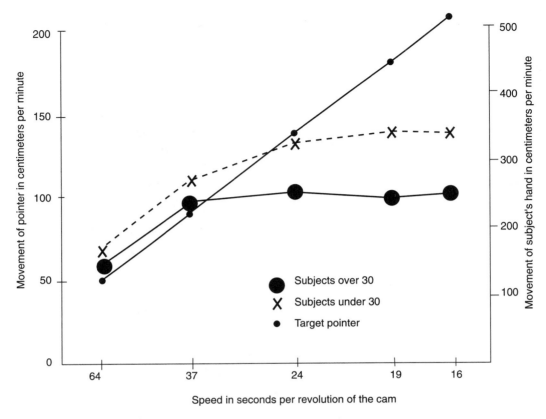

Figure 16.10. Graph showing the ability of young vs. older adults to follow unpredictable target movements of different speeds. (Adapted from Welford AT. Motor skills and aging. In: Mortimer JA, Pirozzolo FJ, Maletta GJ, eds. The aging motor system. NY: Praeger, 1982:159.)

Table 16.1.   Age-Related Slowing in the Performance of Reaching Movements as a Function of Task Complexity[a]

Task	Age-Groups Compared	Percentage Increase[b]
Simple key press or release to light or sound		
Average of 11 studies listed by Welford	twenties with sixties	16%
Ten-choice (Birren, Riegel, and Morrison, 1962)	18–33 with 65–72	
Straightforward relationship		27
With numerical code, mean of 5 studies		50
With verbal code, mean of two studies		45
With color code		94
With part color and part letter code		86
Ten-choice (Kay 1954, 1955)	25–34 with 65–72	
a. Signal lights immediately above response keys		−13 (no errors made)
b. Signal lights 3 ft from keys		26 (−43)
c. As b, but signal lights arranged so that leftmost responded to with rightmost key, and so forth		46 (−19)
d. With numerical code		56 (+138)
e. The difficulties of d and b combined		299 (+464)

[a]Adapted from Welford AT. Motor skills and aging. In: Mortimer JA, Pirozzolo FJ, Maletta GJ, eds. The aging motor system. NY: Praeger, 1962:163.
[b]Percentage changes of errors are shown in parentheses

to the right). Though decrements have been found in performance on many RT tasks, a recent study has also shown that when older adults are not instructed to worry about accuracy on such a task, they demonstrate no decrease in reaching speed (44).

The primary source of the slowing in complex RT tasks is in the first phase of performance, the time to observe the signals and relate them to action, rather than in the second phase, the time to execute the movement (41, 43). When performing more continuous tasks, the second phase, that of movement execution, can overlap to some extent with the first. For example, a person may process the information relating to the next signal while making the first response. This type of task appears to be more difficult for older adults possibly because they need more time to monitor their responses, and thus have difficulty processing other signals simultaneously (41).

For example, older adults (63 to 76 years old) were compared to younger adults (19 to 29 years) on a task where they moved as quickly as possible to one of two alternate endpoints, with one farther away than the other, in the same direction (45). The younger subjects could overlap the time required to choose the endpoint with the initial stages of the movement itself, while the older subjects were less able to do this. Although there is no evidence that the time taken for monitoring increases with age, older adults seem less able to suppress monitoring (41).

What might be reasons for this lack of suppression? It has been hypothesized that suppression of monitoring occurs when the outcome of a task is certain; thus, if there is a possibility of error, monitoring will be more probable. In addition, suppression of monitoring may be possible when movement subunits are coordinated into higher units of performance (41). However, to do this often requires that the subject hold the movement subunits together in working memory while performing the task.

A study tested this ability in older (ages 60 to 81) vs. young (ages 17 to 28) adults. Subjects were asked to perform two serial key pressing tasks, one that had few subunits (12, 12, 12, etc.) and one that was more complex (1234, 32, 1234, etc.). They found that the older adults were slower than the young adults, particularly with the second series (46).

Compensation and Reversibility of Decrements in Reaching Performance

Although decrements in reaching performance may be found in older adults in experimental conditions, they are often not observed in the workplace or in Activities of Daily Living (41). It has been suggested that performance is preserved because many compensatory strategies are used to improve reach and grasp skills. Many of these compensatory strategies used by older adults appear to be unconscious, automatic processes (41). For example, older adults may increase the effort they put into the movement. In the workplace, they may work more continuously with fewer brief pauses. They may also prepare for movements that require speed and accuracy in advance, thus allowing anticipatory processes to aid in performance. In many tasks, they may also make a trade-off between speed and accuracy. Finally, it has also been shown that older adults set higher criteria for responding to RT signals in sensory discrimination tasks (41).

Can the changes in reaching skills that occur with aging be counteracted by practice or training? Yes! Clear improvement has been reported for eye-hand coordination skills in older adults with practice (42, 47). Greatest improvement is seen in more complex tasks. Interestingly, older adults show more improvement with practice than do younger adults on performance of RT tasks (48). This may occur because young adults are closer to their ceiling of performance when starting to learn the task. However, practice does not eliminate the age differences in the performance of these tasks.

Practice also improves performance in older adults related to the perceptual processes involved in eye-hand coordination tasks, such as visual acuity, signal detection, and auditory discrimination (42).

In addition, the effects of practice remain high, even 1 month after practice on eye-hand coordination tasks has ended. One study compared the performance of young (ages 19 to 27) and older (ages 62 to 73) adults on a task that involved fine movements of the hands, signal detection, memory scanning, visual discrimination, and anticipation timing, called "Space Trek." Subjects were given 51 1-hour practice sessions over a period of 2 to 5 months. One month after training ended, there was only a small decrease in performance levels (42).

In another study, older adults (ages 57 to 83) were given practice in eye-hand coordination skills by playing video games, such as PacMan (49). These games involved making fast decisions about changes in the speed and direction of hand movements. Over a 7-week period, scores tripled on the task. In addition, practice on the video games transferred over to other RT tasks that required subjects to quickly select a motor response.

These studies suggest that older adults learn as much, if not more, with practice than young adults, and that they retain the learned skills as well as young adults. In addition, the way subjects improved with practice was similar for the young and older adults; however, the older adults simply learned more slowly. This slower rate of learning of eye-hand coordination skills in older subjects may be due to material taking longer to register in long-term memory (41).

What does this mean in terms of determining the best strategies for teaching eye-hand coordination skills to older adults? Since the time required for registering information in long-term memory lengthens with age, learning needs to be unhurried. Otherwise extra information to be processed during the time required to register information in longer-term memory will simply disrupt the memory process (41).

In teaching eye-hand coordination skills, there are sometimes problems in translating verbal instruction into motor performance. To avoid this, one can use demonstrations. However, in this case, the pace of the demonstration should be under the learner's control. Thus, using slow-motion, self-paced videos in training may help (41).

Active decision making is also an important factor in learning at any age. In a maze study with adults, it was shown that learning took place much faster if the correct pathway was marked, but the subject had to make an active choice (50). This helped subjects of all ages, but it especially helped older adults (41, 50).

It was also shown that using a mixture of mental practice and physical practice when learning a pursuit rotor task was as good as physical practice alone for 65- to 69- and 80- to 100-year-olds (51).

Thus, learning of eye-hand coordination tasks by older adults can be facilitated by using a type of discovery learning, which involves demonstrations that can be self-paced, active learning, and a combination of physical and mental practice (41).

SUMMARY

1. Infants as young as a week old show pre-reaching behaviors, where they reach toward objects that are in front of them. These reaches are not accurate, and the infants do not grasp the object, since an extension synergy controls the arm/hand movements. When the arm is extended, the hand is open. But the reaches are clearly aimed at the object, since they are significantly more accurate than arm movements where the eyes aren't fixated on the object.

2. At about 2 months, the extension synergy is broken up, so that the fingers flex as the arm extends. At this time, head-arm movements become coupled as the infant gains control over the neck muscles.

3. At about 4 months, infants begin to gain trunk stability, along with a progressive uncoupling of head-arm-hand synergies. These changes allow the emergence of functional reach and grasp behavior.

5. From 4 months onward, reaching becomes more refined, with the approach path straightening and the number of segments of the reach being reduced.

6. Visually triggered reaching is dominant in

the newborn, changing to visually guided reaching at about 5 months of age, and returning to visually triggered reaching by 1 year of age, though guided reaching is still available.

7. The development of hand orientation begins to occur at the onset of successful reaching, at about 5 months of age.

8. The pincer grasp develops at about 9 to 10 months of age, along with the development of the pyramidal tract.

9. Reaction time shows a progressive reduction with age, with sharper changes occurring until 8 to 9 years, followed by slower changes until 16 to 17 years.

10. Children from 4 to 6 years make predominantly visually triggered (feed-forward) movements, using little visual feedback. At 7 to 8 years, visual feedback is dominant, leading to poor reaching in the dark, but more accurate reaching with vision present. By 9 to 11 years, there is an integration between feed-forward and feedback movements.

11. Older adults show a slowing in reaching movements, with much of this due to central processing slowing. The slowing in performance on reaching movements is greater for more complex tasks.

12. Part of the slowing may result from an inability to suppress monitoring of movements, due to either uncertainty concerning the accuracy of the movement, or an inability to integrate movement subunits into larger chunks in working memory.

13. Most age-related decrements in reaching performance can be improved with training. Training effects remain high for at least a month after training has ended and also transfer to other reaching tasks.

REFERENCES

1. Twitchell T. Reflex mechanisms and the development of prehension. In: Connolly K, ed. Mechanisms of motor skill development. NY: Academic Press, 1970.

2. McDonnell PM. Patterns of eye-hand coordination in the first year of life. Can J Psychol 1979;33:253–267.

3. Piajet J. The origins of intelligence in children. NY: WW Norton, 1954.

4. White BL, Castle P, Held R. Observations on the development of visually-directed reaching. Child Dev 1964;35:349–364.

5. Bower TGR, Broughton JM, Moore MK. The coordination of visual and tactual input in infants. Perception Psychophysics 1970; 8:51–53.

6. Bower TGR, Broughton JM, Moore MK. Demonstration of intention in the reaching behavior of neonate humans. Nature. 1970; 228:679–681.

7. Dodwell PC, Muir D, Difranco D. Responses of infants to visual presented objects. Science 1976;194:209–211.

8. Hofsten C von. Eye-hand coordination in the newborn. Developmental Psychology 1982; 18:450–461.

9. Vinter A. Manual imitations and reaching behaviors: an illustration of action control in infancy. In: Bard C, Fleury M, Hay L, eds. Development of eye-hand coordination across the lifespan. Columbia, SC: University of South Carolina Press 1990:157–187.

10. Amiel-Tison C, Grenier A. Evaluation neurologique du nouveau-ne et du nourrison. Paris: Masson, 1980.

11. Hofsten C von. Studying the development of goal-directed behavior. In: Kalverboer AF, Hopkins B, Geuze R, eds. Motor development in early and later childhood: longitudinal approaches. Cambridge: Cambridge University Press 1993:109–124.

12. Hofsten C von. Developmental changes in the organization of pre-reaching movements. Developmental Psychology 1984;3;378–388.

13. Paillard J. The contribution of peripheral and central vision to visually guided reaching. In: Ingle DJ, Goodale MA, Mansfield RJW, eds. Analysis of visual behavior. Cambridge, MA: MIT Press, 1982:367–385.

14. Hofsten C von, Fazel-Zandy S. Development of visually guided hand orientation in reaching. J Exp Child Psychol 1984;38:208–219.

15. Hofsten C von, Ronnqvist L. Preparation for grasping an object: a developmental study. J Exp Psychol 1988;14:610–621.

16. Kuypers HGJM. Corticospinal connections: postnatal development in the rhesus monkey. Science 1962;138:678–680.

17. Kuypers HGJM. The descending pathways to the spinal cord, their anatomy and function. In: Eccles JC, ed. Organization of the spinal cord. Amsterdam: Elsevier, 1964.

18. Lawrence DG, Hopkins DA. Developmental aspects of pyramidal motor control in the rhesus monkey. Brain Res 1972;40:117–118.

19. Corbetta D, Mounoud P. Early development of grasping and manipulation. In: Bard C, Fleury M, Hay L, eds. Development of eye-hand coordination across the lifespan. Columbia, SC: University of South Carolina Press 1990:189–213.

20. Hofsten C von, Lindhagen K. Observations on the development of reaching for moving objects. J Exp Child Psychol 1979;28:158–173.

21. Napier JR. The prehensile movements of the human hand. J Bone Joint Surg 1956; 38B:902–913.

22. Forssberg H, Eliasson AC, Kinoshita H, Johansson RS, Westling G. Development of human precision grip I: basic coordination of force. In press.

23. Gibson E, Walker AS. Development of knowledge of visual-tactual affordance of substance. Child Dev 1984;55:453–460.

24. Ruff HA. Infants' manipulative exploration of objects: effects of age and object characteristics. Dev Psychol 1984;20:9–20.

25. Connolly KJ. The development of competence in motor skills. In: Nadeau CH, Halliwell WR, Newell KM, Roberts GC, eds. Psychology of motor behavior and sport. Champaign, IL: Human Kinetics, 1979:229–250.

26. Bayley N. Manual for the Bayley scales of infant development. NY: Psychological Corporation. 1969.

27. Hein A, Held R. Dissociation of the visual placing response into elicited and guided components. Science 1967;158:390–392.

28. Held R, Hein A. Movement-produced stimulation in the development of visually guided behavior. Journal of Comparative and Physiological Psychology 1963;56:872–876.

29. Hay L. Developmental changes in eye-hand coordination behaviors: Preprogramming versus feedback control. In: Bard C, Fleury M, Hay L, eds. Development of eye-hand coordination across the lifespan. Columbia, SC: University of South Carolina Press 1990:217–244.

30. Brown JV, Sepehr MM, Ettlinger G, Skreczek W. The accuracy of aimed movements to visual targets during development: the role of visual information. J Exp Child Psychol 1986;41:443–460.

31. Fitts PM. The information capacity of the human motor system in controlling the amplitude of movement. J Exp Psychol 1954;47; 381–391.

32. Hay L, Bard C, Fleury M. Visuo-manual coordination from 6 to 10: specification, control and evaluation of direction and amplitude parameters of movement. In: Wade MG, Whiting HTA, eds. Motor development in children: aspects of coordination and control. Dordrecht: Martinus Nijhoff, 1986.

33. Rey A. Le freinage volontaire du mouvement graphique chez l'enfant. In: Epreuves d'intelligence pratique et de psychomotricite. Neuchatel: Delachaux & Niestle. 1968.

34. Shumway-Cook A, Woollacott M. The growth of stability: postural control from a developmental perspective. Journal of Motor Behavior 1985;17:131–147.

35. Kerr R. Movement control and maturation in elementary-grade children. Percept Mot Skills 1975;41:151–154.

36. Sugden DA. Movement speed in children. Journal of Motor Behavior 1980;12:125–132.

37. Hay L. Accuracy of children on an open-loop pointing task. Percept Mot Skills 1978; 47:1079–1082.

38. Schellekens JMH, Kalverboer AF, Scholten CA. The microstructure of tapping movements in children. Journal of Motor Behavior 1984;16:20–39.

39. Dellen T Van, Kalverboer AF. Single movement control and information processing, a developmental study. Behav Brain Res 1984; 12:237–238.

40. Hay L. Spatial-temporal analysis of movements in children: motor programs versus feedback in the development of reaching. Journal of Motor Behavior 1979;11:189–200.

41. Welford AT, Motor skills and aging. In: Mortimer JA, Pirozzolo FJ, Maletta GJ, eds. The aging motor system. NY: Praeger, 1982:152–187.

42. Williams H. Aging and eye-hand coordination. In: Bard C, Fleury M, Hay L, eds. Development of eye-hand coordination across the lifespan. Columbia, SC: University of South Carolina Press 1990:327–357.

43. Welford AT. Motor Performance. In: Birren G, Schaie K, eds. Handbook of the psychology of aging. NY: Van Nostrand Reinhold, 1977:3–20.

44. GL Williamson, CI Leiper, NH Mayer. Bea-

ver College Assessment of speed and accuracy of movement in older adults using Fitts' tapping test. Neurosci Abstr 1993;19:556.

45. Rabbit P, Rogers M. Age and choice between responses in a self-paced repetitive task. Ergonomics 1965;8:435–444.

46. Rabbit P, Birren JE. Age and responses to sequences of repetitive and interruptive signals. J Gerontol 1967;22:143–150.

47. Falduto L, Baron A. Age-related effects of practice and task complexity on card sorting. J Gerontol 1986;41:659–661.

48. Jordan T, Rabbitt P. Response times to stimuli of increasing complexity as a function of ageing. Br J Psychol 1977;68:189–201.

49. Clark J, Lanphear A, Riddick C. The effects of videogame playing on the response selection processing of elderly adults. J Gerontol 1987;42:82–85.

50. Wright JM von. A note on the role of "guidance" in learning. Br J Psychol 1957;48:133–137.

51. Surberg PR. Aging and effect of physical-mental practice upon acquisition and retention of a motor skill. J Gerontol 1976;31:64–67.

Chapter 17

ABNORMAL UPPER EXTREMITY MANIPULATION CONTROL

INTRODUCTION

Normal upper extremity function is the basis for fine-motor manipulation skills important to activities such as feeding, dressing, grooming, and handwriting. In addition, upper extremity function plays an important role in gross motor skills such as crawling, walking, the ability to recover balance, and to protect the body from injury when recovery is not possible.

Because upper extremity control is intertwined with both fine and gross motor skills, recovery of upper extremity function is an important aspect of retraining the patient with impaired motor control and falls within the purview of most areas of rehabilitation, including both occupational and physical therapy.

Abnormalities of upper extremity function in the patient with a neurological disability can result from a wide variety of sensory, motor, and cognitive impairments. Thus, assessment and treatment of upper ex-

tremity dysfunction requires an understanding of the problems associated with specific types of neurological impairment, and the way in which these problems affect the key components of upper extremity function.

In previous chapters we suggested the key components of upper extremity function included (*a*) locating a target, requiring the coordination of eye-head movements, (*b*) reaching, involving transportation of the arm and hand in space, (*c*) manipulation, including grip formation, grasp, and release, and (*d*) postural control. In addition, goal-directed upper extremity movements also involve higher cognitive processes necessary for generating and planning an intent to act, and maintaining that intent long enough to carry out the action plan.

As we mentioned in the last two chapters, the research on upper extremity dyscontrol contradicts traditional assumptions that upper extremity function is due to a single controlling system that develops in a proximal to distal manner. This has a number of important implications for clinicians involved in retraining the patient with upper extremity dysfunction. It suggests that neural pathology can affect some aspects of upper extremity function, while leaving others unaffected.

In addition, it suggests that therapy directed at recovery of hand function should occur simultaneously with retraining of shoulder or more proximal components of the movement, rather than waiting to work on hand control until proximal control has been developed, which has been a traditional rehabilitation approach.

This chapter focuses on abnormal upper extremity function as it relates to manipulatory skills. We review problems related to the key components of upper extremity control, incorporating a discussion of sensory, motor, and higher level problems that affect each aspect of upper extremity control. We begin with a review of problems related to locating a target, requiring the coordination of eye-head movements.

TARGET LOCATION PROBLEMS: EYE-HEAD COORDINATION

A critical aspect of manipulatory dysfunction is the inability to locate a target and maintain one's gaze on that target preceding the reach. Remember from the last two chapters that some target location tasks require eye movements alone, while others require a combination of eye-head movement, and still other tasks require a combination of eye-head-trunk movements, depending on the eccentricity of the target in space. This has led researchers to suggest that eye-head coordination is not controlled by a single mechanism, but rather emerges from an interaction of several different neural mechanisms (1).

What types of problems affect the ability to stabilize gaze during different head movements toward a target, and thus potentially affect the accuracy and precision of reaching movements? Problems include (*a*) disruption of visually driven eye movements due to damage within the oculomotor system; (*b*) damage to the vestibular system, which disrupts

vestibulo-ocular reflex control of eye movements in response to head movements; and (*c*) inability to adapt the vestibulo-ocular reflex to changes in task demands due to cerebellar damage (2). All of these types of problems affect the patient's ability to stabilize gaze on an object when moving the head. However, in this chapter, we focus primarily on problems related to visually driven eye movements.

Visual Deficits

Central lesions affecting the processing of visual signals may also disrupt upper extremity motor control in the patient with a neurological deficit. Visual field deficits following a stroke, such as homonymous hemianopia, restrict a patient's ability to see objects in one-half of the visual field (1).

Until recently, pathology causing lesions in the visual cortex of humans was thought to cause total blindness, except for a rudimentary ability to detect changes in visual illumination. However, recently it has been shown that monkeys with lesions in the striate cortex are still able to reach toward objects moving across their visual field (3). It has been hypothesized that these reaching movements may be due to visual processing occurring in subcortical structures, such as the superior colliculus.

Research with humans has now confirmed these findings. When patients were not asked whether they could "see" the object, but simply to move their eyes toward where they thought the object might be, the direction and amplitude of their eye movements were significantly correlated with the position of the targets (4).

More recent experiments have been performed on subjects with hemianopia due to a hemispherectomy on one side (5). Patients with hemianopia were asked to point to the target when it appeared in either their normal visual field or their affected field. When it was in the affected field, they were asked to "guess" where it was, and to point there, since patients said that they couldn't see it. Again, pointing positions in the hemianopic field were definitely correlated with the target positions.

Although subjects were initially very poor at reaching for objects in this manner, their performance improved with training. If they were simply told that the target would appear at a different location for each trial, with practice, they showed a clear and rapid improvement in their abilities (1, 6).

Patients with parietal lesions also show problems with eye movements when these movements are a part of exploratory visual searches or reaching behavior. They may have problems breaking visual fixation (Balint's syndrome) or in optic ataxia; they also may have slowed reaction time for saccades, with the saccades subdivided into staircase patterns (7, 8).

TRANSPORT PROBLEMS

Remember from the previous chapters that research has shown that the transport component of reaching varies, depending on the goal of the task. Thus, the trajectory and duration of the movement used during the transport phase varies, depending on whether the goal is to touch a target or grasp an object, or to grasp and move the object in different ways. We hypothesize that one consequence of an upper motor neuron lesion is the loss of this task-specific flexibility in how movements are organized.

Motor Dyscoordination

As we mentioned earlier, reaching is controlled by a different neural mechanism from that of grasping; hence, patients can have impaired reach but intact grasp, or vice-versa. For many patients who are neurologically impaired, both reach and grasp are affected, reflecting dysfunction in the multiple systems controlling upper extremity function. This section reviews a variety of musculoskeletal and motor constraints that affect reaching.

MUSCULOSKELETAL CONSTRAINTS

Many patients with upper motor neuron lesions develop secondary musculoskeletal impairments due to weakness, spasticity, or the presence of mass patterns. Musculoskeletal impairments limit the ability to move the arm freely in space. Shoulder subluxation is a frequent accompaniment of other primary motor problems in the flaccid stroke patient. Tightness in the chest muscles and ligaments can develop in patients who habitually hold the involved arm in a flexed posture, which includes internal rotation of the shoulder and protraction of the scapula. Tight elbow, wrist, and finger flexors limit the patient's ability to actively extend the hand (9–11).

PAIN AND EDEMA

Another complication that interferes with the recovery of upper extremity function following a stroke is pain and/or swelling in the hemiplegic arm. In addition to shoulder pain, the shoulder-hand syndrome is a recognized concomitant of stroke, which occurs in approximately 15% of all stroke patients. The shoulder-hand syndrome encompasses pain with motion, and loss of range of motion in both the shoulder and the hand. In severe cases, there is pain at rest. If shoulder-hand syndrome is prolonged, it can lead to a "frozen" shoulder. There is no agreement concerning the underlying cause of shoulder pain following stroke, nor is there agreement on methods for treatment (12–15).

WEAKNESS

Neural lesions affecting the ability to generate force are a major limitation in many patients with a neurological impairment. Strength is defined as the ability to generate sufficient tension in a muscle for the purposes of posture and movement (16). Strength results from both properties of the muscle itself and the appropriate recruitment of motor units, as well as the timing of their activation (16, 17). Neural aspects of force production reflect (*a*) the number of motor units recruited, (*b*) the type of units recruited, and (*c*) the discharge frequency (18).

Weakness, or the inability to generate tension, is a major impairment of function in many patients with upper motor neuron lesions. Stroke patients have been shown to have abnormal and reduced firing rates of motor neurons (19). Thus, weakness, or the inability to recruit motor neurons, is a major constraint affecting all aspects of upper extremity function, including the ability to transport, grasp, and release objects.

SPASTICITY

As we mentioned in Chapter 9, the range of muscle tone abnormalities found within patients who have UMN lesions is great. We defined normal muscle tone as the muscle's resistance to being lengthened, or its *stiffness*, and that stiffness or tone is the result of both non-neural and neural components. On the upper end of the tone spectrum is hypertonicity or **spasticity**, often defined as "a motor disorder characterized by a velocity-dependent increase in tonic stretch reflexes (muscle tone)" (20). However, since muscle tone or stiffness is a result of both non-neural and neural components, it has also been emphasized that increased muscle stiffness in spastic hypertonia may be due to changes in the intrinsic properties of the muscle fibers themselves.

Many clinicians view spasticity or disorders of tone to be the most significant impairment constraining function in the patient with upper motor neuron disease (9–11). However, the extent to which spasticity impairs upper extremity function is still unclear.

Results from a study examining the extent to which abnormal stretch reflexes in antagonist muscles impair arm movements in stroke patients raises questions about the extent to which velocity-dependent spasticity limits upper extremity control (21). For example, it has been hypothesized that flexor spasticity in the biceps may prevent effective activation of the triceps and extension of the arm. Results from studies examining upper extremity reaching movements in patients with hemiplegia do not support the hypothesis that the primary constraint on upper extremity reaching is spasticity of the biceps, but rather weakness and inability to recruit motoneurons in the triceps (21).

Other studies examining reaching and other types of movements have found inappropriate "shortening reactions" that constrain upper extremity movements. A shortening reaction is the inappropriate activation of the stretch reflex during shortening contractions of a muscle, thus impairing a patient's ability to move the arm. Inappropriate shortening reactions have been reported in patients following stroke (21) and in patients with Parkinson's disease (22).

It is important to note that none of the studies described denies the fact that spasticity impairs motor control in the patient with neurological deficits. These studies do, however, challenge the assumption that spasticity is the primary impairment to normal motor control (23, 24).

Another effect that spasticity may have on upper extremity motor control relates to stiffness abnormalities during reaching. Remember that in Chapter 16, we explained that the location programming theory hypothesizes that when a person makes an arm movement, the nervous system programs the relative balance of tensions (or stiffness) of two opposing (agonist and antagonist) muscle sets in multiple joints in order to move the arm to a new position in space. Thus, in patients with stiffness control problems, such as spasticity, location programming would be very difficult or impossible.

MASS PATTERNS OF MOVEMENT

The presence of mass patterns of movement is another major limitation of upper extremity function in many patients who have suffered stroke or traumatic brain injury. Normal upper extremity function requires the ability to combine various types of movements, and to use the fingers independently. The upper extremity flexion synergy usually involves abduction, extension, and external rotation of the shoulder, elbow flexion, forearm supination, and flexion of the wrist and fingers. The extensor pattern is forward flexion, adduction, and internal rotation of the shoulder, extension of the elbow, forearm pronation, and extension of the fingers and thumb. More recently, massed patterns of movement have been viewed as invariant co-ordinative structures (27).

DYSCOORDINATION

Studies examining the trajectories of the hemiplegic arm in patients with hemiparesis found that movement amplitudes were smaller, and movement times were longer than in nondisabled subjects, with disruptions of interjoint coordination between the elbow and shoulder (28).

Studies have looked at the contributions of specific brain subsystems to these problems. The cerebellum appears to be important in the programming of ballistic movements (also referred to as open-loop or nonfeed-back-controlled movements). This is because studies have shown that patients with cerebellar disorders show abnormal ballistic arm movements. There is some evidence that slow closed-loop movements may be less affected by cerebellar dysfunction (29–33).

One study examined the ability of 7-year-old children with mild cerebral palsy (either ataxic or athetoid) to reach for a moving object. It was found that the reaches of these movement-impaired children had longer transport phases compared with nondisabled children and thus were less efficient (34). Interestingly, despite their motor impairments, the disabled children were able to reach for and grasp even quickly moving targets. The researchers found that the children aimed their reaches well ahead of the moving targets, suggesting that the children were able to compensate for their movement deficits when planning a reaching movement. They aimed their movements enough ahead of the target so they could sustain accuracy when reaching, despite their movement impairments (34).

MOTOR IMPAIRMENTS AFFECTING THE NONHEMIPARETIC LIMB

Traditionally, researchers have maintained that unilateral cerebral lesions manifest in the limb contralateral to the lesions. Now researchers are also finding subtle deficits affecting the ability to reach on the nonhemiparetic side. By studying reaching in the arm ipsilateral to a lesion, researchers have also been able to understand the contribution of a particular hemisphere to a reaching movement without the confounding influence of the severe sensory and motor loss that occurs in the contralateral limb.

An initial study examining motor problems in the nonhemiparetic limb has suggested that weakness is a contributing factor in reaching problems in this limb as well as the hemiparetic limb (35). Other studies have found that problems in reaching in the nonhemiparetic arm following unilateral hemispheric lesion may involve other factors as well.

In recent studies (36, 37), researchers examined reaching abilities in two groups of patients suffering from unilateral damage to the left or right cerebral hemispheres. Subjects were required to reach quickly and accurately to a small visual target using the arm ipsilateral to the lesion. Both patient groups were found to be less accurate than controls and required more time to complete the reach after the target was illuminated. The researchers found, however, a significant difference between the performance of subjects with right vs. left hemisphere lesions. While the right hemisphere lesioned group took longer to initiate a reach, the movements themselves were similar to those of the control group. In contrast, the left hemisphere lesioned group did not have problems in the time required to initiate the reach, but took much longer to execute the reach itself. Thus, reach was impaired in both groups, but for apparently different reasons. These authors suggest that a lesion in the right hemisphere affects the patient's ability to quickly detect the spatial position of the target (higher level visual processing). In contrast, a lesion in the left hemisphere appears to affect the patient's ability to select an appropriate program (higher level motor processing) to achieve the target position, and/or to modify that program as it is being executed (36, 37).

Sensory Impairments

Both visual and somatosensory impairments may have significant effects on manipulatory function. One common visual system problem affecting the transport phase of reaching is optic ataxia.

OPTIC ATAXIA

Lesions on either side of the posterior parietal area in humans can cause marked eye-hand coordination impairment, or optic ataxia. **Optic ataxia** is defined as the inability to reach for objects in extrapersonal space, in the absence of extensive motor, visual, or somatosensory deficits (1). Patients with optic ataxia typically misreach for objects within the visual field that is contralateral to their lesion.

This disorder was first described by Balint in 1909 (7) using the term "visual disorientation." He noted that the patient could reach normally with his left hand, but when asked to reach with his right hand, he made mistakes in all directions, until he eventually bumped into the object with his hand. He found that the problem was related to visual control of that hand, because if he asked the patient to first point to the object with his left hand, then he could reach accurately with his right hand. On autopsy, it was found that the patient had a lesion in the posterior parietal areas, including the angular gyrus and the anterior occipital lobe on both sides of the brain (1).

Patients with optic ataxia have now been tested carefully in the laboratory setting. It has been found that in the absence of visual feedback concerning their hand movement, patients with unilateral lesions misreach toward the side of the lesion, when they use the hand contralateral to the lesioned hemisphere. Thus, there is always a directional error in reaching.

There are specific motor disorganization problems in these patients as well. It has been hypothesized that their problems relate to programming visually guided goal-directed movements (1). It has been shown that the deceleration phase of reaching is much longer than that in the normal hand, with many small peaks. In addition, these patients have problems with grasp formation. Figure 17.1 shows a reach of a patient with optic ataxia with his

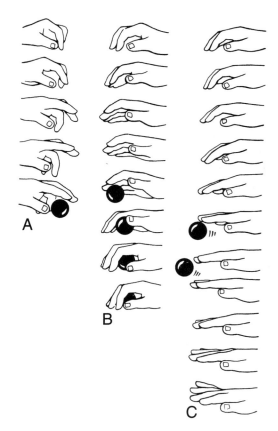

Figure 17.1. Drawing of the grip patterns of a patient with optic ataxia. **A**, Normal hand. **B**, Affected hand, visual feedback. **C**, Affected hand, no visual feedback. (From Jeannerod M. The neural and behavioral organization of goal-directed movements. Oxford: Oxford University Press, 1990:225.)

normal hand (*a*), affected hand with visual feedback (*b*), and (*c*) without vision. Note that even with visual feedback, the affected hand didn't begin to close until the last moment and the terminal grip size was too big. Without visual feedback, grasp formation did not occur.

Why would patients with optic ataxia show no grasp formation? Is it simply a strategy they use because they have so much error in their reach? It has been argued that this isn't the case, because they even show this with visual feedback. Thus, it has been concluded that it results from a specific problem with eye-hand coordination mechanisms responsible for adjusting finger posture to the shape of the object (1).

SOMATOSENSORY LOSS

As noted in earlier chapters, experiments by Sherrington in the late 1800s showed that monkeys that were deafferented on one side of the spinal cord stopped using the affected limb. He thus concluded that sensory feedback was critical to movement control. In contrast, researchers who deafferented both limbs of animals showed that the animals recovered motor function. Movements were initially awkward, but improved within as little as 2 weeks, as long as visual feedback was available (38).

Interestingly, recovery starts with the animals only being able to sweep the object across the floor. Then, a coarse grasp with all four fingers develops, and then a pincer grasp reappears (39). It has been suggested that when unilateral deafferentation occurs, the animals may learn not to use the deafferented limb, or even develop inhibition of the deafferented arm (39). This "learned disuse" hypothesis is supported by the fact that unilaterally deafferented animals recover movement coordination as well as bilaterally deafferented animals if their normal limb remains immobilized so that they have to use the deafferented limb (1).

Also, remember from the chapter on normal eye-hand coordination that experiments on deafferented monkeys showed that, when making single-joint movements, they could reach targets with relative accuracy, even when they could not see the hand. Displacing the forearm just prior to movement onset during a reach also did not significantly disturb pointing accuracy in these deafferented animals. It was thus concluded that single-joint movements depend on changes in muscle activation levels that are programmed prior to movement onset and that no feedback is required for reasonably accurate execution of these movements (40).

In addition, recent experiments on humans after pathological deafferentation have confirmed the results from experiments on monkeys (41). One patient had suffered a severe peripheral sensory neuropathy, so that there was loss of sensation in both the arms and the legs. Light touch, vibration, and temperature sensation were impaired or totally absent in both hands. Tests showed that in spite of these problems, the patient could perform many motor tasks, even without vision. For example, the patient could tap, do fast alternating flexion and extension movements, and draw figures in the air, using only the wrist and fingers (1, 41).

It was also noted that EMG activity during flexion and extension of the thumb was similar to that seen in normal subjects. The subject could also learn new thumb positions with vision and then reproduce those positions without vision. Thus, motor learning was also possible. However, the patient's performance rapidly deteriorated when asked to repeat the movement many times with the eyes closed.

In a second study on patients with peripheral sensory neuropathy, patients could perform repetitive flexion and extension movements of the wrist, with normal EMG activity, as long as the movements were not too fast. At a certain point, however, the intervals between the EMG bursts tended to disappear. It was hypothesized that this was due to the higher level of cocontraction of agonist and antagonist muscles seen in these patients (42).

Patients could also hold a steady posture with their deafferented limb as long as they had visual feedback. However, without visual feedback, large errors were made, and the limb drifted back to its initial position, as shown in Figure 17.2 (42).

What does this information tell us about the role of kinesthetic feedback in reaching? It appears that it is not required for movement initiation and execution. However, it is still important for accurate reaching involving multiple joints. Researchers testing humans with peripheral sensory neuropathy found that patients were able to make accurate movements only if they involved single joints. They showed great problems in performing natural movements used in normal life (43).

IMPAIRMENTS AFFECTING GRASP AND RELEASE

The range of grips required for daily life tasks is great, varying from grips requiring

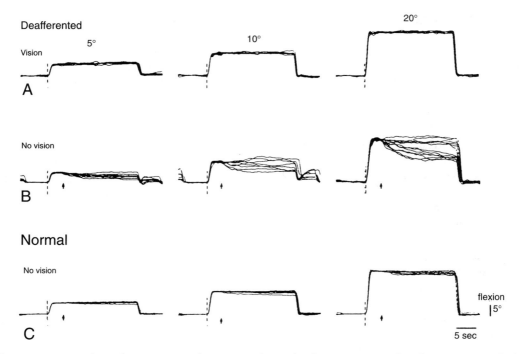

Figure 17.2. Recordings of wrist position of a patient with peripheral sensory neuropathy. The patient was asked to rotate the wrist to reach positions of 5°, 10°, and 20°, against an elastic load. **A,** With vision, the patient had no problems. **B,** Without vision, the position drifted back in the direction of the load. **C,** A normal subject's performance without vision. (Adapted from Sanes JN, Mauritz KH, Dalakas MC, Evarts EV. Motor control in humans with large-fiber sensory neuropathy. Human Neurobiology 1985;4:110.)

great precision, but not much force, to those requiring greater amounts of force, but not much precision. Precision grip involves control of individual finger motions, and is largely carried out by the intrinsic hand muscles (44, 45). In contrast, a power grip appears to involve a generalized coactivation of all the digits, primarily uses the extrinsic hand muscles, and does not require a fine degree of control. The two grips appear to be controlled by different cortical neurons (46, 47).

Motor Problems

PROBLEMS AFFECTING ACTIVATION AND COORDINATION OF AGONIST MUSCLES

Corticomotoneurons play an essential role in precision grip, and their loss due to neural injury results in an inability to recruit distal muscles, particularly the intrinsic hand muscles. Muscle activation bursts can be ab-

sent, delayed, or prolonged in patients with pyramidal tract lesions, affecting the timing and precision of hand movements (48).

Unfortunately, it appears that no other area of the CNS (not even corticomotoneurons in the opposite hemisphere) can substitute for these neurons when they are injured. In addition, there do not appear to be any alternative tracts within the CNS that can substitute for loss of descending corticospinal tracts. This limits the recovery of precision grip in patients with neural lesions affecting the primary motor cortex or its descending tracts (49–51).

Research on reaching behavior in monkeys whose corticospinal system had been lesioned at birth has shown that the distal component of the reach never matures. For example, when area 4 of the motor cortex is lesioned in infancy, a precision grip never develops. Remember from the chapter on development of upper extremity and manipulatory control that precision grip usually develops in monkeys at about 8 months of age, at the time that the pyramidal track matures (1, 52).

Research studies have examined recovery of upper extremity control in adult patients who have had a stroke, with primary damage to the motor cortex areas and the pyramidal pathways. These studies have shown that movement in proximal joints recovers first, with normal force returning in 4 to 6 weeks. However, isolated finger movements were permanently lost in these patients (53). Remember that control of proximal joints involves a different system from that controlling distal muscles.

Other studies examining recovery of upper extremity function in adult stroke patients have found that the shoulder-elbow synergy for transporting the hand to the object showed recovery if the shoulder was passively supported against gravity, but finger movements were always clumsy. The patients could not shape the hand in anticipation of the grasp. Also, the grasp was made by using the palm of the whole hand, rather than by using the pincer grasp with the fingertips (1, 54).

Studies have examined the reaching behavior of developmentally disabled children, including those with hemiplegia or Down syndrome (55–57). In some cases of mild impairment, hemiplegia is not readily identified until about 40 weeks, when the infant first begins to use the pincer grasp and manipulate objects (1). In one child of 23 months, the hand with hemiplegia was used only when the normal hand was immobilized, and even then, it was with great difficulty that the child grasped objects. Figure 17.3, adapted from film records, illustrates the child reaching for a prong from a pegboard with the normal hand and the affected hand, with visual feedback. Note that the normal hand did not anticipate the shape of the object well, but a finger extension/flexion pattern was used. Also, contact of the hand with the object caused the fingers to close around the object, giving an accurate grasp. However, the hemiplegic hand showed an exaggerated opening during the entire movement, with no anticipatory

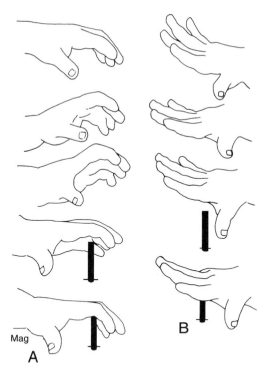

Figure 17.3. Drawing from film records of the reaches of a hemiplegic 23-month-old child reaching for a prong from a pegboard with the normal hand and the affected hand, with visual feedback. **A,** Normal hand. **B,** Affected hand. (From Jeannerod M. The neural and behavioral organization of goal-directed movements. Oxford: Oxford University Press, 1990:72.)

grasp formation. There was a very slight closing of the hand after contact with the object, giving a very clumsy grasp (1).

In a second child of 5 years of age, the hemiplegic hand showed more normal reach and grasp movements. The authors suggest that more normal movement patterns may be the result of many years of rehabilitation training (1). Figure 17.4 depicts film records of her reaching movements with her normal hand (*A*) and her hemiplegic hand (*B, C, D*). Note that reaching in the hemiplegic hand was only affected in relation to the pattern of grip formation. Finger shaping was abnormal, with the index finger extended in an exaggerated manner, and then flexing only slightly, if at all, before contacting the object. Due to these problems, the objects were sometimes dropped during the grasp (1).

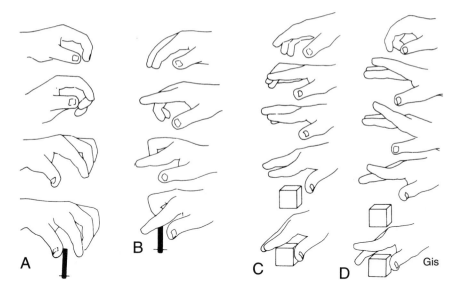

Figure 17.4.   Drawing from film records of the reaches of a hemiplegic 5-year-old child after many years of rehabilitation reaching for a prong from a pegboard with the normal hand and the affected hand, with visual feedback. **A**, Normal hand. **B**, **C**, and **D**, Affected hand. (From Jeannerod M. The neural and behavioral organization of goal-directed movements. Oxford: Oxford University Press, 1990:73.)

INAPPROPRIATE ACTIVATION OF ANTAGONIST MUSCLES

Abnormalities of upper extremity function can result from disturbances to the timing and amplitude of contraction of antagonist muscles. In some patients, for example, those with athetoid cerebral palsy, the antagonist muscle is inappropriately active. Antagonist activation can occur prior to the agonist muscle, causing movement in the wrong direction. Alternatively, antagonist activation can occur simultaneously with the agonist, resulting in decreased amplitude of movement (48).

Surprisingly, in many patients who are neurologically impaired, abnormal coordination of muscles is not found consistently in all types of upper extremity movements. For example, when patients with severe dystonia were asked to wave, muscle activation patterns underlying the alternating wrist flexion and extension movements were normal. In contrast, excessive and inappropriate coactivation of agonist and antagonist muscles was present in these same patients during precision hand movements such as when asked to write their name (58). This may be due to nonpyramidal vs. pyramidal systems controlling these two types of movements.

SENSORY PROBLEMS

Open-loop control or ballistic reaching movements are preprogrammed, and therefore do not require sensory feedback to control the movement. Relatively normal ballistic upper extremity movements have been found in patients with complete limb deafferentation (59). In contrast, closed-loop movements, such as precision hand movements, require continuous sensory inputs, and are significantly impaired in patients with sensory loss (60).

Recent studies have suggested that the control processes involved in precision grip and lift are better described as "discrete event driven control" rather than as a "continuous closed-loop" control (61, 62). As a basis for this hypothesis, research has shown that sensory information is used intermittently at critical times within a precision grip and lift task, rather than continuously.

A precision grip and lift task is organized into distinct phases which are linked together. The pattern of muscle activity used in the different phases of this movement is determined by a combination of previous experience and afferent information (visual and somatosensory) generated during the performance of the task (61, 62).

Tactile input is necessary to determine the appropriate grip force. If grip force is too tight, the object can't be manipulated; if it is too loose, the object will be dropped. In a precision grip, forces for gripping and lifting are generated simultaneously and appear to be very dependent on cutaneous input. When the fingers of neurologically intact subjects are anesthetized, grip forces are often inappropriate to the object being gripped (61).

What happens to eye-hand coordination skills in the patient with a neurological impairment with loss of somatosensation? Experiments have been performed in which the reaching skills of patients with lesions in the somatosensory pathways at brainstem levels and at parietal cortex levels were examined (1). In the patient with the lesion at the brainstem level, the hand ipsilateral to the lesion was affected. When vision was present, the reach was normal, as shown in Figure 17.5*A*, except that it was longer in duration than it was in the normal hand. However, without vision, the grasping movements were critically changed (Fig. 17.5*B* and *C*). Finger grip was either absent altogether, or incomplete. In the first reach the patient made with no visual feedback, there was no grip formation at all,

while in the second reach, there was incomplete grip formation (1).

Patients with central lesions to the parietal lobe, particularly the post-central gyrus and the supramarginal gyrus, show similar patterns for reach and grasp as patients with peripheral sensory problems. In a detailed study on the recovery of reach and grasp in a patient with a parietal lobe lesion, researchers found the patient did not use her right hand spontaneously immediately following her lesion, but later used it in many actions, as long as she had visual feedback. Without visual control, her movements were very awkward. For example, she couldn't sustain repetitive tapping movements unless she could see or hear her fingers moving (1).

In contrast to patients with peripheral deafferentation, who could grip normally as long as visual feedback was present, grip formation was impaired in the patient with a parietal lesion, even with visual feedback present (1). Figure 17.6*A* shows the grasp component of a reach with the patient's normal hand, while Figure 17.6*B* and *C* show the grasp of the affected hand both with and without visual feedback. When she reached with the affected hand with vision, the patient made grasps using the whole palm of the hand. Without visual feedback, only the initial part of the transportation phase was normal. Then the hand seemed to "wander above the object, without a grasp" (1, p 207).

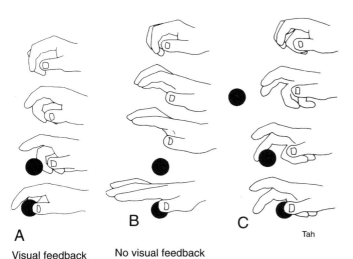

A Visual feedback   **B**   **C**   No visual feedback   Tah

Figure 17.5. Drawing from film records of the grip patterns of a patient with lesion of the somatosensory pathways at the brainstem level. **A**, With vision grasp was normal. **B** and **C**, Without vision, it was absent or incomplete. (From Jeannerod M. The neural and behavioral organization of goal-directed movements. Oxford: Oxford University Press, 1990:205.)

Figure 17.6. Drawing of the grip patterns of a patient with parietal lobe lesions. **A**, Normal hand, no visual feedback. **B**, Affected hand, visual feedback. **C**, Affected hand, no visual feedback. (From Jeannerod M. The neural and behavioral organization of goal-directed movements. Oxford: Oxford University Press, 1990: 208.)

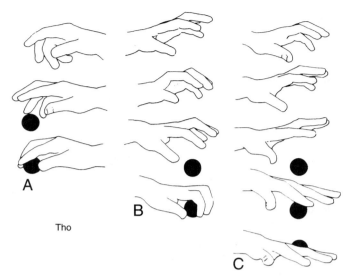

Tho

Thus, loss of sensory information results in abnormal grip and lift forces, and problems in the control of small, fine movements of the hand (41, 61–63).

POSTURAL PROBLEMS

The ability to move our arms purposefully requires good postural control to maintain an appropriate orientation and stability of the body during the performance of upper extremity tasks. In the chapters on normal and abnormal postural control, we reviewed in detail the research on anticipatory postural adjustments that are normally made in advance of potentially destabilizing reaches to prevent or minimize displacement of the body. We also discussed abnormalities in the ability to effectively preprogram these anticipatory postural adjustments seen in a variety of patient populations, thus resulting in slowed and inefficient upper extremity movements. Please refer back to these chapters for more information on problems with postural control as it relates to upper extremity movements.

PROBLEMS WITH ADAPTATION

The ability to adapt upper extremity movements to changes in task and environmental demands is an essential component of

normal upper extremity control. Sensory information is critical to adapting movements and is used to correct errors during the execution of upper extremity movement, ensuring accuracy during the final portions of the movement.

Visual Deficits

The primary function of visual feedback in reaching appears to be related to the attainment of final accuracy. It has been hypothesized that the constancy of thumb position with relation to the wrist during reaching may be part of a strategy of providing clear visual feedback information regarding the endpoint of the limb (64).

Somatosensory Deficits

Is somatosensory input essential for the production of reaching movements? Considerable research (1, 38) has shown that monkeys that were deafferented still were able to perform adequate reaching and grasping movements as soon as 2 weeks after the lesion was made, as long as vision was available. They noted that movements were awkward at first, with animals only sweeping objects along the floor. They then developed a primitive grasp with four fingers together and no thumb, and finally redeveloped a crude pincer grasp a few months after the lesion was made (1).

Other such experiments have shown that deafferented monkeys can still make reasonably accurate single joint pointing movements, even when vision of the arm is occluded, when the pointing task was learned before deafferentation (40). In this case, even displacing the arm before the movement didn't affect terminal accuracy, even though they couldn't see or feel their arm position! Thus, it was concluded that the monkey is capable of using a central motor program to perform reaching movements and that kinesthetic feedback isn't required for achieving reasonable accuracy. However, the animal could not adapt the reaching movement to a change in shoulder position, which thus changed the initial coordinates of the arm in space.

Experiments performed with humans with severe peripheral sensory neuropathy in all four limbs have shown similar results (41). The patient was able to perform a wide variety of hand movements, such as tapping movements, and could draw figures in the air, even with the eyes closed. However, when he was asked to repeat the movement many times with the eyes closed, the performance deteriorated quickly. Thus, apparently, somatosensory information isn't required for arm movement initiation or execution as long as the movements are simple or nonrepetitive. However, if patients have to make complex movements requiring coordination of many joints, or repeat movements, then without visual feedback, they are unable to update their central representations of body space. Accordingly, they show considerable movement "drift" and problems with coordination (1). Although these experiments suggest that certain movements may be carried out without somatosensory feedback, considerable work has also shown the important contributions of sensory feedback to the fine regulation of movement.

Anticipatory Aspects

The ability to move smoothly, grasp, and pick up objects, is a combination of anticipatory action and both intermittent and continuous sensory information about the ongoing events. Anticipatory activity is based on prior knowledge about the task itself, and the movements that need to be made.

An essential component of all reaching movements is proactive visual and somatosensory control, which is responsible for the correct initial direction of the limb toward the target and the initial coordination between limb segments. In addition, visual information about the characteristics of the object to be grasped is used proactively to preprogram the forces used in precision grip.

It has been hypothesized that visual and somatosensory information is used to update proprioceptive and visual body maps, which allows the accurate programming of reaching movements. To determine the influence of updated maps of the body workspace on the accuracy of a reaching movement, experiments were performed to manipulate visual information regarding hand and target positions *prior to movement*. When the subject could not see the hand prior to movement, there were large errors. It was thus concluded that a proprioceptive map of the hand, by itself, was not adequate to appropriately code the hand position in the reaching workspace. This means that somatosensory inputs must be calibrated by vision in order for the proprioceptive map and the visual map to be matched (1). No experiments have yet been performed to determine how often the proprioceptive map needs to be updated by visual inputs to ensure accurate movements.

Loss of motor control resulting in limited ability to move may also affect exploratory aspects of motor control. This reduction of exploratory movements may contribute to impaired upper extremity control by affecting anticipatory aspects of the movement.

APRAXIA

Up until now, our discussion of abnormal upper extremity manipulative control has related to the examination of problems in each of the constituent components. However, the use of the upper extremity in the performance of simple everyday tasks is more than the simple summation of these components. It requires the integration of these components into an action plan. An action plan specifies the conceptual content of the action, along with its hierarchical and sequential organization (65). The left cerebral cortex includes structures specialized for higher-order motor programming or the formation of action plans (66).

One way researchers have studied the nature of these motor programs is by analyzing the types of errors made by patients with left hemisphere damage. Disorders that result from dysfunction of this specialized left hemisphere have been termed apraxias. One type of apraxia that has been studied extensively is ideational apraxia, also referred to as frontal apraxia (67), or frontal lobe executive disorder (68). This is a disorder of the execution of movement that cannot be attributed to weakness, incoordination or sensory loss, or to poor language comprehension or inattention to commands.

To understand this disorder, it is helpful to first appreciate what occurs when a normal adult decides to perform a task. It is hypothesized that the first step involves formulating the *intention* to perform the task and then formulating an *action plan*. The essential requirement of an action plan is that it specifies the *goal* of the action along with the hierarchical and sequential organization of nested actions that are required to achieve the ultimate goal. Intentions, as defined by activated action plans, are an integral feature of all purposeful behavior. It has been hypothesized that the core of the intentional disorder of frontal apraxia is a weakening of the top-down formulation of action plans, that is, an inability to sustain the intent to the completion of the action plan (66).

As a result, irrelevant objects exert a strong influence on the action plan, and this leads to numerous performance errors. Researchers have begun to develop a system for coding performance errors based on this concept of hierarchically organized units of action within an action plan. These studies have enumerated examples of errors during the per-

formance of common activities of daily living, including buttering hot coffee, putting clothes on backwards or inside-out, drinking from an empty cup, skipping key steps during activities such as shaving, toothbrushing, or hairbrushing, using a fork to eat cereal, putting toothpaste on a razor, scrubbing the upper lip and chin with a toothbrush, eating toothpaste, and applying arm deodorant over a shirt (66). In a classic paper, Luria describes the behavior of a frontal apraxia patient who would light a candle and put it in his mouth to perform the habitual movements of smoking a cigarette (67).

SUMMARY

1. Understanding the cause of impairments in eye-hand coordination may be difficult, due to the complexity of the interactions between neural substrates involved in reaching skills.

2. Lesions to the motor cortex areas and the pyramidal pathways following stroke show recovery of function in the proximal joints first, with normal force returning in 4 to 6 weeks. However, recovery of isolated finger movements almost never occurs.

3. Studies on patients with interhemispheric lesions suggest that proximal arm movements are controlled by a diffuse cortical and subcortical uncrossed pathway, while hand movements are controlled only by the contralateral motor cortex.

4. Patients with lesions in the visual striate cortex are still able to reach toward objects moving across their visual field, even though they are considered totally blind, possibly due to subcortical visual processing in the superior colliculus.

5. Patients with peripheral sensory neuropathy can make accurate single joint movements, but show great problems in performing most normal movements. With visual feedback, reaching is reasonably normal, but without vision, finger grip is either absent or abnormal.

6. Lesions on either side of the posterior parietal area can cause optic ataxia or the inability to reach for objects in extrapersonal space (in the absence of extensive motor, visual, or somatosensory deficits).

7. Damage to the left hemisphere may cause

apraxia, a disorder of the execution of movement that can be accounted for neither by weakness, incoordination or sensory loss, nor by poor language comprehension or inattention to commands. The core of this disorder may be a weakening of the top-down formulation of action plans, that is, an inability to sustain the intent to the completion of the action plan. As a result, irrelevant objects exert a strong influence on the action plan, leading to performance errors.

REFERENCES

1. Jeannerod M. The neural and behavioral organization of goal-directed movements. Oxford: Oxford University Press, 1990:283.
2. Martin TA, Keating JG, Goodkin HP, Bastian AJ, Thach WT. Storage of multiple gaze-hand calibrations. Neuroscience Abstracts 1993;19:980.
3. Humphrey NK, Weiskrantz L. Vision in monkeys after removal of the striate cortex. Nature 1969;215:595–597.
4. Peoppel E. Letter to the editor. Nature 1973; 243:231.
5. Perenin MT, Jeannerod M. Visual function within the hemianoptic field following early cerebral hemidecortication in man. I. spatial localization. Neuropsychologia 1978;16:1–13.
6. Zihl J, Werth R. Contributions to the study of "blindsight." II. The role of specific practice for saccadic localization in patients with postgeniculate visual field defects. Neuropsychologia 1984;22:13–22.
7. Balint R. Seelenhamung des "Schauens," optische Ataxie, raumlische Storung des Aufmersamkeit. Monatshr Psychiatr Neurol 1909;25:51–81.
8. Waters RL, Wilson DJ, Savinelli R. Rehabilitation of the upper extremity following stroke. In: Hunter J, Schneider LH, Mackin EJ, Bell JA, eds. Rehabilitation of the hand. St. Louis: CV Mosby, 1978;505–520.
9. Carr JH, Shepherd RB. A motor relearning programme for stroke. Rockville, MD: Aspen, 1983.
10. Davies P. Steps to follow. New York: Springer-Verlag, 1985.
11. Bobath B. Adult hemiplegia: evaluation and treatment. London: William Heinemann Medical Books, 1978.
12. Davis SW, Petrillo CR, Eichberg RD, Chu DS. Shoulder-hand syndrome in a hemiplegic population: a 5-year retrospective study. Arch Phys Med Rehabil 1977;58:353–356.
13. Patridge CJ, Edwards SM, Mee R, Langenberghe HVK van. Hemiplegic shoulder pain: a study of two methods of physiotherapy treatment. Clinical Rehabilitation 1990; 4:43–49.
14. Roy CW. Shoulder pain in hemiplegia: a literature review. Clinical Rehabilitation 1988; 2:35–44.
15. Cailliet R. The shoulder in hemiplegia. Philadelphia: FA Davis, 1980.
16. Smidt GL, Rogers MW. Factors contributing to the regulation and clinical assessment of muscular strength. Phys Ther 1982;62: 1283–1290.
17. Buchner DM, DeLateur BJ. The importance of skeletal muscle strength to physical function in older adults. Annals of Behavioral Medicine 1991;13:1–12.
18. Rogers MM. Musculoskeletal considerations in production and control of movement. In: Montgomery P, Connolly BH, eds. Motor control and physical therapy. Hixson, TX: Chattanooga Group, 1991:69–82.
19. Duncan P, Badke MB. Stroke rehabilitation. Chicago: Year Book, 1987.
20. Lance JW: Symposium synopsis. In: Feldman RG, Young RR, Koella WP, eds. Spasticity: disordered motor control. Chicago: Year Book Medical Publishers, 1980:485.
21. Sahrmann SA, Norton BJ. The relationship of voluntary movement to spasticity in the upper motor neuron syndrome. Arch Neurol 1977;2:460–465.
22. Johnson RH. Disorders of stretch reflex modulation during volitional movements. Brain 1991;114:443–460.
23. Katz R, Rymer Z. Spastic hypertonia: mechanisms and measurement. Arch Phys Med Rehabil 1989;70:144–155.
24. Gordon J. Assumptions underlying physical therapy intervention: theoretical and historical perspectives. In: Carr J, Shepherd R, Gordon J, Gentile AM, Held J, eds. Movement science foundations for physical therapy in rehabilitation. Rockville: Aspen, 1987.
25. Brunnstrom S. Movement therapy in hemiplegia: a neurophysiological approach. New York: Harper & Row, 1970.
26. Gowland C. Staging motor impairment after stroke. Stroke 1990;21(suppl II):II-19–II-21.

27. Kamm K, Thelen E, Jensen J. A dynamical systems approach to motor development. In: Rothstein J, ed. Movement science. Alexandria, VA: American Physical Therapy Association, 1991:11–23.

28. Levin MF, Horowitz M, Jurrius C, Lamothe AG, Feldman AG. Trajectory formation and interjoint coordination of drawing movements in normal and hemiparetic subjects. Neuroscience Abstracts 1993;19:990.

29. Flowers K. Visual "closed loop" and "open loop" characteristics of voluntary movement in patients with Parkinsonism and intention tremor. Brain 1976;99:269–310.

30. Hallet M, Marsden CD. Physiology and pathophysiology of the ballistic movement pattern. In: Desmedt JE, ed. Progress in clinical neurophysiology: motor unit types, recruitment and plasticity in health and disease. Basel: Karger, 1981:331–346.

31. Hallet M, Shahani BT, Young RR. EMG analysis of patients with cerebellar deficit. J Neurol Neurosurg Psychiatry 1975;38:1163–1169.

32. Thach WT. Correlation of neural discharge with pattern and force of muscular activity, joint position and direction of intended next movement in motor cortex and cerebellum. J Neurophysiol 1978;41:654–676.

33. Deecke L, Kornhuber HH. Cerebral potential and the initiation of voluntary movement. In: Desmedt JE, ed. Progress in clinical neurophysiology, vol 1: Attention, voluntary contraction and event-related cerebral potentials. Karger: Basel, 1977:132–150.

34. Forsstron A, von Hofsten C. Visually directed reaching of children with motor impairments. Devel Med Child Neurol 1982;24:653–661.

35. Giulliani C, Genova PA, Purser KE, Light KE. Limb trajectory in non-disabled subjects under two conditions of external constraint compared with the non-paretic limb of subjects with hemiparesis. Neuroscience Abstracts 1993;19:990.

36. Fisk JD, Goodale MA. The effects of unilateral brain damage on visually guided reaching: hemispheric differences in the nature of the deficit. Exp Brain Res 1988;72:425–435.

37. Smutok MA, Grafman J, Salazar AM, Sweeney JK, Jonas BS, DiRocco PJ. Effects of unilateral brain damage on contralateral and ipsilatral upper extremity function in hemiplegia. Phys Ther 1989;69:195–203.

38. Taub E, Berman AJ. Movement and learning in the absence of sensory feedback. In: Freedman SJ, ed. The neurophysiology of spatially oriented behavior. Homewood: Dorey Press, 1968:173–192.

39. Taub E. Motor behavior following deafferentation in the developing and motorically immature monkey. In: Herman RM, Grillner S, Stein DG, Stuart DG, eds. Neural control of locomotion. NY: Plenum Press, 1976:675–705.

40. Polit A, Bizzi E. Processes controlling arm movements in monkeys. Science 1978;201:1235–1237.

41. Rothwell JC, Traub MM, Day BL, Obeso JA, Thomas PK, Marsden CD. Manual motor performance in a deafferented man. Brain 1982;105:515–542.

42. Sanes JN, Mauritz KH, Dalakas MC, Evarts EV. Motor control in humans with large-fiber sensory neuropathy. Human Neurobiology 1985;4:101–114.

43. Jeannerod M. The formation of finger grip during prehension. A cortically mediated visuomotor pattern. Behav Brain Res 1986;19:99–116.

44. Muir RB, Lemon RM. Corticospinal neurons with a special role in precision grip. Brain Res 1983;261:312–316.

45. Muir RM. Small hand muscles in precision grip. A corticospinal prerogative. Exp Brain Res 1985;10:155–173.

46. Hoffman DS. Luschell ES. Precentral cortical cells during a controlled jaw bite task. J Neurophysiol 1980;44:333–348.

47. Fahrer M. Surgical approaches to the nerves of the upper limb. In: Tubiana R, ed. The hand. Philadelphia: WB Saunders, 1988:539–547.

48. Hallett M. Analysis of abnormal voluntary and involuntary movements with surface electromyography. In: Desmedt JE, ed. Motor control mechanisms in health and disease. New York: Raven Press, 1983:907–914.

49. Lawrence DG, Hopkins DA. The development of motor control in the rhesus monkey: evidence concerning the role of corticomotoneuronal connections. Brain 1976;99:235–254.

50. Wise SD, Evarts EV. The role of the cerebral cortex in movement. Trends Neurosci 1981;4:297–300.

51. Passingham R. Perry H, Wilkinson F. Failure

to develop a precision grip in monkeys with unilateral neocortical lesions made in infancy. Brain Res 1978;145:410–414.

52. Kuypers HG. Corticospinal connections: postnatal development in rhesus monkey. Science 1962;138:678–680.

53. Hecaen H, de Ajuriaguerra J. Etude des troubles toniques, moteurs et vegetatifs et de leur recuperations apres ablation limitee du cortex moteur et premoteur. Congres des Medecins Alinenistes et Neurologistes 1948:269–274.

54. Lough S, Wing AM, Fraser C, Jenner JR. Measurement of recovery of function in the hemiparetic upper limb following stroke: a preliminary report. Human Movement Science 1984;3:247–256.

55. Jeannerod M. Mechanisms of visuomotor co-ordination: a study in normal and brain-damaged subjects. Neuropsychologia 1986; 24:41–78.

56. Eliasson AC, Gordon AM, Forssberg H. Basic coordination of manipulative forces in children with cerebral palsy. Dev Med Child Neurol 1991;134:126–154.

57. Cole KJ, Abbs JH Tuner GS. Deficits in the production of grip forces in Down's syndrome. Dev Med Child Neurol 1988; 30:752–758.

58. Rothwell JC, Obeso JA, Day VL, Marsden CD. Pathophysiology of dystonias. In: Desmedt JE, ed. Motor control mechanisms in health and disease. New York: Raven Press, 1983:851–864.

59. Hallet M, Marsden CD. Physiology and pathophysiology of the ballistic movement pattern. In: Desmedt JE, ed. Progress in clinical neurophysiology, vol 9. Motor unit types,

recruitment and plasticity in health and disease. Karger: Basel, 1981:331–346.

60. Fromm C, Evarts E. Relation of motor cortex neurons to precisely controlled and ballistic movements. Neurosci Lett 1977;5:259–265.

61. Johansson RS, Westling G. Roles of glabrous skin receptors and sensorimotor memory in automatic control of precision grip when lifting rougher or more slippery objects. Exp Brain Res 1984;56:550–564.

62. Johansson RS, Westling G. Signals in tactile afferents from the fingers eliciting adaptive motor responses during precision grip. Exp Brain Res 1987;66:141–154.

63. Jeannerod M, Michel F, Prablanc C. The control of hand movements in a case of hemianaesthesia following a parietal lesion. Brain 1984;107:899–920.

64. Wing AM, Frazer C. The contribution of the thumb to reaching movements. Q J Exp Psychol 1983;35A:297–309.

65. Poizner H, Mack L, Verfaellie M, Rothi LJG, Heilman KM. Three-dimensional computer-grapic analysis of apraxia. Brain 1990; 113:85–101.

66. Schwartz MF, Reed ES, Montgomery M, Palmer C, Mayer NH. The quantitative description of action disorganization after brain demage: a case study. Cognitive Neuropsychology 1991;8:381–414.

67. Luria AR. Higher cortical functions in man. NY: Basic Books, 1966.

68. Norman DA, Shallice T. Attention to action: willed and automatic control of behavior. In: Davidson RJ, Schwartz GE, Shapiro D, eds. Consciousness and self-regulation, vol 4. New York: Plenum, 1986.

Chapter 18

ASSESSMENT AND TREATMENT OF THE PATIENT WITH UPPER EXTREMITY MANIPULATORY DYSCONTROL

INTRODUCTION

Mrs. Poirot, our patient from Chapter 15, has been referred for therapy to improve her upper extremity manipulatory control. Remember that 6 weeks ago she had a stroke in the left hemisphere, and has some residual right hemiparesis, with mild spasticity. While in the past, movements of her right arm were confined to a fixed synergy, either flexion or extension, she is now able to move outside the context of these fixed coordinative patterns. Arm function in the hemiparetic arm has begun to return, and she has developed the ability to move her arm, though movements are weak and dyscoordinated. She is also beginning to show some ability to coordinate finger movement for grasp. She also appears to have

417

subtle but distinct problems in coordinating reach and grasp in her nonhemiparetic arm.

Mrs. Poirot has sensory and perceptual problems as well. She has a moderate hemianopsia, decreasing the peripheral visual field on the right. She has decreased cutaneous and proprioceptive sensory function in the hemiparetic arm. Mrs. Poirot's stroke occurred in the left cerebral hemisphere; as a result, she has mild aphasia, affecting primarily her ability to verbally express herself. In addition, she is showing ADL performance errors, which suggests that she has problems related to ideational apraxia.

This combination of sensory and motor impairments will likely affect all aspects of upper extremity control, including eye-head coordination for locating a target, reach, grasp, release, manipulation, and the use of anticipatory postural adjustments before upper-extremity movements.

This chapter presents a task-oriented approach to assessment and treatment of the patient with upper extremity manipulatory control problems. As we noted in Chapter 5, a task-oriented approach reflects a conceptual framework for clinical practice that incorporates four key elements: the clinical decision-making process, hypothesis-oriented clinical practice, a model of disablement, and a systems theory of motor control. An important part of the task-oriented approach is the ability to generate multiple hypotheses about the potential causes of dysfunction in the patient, and systematically test those hypotheses in order to refine one's understanding of the problems contributing to loss of function.

It is important to remember that the development of clinical methods such as a task-oriented approach based on a systems theory of motor control is just beginning. As systems-based research provides us with an increased understanding of normal and abnormal upper extremity control, new methods for assessing and treating problems affecting upper extremity function will emerge.

ASSESSMENT

A task-oriented assessment of upper extremity control evaluates behavior at three levels, including (*a*) objective measurement of functional upper extremity skills, (*b*) evaluation of the key components that form the basis for functional skills, and (*c*) quantification of the underlying sensory, motor, and cognitive impairments that constrain performance of skills at levels 1 and 2. In addition, a thorough assessment must include a review of the patient's medical and social history, as well as a review of current symptoms and concerns.

Since no one test will measure all levels of function, the clinician must assemble a battery of tests that best meets the needs of the type of patient being evaluated, while examining performance in each of these areas (1–4). A three-level assessment allows the clinician to answer the following questions:

1. To what degree can the patient perform functional tasks?
2. What strategies does the patient use to perform the tasks, and can they adapt strategies to changing task conditions?
3. What are the sensory, motor, and cognitive impairments that constrain how they perform the task, and can these impairments or strategies be changed through intervention, thereby improving the level of functional performance, or is the patient performing optimally, given the current set of impairments?

The information gained through assessment is used to develop a comprehensive list of problems, establish short- and long-term goals, and formulate a plan of care for retraining upper extremity control.

Functional Assessment of Upper Extremity Control

A task-oriented approach to evaluating upper extremity function begins with a functional assessment to determine how well a patient can perform a variety of skills that depend on control of the upper extremity. A functional assessment can provide the clinician with information on the patient's level of performance compared to standards established with normal subjects. There are a number of approaches to assessing functional performance related to upper extremity control. Tests can be categorized into ADL scales, physical capacity evaluation tests, and tests that examine hand dexterity and manipulation.

TESTS OF ACTIVITIES OF DAILY LIVING

Standardized Activities of Daily Living (ADL) scales test bathing, dressing, grooming, toileting, feeding, mobility, and continence. Examples of ADL scales include the Katz Index (5), Functional Independence Measure (FIM) (6), PULSES profile (7), and the Barthel Index (8).

Standardized Instrumental Activities of Daily Living (IADL) scales also offer an approach to assessing upper extremity function by examining skills that require environmental interactions, such as telephone usage, traveling, shopping, preparing meals, housework, and finances.

STANDARDIZED TESTS OF MANIPULATION AND DEXTERITY

One of the most common approaches to evaluating upper extremity function focuses on the assessment of manipulation and dexterity. Manipulation refers to general movement of an object in space, or with reference to another object. It can also be used to refer to in-hand manipulation of an object, such as when one modifies or adjusts an object while it remains in the hand (10). Manipulation requires that hand and finger function adapt according to the physical and spatial properties of objects (11).

Manipulation typically involves several categories of skills, including tool-use skills (pencils, pens, scissors), dressing (buttoning, typing), eating skills (use of a knife, opening containers), and other skills such as money handling (12). Performance of these skills requires a variety of hand movements with reference to an object, including pushing, pulling, shaking, and throwing, transferring, and releasing. In addition to hand movements,

these tasks require other key components of upper extremity function, such as eye-head coordination, postural control, and arm transport. When evaluating patients with apparent unilateral involvement, keep in mind that often both sides of the body evidence problems with upper extremity control. Hence, the clinician should assess both sides. Some commonly used tests of hand dexterity and manipulation skills for adults are detailed below.

Jebsen Hand Function Test

The Jebsen Hand Function Test was one of the earliest objective standardized tests of hand function (13). It contains seven timed subtests: writing, card turning, picking up small items, simulated feeding, stacking checkers, picking up light cans and heavy cans (Fig. 18.1). The Jebsen-Taylor test requires that both hands be tested, with the nondominant hand tested first. The test is relatively quick to administer (10 to 15 minutes), and uses inexpensive and readily available materials. In addition, it has established norms against which a patient's performance can be compared (13, 14). The Jebsen-Taylor generally has excellent test-retest reliability, with the exception of writing and feeding subtests, which tend to show practice effects (15).

The purpose of the Jebsen-Taylor test is to assess hand functions that are common to many ADL tests. Studies have found a moderate correlation between scores on the Jebsen-Taylor test and ADL ability as measured by the Klein-Bell ADL Scale (16). However, the correlations have not been high enough to warrant substitution of the Jebsen for an ADL test (16).

Purdue Pegboard Test

The Purdue Pegboard test is another test of finger manipulation and hand dexterity (17). This test is a time-based measure of dexterity, requiring the placement of pins into holes, or the assembly of a group of pins, washers, and collars. There are four subtests that examine prehension in the right, left, and both hands, and a bimanual assembly task.

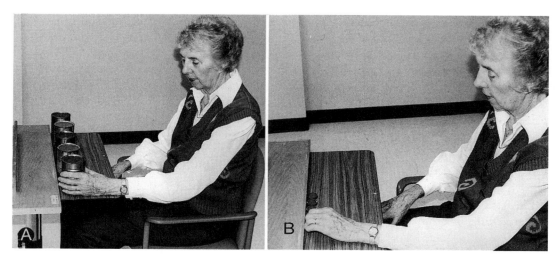

Figure 18.1. Jebsen-Taylor Hand Function Test. Two items from this seven-item test are shown, **A**, lifting light cans, and **B**, stacking checkers.

Thus, the test scores dexterity in each hand tested separately, as well as bimanual dexterity. The patient's performance is compared against standardized normative data. Like all the timed tests, the Purdue does not evaluate the cause of impaired prehension; it only documents that an impairment exists.

Minnesota Rate of Manipulation Test

The Minnesota Rate of Manipulation Test (MRMT) (American Guidance Service) is a standardized test of manual dexterity, and contains five subtests: the placing test, turning test, displacing test, one-hand turning and placing test, and two-hand turning and placing test (18). These are timed tests of dexterity that require the subject to manipulate blocks and place them into a series of holes. The placing and the turning tests are the most commonly administered of the five subtests. The test is standardized, and norms are available.

PHYSICAL CAPACITY EVALUATION

Physical Capacity Evaluation (PCE), alternatively referred to as a functional capacity or work skills evaluation, is another approach to evaluating functional upper extremity control. A Physical Capacity Evaluation involves a comprehensive assessment battery of the patient's functional and physical abilities, and is used to determine the patient's ability to return to work. A detailed discussion of PCE is beyond the scope of this chapter, but a brief review of some of the available tests that evaluate upper extremity control is presented.

A number of commercially available standardized tests examine upper extremity function related to physical work. The Valpar Work Samples (Valpar Work Samples, Valpar Corporation, Tucson) is a standardized test that uses 19 work samples to evaluate reaching, handling, manipulating, and feeding (18). The BTW Work Simulator (Work Simulator, Baltimore Therapeutic Equipment Co., Baltimore, MD) also evaluates upper extremity function through the use of a mechanical device with 18 different tool attachments. Thus, the patient's ability to handle and manipulate tools is quantified and performance compared to normative data (19).

The advantage of functional performance-based assessments, whether ADL, PCE, or hand dexterity, is their ability to quantify functional performance and compare it to established norms. Two limitations of this type of testing include (*a*) tests do not assess how a patient performs the task, that is, the quality of movement used; and (*b*) the tests do not provide insight into why a patient is unable to perform a functional skill, that is, into the underlying impairments that constrain function. This latter point is particularly significant, since a major focus of treatment is directed at trying to resolve underlying impairments and helping patients to recover strategies that will enable them to perform the key components of upper extremity control.

Assessing Key Components of Upper Extremity Control

In previous chapters, we described the second level of a task-oriented assessment as a **strategy assessment**. A strategy assessment is a qualitative examination of the way in which a subject coordinates movements to accomplish specific tasks. It also includes strategies for organizing sensory/perceptual information underlying a particular task. In this chapter, strategy assessment refers to the evaluation of the key elements of upper extremity control that underlie a broad range of functional skills. Ideally, assessment of upper extremity control would evaluate these key elements separately. Thus, standardized tests would allow the evaluation of the following key components in patients with upper extremity dysfunction: (*a*) eye-head coordination, (*b*) postural control (weightbearing on arms for support, as well as postural adjustments in the legs and trunk, which support reaching movements), (*c*) arm and hand transport, (*d*) grasp and release (fine pincer and power grasp), and (*e*) manipulation skills, including in-hand manipulation as well as bilateral manipulation skills. In addition, tests would assess the patient's ability to adapt these components to changes in task and environmental demands. For example, they would assess the ability to adapt grasp to objects of different size, shape, weight, and texture.

There is a great need for standardized assessment tests that isolate and evaluate key components of upper extremity manipulatory function. The development of such tests would allow clinicians to isolate and quantify problems in key components and suggest directions for clinical intervention.

LOCATING A TARGET—EYE-HEAD COORDINATION

Research has shown that when an object to be grasped appears in the peripheral visual field, there is normally a predictable sequence of movements. The eyes reach the target first, then the head, and finally the arm. Locating an object to be grasped requires various combinations of eye, head, and trunk motion, depending on the location of the object with reference to the visual field (20). Apparently, these task-specific movements of the eye, head, and/or trunk are controlled by different systems. Thus, evaluating eye-head coordination underlying the ability to locate an object to be grasped requires the assessment of three systems: eye movements to a target close to the central visual field; eye and head movements to a target located in the periphery; and eye, head, and trunk movements to locate a target, which is even more eccentric (20).

A clinical approach to assessing eye-head coordination has been proposed based on this understanding of the separate systems controlling eye-head movements (21, 22). Eye movements used to locate targets presented within the central visual field are assessed first. The patient is asked to keep the head still and move only the eyes. Both saccadic eye movements to fixed targets and smooth pursuit eye movements used to track moving targets are tested. This is shown in Figure 18.2. The patient's ability to locate the target with the eyes and maintain a stable gaze on the target for 15 seconds is assessed (22). Eye movements are graded subjectively according to a three-point scale: intact, impaired, or unable. In addition, any subjective complaints related to blurred or unstable vision reported by the patient are recorded. In assessing our patient, Mrs. Poirot, you might note that she has difficulty making accurate eye movements to targets that are presented in her right visual field. She also has difficulty tracking moving targets.

Next, the patient's ability to locate and

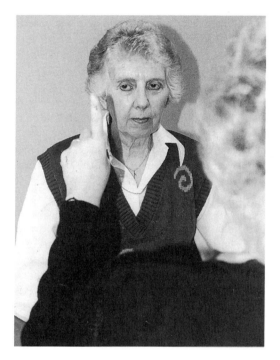

Figure 18.2. Testing the patient's ability to make saccadic eye movements to locate and maintain gaze on a target located within the near peripheral field.

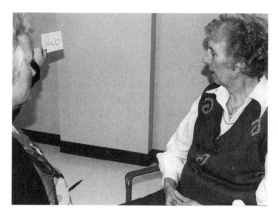

Figure 18.3. Testing eye-head coordination. The patient's ability to make coordinated eye-head movements to locate a target in the far peripheral visual field is shown.

stabilize gaze on targets presented in the peripheral visual field is assessed. This is shown in Figure 18.3. The coordination of combined eye-head movements is graded subjectively using the three-point scale just presented. Patients should be able to localize a target with the eyes and maintain a stable gaze on that target while the head is moving. We note that Mrs. Poirot is able to make coordinated eye-head movements to targets located in her left periphery, but is unable to coordinate eye-head movements to targets presented on her right.

Finally, the patient's ability to make eye-head-trunk movements necessary to locate targets oriented in the far periphery is assessed. In the case of Mrs. Poirot, you may note that she evidences a similar inability to make coordinated eye, head, and trunk movements to targets presented in her far right visual field.

Patients are tested initially in the seated position; however, depending on the patient's

abilities, eye-head coordination may be tested in standing and during walking as well (22).

EYE-HAND COORDINATION

Tests of visuomotor coordination evaluate the coordination between vision and arm movements. With the growing use of personal computers, many tests have been computerized, using a joystick and computerized video graphics to examine the ability to track still or moving visual targets presented on a computer screen (23). Computerized visual tracking tests allow the objective quantification of errors in eye-hand coordination. Unfortunately, they do not distinguish between errors that result from an inability to visually locate and maintain a stable gaze on the target and movement errors in controlling the joystick.

REACH AND GRASP

Reach and grasp is a sensory-motor skill with higher level adaptive components as well. Locating a target in space requires visual pathways including areas from the visual cortex to the parietal lobe, the so-called "where" pathways (see Chapter 3 for further information on these pathways). This information is then used to form an action plan that allows coordinated movements of the eyes, head, and hand in space.

The motor plan is task-dependent. When the task involves pointing, the arm and the hand are controlled as a unit. In contrast, when the task involves grasping an object, the arm that is involved in the transport part of the movement is controlled separately from the hand, which is involved in the grasp portion of the movement. While these two components are controlled separately, they are linked spatially and temporally.

Grasp formation begins during the transport phase of movement. We are not aware of any standardized tests that evaluate and document specific movement strategy problems related to the organization and coordination of the different components of movements involved in reach and grasp. The following sections offer suggestions to help the clinician think about ways to assess movement strategies used in reach and grasp. We too await the development of standardized systematic assessment tools for assessing reach and grasp.

Transport Phase of Reach

Remember from previous chapters that reaching is task-dependent. Thus, the characteristics of the movement (for example, how fast one moves or how straight the trajectory is) depend on the nature of the task being performed. Therefore, when assessing the transport phase of reaching, the clinician will want to use a variety of tasks. For example, tasks could include pointing at a target, reaching for and grasping a target, or reaching, grasping, and lifting a target. Though these tasks use a variety of grasp components, only the transport phase will be observed at this point.

In addition, one will want to locate the targets at different places relative to the patient's body, for example, ipsilateral to the reaching arm vs. on the contralateral side of the body, and close to the patient vs. far away (within arm's reach or requiring forward lean of the trunk).

What should the clinician be looking at in order to assess the efficiency of the trans-

port phase of reach? First, one can look at the accuracy of the transport phase itself. In addition, one can look at the duration of transport, determining the time it takes for the patient to get to the target. Yet, the greatest insight comes from observing the movement profile itself, including the relative coordination among the segments of the upper extremity making the movement.

What modifications would you expect to see in Mrs. Poirot's transport phase of a reaching movement when she performs various types of tasks? Normally, when you grasp and lift an object, the movement speed will be faster than if you simply point at an object, since the momentum of the transport phase can be used to assist the lifting of the object. You should ask yourself: does the patient continue the momentum during the entire reaching movement? Does the patient slow the movement unnecessarily in order to grasp the object prior to the lift? During a reach and grasp task, involving a stationary target, does the patient show clear acceleration and deceleration of the movement profile, slowing the movement appropriately in order to grasp the object rather than knocking it over?

To assist in improving the ability to analyze the different characteristics of the transport phase, videotaping the movements may be helpful. Videotaping allows the clinician to view the movement over and over, analyzing its various components. In addition, the ability to slow the videotape and stop the film as necessary can facilitate the clinician's ability to understand the movement profile. Use of videotaping can be helpful to understanding the movement, but it is time-consuming, and for that reason is not often used on a routine basis in the clinic.

Remember from Chapter 15 that there is a relationship between movement speed, distance, and accuracy; this is represented by Fitts' law (24). Thus, when subjects are asked to move with greater accuracy, they slow down. Clinicians who are assessing task-dependent movements involved in reaching should examine the relationship between the patient's movement speed and accuracy. For example, one approach to examining this trade-off between speed and accuracy would be to have the patient hold a pencil and time how long it takes the patient to move the pencil point back and forth 10 times between two circles, drawn on a piece of paper. One could tell the patient to move as fast as possible while attempting to place the pencil point within the circle. Accuracy is determined by the number of dots outside the two circles. The difficulty of the task can be varied by how large the circles are, and how far apart they are. This gives the clinician insight into the patient's ability to make accurate movements and how he or she improves performance with respect to speed and accuracy over time. We might anticipate that Mrs. Poirot will show impairments in movement time and accuracy in both her arms, with deficits more pronounced in the hemiparetic arm.

Finally, during the process of assessing reach, the clinician will want to look at the patient's ability to use visual information to correct the accuracy of a reach. One approach could use prism glasses to offset the visual image that the subject sees. During the course of a reach, once the hand comes into view, the person perceives the error between the hand position and the perceived target position and uses visual cues to update the movement path to reach the target accurately. Using this type of test, we would expect that Mrs. Poirot would be unable to use visual feedback and therefore would be unable to correct the movement path, thus making inaccurate reaches.

Grasp

The same types of tasks that were used to evaluate the transport portion of a reach and grasp movement can be used to assess grasp. Now the clinician will focus on evaluating the characteristics of the grasp portion of the movement. Again, videotaping a patient's performance will assist the clinician in identifying problems related to hand orientation and grasp formation. In addition to the tasks mentioned earlier, the clinician might want to structure tasks that include gripping objects of different orientation, gripping objects of different sizes and shapes, gripping objects of different weights, gripping and lifting objects, vs. gripping and throwing objects, vs. gripping and fitting objects into holes. Finally, the clinician might want to assess the patient's ability to reach and grasp not only stationary objects but those that are moving at various speeds.

What should the clinician watch for when assessing grasp? It will be important to observe the orientation of the hand and the shape of the fingers relative to the thumb during the reach. One should ask: At what point in the movement trajectory does the hand open maximally, and then begin to close in anticipation of a grasp? It is also important to observe the position of the thumb during the course of the movement. Does it remain in a stable position during the course of the movement, thereby serving as a reference point for the reach and grasp?

Remember that grip formation takes place during the transportation phase and is anticipatory of the characteristics of the object to be grasped. Some problems you might expect to see in patients who have impaired grasp formation are (a) an absence of anticipatory hand shaping during the transport phase of the movement, (b) a hand that does not close appropriately in relation to the object to be grasped, or alternatively closes too soon, or (c) an inability to alter the hand shape to accommodate objects of different shapes and sizes.

Questions that should be asked concerning the patient's performance are: What type of grip does the patient use? Does the patient vary the number of fingers used during grasp, depending on weight and size characteristics of the object to be lifted? Does the patient show errors in slip or in pushing the object to be gripped into the surface? Our patient, Mrs. Poirot, makes frequent errors in programming grip and lift forces, as evidenced by the fact that objects frequently slip from her grasp when she is trying to lift. Also, she sometimes uses too much force when lifting a paper cup, causing compression of the sides of the cup and spilling of the liquid inside. This suggests errors in the programming of grip and lift forces.

IN-HAND MANIPULATION SKILLS

In-hand manipulation is defined as the process of adjusting objects within the hand after grasp. The In-Hand Manipulation Skills (TIME) test evaluates in-hand manipulation skills based on Exner's Classification system (10). This test examines the following categories of in-hand manipulation skills: (*a*) translation, that is, moving an object from the fingers to the palm and back, as when picking up a coin and moving it to the palm; (*b*) shift, defined as adjusting the position of an object held near the DIP joints of the fingers with the thumb opposed, for example, moving a pen so it is held closer to the point for easier writing; (*c*) rotation (simple or complex) involving rotating an object, stabilizing, and then moving the object, for example, turning a paper clip so it can be used.

POSTURAL CONTROL

Examining the ability of the patient to control the body's position in space during the execution of upper extremity movements is an important part of assessing upper extremity manipulatory control. There are several ways one could assess the relationship between postural control and manipulation skills. One approach would be to keep the manipulation task constant and vary the postural conditions. For example, one could ask a patient to reach for a target while sitting in a chair with support, vs. a chair with no back support, vs. standing on a firm surface or a moving surface. The clinician would observe the patient's ability to maintain stability and the patient's ability to maintain the efficiency and accuracy of the reaching task, as postural conditions become more stringent.

An alternative approach to examining the relationship between posture and upper extremity control would be to maintain a constant postural condition, such as standing unsupported, and to vary the destabilizing characteristics of the upper extremity task. For example, lifting a light object slowly while standing is less destabilizing to the body's position in space than lifting a heavy object quickly. For further ideas, refer to the chapter on clinical assessment of postural control.

ASSESSING PLANNING AND SEQUENCING OF ACTIVITIES OF DAILY LIVING

As you remember from Chapter 17, deficits in executive control can impair a patient's ability to carry out functional ADL activities. This causes the patient to produce frequent errors resulting from misuse of objects, to perform actions out of sequence, and to perseverate on tasks. Tasks that require planning and organization over time are most frequently affected. These types of problems have been referred to as frontal apraxia by Luria (25–28).

It has been suggested that to evaluate these types of performance errors, you need a descriptive theory that will allow you to pick out units of action and define their properties at different levels of organization. Such a descriptive theory of action has been suggested, and is the basis for an action coding system that allows the identification and documentation of performance errors associated with ADL (26).

This action coding system takes commonly performed ADL and breaks them down into their constituent parts, hierarchically organizing them and identifying those units that are critical to achieving the goal (26).

At the lowest level of the action hierarchy are what the authors refer to as A1 level and A1 crux level acts. Multiple A1 level acts are then combined into A2 level acts, which are basic task subgoals. For example, when sugaring a cup of coffee to drink, opening the sugar is considered an A1 level action, pouring the sugar into the coffee is considered a critical or A1 crux level of action, and stirring the coffee is another A1 action. The aggregation of all these level A1's form the basic A2 task subgoal of putting the sugar into the coffee (26).

This type of action coding system allows identification of the type and frequency of errors when performing a task. For example, a patient might attempt to pour sugar into his coffee prior to opening the sugar packet. Or, the patient might stir hot water with his spoon prior to putting in the coffee. Or, the patient could reach for the sugar and get distracted by the butter, which is nearby, and does not satisfy the A1 crux, or the goal of the task (26).

When applying this type of analysis to Mrs. Poirot's ADL skills, we might expect to see frequent errors in sequencing her performance and to be frequently distracted and unable to fulfill the goal of the task.

This approach to evaluating ADL performance errors is now under development. It offers great potential for clinicians in identifying and documenting higher level problems affecting the planning and execution of upper extremity tasks.

Assessing Impairments Affecting Upper Extremity Function

The third level of assessment of upper extremity control examines the sensory, motor, and cognitive subsystems and processes involved in the generation of task-specific movement. These include measurement of musculoskeletal and neuromuscular limitations, including range of motion, strength, spasticity, mass patterns, assessment of sensory impairments, and evaluation of cognitive and perceptual limitations. Since assessment of these underlying systems has been discussed in detail in previous clinical chapters, only a brief review of strategies for assessing impairments specific to upper extremity control is presented.

RANGE OF MOTION

Since mobility in the hand and arm is necessary to upper extremity function, evaluating and documenting limitations in active and passive joint motion in upper extremity joints are important for understanding performance limitations. Limitation in joint motion can be documented using goniometric recordings. Decreased motion is often an indirect effect of neurological lesion, associated with paresis, mass flexion patterns, or spasticity.

The American Society for Surgery of the Hand (29) recommends a composite measure to represent joint motion of the fingers and thumb. Total active motion (TAM) is the sum of active flexion measurements of the metacarpophalangeal, proximal, and distal interphalangeal joints, minus the active extension deficits of the same joints. Total passive motion (TPM) is calculated in the same way, using passive measurements. Total motion measures provide a single value that represents the total active motion of a digit. This approach to measurement is discussed more fully elsewhere (2).

STRENGTH

The ability to generate force is fundamental to moving the arm for upper extremity function. Generally, the ability to generate force is evaluated through manual muscle testing, which examines strength during a concentric voluntary contraction. As described in previous chapters, strength testing in the patient with an upper motor neuron lesion is controversial (review Chapters 10 and 14).

Among the concerns related to strength testing in patients with neurological disorders is whether the ability to generate force during a manual muscle test accurately predicts the muscle's capacity to function properly during a task-dependent movement. While there is no universal agreement on many of the issues related to strength testing, it continues to be considered an essential part of an evaluation of upper extremity function. It is particularly important to evaluate strength of both the extrinsic and intrinsic muscles of the hand. Strength of pinch and grasp can be measured using manual muscle tests.

An objective measurement of grip strength can be determined using a dynamometer, shown in Figure 18.4 (Jamar Dynamometer, Asimow Engineering Co, Los

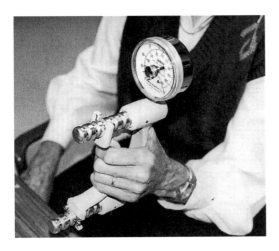

Figure 18.4. A Jamar dynamometer can be used to objectively measure grip strength.

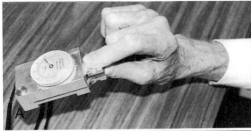

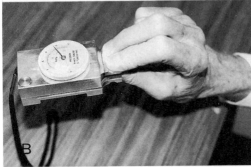

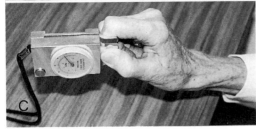

Figure 18.5. Use of a pinch meter to measure precision grip strength. Three types of pinch are assessed: **A**, tip-to-tip, **B**, three-point chuck, and **C**, key or lateral grip.

Angeles) (30–32). The use of a dynamometer allows grip strength to be evaluated at various hand widths. This is important because grip strength varies according to the size of the object being grasped (2, 33). Normative tables for grip function are available (34–35).

Dynamometer testing requires that the patient have sufficient grip strength to grasp the dynamometer. In cases of very weak grip, a bulb dynamometer, or a blood pressure cuff rolled to 5 cm and inflated to 5 mm Hg, can be used to document grip strength. Change in the millimeters of mercury is recorded as the power of grip (33).

Electronic pinch meters (Pinch Gauge, B&L Engineering, Santa Fe Springs, CA) can be used to measure strength of pinch (33). Usually, three types of pinch are assessed: (*a*) tip-to-tip (thumb tip to index finger tip), (*b*) thumb pulp to index and long finger pulp (3-point chuck), and (*c*) thumb pulp to lateral aspect of index finger (key or lateral grip). These are shown in Figure 18.5. The mean of three trials is compared to norms that are specific to the type of pinch meter used.

ABNORMAL SYNERGIES

In the patient who has suffered a stroke, a major constraint on the ability to move the shoulder, elbow, and hand voluntarily is the presence of abnormal synergies of movement (36, 37). Determining the degree to which a patient is constrained by abnormal synergies is still considered by many clinicians an important part of assessing upper extremity control in stroke patients (38).

The assessment scale shown in Table 18.1 was proposed by Signe Brunnstrom (36) and is based on proposed stages of recovery as indicated by the degree to which voluntary control is constrained by abnormal synergistic movement. This approach to assessment is the basis for the more recent test, the Fugl Myer Measurement of Physical Performance used to quantify movement disorders in the patient who has had a stroke (37).

SENSATION

Sensation testing is a critical part of evaluating hand function because degree of sen-

Table 18.1.   Hemiplegia—Classification and Progress Record. Upper Limb—Test Sitting[a]

Name_____Age_____Date of onset_____Side affected_____

Date

_____ Passive motion sense, shoulder_____elbow_____

_____ pron.-supin._____wrist flex.-ext._____

_____ 1. NO MOVEMENT INITIATED OR ELICITED_____

_____ 2. SYNERGIES OR COMPONENTS FIRST APPEARING. Spasticity developing_____

_____   Flexor synergy_____

_____   Extensor synergy_____

_____ 3. SYNERGIES OR COMPONENTS INITIATED VOLUNTARILY. Spasticity marked_____

FLEXOR SYNERGY		Active Joint Range			Remarks
Shoulder girdle	Elevation				
	Retraction				
Shoulder joint	Hyperextension Abduction				
	Ext. rotation				
Elbow	Flexion				
Forearm	Supination				
EXTENSOR SYNERGY					
Shoulder	Pectoralis major				
Elbow	Extension				
Forearm	Pronation				
4. MOVEMENTS DEVIATING FROM BASIC SYNERGIES Spasticity decreasing	Hand to sacral region				
	Raise arm forw.-horiz.				
	Pron.-supin. elbow at 90°				
5. RELATIVE IN-DEPENDENCE OF BASIC SYNERGIES Spasticity waning	Raise arm side-horiz.				
	Raise arm over head				
	Pron.-supin. elbow extended				
6. MOVEMENT COORDINATION NEAR NORMAL. Spasticity minimal					

[a]From Brunnstrom S. motor testing procedures in hemiplegia: based on sequential recovery stage. Phys Ther. 1966; 46: 357–375.

sibility has been shown to be a valid predictor of recovery of hand function (39–41). Sensory testing includes two-point discrimination, cutaneous sensation (monofilament test), stereognosis, vibration, proprioception (or position sense), thermal (head/cold), and pain (pin-prick).

A hierarchy of sensory testing in the upper extremity has been suggested (2). The simplest level of sensory function is the ability to discriminate a single point touch-pressure stimulus. Touch-pressure sensibility can be assessed objectively by using calibrated nylon monofilaments (42–43). The use of gradu-

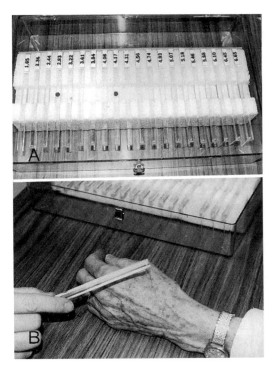

Figure 18.6. The use of graduated nylon monofilaments to test touch/pressure sensibility. **A,** A standardized series of graduated monofilaments is used to test **B,** touch pressure.

ated nylon monofilaments (Fig. 18.6) is considered one of the most reliable and valid tests of sensory capacity and its relationship to functional abilities. A detailed description of sensory testing and norms using graduated monofilaments may be found in a review by Levin and colleagues (41).

The next level in the proposed sensory hierarchy is two-point discrimination. This test examines the patient's ability to detect two stimuli applied simultaneously to the upper extremities. The ability to detect still and moving stimuli is tested. Reliability can be increased by using a commercial two-point discriminator testing instrument (2). Two-point discrimination tests can be important predictors of recovery of hand function. Studies have shown that an inability to discriminate between two points applied simultaneously to the fingertips 1 cm apart is predictive for poor recovery of hand function (44). Recovery of hand function can be im-

proved if patients can learn to substitute vision for impaired tactile sensation (44).

The ability to discriminate textures is proposed as the next level of sensory/perceptual hierarchy. This includes the ability to distinguish the roughest, smoothest, and most irregular textures. Finally, at the top of the proposed sensory/perceptual hierarchy is object recognition, representing the most complex of the sensory/perceptual skills (2).

EDEMA AND PAIN

Upper extremity edema is a common problem in many types of patients and is attributed to an inadequate pumping mechanism acting on the venous and lymphatic systems; this reduces the functional abilities of the hand by restricting motion. Edema can be measured using circumferential assessment (measurement of the circumference of the hand) or through volumetric assessment (44, 45).

Volumetric assessment measures the water displaced when a limb is immersed. There are numerous commercially available volumeters consisting of a plastic tank with a dowel centered in the lower third of the container to control the depth of hand immersion. A spout at the top of the container allows the displaced water to collect in a 500-ml graduated cylinder (46). There are significant differences between dominant and nondominant hands, suggesting that clinicians should not compare volume measurement of affected and unaffected arms. Instead, volume of the impaired extremity should be compared to itself over time (44).

Volumetric assessment of upper extremity edema can be carried out in sitting or in standing, and shows high test-retest reliability. However, volumes are lower in sitting than in standing, suggesting the importance of maintaining a consistent position during testing. Best reliability in testing is found when volumetric assessment is performed in the seated position (44).

Another complication that interferes with the recovery of upper extremity function is pain. Assessment of pain usually involves questioning the patient about the location and extent of pain symptoms, determining whether pain is constant or intermittent, and whether it is present at rest or only when the patient moves. Intensity of pain is determined by asking the patient to grade the intensity of the pain on a subjective scale, for example, on a scale of 0 to 5 or 0 to 10 (47–49).

In summary, a comprehensive assessment of upper extremity function requires a battery of measures that examine performance at many different levels. Further information on guidelines for assessment of hand function can be found through the American Society for Surgery of the Hand (29) and the American Society of Hand Therapists (50).

TRANSITION TO TREATMENT

Developing therapeutic strategies to retrain upper extremity control in the patient with neurological dysfunction begins with the identification of a comprehensive list of patient problems, including both the functional limitations, or disabilities, as well as the specific impairments that constrain function (51). As mentioned in Chapter 5, when identifying impairments, it is important from a therapeutic standpoint to distinguish permanent impairments from those that are temporary and thus potentially amenable to treatment.

From a comprehensive list, the therapist and patient identify priority problems that will become the focus for initial intervention strategies (52). Thus, a list of short- and long-term treatment goals that are objective and measurable are established and a specific treatment plan is formulated for each of the problems identified.

Short-Term Goals

Short-term goals should be described in objective and measurable terms. They may be described in terms of resolving impairments and recovery of key components of upper extremity control, including (*a*) eye-head coordination, (*b*) postural control (weightbearing on arm for support, as well as trunk control for reaching movements), (*c*) arm and hand transport, (*d*) grasp and release (fine pincer and power grasp), (*e*) manipulation skills, including in-hand manipulation as well as bilateral manipulation skills. In addition, short-term goals may be described in terms of interim steps to achieving independence in a functional task.

Long-Term Goals

As proposed in Chapter 5, long-term goals should be objective and measureable, and can be expressed in terms of recovery of functional capacity of the upper extremity, related to either ADL, work, or use of the upper extremity in posture and mobility tasks.

TREATMENT

The goals of a task-oriented approach to retraining the patient with upper extremity manipulatory dyscontrol include (*a*) resolve or prevent impairments; (*b*) develop strategies related to the recovery of the key components of upper extremity control, including eye-head coordination, postural control, arm and hand transport, grasp and release (fine pincer and power grasp), and manipulation skills (in-hand as well as bilateral skills), and (*d*) retrain functional tasks, including the capacity to adapt strategies so that functional tasks can be performed in changing environmental contexts.

The therapeutic techniques used to retrain upper extremity control will vary, depending on the particular constellation of problems facing each patient. For example, retraining ADL skills in a patient with hemiplegia may require passive mobilization of proximal (trunk, scapula, and shoulder complex) and distal structures to remediate musculoskeletal impairments. The presence of weakness and neuromuscular dyscontrol may require clinical techniques to facilitate active movement necessary for transporting the arm and hand in space. Sensory reeducation may be used to improve sensibility. For those patients constrained by impaired eye-head coordination, a program to improve visual location and gaze stabilization may be appropriate. Finally, strategies to retrain grasp and release capability in the hand will likely be needed.

Is Proximal Control a Prerequisite for Retraining Hand Function?

Current research examining the neural basis for reach and grasp has a number of important implications for clinicians when retraining upper extremity control in the patient with a neurological lesion. Research on normal reaching suggests that proximal functions including posture, arm, and hand transport, are controlled by different mechanisms from those controlling distal functions related to grasp and release. In addition, studies have shown that CNS lesions can have a selective effect on transport versus manipulation aspects of upper extremity function. Because these two aspects of upper extremity function are controlled separately, they may recover at different rates (53).

In addition, the degree to which recovery occurs is dependent on the extent to which other areas of the CNS can substitute for those parts of the CNS that are injured. Proximal functions involving the transport phase and/or stability, may be easily substituted by other neural mechanisms. In contrast, lesions affecting precision movements of the hand may find no substitute in the CNS, and thus recovery may be limited.

On a hopeful note, research suggests that training can help improve hand function despite lesions to areas thought to be critical to these movements. Cortically controlled hand movements require more attention and active participation of the subject than do automatic movements (58, 59). In addition, cortically induced movements require long periods of training and are very labor-intensive (53, 60).

Thus, it does not appear that control over proximal body segments is a necessary precursor to working on distal hand function, suggesting that the two can be worked on simultaneously, rather than sequentially (53). It may not be necessary to wait for proximal control to emerge before working on hand function, since the two systems controlling them are different.

Treating at the Impairment Level

The goal of treatments aimed at the impairment level is to correct those impairments that can be changed, and prevent the development of secondary impairments. Alleviating underlying impairments enables the patient to resume using previously developed strategies for upper extremity control. When permanent impairments make resumption of previously used strategies impossible, new strategies will have to be developed.

Treatment strategies aimed at modifying sensory and motor impairments were presented in detail in Chapters 10 and 14. A brief discussion of some treatment suggestions often used in modifying impairments in the upper extremity are presented below (61–63).

REDUCING MUSCULOSKELETAL IMPAIRMENTS

An important part of retraining upper extremity control is reducing the musculoskeletal constraints that develop secondary to other impairments such as paresis or spasticity. Passive and active exercises are used to mobilize structures essential to upper extremity control, including both proximal structures such as the trunk, scapula, and shoulder musculature, as well as distal structures involving the hand and wrist.

Many sources describe in detail approaches to mobilizing the trunk, scapula, and shoulder structures in the patient with a neurological impairment (37, 61–65). These techniques, however, have yet to be validated through controlled research. For example, Figure 18.7 shows one approach to mobilizing musculoskeletal structures in the trunk, arm, and hand (63). In this approach, the patient is in the supine position, and rotates the shoulders and hips in the opposite direction to lengthen the trunk (63). This approach is used to elongate trunk, arm, and hand muscles that have shortened because of paresis or spasticity.

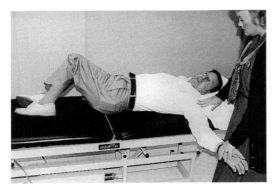

Figure 18.7. Counter-rotation between the shoulders and hips results in elongation of the trunk and is used to reduce muscle tightness in trunk muscles.

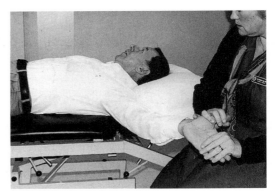

Figure 18.8. Passive extension of the wrist and hand to reduce tightness in the upper extremity.

Elongating tight wrist and hand flexors is often considered a necessary part of retraining upper extremity control in the patient with a neurological deficit. Hemiplegic patients who habitually hold the involved upper extremity in mass flexion develop tightness of these structures, which limits return of active movement. Figure 18.8 gives an example of how the wrist and hand can be brought into extension passively in order to lengthen tight muscles (61–63).

Other approaches to remediating musculoskeletal constraints include the use of plaster casts, splints, and orthoses to increase range of motion and mobility of arm and hand structures (66–72).

The use of splints, whether passive or dynamic, will not be covered within the context of this book. The reader is referred to other texts that discuss splints in detail (64, 66, 72–76). The use of upper extremity weightbearing activities that stretch hand and arm structures has also been suggested as an approach to reducing musculoskeletal limitations (37, 61–63). Upper extremity weightbearing activities include having the patient practice maintaining body weight through an extended arm placed to the side (Fig. 18.9A), to the back (Fig. 18.9B), and to the front of the body (Fig. 18.9C). In addition, weightbearing through an extended arm can be practiced in the standing position (Fig. 18.10).

While these activities are routinely suggested as part of most upper extremity retraining programs, it is important to note that research validating the effectiveness of these techniques has not yet been done.

SENSORY REEDUCATION

A number of reports have been published that recount approaches to retraining sensibility in patients with peripheral and central neural injuries resulting in decreased sensation (77–79). How much can functional sensation be improved following a peripheral or central lesion affecting sensibility? The answer is: we don't know.

Several authors have recommended that sensory reeducation programs focus on both discriminative and protective sensory functions (39, 78–81). Early training focuses on the detection and localization of moving and stationary light touch stimuli. As patients learn to perceive constant and moving touch, sensory reeducation focuses on learning to discriminate size and shape, object recognition, and two-point discrimination. A large part of the training makes use of higher cortical functions, including attention, learning, and memory, to facilitate sensory detection, recognition, and localization (78). Tactile retraining generally occurs both with and without vision.

Since the patient with decreased sensibility will not experience discomfort or pain, an important part of sensory reeducation is teaching patients strategies to protect the

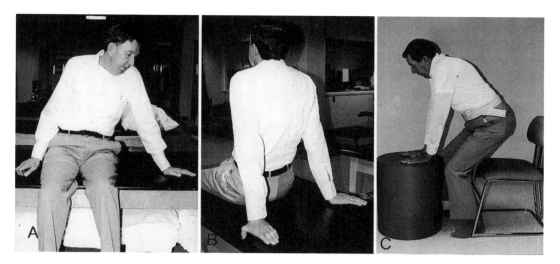

Figure 18.9. Upper extremity weightbearing activities. Retraining upper extremity weightbearing **A**, to the side; **B**, to the rear; and **C**, forward.

limb with decreased sensation from noxious and injurious stimuli (80). To protect the hand and arm from injury, a series of guidelines have been recommended and are summarized in Table 18.2.

It is unclear whether sensory reeducation teaches patients how to use the remaining sensibility to their advantage or whether it actually alters the physiological basis for sensation (39). For example, since it is known that moving stimuli are more detectable than stationary stimuli, the patient can be taught to move the hand to achieve a moving stimulus, and thus improve the chances for sensory awareness. Alternatively, vision can be used to compensate for deficits in tactile sensation; thus, the patient can be taught to look at the hand when reaching or grasping for an object (39).

Investigators involved in retraining sensory function report that the capacity to adapt to impaired sensibility is dependent on the patient's motivation as well as training. Those patients who were willing to use the impaired limb were better able to recover function. For a more complete discussion of methods for sensory reeducation, the reader is referred to articles by Callahan (79) and Bell-Krotoski and colleagues (39).

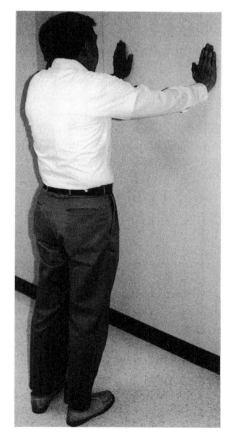

Figure 18.10. Upper extremity weightbearing can also be trained in the standing position.

Table 18.2. Protective Strategies for Patients with Decreased Sensibility in the Upper Extremity[a]

1. Avoid exposure to thermal extremes and sharp objects.
2. Do not use excessive force when gripping a tool or object.
3. Build up small handles in order to distribute force and avoid localized increase in pressure.
4. Avoid tasks that require the use of a uniform grip over long periods of time.
5. Change tools frequently to alter grip and to rest tissues.
6. Observe skin for signs of stress.
7. Treat blisters and lacerations quickly and with care to avoid infection.
8. Maintain daily skin care including soaking, and oil massage to maintain optimal skin condition.

[a]Adapted from Brand PW. Management of sensory loss in the extremities. In: Omer E, Spinner M, eds. Management of peripheral nerve problems. Philadelphia: WB Saunders, 1980:262–272.

Retraining Key Components of Upper Extremity Control

A task-oriented approach to retraining involves more than just the resolution of impairments when possible. Ideally, patients should be guided to recover or develop sensory and motor strategies that are effective in performing the key components of upper extremity control. Since research has shown that key components such as reaching and grasping are driven by the nature of the task, retraining these key components must be done within the context of purposeful tasks. Therefore, we are combining a discussion of the two levels of training, the strategy and the adaptive task level, into one section.

RETRAINING EYE-HEAD COORDINATION

An important part of regaining upper extremity control is retraining eye-head coordination, which is essential to locating and stabilizing gaze on a target or object to be grasped. Problems that affect the ability to locate objects and stabilize gaze potentially affect the accuracy and precision of reaching movements. Since different control mechanisms underlie the movements of eyes, head, and trunk, these systems need to be trained separately and in combination.

A progression of exercises for retraining eye-head coordination and gaze stabilization in patients with vestibular dysfunction has been proposed by Susan Herdman, a physical therapist and David Zee, M.D., from Johns Hopkins University Medical School (21, 82). These exercises have been used successfully to retrain eye-head coordination problems in patients with central neurological disorders (83).

This approach is reviewed in Table 18.3 and begins with exercises to retrain saccadic and smooth-pursuit eye movements while the head is still (21, 82). Exercises are progressively given to retrain coordinated eye movements in conjunction with head movements to targets located in the peripheral visual field. Also practiced are exercises to maintain a stable gaze on an object moving in phase with the head. Finally, movements involving eye, head, and trunk motions are practiced as patients learn to locate targets oriented in the far periphery. Exercises are practiced in sitting, standing, and walking.

Research in the field of retraining visual perception in patients with central neural lesions is just beginning. Traditionally, strategies to assist patients with visual field deficits, such as homonymous hemianopsia, involved teaching patients to consciously scan the space represented by the impaired visual field.

Until recently, it was thought that lesions to the visual cortex resulted in permanent impairments to the visual system. However, as described in the previous chapter, patients with lesions in central visual structures are able to make fairly accurate eye movements and/or reaching movements to targets when told to move toward where they thought the object might be (84–85). Initially, patients were very poor at reaching for objects in this manner; however, their performance improved with practice (20).

These studies raise many questions about the potential for retraining visual function in the patient with impaired visual perception due to central neural lesions. Re-

Table 18.3.   Eye-Head Coordination Exercises for Gaze Stabilization[a]

Stage I. Eye Exercises

A. Exercises to improve visual following (smooth pursuit)
   1. Sit in a comfortable position; do not move your head.
   2. Hold a small target (about 2″ × 2″, like a matchbook cover) containing written material at arm's length in front of you.
   3. Keep your head still.
   4. Move your arm slowly from side to side (about 45°). Try to keep the words in focus as you move.
   5. Move your arm to the left, then right, then center. Rest for 3 seconds. Repeat 5 times.
   6. Move your arm up and down about 30°. Move your arm up, then down, then center. Rest for 3 seconds. Repeat 5 times.

B. Exercises to improve gaze redirection (saccade)
   1. Sit in a comfortable position; do not move your head.
   2. Hold two small targets (2″ × 2″) one in each hand, about 12″ apart in front of you.
   3. Move your eyes only from one target to the other.
   4. Move right, move left. Stop and rest.
   5. Repeat 5 times.
   6. Hold the two targets in front of you vertically, above and below the midline. Keep your head still; move your eyes only from one target to the other.
   7. Move eyes up, eyes down. Stop and rest.
   8. Repeat 5 times.

Stage II. Head Exercises

A. Move head, object still
   1. Side-to-side movements: Hold at arm's length a small target (like a matchbook). Try to keep the words in clear focus; move your head slowly from side to side. Move head to the right, move head left, move head to the center. Rest. Repeat 5 times.
   2. Up and down movements: Repeat, but move your head up and down while keeping your eyes on the target held in front of you. Move head up, move head down, come to the center. Stop and rest. Repeat 5 times.
   3. To progress yourself, move your head at faster and faster speeds, until you can no longer read the words. Repeat using a target that is attached to the wall, 6 feet away.
   4. Practice both (1) and (2) with your eyes closed. You should try to visualize in your mind the target, and focus on it as though your eyes were open.

Stage III. Eye-Head Exercises

A. Move eyes and head to stationary objects
   1. Side-to-side movements: Hold two small targets (2″ × 2″), one in each hand, about 36″ apart in front of you. Move your head and eyes to look at first, one target, then the other. Try to clearly focus on the words on each target each time you move your head and eyes. Look left, look right, then rest. Repeat 5 times.
   2. Up-and-down movements: Hold the two targets in front of you vertically, above and below the midline, about 36″ apart. Move your head and eyes to look at first, one target, then the other. Try to clearly focus on the words on each target each time you move your head and eyes. Look left, look right, then rest. Repeat 5 times.
   3. To progress yourself, repeat (1) and (2) moving your head at faster and faster speeds, until you can no longer read the words. Repeat, using a target that is attached to the wall, 6 feet away.

B. Move eyes and head and object in phase together
   1. Side-to-side movements: Hold a small target (about 2″ × 2″, like a matchbook cover) containing written material at arm's length in front of you. Move your arm and head together from side to side. Try to keep the words in clear focus while you move your arm and head together slowly from side to side (about 45°). Move left, move right, move center, and rest. Repeat 5 times.
   2. Up-and-down movements: Hold a small target (about 2″ × 2″, like a matchbook cover) containing written material at arm's length in front of you. Move your arm and head together up and down. Try to keep the words in clear focus while you move your arm and head together slowly up and down (about 30°). Move up, move down, move center, and rest. Repeat 5 times.
   3. To progress yourself, repeat (1) and (2) moving your head at faster and faster speeds, until you can no longer read the words. Repeat, using a target which is attached to the wall, 6 feet away.

[a]From Zee DS. Vertigo. Current therapy in neurologic disease. 1985:1–13.

search is needed to develop new strategies for retraining visual impairments, and to test the efficacy of these strategies on recovery of visual localization of targets in space.

RETRAINING THE TRANSPORT PHASE OF REACH

Transport requires the ability to move the arm in a coordinated way in all directions. It includes transporting the hand to an object to be grasped, as well as transporting the grasped object to a new location.

When a neurological lesion results in paresis and the inability to recruit motor neurons for active movement, retraining upper extremity movement control often begins with therapeutic strategies used to facilitate active motion by the patient. Several authors have laid out a progression of activities for retraining arm function primarily in stroke patients, which include retraining control of arm movements underlying the transport phase of upper extremity function (37, 61–63, 65).

Most of these suggestions relate to practicing control of isolated joint movements in supine, sitting, and standing. For example, retraining active control of arm movements is often begun in the supine position with the

shoulder flexed and the elbow extended (Fig. 18.11A). This position minimizes the amount of force the patient must generate to move the arm actively against gravity. In some cases, gravity can assist motion. For example, as shown in Figure 18.11B, when the patient is asked to touch his hand to his nose (or shoulder or head), gravity assists elbow flexion, while the patient eccentrically activates the triceps to control the descent of the hand.

Other seated activities involve exercises to regain concentric and eccentric contraction of shoulder flexors. The patient is asked to sit with the arm supported on a table (Fig. 18.12) and lift the arm, then drop the arm back to the surface. Shoulder horizontal abduction can be practiced by asking the patient to reach for the opposite shoulder with support given under the elbow as needed.

These exercises are based on the assumption that practicing activation of isolated muscles will carry over to functional tasks, including transport skills involving the arm and hand. As is true for most clinical intervention techniques, therapeutic strategies for retraining arm function are based on clinical observations, and have yet to be validated through controlled studies.

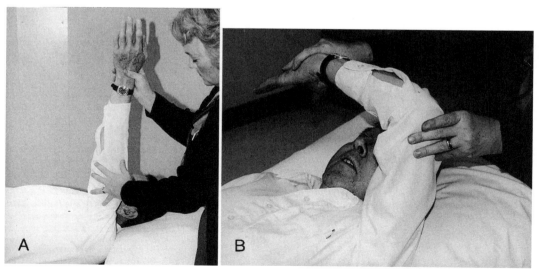

Figure 18.11.   Early retraining of active arm movement. Use of the supine position when retraining active control of the upper extremity can eliminate **A**, the effects of gravity; or **B**, alternatively make use of gravity to assist movement.

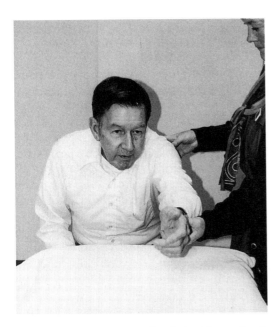

Figure 18.12. Practicing isolated shoulder motion in the sitting position.

Biofeedback and Functional Electrical Stimulation

Biofeedback and functional electrical stimulation (FES) have been used to facilitate motion in paretic limbs (86, 87). In one study, experimenters compared two different biofeedback approaches to retraining functional control of shoulder, elbow, and the distal upper extremity in 20 chronic stroke and six head-injured patients (1 to 7 years postinjury) (87). All patients had some ability to initiate voluntary wrist and finger extension and thumb abduction movements. Ten patients used a "motor copy" approach, in which patients attempted to activate muscles in the involved side using, as a reference, output from the noninvolved extremity. Ten patients used "targeted training," which required the patient to reduce activity in a spastic muscle and recruit activity in the antagonist muscle.

The study found that both approaches were equally effective in making changes in upper extremity function in patients with a chronic neurological lesion; however, the timing of those changes was different, since the motor copy group tended to show their improvements later than did the targeted training group (87).

Adaptive Positioning

Adaptive positioning, particularly modifying seat posture, has traditionally been considered an important approach to improving upper extremity control in the patient with a neurological impairment. Adaptive seating programs are based on three assumptions: (*a*) adaptive seating will reduce abnormal muscle tone; (*b*) improved muscle tone will improve the ability to stabilize posture; and (*c*) increased postural stability will increase the ability to control the upper extremity (88–91).

Several studies have examined the effect of altered seat angles on arm movements in children with and without cerebral palsy. While one study reported faster arm movements in cerebral palsy children with a backrest of 90° (92), most studies have not found that seating posture made a difference on immediate reaching movements, as measured through kinematic analysis of upper extremity movements (89, 93). These results do not rule out a long-term effect of altered seating posture on reaching.

Quite possibly, the effects of positioning are specific to the type of upper extremity task being performed. One study compared the effects of seating and prone standing in subjects with cerebral palsy on the Jebsen-Taylor Hand Function Test (94). This study examined the effects of positioning on the time required to complete eight simulated functional tasks on the Jebsen-Taylor test, and found that some subtests were performed faster in the seated position (small objects subtest), while other subtests were performed faster in the prone standing position (simulated feeding). The authors report the most atypical grasping patterns occurred during the simulated feeding subtest. These results suggest that the effects of positioning may be task-specific (94).

Retraining Task-Dependent Characteristics of Reach

Since the characteristics of the transport phase vary according to the task to be performed, it is important to structure retraining so that the patient learns to modify the movements used to transport the arm and hand in space in a task-dependent way. The following list offers various possible ways to retrain reaching based on research examining the characteristics of transport movements during upper extremity tasks. It is important to remember that these suggestions, like other suggestions made throughout this chapter, have yet to be validated through experimental testing.

1. Since the transport phase of movements such as pointing, reaching, and grasping, and reach, grasp, and moving an object have very different movement characteristics, one cannot train a patient in one task and expect that the performance skills will automatically carry over to the transport phase of the other reaching tasks. Therefore, we suggest that training needs to be specific to each of these task types.

2. It has been shown that visual feedback is important when making corrections during a movement for increased accuracy. Thus, training patients to become proficient in using visual information to correct ongoing movements is essential to retraining upper extremity control. To do this, the clinician should have the patient practice slower movements, drawing the patient's attention to visual cues relating hand movement, particularly thumb position to target location.

3. By asking the patient to move quickly in one motion to targets placed at various distances, the clinician can assist the patient in learning to modulate the initial forces needed to move the arm towards a target. In this way, the patient learns to program forces appropriately for quick and accurate movements.

4. Research also suggests that the ability to move to a new position in space without the use of visual feedback is important when making reaching movements. This can be accomplished through

modulation of stiffness in the agonist and antagonist muscles around the joints (refer back to the discussion of location programming in Chapter 15). By giving patients tasks requiring location programming, the clinician can assist the patient in learning to modulate levels of stiffness in the upper extremity. One approach might be to place the patient at a table where he/she could locate the target visually but not be allowed to see his/her hands. The clinician would determine if they could still be accurate in locating the target in space, based on programming stiffness of the agonist and antagonist muscles.

RETRAINING GRASP

Every day we are called upon to handle a great variety of objects that vary in size, shape, weight, and texture. Hand function requires the ability to grasp, release, and manipulate objects, as well as the capacity to adapt how we grasp in response to characteristics of the object to be grasped.

Often, retraining grasp function in the patient with paresis and dyscontrol begins with retraining a power grasp, then moves to progressively more precise grips (95). A power grasp utilizes a symmetrical grasp pattern and allows for cylindrical hold on objects.

When retraining power grasp, patients are often assisted in molding the hand to the shape of variously sized cylindrical objects with a symmetrical finger flexion pattern, with thumb opposed. Power grasp is practiced in both the vertical and horizontal planes. In addition, a power grip is critical to holding assistive mobility devices. This is shown in Figure 18.13.

It has been recommended that grasp retraining progress to teaching patients a succession of more precise grips. For example, patients are taught to grip using a three-jaw chuck pattern involving the thumb opposed to two fingers (95). Finally, a pincer grip (either tip-to-tip or lateral), which involves index finger and thumb opposition, is taught (refer back to Fig. 18.5 to review these grips).

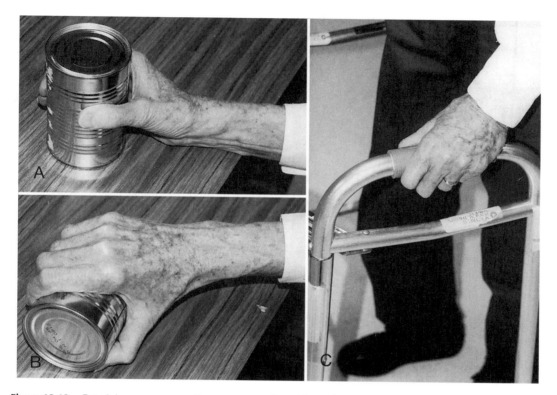

Figure 18.13.   Retraining power grasp. Power grasp used to pick up object oriented **A**, vertically; **B**, horizontally; **C**, in power grip on an assistive device for locomotion.

Retraining Task-Dependent Changes in Grasp

Research has shown that many of the elements of grasp, including how we orient and shape our hand and the amount of force we use to grip is preprogrammed, that is, determined before we even touch the object to be grasped. Hand orientation, shape, and force characteristics are determined based on our previous experience with grasping objects, in conjunction with our ability to perceive relevant cues about the object to be grasped. These two factors are used to program hand shape and force characteristics of grip (96–98).

ACTIVE LEARNING MODULE

You can see this for yourself. Your task is to pick up a glass and pour water in it from a pitcher held in the other hand. Place a cup in front of you, as shown in Figure 18.14A. Now reach for the cup and grasp it in preparation for pouring water into it. Notice the orientation of the hand and the movement you use to pick up the glass for this task. Now turn the glass over, as shown in Figure 18.14B. Your task is identical, to pour water into the glass without setting it down. Notice how you modify the orientation of your hand and the movement you use to accomplish the task.

Thus, an important part of regaining functional recovery of upper extremity control requires learning to modify grasp strategies for changing task demands. Retraining the ability to adapt grasp should address both motor and perceptual aspects of the task. This is because recovery of effective grip requires control over extrinsic and intrinsic muscles of the hand, as well as the ability to discriminate perceptual cues critical to preprogramming hand shape and force.

Errors in grasp, including gripping too

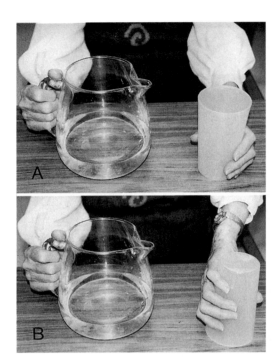

Figure 18.14. Modifying reach to changing task demands. **A**, Reaching for a cup when it is oriented right-side up. **B**, Changes in orientation of the hand when reaching for a cup that is inverted.

loosely and letting objects slip, or gripping too tightly and crushing objects, result from inappropriate force control. However, it is not always easy to determine if errors are the result of poor control over muscles, or alternatively, from errors in perceiving characteristics of the object to be gripped and thus programming force incorrectly.

Attending to Relevant Perceptual Cues

Modifying the shape of the hand and the force used to grasp are done in anticipation of the grasp, based on previous experience and relevant perceptual cues. Thus, an essential part of retraining hand function is helping patients relearn the capacity to discriminate perceptual cues, which are critical to programming hand shape, and force characteristics of grasp.

This could be accomplished by helping patients explore objects both visually and with their hands, drawing their attention to object characteristics that are important in correctly programming hand shape and force. Prior to actually grasping and lifting an object, asking patients questions about their perceptions regarding essential characteristics of an object is another way to help patients attend to relevant perceptual cues related to the task. For example, the clinician could ask: "Do you think that object is heavy or light? Is it slippery or not?"

Though research suggests that retraining perceptual aspects of grip is important to the recovery of control, strategies for such retraining are just emerging and have yet to be tested experimentally.

RELEASE

To achieve a functional grasp, patients not only must be able to grasp, but release objects. For many patients with neurological lesions, a power grasp is accomplished by using a mass pattern of flexion. While this pattern is successful in creating grasp, the patient is unable to actively extend the fingers and release the grasp without the assistance of the other hand. Alternatively, a patient may use wrist flexion to passively extend the fingers and thus accomplish release (64, 95).

Rhoda Erhardt, an occupational therapist, has published an extensive assessment form that describes a developmental sequence for releasing objects (95). This sequence has been used as the basis for a program to retrain release in the adult patient with a neurological impairment (64). The suggested sequence begins with learning to release an object that is externally stabilized. This approach is based on the observation that children learn to release an object externally stabilized on a supporting surface prior to learning to release objects in space (95).

Thus, patients are taught to release objects that are stabilized either by the patient's other hand, by the therapist's hand, or by a supporting surface. This is followed by learning to release objects that are not supported. Patients practice releasing an object using a pattern of finger extension with the wrist in neutral, as opposed to release resulting from wrist flexion, producing mechanical extension of the fingers.

IN-HAND MANIPULATION

An important part of recovery of hand function is helping patients regain the ability to manipulate objects within the hand itself, without setting the object down or transferring it to the opposite hand.

⊚ *ACTIVE LEARNING MODULE*

You can see this for yourself. Pick up a pencil and begin to write. Now, alter the position of the pencil so you can erase. In-hand manipulation skills enable you to change the position of the pencil in your hand without using the other hand, or setting the pencil down to alter your grip.

Patients learning to regain in-hand manipulation skills practice "intrinsic movements," which allow objects of various sizes and shapes to be moved within the hand itself. Movements practiced include (*a*) moving an object from the fingers to the palm and back, called translation, (*b*) rotating an object end over end, referred to as rotation, and (*c*) adjusting the position of an object held near the distal joints of the fingers with the thumb opposed, referred to as shift (99, 100).

POSTURAL CONTROL

As noted earlier, postural control is an important aspect of upper extremity control. Postural dyscontrol can be a contributing factor to problems related to upper extremity dysfunction. Therefore, treatment of postural disorders is considered a key component of retraining upper extremity control. This topic was covered in detail in Chapter 10, and the reader is urged to review concepts related to retraining postural activity associated with upper extremity movement.

RETRAINING PROBLEMS IN PLANNING AND SEQUENCING ACTIVITIES OF DAILY LIVING SKILLS

For many patients, limitation in the recovery of independence in ADL skills is not so much related to specific movement coordination and sensory disorders, as it is to problems in the planning and sequencing of everyday acts. The treatment of these types of problems is a complex issue and beyond the scope of this chapter.

Learned Disuse

A major constraint on recovery of arm function may be the unwillingness of patients to use an impaired upper extremity when the nonimpaired extremity is available. Thus, "learned disuse" in both primates and humans often follows sensory or motor loss affecting one side of the body (101–103). Researchers have known for many years that restraining the intact limb in monkeys will force the animal to use the impaired arm (104, 105). This knowledge has led to the development of "forced-use" paradigms to encourage the use of a chronically impaired upper extremity (106, 107).

In these research studies, hemiplegic patients (1 to 5 years poststroke or head-injured) were required to wear slings restraining the nonimpaired arm during waking hours for 14 days. In each case, patients spent 6 to 7 hours a day practicing tasks that required upper extremity function (eating, throwing a ball, writing, pushing a broom, manipulating checkers and pegs).

Results suggested that motor ability was significantly improved following restraint of the noninvolved arm in chronic stroke patients. Patients involved in the forced-use paradigm significantly improved ADL abilities compared to a control group, and improvements were sustained 1 to 2 years postintervention (106, 107).

Forced-use paradigms are still at a research stage in development. It is not clear if and how they might be used in retraining upper extremity control in the patient with an upper motor neuron lesion. Criteria need to be established for patients for whom this approach might be appropriate. Many patients are excluded from this type of treatment due to imbalance, and the need to use the unimpaired upper extremity for balance control and to prevent falls (106).

One important and encouraging aspect of these forced-use studies is the awareness that motor improvements are possible even in chronically impaired patients who are 1 to 5 years post-onset.

SUMMARY

1. Retraining control of the upper extremity is important to most areas of rehabilitation including physical and occupational therapy. While both areas of therapy retrain upper extremity control, physical therapists tend to focus on postural and mobility aspects of upper extremity function, while occupational therapists tend to function on ADL aspects, including the recovery of fine motor hand skills.

2. A task-oriented approach to assessment of upper extremity function requires a battery of tests that measure (a) functional performance, either ADL or work-related; (b) key components of control, including eye-head coordination, posture, transport, grasp and release, and manipulation; and (c) underlying sensory, motor, and cognitive impairments, including range of motion, strength, sensation, volume, and coordination.

3. Preparing treatment plans to retrain upper extremity control requires the identification of a comprehensive list of patient problems, including the functional limitations, or disabilities, as well as the specific impairments that constrain function. From this list, short- and long-term treatment goals are established, and therapeutic strategies are developed to meet those goals.

4. A task-oriented approach to retraining upper extremity control seeks to minimize impairments while maximizing the patient's capacity for function. Retraining involves the development of therapeutic strategies to (a) remediate as many sensory, motor, and cognitive impairments as possible, (b) generate strategies to achieve the key components of upper extremity control, and (c) develop the capacity to perform functional tasks under a variety of environmental contexts. This requires the development of adaptive capacity.

5. Research suggests that the development of control over proximal body segments is not a necessary precursor to the emergence of distal hand function. Proximal and distal segments of the upper extremity appear to be controlled separately, and therefore can be retrained simultaneously, rather than sequentially.

6. Hand function requires the ability to grasp, release, and manipulate objects, as well as the capacity to adapt how we grasp in response to characteristics of the object to be grasped. Many elements of grasp, including hand shape and force characteristics, are preprogrammed using previous experience and relevant perceptual cues about the object to be grasped. Thus, retraining hand function requires attention to both motor and perceptual aspects of the task.

7. Sensory reeducation programs focus on several aspects of sensory function including discrimination and protective sensory functions. It is unclear whether sensory reeducation teaches the patient how to use the remaining sensibility to their advantage, or whether it actually alters the physiological basis for sensation. It is clear, however, that the capacity to adapt to impaired sensibility is dependent on the patient's motivation as well as training. Studies have shown that those patients who were willing to use the impaired limb were better able to recover function.

8. A major constraint on recovery of arm function may be the unwillingness of patients to use an impaired upper extremity when the nonimpaired extremity is available. Results from studies examining "forced-use" paradigms suggest that motor ability can be significantly improved by limiting the hemiplegic patient's use of the noninvolved arm. One important and encouraging aspect of these forced-use studies is the awareness that motor improvements are possible even in chronically impaired patients who are 1 to 5 years post-onset.

REFERENCES

1. Smith HD. Assessment and evaluation: an overview. In: Hopkins HL, Smith HD, eds. Willard and Spackman's occupational therapy, 8th ed. Philadelphia: JB Lippincott, 1993:158–165.

2. Fess EE. Documentation: essential elements of an upper extremity assessment battery. In: Hunter JM, ed. Rehabilitation of the hand, 2nd ed. St. Louis: CV Mosby, 1990:53–81.

3. Bear-Lehman J, Abreu BC. Assessing the

hand: issues in reliability and validity. Phys Ther 1989;12:1025–1033.

4. Caldwell CB, Wilson DJ, Braun RM. Evaluation and treatment of upper extremity in the hemiplegic patient. Clin Orthop Rel Res 1969;63:69–93.

5. Katz S, Downs TD, Cash HR, Grotz RC. Progress in development of the index of ADL. Gerontologist 1970;1:20–30.

6. Keith RA, Granger CV, Hamilton BB, Sherwin FS. The functional independence measure: a new tool for rehabilitation. In: Eisentberg MG, Grzesiak RC, eds. Advances in clinical Rehabilitation, vol 1. New York: Springer-Verlag, 1987:6–18.

7. Granger CV, Albrecht GL, Hamilton BB. Outcome of comprehensive medical rehabilitation: measurement of PULSES profile and the Barthel index. Arch Phys Med Rehabil 1979;60:145–154.

8. Mahoney RI, Barthel DW. Functional evaluation: the Barthel index. Md Med J 1965; 14:61–65.

9. Lawton MP. The functional assessment of elderly people. J Am Geriatr Soc 1971; 19:465–481.

10. Exner CE. Development of hand functions. In: Pratt PN, Allen AS, eds. Occupational therapy for children. St Louis: CV Mosby, 1989.

11. Corbetta D, Mounoud P. Early development of grasping and manipulation. In: Bard C, Fleury M, Hay L, eds. Development of eye-hand coordination across the lifespan. Columbia, SC: University of South Carolina Press, 1990:188–216.

12. Swanson AB, Goran-Hagert C, Swanson, GD. Evaluation of impairment of hand function. In: Hunter JM, Schneider LH, Mackin EJ, Bell JA, eds. Rehabilitation of the hand. St. Louis: CV Mosby, 1978:31–69.

13. Jebsen RH, Taylor N, Trieschmann RB, Trotter MJ, Howard L. An objective and standard test of hand function. Arch Phys Med 1969;50:311–319.

14. Agnew PJ, Maas F. Hand function related to age and sex. Arch Phys Med Rehabil 1982;63:269–271.

15. Stern EB. Stability of the Jebsen-Taylor hand function test across three test sessions. Am J Occup Ther 1992;7:647–649.

16. Lynch KB, Bridle MJ. Validity of the Jebsen-Taylor hand function test in predicting

activities of daily living. Occup Ther J Res 1989;5:316–318.

17. Tiffin J. Purdue pegboard examiner manual. Chicago: Science Research Associates, 1968.

18. Baxter-Petralia P, Bruening LA, Blackmore SM, McEntee PM. Physical capacity evaluation. In: Hunter JM, et al., eds. Rehabilitation of the hand. St Louis: CV Mosby, 1990:93–108.

19. Curtis RM, Engalitcheff J Jr. A work simulator for rehabilitating the upper extremity—preliminary report. J Hand Surg 1981; 6:499–510.

20. Jeannerod M. The neural and behavioral organization of goal-directed movements. Clarendon Press: Oxford, 1990.

21. Herdman S. Assessment and treatment of balance disorders in the vestibular-deficient patient. In: Duncan P, ed. Balance: proceedings of the APTA Forum. Alexandria, VA: APTA, 1989.

22. Shumway-Cook A, Horak F. Rehabilitation of the patient with vestibular deficits. Neurol Clin 1990;8:441–457.

23. Behbehani K, Kondraske G, Richmond JR. Investigation of upper extremity visuomotor control performance measures. IEEE Trans Biomed Eng 1988;7:518–525.

24. Fitts PM. The information capacity of the human motor system in controlling the amplitude of movement. J Exp Psychol 1954; 47:381–391.

25. Poizner H, Mack L, Verfaellie M, Rothi LJG, Heilman KM. Three-dimensional computergrapic analysis of apraxia. Brain 1990;113:85–101.

26. Schwartz MF, Reed ES, Montgomery M, Palmer C, Mayer NH. The quantitative description of action disorganization after brain damage: a case study. Cognitive Neuropsychology 1991;8:381–414.

27. Luria AR. Higher cortical functions in man. NY: Basic Books, 1966.

28. Norman DA, Shallice T. Attention to action: willed and automatic control of behavior. In: Davidson RJ, Schwartz GE, Shapiro D, eds. Consciousness and self-regulation, vol 4. New York: Plenum, 1986.

29. American Society for Surgery of the Hand. The hand: examination and diagnosis. New York: Churchill Livingstone, 1983.

30. Bechtol CO. Grip test use of dynamometer

with adjustable hand spacing. JAMA 1954; 36:820–824.

31. Schmidt RT, Toews J. Grip strength as measured by the Jamar dynamometer. Arch Phys Med Rehabil 1970;5:321–327.

32. Fike ML, Rousseau E. Measurement of adult hand strength: a comparison of two instruments. Occupational Therapy Journal of Research 1982;2:43–49.

33. Fess EE, Harmon KS, Strickland JW, Steichen JB. Evaluation of the hand by objective measurement. In: Hunter JM, Schneider LH, Mackin EJ, Bell JA, eds. Rehabilitation of the hand. St. Louis: CV Mosby, 1978:70–93.

34. Kellor M, Frost J, Silverberg N, et al. Hand strength and dexterity: norms for clinical usage. Am J Occup Ther 1971;25:77–83.

35. Mathiowetz v, Kashaman N, Valland G et al. Grip and pinch strength: normative data for adults. Arch Phys Med Rehabil 1985; 66:69–74.

36. Brunnstrom S. Motor testing procedures in hemiplegia: based on sequential recovery stages. Phys Ther 1966;46:357–375.

37. Duncan P, Badke MB. Stroke rehabilitation: the recovery of motor control. Chicago: Year Book, 1987.

38. Gowland C. Staging motor impairment after stroke. Stroke 1990;21(suppl II):II-19–II-21.

39. Bell-Krotoski J. Weinstein S, Weinstein C. Testing sensibility, including touch-pressure, two-point discrimination, point localization, and vibration. J Hand Therapy 1993;2:114–123.

40. Bell JA. Sensibility evaluation. In: Hunter JM, Schneider LH, Mackin EJ, Bell JA, eds. Rehabilitation of the hand. St. Louis: CV Mosby, 1978:273–291.

41. Levin S, Pearsall G, Ruderman R. Von Frey's method of measuring pressure sensibility in the hand: an engineering analysis of the Weinstein-Semmes pressure aesthesiometer. J Hand Surg 1978;3:211.

42. Semmes J, Weinstein S, Ghent L, Teaber HL. Somatosensory changes after penetrating brain wounds in man. Cambridge: Harvard University Press, 1960.

43. Werner JL, Omer GE. Evaluation cutaneous pressure sensation of the hand. Am J Occup Ther 1070;24:347–356.

44. Waters RL, Wilson DJ, Savinelli R. Rehabilitation of the upper extremity following stroke. In: Hunter JM, Schneider LH, Mackin EJ, Bell JA, eds. Rehabilitation of the hand. St. Louis: CV Mosby, 1978:505–520.

45. Stern EB. Volumetric comparison of seated and standing test postures. Am J Occup Ther 1991;801–805.

46. Waylett J, Seibly D. A study to determine the average deviation accuracy of a commercially available volumeter. J Hand Surg 1981;6:300–313.

47. Partridge CJ, Edwards SM, Mee R, Langenberghe HVK van. Hemiplegic shoulder pain: a study of two methods of physiotherapy treatment. Clinical Rehabilitation 1990; 4:43–49.

48. Roy CW. Shoulder pain in hemiplegia: a literature review. Clinical Rehabilitation 1988; 2:35–44.

49. Cailliet R. The shoulder in hemiplegia. Philadelphia: FA Davis, 1980.

50. American Society of Hand Therapists. Clinical assessment recommendations. Garner, NC: American Society of Hand Therapists, 1981.

51. International classification of impairment, disabilities and handicaps: a manual of classification relating to the consequences of disease. Geneva: World Health Organization, 1980.

52. O'Sullivan, S. Clinical decision making: planning effective treatments. In: O'Sullivan S, Schmitz T. Physical rehabilitation: assessment and treatment. 2nd ed. Philadelphia: FA Davis, 1988:1–8.

53. Pehoski C. Central nervous system control of precision movements of the hand. In: Case-Smith J, Pehoski C, eds. Development of hand skills in children. Rockville, MD: American Occupational Therapy Association, 1992:1–11.

54. Growden JH, Chambers WW, Liu CN. An experimental study of cerebellar dyskinesia in the rhesus monkey. Brain 1967;90:603–630.

55. Lawrence DG, Hopkins DA. The development of motor control in the rhesus monkey: evidence concerning the role of corticomotoneuronal connections. Brain 1976; 99:235–254.

56. Schwartzman RJ. A behavioral analysis of complete unilateral section of the pyramidal tract at the medullary level in macaca mulatta. Ann Neurol 1978;4:234–244.

57. Chapman C, Wiesendanger M. Recovery of function following unilateral lesions of the bulbar pyramid in the monkey. Electroencephalogr Clin Neurophysiol 1982;53:374–387.

58. Evarts EV. Role of motor cortex in voluntary movements in primates. In: Brookhart JM, Mountcastle VB, eds. Handbook of physiology, section I. Volume II, Motor control. Bethesda, MD: American Physiological Society, 1981.

59. Wise SD, Evarts EV. The role of the cerebral cortex on movement. Trends Neurosci 1981;4:297–300.

60. Asanuma H, Arissian S. Direct and indirect sensory input pathways to the motor cortex: its structure and function in relating to learning motor skills. J Physiol 1984;39:1–19.

61. Bobath B. Adult hemiplegia: evaluation and treatment. London: Wm Heinemann Medical Books, 1970.

62. Carr J, Shepard R. Motor relearning programme for stroke. Rockville, MD: Aspen, 1983.

63. Davies P. Steps to follow. New York: Springer-Verlag, 1985.

64. Boehme R. Improving upper body control. Tucson, AZ: Therapy Skill Builders, 1988.

65. Voss D, Ionta M, Myers B. Proprioceptive neuromuscular facilitation: patterns and techniques. 3rd ed. Philadelphia, Harper & Row, 1985.

66. Fess EK, Gettle D, Strickland J. Hand splinting: principles and methods. St. Louis: CV Mosby, 1981.

67. Cusick B, Sussman M. Short leg casts: their role in the management of cerebral palsy. Phys Occup Ther Ped 1982;3/4:93–110.

68. Yasukawa A. Upper-extremity casting: adjunct treatment for the child with cerebral palsy. In: Case-Smith J, Pehoski C, eds. Development of hand skills in children. Rockville, MD: American Occupational Therapy Association, 1992:111–123.

69. Smith LH, Harris SR. Upper extremity inhibitive casting for a child with cerebral palsy. Phys Occup Ther Ped 1985;5:71–79.

70. Cruickshank DA, O'Neill DL. Upper extremity inhibitive casting in a boy with spastic quadriplegia. Am J Occup Ther 1990; 6:552–555.

71. Law M, Cadman D, Rosenbaum P, Walter S, Russell D, DeMatteo C. NDT therapy and upper extremity inhibitive casting for children with CP. Dev Med Child Neurol 1991;33:379–387.

72. Cannon N. Manual of hand splinting. New York: Churchill Livingstone, 1985.

73. Lindholm L. Weight-bearing splint: a method for managing upper extremity spasticity. Physical Therapy Forum 1985;5:3.

74. Malick M. Manual on static hand splinting. Pittsburgh: Harmarville Rehab Center, 1980.

75. Neuhaus BE, Ascher B, Coullon M, et al. A survey of rationales for and against hand splinting in hemiplegia. Am J Occup Ther 1981;35:83–95.

76. Zizlis J. Splinting of the hand in a spastic hemiplegic patients. Arch Phys Med Rehabil 1964;1:41–43.

77. Maynard CJ. Sensory reeducation following peripheral nerve injury. In: Hunter JM, Schneider LH, Mackin EJ, Bell JA, eds. Rehabilitation of the hand. St. Louis: CV Mosby, 1978:318–323.

78. Dellon AL, Curtis RM, Edgerton MT. Reeducation of sensation in the hand following nerve injury. Plast Reconstr Surg 1974; 53:297–305.

79. Callahan AD. Sensibility testing: clinical methods. In: Hunter JM, Schneider LH, Mackin EJ, Callahan AD, eds. Rehabilitation of the hand. St. Louis: CV Mosby, 1990:600–602.

80. Brand PW. Management of sensory loss in the extremities In: Omer E, Spinner M, eds. Management of peripheral nerve problems. Philadelphia: WB Saunders, 1980:862–872.

81. Vinogrand A, Taylor E, Grossmand S. Sensory retraining of the hemiplegic hand. Am J Occup Ther 1962;5:246–256.

82. Zee DS. Vertigo. Current therapy in neurological disease. Philadelphia: BC Decker, 1985.

83. Shumway-Cook, unpublished observations.

84. Peoppel E. Letter to the editor. Nature 1973;243:231.

85. Perenin MT, Jeannerod M. Visual function within the hemianoptic field following early cerebral hemidecortication in man. I. spatial localization. Neuropsychologia 1978;16:1–13.

86. Kraft GH, Fitts S, Hammond MC. Techniques to improve function of the arm and hand in chronic hemiplegia. Arch Phys Med Rehabil 1992;73:220–227.

87. Wolf SL, LeCraw DE, Barton LA. Comparison of motor copy and targeted biofeedback training techniques for restitution of upper extremity function among patients with neurologic disorders. Phys Ther 1989; 69:719–735.

88. McPherson J. Schild R, Spaulding SJ, Barsamian, Transon C, White SC. Analysis of upper extremity movement in four sitting positions: a comparison of persons with and without cerebral palsy. Am J Occup Ther 1991;2:123–129.

89. Shellenkens JM, Scholten CA, Kalverboer AF. Visually guided hand movements in children with minor neurological dysfunction: response time and movement organization. J Child Psych Psychiatry 1983; 24:89–102.

90. Kluzik J, Fetters L, Coryell J. Quantification of control: a preliminary study of effects of neurodevelopmental treatment on reaching in children with spastic cerebral palsy. Phys Ther 1990;2:65–78.

91. Waksvik K, Levy R. An approach to seating for the cerebral palsied. Can J Occup Ther 1979;46:147–152.

92. Nwaobi OM, Brubaker CE. Cusick B, Sussman M. Electromyographic investigation of extensor activity in cerebral palsied children in different seating positions. Dev Med Child Neurol 1983;25:175–183.

93. Seeger BR, Caudrey DJ, O'Mara NA. Hand function in cerebral palsy: the effect of hip flexion angle. Dev Med Child Neurol 1984; 26:601–606.

94. Noronha J, Bundy A, Groll J. The effect of positioning on the hand function of boys with cerebral palsy. Am J Occup Ther 1989; 43:507–512.

95. Erhardt RP. Developmental hand dysfunction: theory, assessment and treatment. Tucson, AZ: Therapy Skill Builders, 1982.

96. Fisk JD. Sensory and motor integration in the control of reaching. In: Bard C, Fleury M, Hay L, eds. Developmental of eye-hand coordination across the lifespan. Columbia,

SC: University of South Carolina Press, 1990:75–98.

97. Forssberg H, Eliasson AC, Kinoshita H, Johansson RS, Westling G. Development of human precision grip: basic coordination of force. Brain Res 1991;85:451–457.

98. Westling G, Johansson RS. Factors influencing the force control during precision grip. Exp Brain Res 1984;53:277–284.

99. Elliot J, Connolly K. A classification of manipulative hand movements. Dev Med Child Neurol 1984;26:283–296.

100. Exner CE. In-hand manipulation skills. In: Case-Smith J, Pehoski C, eds. Development of hand skills in the child. Rockville, MD: American Occupational Therapy Association, 1992:35–45.

101. Seligman ME, Maier S. Failure to escape traumatic shock. J Exp Psychol 1967;74:1–9.

102. Taub E. Motor behavior following deafferentation in the developing and motorically mature monkey. In: Herman R, Grillner S, Ralston JH, Stein PSG, Stuart D, eds. Neural control of locomotion. New York: Plenum, 1976.

103. Rothwell JC, Traub MM, Day BL, Obeso JA, Thomas PK, Marsden CS. Manual motor performance in a deafferented man. Brain 1982;105:515–542.

104. Knapp HD, Taub E, Berman J. Movements of monkeys with deafferented forelimbs. Exp Neurol 1963;7:305–315.

105. Taub E, Berman AJ. Avoidance conditioning in the absence of relevant proprioceptive and exteroceptive feedback. J Comp Physiol Psychol 1963;56:1012–1016.

106. Wolf SL, Lecraw DE, Barton LA, Jann BB. Forced use of hemiplegic upper extremities to reverse the effect of learned nonuse among chronic stroke and head injured patients. Exp Neurol 1989;104:125–132.

107. Taub E, Miller NE, Novack TA, et al. Technique to improve chronic motor deficit after stroke. Arch Phys Med Rehabil 1993; 74:347–354.

Appendix A. Postural Control Assessment Form

Patient: _____ Sex _____ Age: _____

Telephone: _____ Date: _____/ _____/ _____

Referring physician: _____ Therapist: _____

I. HISTORY

A. Social History

Living Situation:

_____ Home _____ Retirement Center _____ Nursing Home

Lives With:

_____ Alone _____ Spouse _____ Friend _____ Paid assistant

B. Medical History

Date of Onset of Condition:

Diagnosis:

Co-morbidities: _____ (number)

List:

C. Fall/Imbalance History

How many falls?

0_____ No history of falls

1_____ Has fallen 1–2 times in last year

2_____ Has fallen 1–2 times in six months

3_____ Has fallen 1–2 times in the last six weeks

When was your most recent fall? _____

Did the fall occur inside or outside? _____

How did fall occur? _____

Injuries resulting from fall? _____

Dizziness during fall? _____

How often do you lose your balance, ie. trip slip or stumble?

0_____ No history of imbalance

1_____ Has imbalance monthly

2_____ Has imbalance weekly

3_____ Has imbalance daily

D. CURRENT MEDICATIONS

No of meds: _____ Types:

E. BLOOD PRESSURE

Take patient's blood pressure in the supine position, again after moving into the seated position, and again after standing.

B/P Supine: _____ B/P Sitting: _____ B/P Standing: _____

447

II. PERFORMANCE BASED FUNCTIONAL MEASURES OF BALANCE

A. Functional Balance Scale

(Reprinted with permission: Berg K, Measuring balance in the elderly: Validation of an instrument [Dissertation]. Montreal, Canada: McGill University, 1993.)

1. Sitting to standing

Instruction: Please stand up. Try not to use your hands for support.

Grading: Please mark the lowest category which applies.

    (4) able to stand, no hands and stabilize independently

    (3) able to stand independently using hands

    (2) able to stand using hands after several tries

    (1) needs minimal assist to stand or to stabilize

    (0) needs moderate or maximal assist to stand

2. Standing unsupported

Instruction: Stand for two minutes without holding.

Grading: Please mark the lowest category which applies.

    (4) able to stand safely 2 min

    (3) able to stand 2 min with supervision

    (2) able to stand 30 sec unsupported

    (1) needs several tries to stand 30 sec unsupported

    (0) unable to stand 30 sec unassisted

IF SUBJECT ABLE TO STAND 2 MIN SAFELY, SCORE FULL MARKS FOR SITTING UN-SUPPORTED. PROCEED TO POSITION CHANGE STANDING TO SITTING.

3. Sitting unsupported feet on floor

Instruction: Sit with arms folded for two minutes.

Grading: Please mark the lowest category which applies.

    (4) able to sit safely and securely 2 min

    (3) able to sit 2 min under supervison

    (2) able to sit 30 sec

    (1) able to sit 10 sec

    (0) unable to sit without support 10 sec

4. Standing to sitting

Instruction: Please sit down.

Grading: Please mark the lowest categroy which applies.

    (4) sits safely with minimal use of hands

    (3) controls descent by using hands

    (2) uses back of legs against chair to control descent

    (1) sits independently but has uncontrolled descent

    (0) needs assistance to sit

5. Transfers

Instruction: Please move from chair to bed and back again. One way toward a seat with armrests and one way toward a seat without armrests.

Grading: Please mark the lowest category which applies.

    (4) able to transfer safely with only minor use of hands

    (3) able to transfer safely with definite need of hands

    (2) able to transfer with verbal cueing and/or supervision

    (1) needs one person to assist

    (0) needs two people to assist or supervise to be safe

6. Standing unsupported with eyes closed

Instruction: Close your eyes and stand still for 10 sec.

Grading: Please mark the lowest category which applies.

    (4) able to stand 10 sec safely

    (3) able to stand 10 sec with supervision

    (2) able to stand 3 sec

    (1) unable to keep eyes closed 3 sec but stays steady

    (0) needs help to keep from falling

7. Standing unsupported with feet together.

Instruction: Place your feet together and stand without holding.

Grading: Please mark the lowest category which applies.

    (4) able to place feet together indep and stand 1 min safely

    (3) able to place feet together indep and for 1 min with supervision

    (2) able to place feet together indep but unable to hold for 30 sec

    (1) needs help to attain position but able to stand 15 sec feet together

    (0) needs help to attain position and unable to hold for 15 sec

THE FOLLOWING ITEMS ARE TO BE PERFORMED WHILE STANDING UNSUPPORTED

8. Reaching forward with outstretched arm

Instruction: Lift arm to 90 degrees. Stretch out your fingers and feach forward as far as you can. (Examiner places a ruler at end of fingertips when arm is at 90 degrees. Fingers should not touch the ruler while reaching forward. The recorded measure is the distance forward that the fingers reach while the subject is in the most forward lean position.)

Grading: Please mark the lowest category which applies.

    (4) can reach forward confidently >10 inches

    (3) can reach forward >5 inches safely

    (2) can reach forward >2 inches safely

    (1) reaches forward but needs supervision

    (0) needs help to keep from falling

9. Pick up object from the floor

Instruction: Pick up the shoe/slipper which is placed in front of your feet

Grading: Please mark the lowest category which applies.

(4) able to pick up slipper safely and easily

(3) able to pick up slipper but need supervision

(2) unable to pick up but reaches 1–2 inches from slipper and keeps balance indep

(1) unable to pick up and needs supervison while trying

(0) unable to try/needs assist to keep from falling

10. Turning to look behind/over left and right shoulders.

Instruction: Turn to look behind you over/toward left shoulder. Repeat to the right.

Grading: Please mark the lowest category which applies.

(4) looks behind from both sides and weight shifts well

(3) looks behind one side only; other side shows less weight shift

(2) turns sideways only but maintains balance

(1) needs supervision when turning

(0) needs assist to keep from falling

11. Turn 360 degrees

Instruction: Turn completely around in a full circle. Pause. Then turn a full circle in the other direction.

Grading: Please mark the lowest category which applies.

(4) able to turn 360 safely in <4 sec each side

(3) able to turn 360 safely one side only in < 4 sec

(2) able to turn 360 safely but slowly

(1) needs close supervision or verbal cueing

(0) needs assistance while turning

DYNAMIC WEIGHT SHIFTING WHILE STANDING UNSUPPORTED

12. Stool touch

Instruction: Place each foot alternately on the stool. Continue until each foot has touched the stool four times.

Grading: Please mark the lowest category which applies.

(4) able to stand indep and safely and complete 8 step in 20 sec

(3) able to stand indep and complete 8 steps in >20 sec

(2) able to complete 4 steps without aid with supervision

(1) able to complete >2 steps needs minimal assist

(0) needs assistance to keep from falling/unable to try

13. Standing unsupported, one foot in front

Instruction: (Demonstrate to subject) Place one foot directly in front of the other. If you feel that you cannot place your foot directly in front, try to step far enough ahead that the heel of your forward foot is ahead of the toes of the other foot.

Grading: Please mark the lowest category which applies.

    (4) able to place foot tandem indep and hold 30 sec

    (3) able to place foot ahead of other indep and hold 30 sec

    (2) able to take small step indep and hold 30 sec

    (1) needs help to step but can hold 15 sec

    (0) loses balance while stepping or standing

14. Standing on one leg

Instruction: Stand on one leg as long as you can without holding.

Grading: Please mark the lowest category which applies.

    (4) able to lift leg indep and hold >10 sec

    (3) able to lift leg indep and hold 5–10 sec

    (2) able to lift leg indep and hold = or > 3 sec

    (1) tries to lift leg; unable to hold 3 sec but remains standing indep

    (0) unable to try or needs assist to prevent fall

**TOTAL SCORE _____ / 56 **

III. STRATEGY ASSESSMENT

A. Seated postural control

1. *Alignment*: eo _____ ec _____

   Ask patient to sit up as straight as they can.

   2 = Normal alignment of body segments

   1 = Partial correction towards normal alignment

   0 = Abnormal alignment of body segments, ie lateral asymmetry, excessive rotation of the pelvis, kyphosis, or forward flexion of the head, or inabilty to sustain vertical.

2. *Active Weight Shifts*: eo _____ ec _____

   Ask patient to shift weight to one side, as far as they can without losing their balance. Perform one side then the other, first with eyes open, then with eyes closed.

   2 = Normal is defined as the patient's ability to shift weight symmetrically, elongate trunk on weight bearing side, re-establish vertical with and without vision, not dizzy.

   1 = Able to partially complete

   0 = Abnormal, inability to shift weight, asymmetrical weight shift, inability to re-establish vertical.

B. Stance postural control

1. Alignment: Eyes open _____ Eyes Closed _____ Base of Support _____

    Ask patient to stand up as straight as they can, measure base of support at mid foot.

    2 = Normal alignment of body segments, vertical line of gravity at tragus, shoulder, hip, knee and just ant to malleoli, even between both feet.

    1 = Partially able to assume normal alignment

    0 = Abnormal alignment, ie, center of mass laterally displaced, or displaced forward or backward, or excessive rotation of the pelvis, thoracic kyphosis, or forward flexion of the head, cannot sustain a vertical position.

2. Movement Strategies:

    a. Self Initiated Sway Strategy: _____

        Ask patient to sway forward and backward, but not take a step.

        2 = Normal, ankle centered sway, inverted pendulum movement of body with good range forward and backwards.

        1 = Partial ankle strategy, reduced range

        0 = Abnormal is inability to sway about the ankles, controlling the knees and hips in a neutral position.

    b. Reactive Balance Strategy

        Within base of support _____

        Holding patient at the hips, therapist displaces patient small distance by pushing/pulling at hips. Instruction: "Let me move you, try not to take a step, but keep your balance."

        2 = Normal, ankle centered sway, inverted pendulum movement of body with good range forward and backwards.

        1 = Partial ankle strategy, reduced range

        0 = Abnormal is inability to sway about the ankles controlling the knees and hips in a neutral position.

        Outside base of support _____

        Therapist displaces patient's center of mass outside base of support. Instruction: "Let me move you; you might have to take a step, it's OK."

        2 = Ability to take a step with either foot, normal range

        1 = Step with one foot only, or altered range

        0 = Abnormal is inability to take a step to keep from falling.

3. Sensory Strategies

    Clinical Test of Sensory Interaction in Balance:

    Time—30 Sec. Sway 1 = normal sway, 0 = Abnormal (asymmetric or excessive sway)

	Trial 1		Trial 2	
	Time	Sway	Time	Sway
Eyes open, firm surface	_____	_____	_____	_____
Eyes closed, firm surface	_____	_____	_____	_____
Visual dome, firm surface	_____	_____	_____	_____
Eyes open, foam surface	_____	_____	_____	_____
Eyes closed, foam surface	_____	_____	_____	_____
Visual dome, foam surface	_____	_____	_____	_____

IV. SYSTEMS ANALYSIS

A. Mental Status

MINI MENTAL TEST (Mental Status)

1. What is the date today?   _____/_____/_____

2. What day of the week is it? _____

3. What is the name of this place? _____

4. What is your telephone number? _____

or What is your address? _____

5. How old are you? _____

6. When were you born? _____

7. Who is the President of the US now? _____

8. Who was the President before him? _____

9. What was your Mother's maiden name? _____

10. Subtract 3 from 20 and keep subtracting 3 from each new number, all the way down

(20, 17, 14, 11, 8, 5, 2).

_____ Total Number of Errors

0 _____ Oriented at all times (0–2 errors on MM test)

1 _____ Mild intellectual impairment (3–4 errors)

2 _____ Moderate intellectual impairment (5–7 errors)

3 _____ Severe intellectual impairment (8–10 errors)

B. MUSCULOSKELETAL SYSTEM

1. Strength	Right	Left
Gastroc/soleus	_____	_____
TA	_____	_____
Quads	_____	_____
Hamstrings	_____	_____
Hip Flexor	_____	_____
Hip Extensors	_____	_____
Abductors	_____	_____
Adductors	_____	_____
Trunk (partial sit up)		_____

B. MUSCULOSKELETAL SYSTEM—*continued*

2. Range of motion   Right   Left

     Hip   _____   _____

     Knee   _____   _____

     Ankle   _____   _____

     Cervical   _____

     Trunk   _____

     Scoring:

     0 = ankylosed

     1 = moderate hypomobility

     2 = mild hypomobility

     3 = normal

     4 = mild hypermobility

     5 = moderate hypermobility

     6 = severe hypermobility

3. Muscle Tonus: _____

     0 = No increase in muscle tone

     1 = Slight increase in muscle tone, manifested by a slight catch and release or by minimal resistance at the end of the range of motion when the affected part(s) is moved in flexion or extension

     1+ = Slight increase in muscle tone, manifested by a catch, followed by minimal resistance throughout the remainder (less than half) of the ROM

     2 = More makred increase in muscle tone through most of the ROM, but affected part(s) easily moved

     3 = Considerable increase in muscle tone, passive movement difficult

     4 = Affected part(s) rigid in flexion or extension.

4. Pain: _____

5. Cerebellar Coordination:

     Finger to nose: _____

     Pronation/supination: _____

     Heel to shin: _____

     Tremor:

Scoring: 5 = normal, 4 = minimal impairment, 3 = moderate impairment, 2 = severe impairment, 1 = cannot perform.

3. *Peripheral Sensibility*

Test the following senses. Score N if intact, A if abnormal

     Proprioception: _____

     (Great Toe, Ankle)

The following is by subject report:

Central visual acuity _____

Peripheral visual acuity _____

Depth Perception _____

EVALUATION SUMMARY:

Problems:

Functional Level of Performance:

Strategies For Postural Control:

Alignment

Movement

Sensory

Impairments:

Cognitive

Musculoskeletal

Neuromuscular

Sensory

PLAN:

Short Term Goals: (Expressed in temrs of underlying impairments, or interim steps towards a long term goal)

Long Term Goals: (Expressed in terms of functional skills).

Frequency of Treatment: Duration:

Treatment Plan:

GLOSSARY

Action potential—the dramatic jump in voltage across the cell membrane that is observed when a neuron is excited.

Adaptation requirement—one of the three major requirements for successful locomotion reflecting the ability to adapt gait to meet the goals of the animal and the demands of the environment.

Adaptive postural control—modifying sensory and motor systems in response to changing task and environmental demands.

Agnosia—the inability to recognize. Lesions in the parietal lobe often cause agnosia or neglect of the contralateral side of the body, objects, and drawings.

Alpha-motor neurons—motor neurons within the spinal cord that innervate skeletal muscle fibers.

Anticipatory postural control—pretuning sensory and motor systems in expectation of postural demands based on previous experience and learning.

Assessment—the systematic acquisition of information that is relevant and meaningful in providing the clinician with a comprehensive picture of the patient's abilities and problems.

Associative stage—in the Fitts-Posner description of motor learning, this is the second stage. By this time, the person has selected the best strategy for the task and begins to refine the skill.

Asymmetric tonic neck reflex—produces a change in the position of the arms in response to change in head position. Turning the head produces extension in the *face* arm, and flexion in the *skull* arm.

Autonomous stage—in the Fitts-Posner description of motor learning, this is the third stage. In this stage, there is automaticity in the skill, and a low degree of attention is required for its performance.

Body-on-body righting reaction—keeps the body oriented with respect to the ground regardless of the position of the head.

Body-on-head righting reaction—orients the head in response to proprioceptive and tactile signals from the body in contact with a supporting surface.

Cadence—the number of steps per unit of time, usually reported as steps per minute.

Classical conditioning—a form of association learning. An initially weak stimulus (the conditioned stimulus) becomes highly effective in producing a response when it becomes associated with another stronger stimulus (the unconditioned stimulus). After repeated pairing of the conditioned and the unconditioned stimulus, one begins to see a conditioned response (CR) to the CS.

Clinical decision-making process—a procedure for gathering information essential to developing a plan of care consistent with the problems and needs of the patient.

Closed-loop process—motor control processing in which sensory feedback is used for the ongoing production of skilled movement.

Cognitive processes—in this book, we define cognitive processes broadly, to include higher level neural processes such as planning, attention, motivation, and emotional aspects of motor control that underlie the establishment of intent or goals. It is difficult to make a distinction between higher-level perceptual/motor processing and cognitive processing, since there is a gradual transition and overlap between the processing levels.

Cognitive stage—in the Fitts-Posner description of motor learning, this is the first stage in the process. In it, the learner is concerned with understanding the nature of the task, developing strategies that could be used to carry out the task, and determining how the task should be evaluated.

Compensation—behavioral substitution, that is, alternative behavioral strategies are adopted to complete a task.

Conceptual framework—a logical structure that helps the clinician organize clinical practices related to assessment and treatment into a cohesive and comprehensive plan.

Coordinative structure—neural commands that are temporally grouped, so that signals are sent to muscles in a coherent fashion. This reduces the degrees of freedom to be controlled by the nervous system by constraining groups of muscles to act within functionally coherent units (the term synergy is often used as a synonym).

Decerebrate locomotor preparation—animal experimental preparation that leaves the spinal cord, brainstem, and cerebellum intact. An area in the brainstem, called the mesencephalic locomotor region, appears to be important in the descending control of locomotion. Decerebrate cats will not normally walk on a treadmill, but will begin to walk normally when tonic electrical stimulation is applied to the mesencephalic locomotor region.

Declarative learning—The process of learning knowledge that can be consciously recalled and thus requires processes such as awareness, attention, and reflection.

Decorticate locomotor preparation—animal experimental preparation with only the cerebral cortex removed. In this preparation, an external stimulus is not required to produce locomotor behavior, and the behavior is reasonably normal goal-directed behavior.

Degrees of freedom problem—a motor control problem involving how to control the many different joints and muscles of the body.

Denervation supersensitivity—occurs when neurons show a loss of input from another brain region. The postsynaptic membrane of a neuron becomes hyperactive to a released transmitter substance.

Distributed practice—a training session in which the amount of rest between trials equals or is greater than the amount of time for a trial.

Excitatory postsynaptic potential (EPSP)—the change in membrane potential in the postsynaptic cell (typically depolarizing) made by the excitatory transmitter substance released from the presynaptic neuron.

Excitatory summation—occurs when a series of excitatory postsynaptic potentials (EPSPs) continue to build up depolarization to the threshold voltage for the action potential in the next neuron.

Extrinsic feedback—information that supplements intrinsic feedback (e.g., when you tell a patient that he/she needs to pick up his/her foot higher to clear an object while walking).

Flexor withdrawal reflex—a cutaneous reflex caused by a sharp focal stimulus, producing withdrawal, or flexion, and causing protection from injury. The typical pattern of response is ipsilateral flexion and contralateral extension, which allow the support of body weight on the opposite limb. The reflex is mediated by group III and IV afferents.

Forced-use paradigm—a therapeutic approach in which hemiplegic patients are forced to use their hemiplegic arm (the intact side is re-strained) to facilitate the return of function in that arm.

Frozen gait pattern—a gait pattern of patients with Parkinson's disease, characterized by an inability to generate sufficient momentum so that forward progression is arrested.

Gamma-motor neurons—motor neurons from the spinal cord that innervate the muscle spindle muscle fibers.

General static reactions (called attitudinal reflexes)—involve changes in position of the whole body in response to changes in head position.

Glabrous skin—hairless skin.

Habituation—a decrease in responsiveness that occurs as a result of repeated exposure to a nonpainful stimulus. (see *synaptic defacilitation.*)

Intrafusal muscle fibers—Specialized muscle fibers found in muscle spindles (extrafusal fibers are normal skeletal muscle fibers).

HAT—head, arm, neck, and trunk segments that comprise the unit that must be balanced above the legs during locomotion.

Hierarchical processing—a system of neural processing in which higher levels of the brain are concerned with issues of abstraction of information. For example, higher brain centers integrate inputs from many senses, and interpret incoming sensory information.

Hypothesis—a hypothetical explanation about the cause or causes of a problem.

Hypothesis-oriented clinical practice—a process used to systematically test assumptions about the nature and cause of a patient's problems.

Inertia—the tendency to remain at rest; the inability to move spontaneously.

Intrinsic feedback—feedback that comes to the individual through the various sensory systems as a result of the normal production of the movement (e.g., visual information concerning whether a movement was accurate, somatosensory information concerning the position of the limbs as one was moving).

Joint-based planning—one possible way the CNS could control movements toward a target, by using joint angle coordinates to program movements.

Knowledge of performance (KP)—feedback relating to the movement pattern that the performer has made.

Knowledge of results (KR)—a form of extrinsic feedback. It has been defined as verbal (or its equivalent) terminal feedback about the *out-*

come of the movement, in terms of the movement's goal.

Labyrinthine righting reaction—orients the head to an upright vertical position in response to vestibular signals.

Landau reaction—combines the effect of the labyrinthine, optical, and body-on-head righting reactions.

Learning—the process of acquiring knowledge about the world.

Local static reactions—stiffen the animal's limb for support of body weight against gravity.

Long-term memory—continuum of processes involving information storage. Initial stages reflect functional changes in the efficiency of synapses. Later stages reflect structural changes in synaptic connections. These memories are less subject to disruption.

Long-term potentiation (LTP)—similar to sensitization. In the hippocampus, LTP occurs when a weak and an excitatory input arrive at the same region of a neuron's dendrite. The weak input is enhanced if it is activated in association with the strong one. LTP appears to require the simultaneous firing of both pre- and postsynaptic cells. After this occurs, LTP is maintained through an increase in presynaptic transmitter release.

Massed practice—a session in which the amount of practice time in a trial is greater than the amount of rest between trials.

Memory trace—within Adam's closed-loop theory of motor control, the memory trace is used to select and initiate a movement.

Model of brain function—model of brain function, related to motor control, is a simplified representation of the structure and function of the brain as it relates to the coordination of movement.

Model of disablement—an approach to ordering the effects of disease, enabling the clinician to develop a hierarchical list of problems towards which treatment can be directed.

Monosynaptic reflex—the simplest reflex pathway, consisting of a sensory neuron, the Ia afferent neuron from the muscle spindle, an interneuron, the Ia inhibitory interneuron, and a motor neuron, the α-motor neuron to the same muscle. The muscle contracts in response to stretch of the muscle spindle and activation of the Ia afferent neuron.

Motor learning—the study of the acquisition and/or modification of movement; a set of processes associated with practice or experience leading to relatively permanent changes in the capability for producing skilled action. It emerges from a complex of perception-cognition-action processes. Involves the search for a task solution, which emerges from an interaction of the individual with the task and the environment.

Motor program—the term may be used to identify a central pattern generator (CPG), that is, a specific neural circuit like that for generating walking in the cat. In this case, the term represents neural connections that are stereotyped and hardwired. The term is also used to describe higher-level hierarchically organized neural processes that store the rules for generating movements so that tasks can be performed with a variety of effector systems.

Muscle tone—the force with which a muscle resists being lengthened.

Neck-on-body righting reaction—orients the body in response to cervical afferents, which report changes in the position of the head and neck.

Neuronal shock (diaschisis)—the short-term loss of function in neuronal pathways at a distance from the lesion itself.

Operant conditioning—the process of learning to associate a certain response, from among many that have been made, with a consequence. Behaviors that are rewarded tend to be repeated, while behaviors followed by aversive stimuli are reduced in number.

Optical righting reaction—contributes to the reflex orientation of the head using visual inputs.

Parachute or protective responses—protect the body from injury during a fall.

Parallel distributed processing—neural processing in which the same signal is processed simultaneously among many different brain structures, though for different purposes.

Perceptual trace—within Adam's closed-loop theory of motor control, the perceptual trace is considered an internal reference of correctness built up over a period of practice.

Performance-based functional measures—assessment tools that focus on measuring performance on functional tasks.

Plasticity—the ability to show modification or change. Short-term functional plasticity refers to changes in the efficiency or "strength" of synaptic connections. Structural plasticity refers to changes in the organization and numbers of synaptic connections.

Postural control—regulating the body's position in space for the dual purposes of stability and orientation.

Postural fixation reactions—used to recover from perturbations other than to the supporting surface.

Postural motor strategies—the organization of movements appropriate for controlling the body's position in space.

Postural orientation—the ability to maintain an appropriate relationship between the body segments, and between the body and the environment for a task.

Postural stability—the ability to maintain the position of the body, and specifically, the center of body mass (COM), within specific boundaries of space, referred to as stability limits.

Postural tone—increased level of activity in antigravity muscles that helps maintain the body vertically against the force of gravity.

Procedural learning—the process of learning tasks that can be performed automatically without attention or conscious thought, like a habit.

Progression requirement—one of the three major requirements for successful locomotion, reflecting the need for a basic locomotor pattern that can move the body in the desired direction.

Propulsive gait pattern—gait pattern of patients with Parkinson's disease, characterized by an inability to restrain momentum, leading to uncontrolled progression.

Reactive synaptogenesis (collateral sprouting)—process in which neighboring normal axons sprout to innervate synaptic sites that were previously activated by the injured axon.

Recall schema—within Schmidt's Schema theory, when initiating a movement, it is used for the selection of a specific response. Inputs to this schema include the initial conditions, desired goal of the movement, and the abstract memory of previous response specifications in similar tasks.

Receptive field—the specific area of skin, retina, etc., to which a cell is sensitive when the skin or retina is stimulated. The receptive field can be either excitatory or inhibitory.

Recognition schema—within Schmidt's Schema theory, this is used for the evaluation of a response. The sensory consequences and outcomes of previous movements are combined with the current initial conditions to create a representation of the expected sensory consequences.

Recovery—stringent definition requires achieving the functional goal in the same way it was performed preinjury, that is, using the same processes utilized prior to the injury. Less stringent definitions include the ability to achieve task goals using effective and efficient means, but not necessarily those used preinjury.

Recovery of function—the reacquisition of movement skills lost through injury.

Recurvatum—hyperextension, which occurs when the knee has sufficient mobility to move posteriorly past neutral.

Reflex—a stereotyped muscle response to a sensory stimulus. The simplest reflex pathway is the monosynaptic stretch reflex pathway, consisting of a sensory neuron, the Ia afferent neuron from the muscle spindle, an interneuron, the Ia inhibitory interneuron, and a motor neuron, the α-motor neuron to the same muscle. The muscle contracts in response to stretch of the muscle spindle and activation of the Ia afferent neuron.

Regenerative synaptogenesis—process of sprouting of injured axons.

Response-produced feedback—all the sensory information that is available as the result of a movement that a person has produced.

Resting potential—the neuron, when it is at rest, always has a negative electrical charge or potential on the inside of the cell, with respect to the outside. This is called the resting potential.

Righting reactions—allow the animal to assume or resume a species specific orientation of the body with respect to its environment.

Schema—an abstract representation stored in memory following multiple presentations of a class of objects.

Segmental static reactions—involve more than one body segment, and include the flexor withdrawal reflex, and the crossed extensor reflex.

Self-organizing system—a system that can spontaneously form movement patterns that arise simply from the interaction of the different parts of the system.

Sensitization—an increased responsiveness following a threatening or noxious stimulus.

Sensorimotor strategies—reflect the rules for coordinating sensory and motor aspects of postural control.

Sensory strategies—organize sensory information from visual, somatosensory, and vestibular systems for postural control.

Short-term memory—"working" memory, which has a limited capacity for information storage and lasts for a few moments only. This reflects momentary attentional processes.

Spared function—used to describe a function that is not lost following injury.

Spasticity—a motor disorder characterized by a

velocity-dependent increase in tonic stretch reflexes (muscle tone) with exaggerated tendon jerks, resulting from hyperexcitability of the stretch reflex (it is one component of the upper motor neuron syndrome).

Spatial summation—summation that produces depolarization because of the simultaneous action potentials of multiple cells synapsing on the same postsynaptic neuron.

Spinal locomotor preparation—animal experimental preparation in which lesions are made at the low spinal level, to allow the observation of only the hind limbs, or at the high spinal level, to allow the observation of all four limbs as part of the preparation. For this preparation, one needs an external stimulus, for example, an electrical or pharmacological stimulus, to produce locomotor behavior.

Stability limits—boundaries of an area of space in which the body can maintain its position without changing the base of support.

Stability requirement—one of the three major requirements for successful locomotion, reflecting the ability to maintain stability, including the support of the body against gravity.

Step length—the distance from the foot-strike of one foot to the foot-strike of the other foot. For example, the right step length is the distance from the left heel to the right heel when both feet are in contact with the ground.

Strategy—a plan for action; an approach to organizing individual elements within a system into a collective structure.

Stride length—the distance covered by the same foot from one heel-strike to the next heel-strike.

Support moment—the algebraic sum of the joint moments at the hip, knee, and ankle, during the stance phase of the step cycle. The support moment is an extensor torque. This net extensor torque keeps the limb from collapsing while bearing weight, allowing stabilization of the body and thus accomplishing one of the requirements of locomotion.

Symmetric tonic neck reflex—changes the position of the limbs in response to a change in head position. When the head is extended, extensor activity predominates in the upper extremities,

while flexor activity predominates in the lower extremities. Flexion of the head reverses this; thus, there is an increase in flexion in the upper extremities and extensor activity in the lower extremities.

Synaptic defacilitation or habituation—when a neuron that has been activated over a period of time releases less transmitter, often due to transmitter depletion, and is less effective in influencing the postsynaptic neuron.

Synaptic facilitation—when a neuron that is activated over a short period of time begins to release more transmitter with each action potential and therefore more easily depolarizes the next cell.

Synaptic transmission—in chemical synaptic transmission, each action potential in a neuron releases a small amount of transmitter substance. It diffuses across the cleft and attaches to receptors on the next cell, which open up channels in the membrane and depolarize the new cell. If the depolarization is sufficient, an action potential will be activated.

Synergy—functional coupling of groups of muscles such that they are constrained to act together as a unit (synonym: coordinative structure).

Task-oriented approach—a therapeutic approach to retraining the patient with movement disorders, based on a systems theory of motor control.

Temporal summation—summation that results in depolarization because of synaptic potentials from a presynaptic neuron that occur close together in time.

Theory of motor control—a group of abstract ideas about the nature and cause of movement. Theories are often, but not always, based on models of brain function.

Tilting reactions—used for controlling the center of gravity in response to a tilting surface.

Tonic labyrinthine reflex—produces a change in body posture in response to vestibular inputs, signaling head position with respect to gravity. When the body is in supine position, extensor muscles are facilitated; conversely, the prone position results in facilitation of flexor muscles.

INDEX

Page numbers in *italics* denote figures; those followed by "t" denote tables.